Infectious Disease Management in Animal Shelters

Infectious Disease Management in Animal Shelters

Second Edition

Edited by

Lila Miller, BS, DVM
Vice President, Shelter Medicine (retired)
American Society for the Prevention of Cruelty to Animals (ASPCA)
New York, NY, USA

Stephanie Janeczko, DVM, MS, DABVP (Shelter Medicine and Canine/Feline Practice), CAWA
Vice President, Shelter Medicine Services
Director, Julie Morris Shelter Medicine Residency Program
American Society for the Prevention of Cruelty to Animals
New York, NY, USA

Kate F. Hurley, DVM, MPVM, DABVP (Shelter Medicine Practice)
Director, UC Davis Koret Shelter Medicine Program
Assistant Clinical Professor
Shelter Medicine and Small Animal Population Health
School of Veterinary Medicine
University of California
Davis, CA, USA

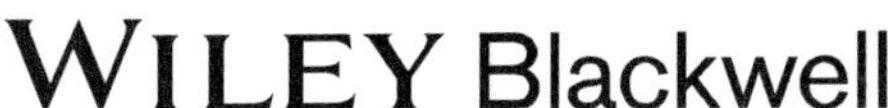

This edition first published 2021

Registered Office
John Wiley & Sons, Inc., 111 River Street, Hoboken, NJ 07030, USA

Editorial Office
111 River Street, Hoboken, NJ 07030, USA

For details of our global editorial offices, customer services, and more information about Wiley products visit us at www.wiley.com.

Wiley also publishes its books in a variety of electronic formats and by print-on-demand. Some content that appears in standard print versions of this book may not be available in other formats.

Library of Congress Cataloging-in-Publication Data

Names: Miller, Lila, editor. | Janeczko, Stephanie, editor. | Hurley, Kate, editor.
Title: Infectious disease management in animal shelters / edited by Lila Miller, Stephanie Janeczko, Kate F. Hurley.
Description: Second edition. | Hoboken, NJ : Wiley-Blackwell, 2021. | Includes bibliographical references and index.
Identifiers: LCCN 2021007215 (print) | LCCN 2021007216 (ebook) | ISBN 9781119294351 (paperback) | ISBN 9781119294375 (adobe pdf) | ISBN 9781119294368 (epub)
Subjects: MESH: Communicable Diseases–veterinary | Communicable Disease Control | Animal Diseases–prevention & control | Animal Welfare
Classification: LCC SF781 (print) | LCC SF781 (ebook) | NLM SF 781 | DDC 636.089/69–dc23
LC record available at https://lccn.loc.gov/2021007215
LC ebook record available at https://lccn.loc.gov/2021007216

Cover Design: Wiley
Cover Image: © (clockwise from left): Courtesy of Stephanie Janeczko; Courtesy of Sandra Newbury; Courtesy of Bridget Chariton; Courtesy of Jennifer Graham

Set in 9.5/12.5pt STIXTwoText by SPi Global, Pondicherry, India

SKY10096815_012225

This textbook is dedicated to the memory of Julie Morris, an animal welfare visionary who was one of the first to recognize the importance of integrating veterinary medicine directly into animal sheltering to improve and save the lives of homeless animals. Her early support of shelter veterinarians and shelter medicine training and programs was responsible for many of the advancements in the field, including this textbook. She is missed tremendously as a mentor, colleague, friend, and leader by the editors of this text and by many others.

Contents

Contributors

Elizabeth A. Berliner, DVM, DABVP (Shelter Medicine Practice, Canine and Feline Practice)
Associate Clinical Professor of Shelter Medicine
Swanson Endowed Director, Maddie's Shelter Medicine Program
Cornell University College of Veterinary Medicine
Ithaca, NY, USA

Dwight D. Bowman, MS, PhD, DACVM (Hon), Delta Omega (Hon)
Director of Master of Professional Studies (MPS) - Veterinary Parasitology
Professor of Parasitology
Cornell University College of Veterinary Medicine
Ithaca, NY, USA

Catherine M. Brown, DVM, MSc, MPH
State Epidemiologist and State Public Health Veterinarian
Massachusetts Department of Public Health
Jamaica Plain, MA, USA

Brian A. DiGangi, DVM, MS, DABVP (Canine & Feline Practice, Shelter Medicine Practice)
Senior Director, Shelter Medicine
American Society for the Prevention of Cruelty to Animals (ASPCA)
New York, NY, USA

Erin Doyle, DVM, DABVP (Shelter Medicine Practice)
Senior Director, Shelter Medicine & Residency Programs
American Society for the Prevention of Cruelty to Animals (ASPCA)
Needham, MA, USA

Virginia R. Fajt, DVM, PhD, DACVCP
Clinical Professor
Texas A&M University
College Station, TX, USA

Jennifer Graham, DVM, DABVP (Avian / Exotic Companion Mammal), DACZM
Associate Professor of Zoological Companion Animal Medicine
Department of Clinical Sciences
Cummings School of Veterinary Medicine at Tufts University
Grafton, MA, USA

Brenda Griffin, DVM, MS, DACVIM, DABVP (Shelter Medicine Practice)
Adjunct Associate Professor
College of Veterinary Medicine, University of Florida
Gainesville, FL, USA

Kate F. Hurley, DVM, MPVM, DABVP (Shelter Medicine Practice)
Director, UC Davis Koret Shelter Medicine Program
UC Davis School of Veterinary Medicine
Davis, CA, USA

Stephanie Janeczko, DVM, MS, DABVP (Shelter Medicine and Canine/Feline Practice), CAWA
Vice President, Shelter Medicine Services
American Society for the Prevention of Cruelty to Animals (ASPCA)
New York, NY, USA

Cynthia Karsten, DVM, DABVP (Shelter Medicine Practice)
Outreach Veterinarian, UC Davis Koret Shelter Medicine Program
UC Davis School of Veterinary Medicine
Davis, CA, USA

S. Emmanuelle Knafo, DVM, Dipl. ACZM (Zoological Medicine)
Avian and Exotics Department
Red Bank Veterinary Hospital
Tinton, NJ, USA

Laurie J. Larson, DVM
Director, CAVIDS Titer Testing Service
University of Wisconsin School of Veterinary Medicine
Madison, WI, USA

Julie K. Levy, DVM, DACVIM, DABVP (Shelter Medicine Practice)
Fran Marino Endowed Professor of Shelter Medicine Education
Maddie's Shelter Medicine Program
College of Veterinary Medicine
University of Florida
Gainesville, FL, USA

Annette Litster, BVSc, PhD, FANZCVS (Feline Medicine), MMedSci (Clinical Epidemiology)
Senior Veterinary Specialist
Zoetis Petcare
Chicago, IL, USA

Araceli Lucio-Forster, PhD
Lecturer
Cornell University College of Veterinary Medicine
Ithaca, NY, USA

Lila Miller, BS, DVM
Vice President, Shelter Medicine (retired)
American Society for the Prevention of Cruelty to Animals (ASPCA)
New York, NY, USA

Sandra Newbury, DVM, DABVP (Shelter Medicine Practice)
Director, University of Wisconsin Shelter Medicine Program
Associate Professor, Department of Medical Sciences
University of Wisconsin-Madison School of Veterinary Medicine
Madison, WI, USA

Jeanette O'Quin, DVM, MPH, DACVPM, DABVP (Shelter Medicine Practice)
Assistant Professor
The Ohio State University
Columbus, OH, USA

Patricia A. Pesavento, DVM, PhD, DIP ACVP
Professor, Department of Pathology, Microbiology, and Immunology
School of Veterinary Medicine, UC Davis
Davis, CA, USA

Janet Scarlett, DVM, MPH, PhD
Emerita Professor of Epidemiology
Founder and Former Director, Maddie's Shelter Medicine Program
Cornell University College of Veterinary Medicine
Ithaca, NY, USA

Ronald D. Schultz, PhD
Emeritus
University of Wisconsin School of Veterinary Medicine
Madison, WI, USA

Martha Smith-Blackmore, DVM
Adjunct Assistant Clinical Professor
Cummings School of Veterinary Medicine at Tufts University
North Grafton, MA;
Veterinary Medical Director
City of Boston Animal Care and Control
Boston, MA, USA

Helen Tuzio, DVM, DABVP [Feline Practice], CVA
Clinical Associate Professor
Long Island University - College of Veterinary Medicine
Brookville, NY, USA

G. Robert Weedon, DVM, MPH
TLC PetSnip, Inc.
Lakeland, FL;
Retired Clinical Assistant Professor and Service Head
College of Veterinary Medicine, University of Illinois
Urbana, IL, USA

Preface

The first shelter medicine textbook, *Shelter Medicine for Veterinarians and Staff*, was published in 2004, five years after the first formal shelter medicine course at a veterinary college was taught at Cornell University in 1999. The preface to the 2009 first edition of *Infectious Disease Management in Animal Shelters* stated that "shelter medicine is a relatively new specialty area in veterinary medicine." Much has changed in the past 12 years, with perhaps the most significant change being that the evolution of shelter medicine resulted in it being recognized as a veterinary specialty in 2014. In addition, there are many shelter medicine classes offered as part of the core and elective curriculum of veterinary colleges, as well as internships and residency programs. The animal welfare field has acknowledged and embraced the foundational role that shelter medicine's core principles of population management, capacity for care, preventive medicine and infectious disease control play in the success of the field as a whole, and their importance in improving and saving individual animal lives. A broad range of animal welfare, veterinary, and even public health organizations have embraced the inclusion of shelter medicine and shelter considerations in guidelines for general management and disease control.

Despite numerous advances in the field, the need for these core foundational strategies persists and the purpose of this textbook remains the same as the first edition, i.e., to provide detailed, useful information regarding fundamental principles of disease control and specific management of the most important diseases encountered in dogs and cats in shelters. The information in this text is based on the authors' own substantial, practical experience working with shelter populations, as well as the latest research and evidence-based medicine. While the emphasis throughout is on strategies for the prevention of illness and mitigation of disease spread, pragmatic information on treatment and considerations for adoption are also included. Reflecting on the dynamic nature of sheltering organizations, the populations they serve, and the environment we live in, this edition contains a new chapter on exotic companion mammals. The chapters on vector-borne, bacterial and protozoal gastrointestinal diseases have been removed, and the zoonosis chapter has been streamlined and no longer includes abbreviated descriptions of the various zoonotic diseases. The editors recognized that an expanding wealth of resources are available to veterinary and sheltering professionals, and other textbooks and websites are available that can provide the latest up-to-date details about disease pathogenesis, diagnostic testing and individual animal treatment protocols. The reader is encouraged to use those resources along with this text. Readers are also encouraged to pay particular attention to the introduction, wellness, sanitation and outbreak management chapters, as this information is useful in all shelter situations. As in any practice, final decisions regarding the selection of treatment protocols, compliance with state, federal and local regulations, safe drug use and shelter practices are the responsibility of the veterinarian. The editors hope that this textbook will contribute to the continued improvement of animal health and welfare and the ongoing elevation of sheltering practices across the field.

Acknowledgments

The editors would like to thank Wiley Blackwell, all our contributing authors, the ASPCA, the UC Davis Koret Shelter Medicine Program and our families, friends and countless colleagues for their support, patience and understanding as we worked to complete this second edition of *Infectious Disease Management in Animal Shelters* textbook. Contrary to what one might think, editing a second edition is not necessarily easier than the first.

Special thanks must go to Erin Doyle for stepping in to write a chapter and Elise Gingrich for assisting with editing two chapters late in the process of completing this textbook. Brian DiGangi deserves particular recognition for not only helping edit this textbook, but for agreeing to co-author an additional chapter at the last minute while editing another shelter medicine textbook. Finally, we would like to acknowledge Jennifer Calder, the co-author of the zoonosis chapter in the first edition. After starting work to revise the chapter for this second edition, Jennifer had to step down to focus on her position as Director of Health of the City of Stamford, Connecticut to manage the COVID 19 pandemic.

1

Introduction to Infectious Disease Management in Animal Shelters

Kate F. Hurley[1] *and Lila Miller*[2]

[1] *UC Davis Koret Shelter Medicine Program, UC Davis School of Veterinary Medicine, Davis, CA, USA*
[2] *American Society for the Prevention of Cruelty to Animals (ASPCA), New York, NY, USA*

1.1 Why This Book?

Though many excellent veterinary texts on infectious disease have been published over the years, the first edition of this book was published in 2009 to fill a gap in understanding the specific challenges and solutions regarding infectious disease management in shelters. The risks in this context are abundant. Animals entering shelters are often unvaccinated, suffering from parasite infestation, poor nutrition and a variety of other stressors. Shelters house lost, unwanted and abused animals spanning every life stage, from neonates to geriatric pets, each with their own unique risks and requirements. Limited resources and outdated facilities, still found at many shelters, increase the difficulty of keeping these vulnerable populations healthy.

At the same time, the potential rewards of successful disease management in shelters are even greater than the challenges. Infectious disease in shelters has historically been a leading cause for euthanasia. But, in addition to being literally lifesaving, successfully treating individual animals, managing outbreaks, and most especially, preventing disease increases animals' welfare. Prevention of illness can also conserve precious resources and free up space in the shelter that would otherwise be occupied by sick animals. In turn, the improved public confidence that a healthy population tends to generate can lead to greater support of the shelter, higher adoption rates, and an increased capacity to invest in programs to decrease shelter admission and keep pets healthy and safe with their families.

1.1.1 Fundamentals of Disease Control in Shelters

Though some unique considerations exist for shelters, the fundamentals of disease management rest on a familiar foundation. In veterinary medicine, it is customary to think about the "disease triad" that describes the interaction of pathogen, host and environment in determining whether disease occurs. Introduction of pathogens into a shelter is virtually inevitable; therefore, efforts focus on supporting animals' immunity and limiting disease spread within the environment.

This text will provide strategies to accomplish each of these goals with respect to specific pathogens commonly encountered in shelters, as well as general information on methods to support immunity and limit environmental

Infectious Disease Management in Animal Shelters, Second Edition.
Edited by Lila Miller, Stephanie Janeczko, and Kate F. Hurley.

spread (e.g. see Chapter 2 on Wellness, Chapter 9 on Canine and Feline Vaccinations and Immunology, Chapter 8 on Sanitation and Chapter 6 on Outbreak Management). The reader will find information that reflects the ways in which shelter-specific considerations result in recommendations that vary from the approach that might be recommended in another context.

For instance, maternally derived antibodies (MDA) in juvenile animals have both good and bad consequences: they provide initial protection against disease but also potentially block vaccines. Initial levels of MDA will determine the age at which vaccines can overcome this interference, and this information has historically guided vaccine recommendations for pet puppies and kittens born to vaccinated dams. However, it is now known that many juvenile animals entering shelters were either born to unvaccinated dams and therefore received no MDA (and therefore no potential for MDA interference); or were born to mothers who survived field strain infection and may have transmitted high levels of MDA (Lechner et al. 2010). This means vaccines may be effective either earlier or later in comparison to offspring of a vaccinated dam with an intermediate level of MDA to transmit. This, coupled with the higher disease exposure risk common to shelters, leads to the recommendation to start vaccination earlier and continue longer for puppies and kittens in a shelter environment.

Another example can be found in the treatment recommendations for dermatophytosis. Often a self-limiting disease of little consequence in privately owned pets, this zoonotic and environmentally persistent (and resistant) pathogen has historically been the cause of euthanasia in many shelters. However, protocols that limit environmental contamination through effective topical, as well as systemic treatment, have been developed to allow this condition to be managed successfully at an increasing number of shelters (Newbury et al. 2011).

1.1.2 The Production Medicine Model

For all its benefits, infectious disease control is only one goal of a successful shelter medical program. The production medicine model, developed in the context of commercial animal husbandry enterprises, proves surprisingly applicable here. The successful livestock veterinarian understands their role extends beyond treatment or even prevention of disease. Rather, they provide guidance to help the production system reach a variety of goals, which may include such things as providing a healthy, safe food product, ensuring that the enterprise is financially sustainable, providing good welfare and maintaining compliance with relevant regulations. None of these goals may be reached at the expense of another.

Similarly, the shelter practitioner must approach the task of disease control with an understanding of the mission of the organization, its goals, requirements and priorities. The true art of shelter medicine involves balancing risks to best serve overall objectives, especially those that are potentially in conflict with one another. Balancing isolation and confinement for infectious disease control with allowing exercise, social interaction and contact with adopters is just one example.

The recommendations in this text aim to highlight some of the ways in which risk and reward balance in a shelter vary in comparison to other contexts. Methods are suggested to mitigate risks while maximizing the shelter's ability to meet their goals. Paradoxically, veterinarians can sometimes best contribute to overall shelter success by recommending practices that are seemingly *less* cautious rather than more when it comes to infectious disease control. For instance, routine quarantine of healthy-appearing incoming animals is commonly recommended in herd-health contexts to screen for animals that may be incubating disease. However, the increased length of stay (LOS) this practice entails, along with the increased population density as well as the cost and staff burden that results, often undermine other goals of the shelter such as judicious use of limited resources and rapid movement of healthy animals into adoptive homes. Alternative strategies to limit disease introduction, without the need for quarantine, include accurate history taking when possible, the performance of careful intake exams and vaccination, daily rounds and monitoring, optimized sanitation procedures and appropriate and prompt use of diagnostic testing. These topics are covered in more detail in Chapter 2 on Wellness and elsewhere in this text.

1.1.3 What's New in the Second Edition?

As with any subject, the understanding of infectious disease management has evolved in the decade since the publication of the first edition. Ongoing research has refined the profession's knowledge of complex and emerging diseases such as feline leukemia and canine influenza, leading to updated recommendations for diagnostic testing and management in shelter animals. Practical field experience has also honed understanding of the best ways to manage long-standing problems. For instance, at the time of publication of the first text, the use of antibody titers and RT-PCR (reverse transcription- polymerase chain reaction) testing for the management of canine distemper outbreaks was relatively new. These methods have now been proven effective in managing many shelter outbreaks, leading to expanded opportunities for non-lethal responses to this potentially devastating illness.

Alongside these advances in understanding disease management, new products have also led to expanded opportunities to preserve shelter animal health. For instance, accelerated hydrogen peroxide (Rescue™) has become a widely used disinfectant in shelters over the last 10 years. This product's reliability against viruses, safety, rapid action, multiple uses and relatively good penetration into organic matter have allowed more efficient sanitation strategies as well as more flexible use of housing materials. Another example is the development of "portals" to conjoin two cages into one more spacious double-compartment unit, allowing segregation of eating and resting areas from those used for elimination. The reduced handling and disease transmission associated with double-compartment housing, along with reduced stress, have led to reported reductions in feline upper respiratory infections (URI) of 70% or more at some shelters (CFHS 2018; Karsten et al. 2017).

The second example above highlights the impact of a growing body of shelter-specific research that extends well beyond the traditional arsenal of infectious disease management tools. The development of the portal was based on the finding that the risk for feline URI was dramatically lessened by the provision of >8 ft^2 floor space in cage housing during the first week of care (Wagner et al. 2018). Another study documented improved immunity and decreased feline URI risk associated with consistent, gentle human interaction with cats (Gourkow and Phillips 2015). The importance of such non-traditional approaches to disease management is reflected in Chapter 2 on Wellness and elsewhere throughout this text.

1.2 The Growth of Shelter Medicine

While scientific advances have been significant, one of the most dramatic developments regarding disease control in shelters has been the rapid evolution of the field of shelter medicine itself. The original edition of this book was published within a decade of such milestones as the first formal course in shelter medicine (taught at Cornell University in 1999), the establishment of the first Shelter Medicine residency training program at UC Davis in 2001, and the founding of the Association of Shelter Veterinarians (ASV) in that same year. Many veterinary colleges have since incorporated shelter medicine classes and shelter externship opportunities into their core and elective curricula.

In the decade since then, the rapid expansion of shelter medicine has been a striking development within veterinary medicine as well as within the field of animal sheltering. From a disease control perspective, a major milestone was reached with the publication of the ASV Guidelines for Standards of Care in Animal Shelters in 2010. This document addressed everything from shelter management, policy and record-keeping; through population management, facility design and sanitation; to the maintenance of physical and behavioral health of animals. The guidelines provide a powerful foundation for any program to maintain shelter animal health because all these elements are interrelated.

In addition to the ASV shelter guidelines, there has been an explosion of resources regarding virtually every aspect of shelter animal care and management. Along with a second edition of the seminal textbook "Shelter Medicine for Veterinarians and Staff," veterinary guidelines and/or textbooks now exist addressing data collection and interpretation in shelters; animal behavior for shelter veterinarians and staff, forensic medicine; high quality, high volume spay/neuter, and more. Websites maintained by shelter medicine programs at various veterinary colleges (e.g. UC Davis, Cornell, the University of Florida, University of Wisconsin) and organizations such as the American Society for the Prevention of Cruelty to Animals (ASPCA) and Maddies' Fund are just a few of the resources that provide useful and practical information for shelter medicine professionals.

The development of shelter medicine as a veterinary specialty has accompanied this proliferation of resources and research. The American Board of Veterinary Specialties conferred provisional recognition of shelter medicine as a specialty within the American Board of Veterinary Practitioners (ABVP) in 2014, and the first diplomates were certified the following year. As more veterinarians seek and attain board certification in shelter medicine, the pool of research and expert consultants to support successful disease-control programs in shelters will continue to grow.

1.2.1 Continued Advances in Animal Shelter Management

Advances in shelter medicine over the last decade have paralleled and supported the rapid evolution of animal-shelter management and community policy concerning abused, homeless and free-roaming dogs and cats. These changes, in turn, have resulted in substantially improved outcomes for shelter animals in many regions. A national database, Shelter Animals Count, (www.shelteranimalscount.org) has been developed to document these trends within the United States. Improvements to cat outcomes have been particularly striking. In 2018, the Million Cat Challenge (www.millioncatchallenge.org) announced that over 1,300 member shelters increased life-saving success compared to each shelter's baseline by over 1.1 million cats in the four years from 2014 to 2018.

With improved outcomes, a positive cycle has been created that further supports successful programs to control disease. Though the belief that euthanasia should be reserved for dangerous or suffering animals is a widely shared value, historically, the number of live outcomes has failed to keep pace with the rate at which healthy animals were admitted to many shelters. This created a painful dilemma: either euthanize healthy animals to create space or permit crowding and allow the resultant disease to take its toll. Non-lethal methods to balance shelter intakes with live outcomes are therefore a potent tool to maintain shelter animal health and welfare.

The practice of "Return to Field" (RTF) (also sometimes called Shelter/Neuter/Return), widely implemented in US shelters over the last decade, provides an example of this phenomenon. (Spehar and Wolf 2019). These programs involve sterilizing, vaccinating and returning cats to the location of origin, and are differentiated from traditional Trap/Neuter/Return (TNR) programs in that they target cats admitted to the shelter as part of normal animal control services, versus specifically captured with the intent to have the cat sterilized. Analysis of one of the first large-scale RTF programs demonstrated not only a reduction in euthanasia of over 75%, but also a 99% decrease in the number of cats euthanized for URI. With an additional outlet for healthy cats other than adoption, shelter managers are far less likely to face a choice between crowding or euthanasia – and the impact on feline health can be dramatic.

1.3 Capacity for Care: Blending Shelter Medicine and Management

The foregoing examples demonstrate the synergy that occurs when shelter health and shelter management practices work in support of each other. The most effective infectious disease control program will address the overall functioning of the shelter as a system, balancing animal intake with the organization's ability to provide appropriate care and find suitable outcomes. The success of this approach has been demonstrated in a shelter management model known as "Capacity for Care," which has been linked to decreased disease and euthanasia and increased live release rates (Karsten et al. 2017). Though piloted with an emphasis on cats, this model applies equally to dogs and involves optimizing the number of animals housed at any one time; actively managing the LOS of animals in the shelter; providing housing for each animal that meets or exceeds the ASV Guidelines for Standards of Care in Animal Shelters and using methods such as scheduled admission and removing barriers to adoption to maintain the population within the organization's humane capacity without resorting to increased euthanasia (CFHS 2016).

Whether used under the formal umbrella of the Capacity for Care management model or otherwise, these practices, when combined, represent an integrated approach that powerfully supports animal health and limits environmental disease transmission. Under these conditions, it is realistic to expect the spread of serious infectious disease to be a relatively rare event. The shelter practitioner can then turn their attention to the chapters within this text that focus on methods to treat animals that enter the shelter already infected, or to improve the health of animals in the community.

Conversely, when housing is poor, LOS prolonged, or animal care is otherwise compromised because shelter capacity is exceeded, even the best vaccination, segregation and sanitation practices will be insufficient. In the face of repeated outbreaks or high levels of endemic disease, the reader is encouraged to revisit this chapter and access other resources – including the numerous guidelines, texts, and consulting services now available – to bring the shelter population into greater balance with the organization's ability to provide care.

1.3.1 Right-Sizing the Population

The ASV Guidelines for Standards of Care caution that "Every sheltering organization has a maximum capacity for care, and the population in their care must not exceed that level" (Newbury et al. 2010). The "right-size" for the shelter population at any one time can be defined as that which maximizes the number of animals served while not exceeding the organization's capacity to provide humane care. Limits on capacity include the number of adequately sized housing units, staffing level, and availability of specialized medical and behavioral care where needed.

Some of these numbers are relatively straightforward to determine. For example, in order to generate an estimated maximum population that can be accommodated, housing units can simply be counted, while total staff time available for daily animal care can be divided by the amount of time required for care on a per animal basis. The National Animal Care and Control Association (NACA) and Humane Society of the United States suggests a minimum of 15 minutes per animal per day for cleaning and feeding as a general guideline (NACA 2009). However, as expectations for care increase and shelter admissions shift toward animals requiring more medical and behavioral care, the time required per animal is better calculated based on direct observation and documentation of average care needs.

Even when housing numbers and staff time are ample, it may still be advantageous to maintain the population below the maximum that can be physically accommodated (Swanson 2015). Rather, the ideal size of the population is driven by the average daily expected throughput (intake or outcome) of animals multiplied by the target LOS to the best possible outcome. The "average daily throughput" should generally be based on monthly intake and outcome estimates based on past performance and, ideally, should be calculated separately by species and age of animals (juvenile versus adult).

Though calculations should ultimately be made separately for holding areas and other common pathways such as animals awaiting transfer to partner agencies, the ideal number of animals available for adoption provides a straightforward illustration and can be a good place to start. This number has sometimes been described as "Adoption Driven Capacity." For instance, if a shelter expects to perform 60 adult cat adoptions in one month, based on historical trends and aims to keep the LOS for cats at no more than 15 days, the calculation for the ideal number of cats awaiting adoption is as follows:

Sixty cats adopted per month/30 days in a month = ~two cats adopted on average each day. Two cats adopted each day × 15 days target LOS per cat to adoption = 30 cats on average that should be available for adoption at any given time.

Doubling the number of cats available from 30 to 60 would mean that cats stay twice as long on average unless the increased population somehow bring in twice the number of adopters. Conversely, reducing the number of cats awaiting adoption from 30 to 20 (for instance via a one-time adoption promotion event) would lower the average LOS from 15 days to 10 (20 cats available for adoption/two adoptions on average per day). The benefits this population decrease could have, in terms of staff time and resource allocation, as well as the direct health effects of reduced population density and shorter LOS, will be apparent to the reader.

This example is provided only as a brief illustration. Detailed instructions on "right-sizing" shelter populations are beyond the scope of this chapter but can be found elsewhere, often under the heading "Capacity for Care" (CFHS 2018; Karsten et al. 2017). Suffice to say that performing these calculations and developing strategies to right-size the shelter population and maintain it at that level are a vital component of a successful shelter health and infectious disease control program.

1.3.2 Length of Stay (LOS)

Reducing the LOS in shelters is an end in itself, provided that it does not come at the expense of successful life-saving outcomes. From a welfare perspective, even the best shelter housing does not replicate the experience of being in a home. Meeting an animal's behavioral needs becomes more challenging the longer they remain in confinement. Studies have also documented an increased risk of shelter-acquired disease as LOS increases (Dinnage et al. 2009; Edinboro et al. 2004). Behavioral deterioration and illness in turn can lead to yet longer stays, triggering a negative cycle that can be difficult to reverse. To avoid this, pro-active plans and consistent checkpoints should be in place, and LOS should be reported and evaluated on a regular basis as a vital indicator of shelter animal and system health.

1.3.2.1 Pathway Planning and Daily Rounds

In addition to right-sizing the population as described above, methods to reduce the LOS include active "pathway planning" toward the best possible outcome for each animal from the moment of admission (or even more ideally, before the animal is admitted), and performing daily population rounds to keep each animal on track. The daily rounds team should include staff members able to assess and resolve clerical-/client-service issues (such as administrative paperwork and client-contact concerns) as well as animal care, medical and behavioral issues. The daily assessment should include an evaluation of the following:

- Paperwork/computer record (including any signage on the animal's housing unit)
- Animal location within the facility and with regard to availability status (e.g. moving animals to adoption at the end of required holding periods)
- Animal health and demeanor, taking steps as needed to address medical and behavioral concerns, reduce stress and improve comfort (e.g. moving a stressed dog to a quieter ward)
- Actions required to move the animal toward the best possible outcome, such as scheduling surgery, contacting rescue, promoting adoption, etc.

The daily rounds team is not expected to both identify and accomplish all needed actions. Rather, daily rounds are a time to capture and assign tasks to the appropriate staff members. While it may seem daunting at first, rounds will more than repay the time it requires to complete them by identifying and removing bottlenecks to animal flow, resolving issues before they cause delays, and noticing and addressing animals' needs to prevent, or at least mitigate, health and behavioral risks. Ultimately, daily rounds save substantial staff time and reduce costs overall.

1.3.2.2 Fast Track Management and Open Selection

A common concern around reducing LOS is that animals will not have time to find their perfect match, especially those with more extensive needs or that are simply a little less likely to appeal to the average adopter. It's important to remember that arbitrary time limits are not a method to reduce the LOS, nor is rushing to euthanasia ever a solution unless an animal is irremediably suffering. Fortunately, such measures are not needed: programs to reduce LOS are designed to benefit *all* animals passing through the shelter, regardless of their perceived adoptability.

One way to ensure sufficient resources for those animals that require more of an investment is to capitalize fully on the potential of some animals to move through the shelter system very quickly. Fast Track management and Open Selection are two well-described methods to accomplish this. The purpose of introducing them here is to familiarize the reader with the concepts and terminology should they wish to pursue more information, which is widely available in publications and web-based sheltering resources.

1.3.2.2.1 Fast Track Management

Fast Track management involves identifying those animals that, as noted above, have the potential to move rapidly through the shelter to adoption. While each shelter should identify what makes an animal "fast track" based on their own records and experience, for most shelters, this will include puppies, kittens, and friendly, healthy, non-geriatric animals, especially those with an unusual breed/appearance, a compelling story, or physical features such as one eye or extra toes that make them appear to be most adoptable.

At its most basic, Fast Track management simply means that these animals "skip to the head of the line" to be processed first. In other words, rather than processing animals in order of intake date, the most adoptable animals get the first spot available in surgery or on the adoption floor. While this may initially seem unfair, Fast Track management tends to benefit "slow track" animals equally, if not more. By moving the fast trackers through quickly, population density is reduced, leaving more space and time to care for, enrich and promote the slow trackers; all of which also helps them move through the shelter more quickly. In fact, some shelters have reported greater decreases in LOS for slow trackers than for fast trackers following a shift to this management method. Additional resources on this subject can be found in the textbook "Shelter Medicine for Veterinarians and Staff" and by searching online for the term Fast Track management in animal shelters (Newbury and Hurley 2012). At the time of publication, two excellent resources on this subject could be found at (https://www.animalsheltering.org/magazine/articles/life-fast-lane) and https://www.sheltermedicine.com/library/resources/?r=fast-track-slow-track-flow-through-planning.

1.3.2.2.2 Open Selection

Open Selection simply refers to the practice of allowing potential adopters to view, interact with and select animals during their holding period. It is appropriate for any potentially adoptable animal, without valid identification or other indicators, that they are likely to be reclaimed. By allowing Open Selection, the legal hold on a stray animal can serve the double purpose of allowing animals to be considered for adoption at the same time as awaiting possible reclaim, with the benefit that the potential adopters themselves will then indicate which animals are truly "Fast Track." By definition, any animal selected for adoption during its hold period has the potential to move quickly through the system and should be prioritized for surgery or any required procedures as soon as they can legally be performed.

Logistically speaking, depending on the housing setup, Open Selection animals can be directly housed in adoption areas with signage indicating that they are not yet available, or visitors can be allowed into stray holding areas. Either way, a simple system should be developed to document holds and determine priority, if more than one potential adopter is interested. Open Selection alone can have a surprisingly big impact on lowering the LOS and reducing population density, sometimes opening the door for more resource-intensive interventions such as daily rounds or housing improvements. This is especially true where a long stray hold inevitably prolongs LOS or when lack of room in adoptions or lack of staff for needed procedures (such as testing or surgery) leaves animals to languish in the shelter past their date of availability.

1.3.2.3 Other Methods to Reduce the Length of Stay

In addition to the methods outlined above, shelter managers and veterinarians should work together with policymakers and other stakeholders, as needed, to reduce unproductive LOS at every opportunity. This is by no means an exhaustive list, but some methods may include:

- Reduce or eliminate stray-holding periods, especially for animals unlikely to be reclaimed
  - In most shelters, reclaim – or at least initial contact with an owner – tends to occur within the first few days of impound. Holding periods beyond this tend to delay progress along other lifesaving pathways.
- Eliminate voluntary intake quarantine periods for healthy appearing animals (as described earlier in this chapter).
  - This includes eliminating holds for puppies and kittens awaiting second vaccines. The best protection for young animals is to practice excellent biosecurity when handling and housing in a shelter, and to move them out into homes (permanent or foster) as quickly as possible.
  - Intake quarantine may still be indicated for animals with an extraordinarily high risk of serious disease, such as transfers from a shelter experiencing an active parvovirus or distemper outbreak or victims of animal hoarding.
- Eliminate bottlenecks associated with procedures that can only be performed by specialized staff, especially those that are difficult

to interpret or provide limited additional information to adopters.
  - Consider allowing feline leukemia virus (FeLV) and feline immunodeficiency virus (FIV) testing to be performed by the adopter's veterinarian with the opportunity for more in-depth conversation and follow-up about the implications and uncertainties of test interpretation and prognosis in a healthy cat.
  - Consider replacing formal behavior evaluations in dogs with a holistic assessment of the dog's history and behavior throughout the shelter stay. Some shelter medicine and behavior experts have raised questions about the validity of non- peer-reviewed behavior evaluations of shelter animals for adoption (Patronek and Bradley 2016).
- Perform spay/neuter surgery on healthy, robust kittens at 1.5 pounds rather than waiting until they reach 2 pounds.
  - Though 2 pounds/1 kg have been common cut-offs for surgical weight in kittens, there is no scientific basis for this tradition and 1.5 pounds is considered acceptable from both a surgical and developmental perspective (ASV 2016).
  - The same surgical, anesthetic, before- and after-care precautions should be used as for pediatric spay/neuter in 2-pound kittens.
  - This can be especially helpful in reducing LOS when foster options are limited and kittens must spend time in the shelter awaiting either a foster home or surgery.

1.3.3 The Importance of Good Housing

For both dogs and cats, shelter housing plays a pivotal role in determining disease risks and spread. The quality and setup of the housing unit will impact every aspect of the animal's experience, from how well they eat and sleep to the quality of the air they breathe. In turn, these factors will in large part determine the animal's susceptibility to disease. Something as simple as separate areas for feeding/resting versus elimination can have a profound effect on animal health and well-being.

The elements of adequate housing to support shelter animal health are described in more detail in Chapter 2 on Wellness, as well as in the ASV Guidelines for Standards of Care in Animal Shelters and other resources. For instance, a comprehensive description of cat-housing considerations in shelters was recently published at the time of this writing. As shelter housing best practices evolve, they should be given priority and attended to meticulously. Though animal health can be preserved even in a dilapidated facility, if the housing units themselves impede an animal's ability to exhibit normal behaviors, are cramped or poorly ventilated and exacerbate noise or stress, infectious disease control will be an ongoing struggle.

1.3.4 Balancing Intake and Positive Outcomes

Right-sizing the population, actively managing LOS and providing high-quality housing will go a long way toward maintaining a shelter population within the organization's capacity to provide care. However, there may still be times when the incoming population exceeds the organization's ability to provide appropriate outcomes. While even the most successful shelter health program may not be sufficient to fully remedy such an imbalance – especially when substantial funding or policy barriers to life-saving programs exist – interventions other than euthanasia are more likely to be effective and accepted, as well as being an end in themselves.

Fortunately, it is increasingly recognized that methods to regulate intake and increase live outcomes are appropriate for shelters of all types, whether publicly funded/municipal or private/non-profit and regardless of the terminology by which they are described (e.g. "Open admission," "Adoption guarantee" or "No-kill"). For instance, at the time of publication of the first edition of this text, scheduling intake, in coordination with available space, was a relatively uncommon practice at municipal shelters. However, it is now more widely recognized that this represents a responsible policy and indeed a best practice to better serve both animals and the public.

This does not mean that intake is limited, only that it is coordinated with available space in order to maintain safe and humane conditions in the shelter. For instance, the intake of an animal presented on a Friday might be deferred until after an adoption event over the weekend in order to make space without resorting to euthanasia. In fact, just as public health is often best served by preventive programs designed to keep people *out* of hospitals, more shelters and communities are investing in safety net programs that serve many animals without requiring shelter entry at all (HSUS 2012).

On the other side of the equation, more strategies have been developed to increase live outcomes for those animals that do enter the shelter's care. For instance, high fees and restrictive policies were once widely considered imperative to protect animals from ill-prepared or uncaring adopters. However, it is now known that animals adopted through a conversational rather than a strict, policy-based adoption process, acquired without a fee and even received as gifts receive equal levels of care and enjoy equal levels of owner attachment (Weiss and Gramman 2009; Weiss et al. 2014). The negative consequences of high adoption fees should never be underestimated: the resultant increases in LOS, crowding and subsequent illness and even euthanasia far outweigh any adoption revenue that would have been gained. Fee-waived events, adoption promotions and a welcoming adoption process are as integral to maintaining animal health in shelters as any medical treatment or vaccine.

Finally, as described earlier in this chapter in the case of RTF, shelter animal health as well as outcomes can be dramatically improved when adoption is not the only live pathway out. Transport programs provide an interim solution to move animals from higher to lower risk shelters, and detailed guidelines and regulations have been developed to minimize the risk associated with this practice by various states, the ASV and National Federation of Humane Societies, among others (National Federation 2019; Newbury et al. 2010). Ideally, in the longer term, shelters and communities will continue to explore and expand other avenues for increasing live outcomes. In addition to RTF, this includes increasing the number of animals reunited with their owners through non-punitive approaches mirroring the "adopters welcome" approach that has enjoyed such success by not only encouraging members of the community to adopt shelter animals, but by also offering ongoing support (http://www.animalsheltering.org/topics/adoptions).

1.4 Conclusion

When the first edition of this book was published in 2009, the urgency of bringing a systematic and tailored approach to infectious disease control in shelters was clearly evident. The focus in the first text was on the management of individual diseases and included chapters on vector-borne, dermatologic and gastrointestinal (GI) diseases. Those chapters have been eliminated in this edition because the information is available elsewhere and has not changed substantially. As shelter medicine and the profession of animal sheltering continue to evolve, the rewards of population-oriented strategies have become ever-more apparent and thus have received more attention in this second edition. By combining the traditional methods of veterinary science with a growing understanding of the unique needs and opportunities in this complex field, the holistic vision of the shelter practitioner as an essential cog in the "Production Medicine" model – where the "product" is healthier animals, shelters and communities, with more animals leaving shelters alive and fewer needing to enter the shelter at all, is closer to being realized.

References

ASV (Association of Shelter Veterinarians) (2016). The Association of Shelter Veterinarians' 2016 Veterinary Medical Care Guidelines for Spay-Neuter Programs. *Journal of the American Veterinary Medical Association* 249 (2): 165–188.

CFHS (Canadian Federation of Humane Societies) (2018). Capacity for Care Case Studies Update. In: Capacity for Care Case Studies, 1–26. Canadian Federation of Humane Societies.

Dinnage, J., Scarlett, J.M., and Richards, J.R. (2009). Descriptive epidemiology of feline upper respiratory tract disease in an animal shelter. *Journal of Feline Medicine and Surgery* 11: 816–825.

Edinboro, C.H., Ward, M.P., and Glickman, L.T. (2004). A placebo- controlled trial of two intranasal vaccines to prevent tracheobronchitis (kennel cough) in dogs entering a humane shelter. *Preventive Veterinary Medicine* 62: 89–99.

Gourkow, N. and Phillips, C.J. (2015). Effect of interactions with humans on behaviour, mucosal immunity and upper respiratory disease of shelter cats rated as contented on arrival. *Preventive Veterinary Medicine* 121 (3–4): 288–296.

HSUS (Humane Society of the United States) (2012). Pets for Life survey.

Karsten, C.L., Wagner, D.C., Kass, P.H. et al. (2017). An observational study of the relationship between capacity for care as an animal shelter management model and cat health, adoption and death in three animal shelters. *The Veterinary Journal* 227: 15–22.

Lechner, E.S., Crawford, P.C., Levy, J.K. et al. (2010). Prevalence of protective antibody titers for canine distemper virus and canine parvovirus in dogs entering a Florida animal shelter. *Journal of the American Veterinary Medical Association* 236 (12): 1317–1321.

National Animal Care and Control Association (NACA) (2009). Determining Kennel Staffing Needs. http://www.nacanet.org/kennelstaffing.html (accessed 17 July 2019).

National Federation of Humane Societies (2019). Companion Animal Transport Programs – Best Practices Overview. http://www.humanefederation.org/TransferBestPractice.cfm (accessed 17 July 2019).

Newbury, S. and Hurley, K. (2012). Population Management. In: Shelter Medicine for Veterinarians and Staff (eds. L. Miller and S. Zawistowski), 93–114. Ames: Blackwell Publishing.

Newbury, S., Blinn, M.K., Bushby, P.A. et al. (2010). ASV Guidelines for Standards of Care in Animal Shelters. https://www.sheltervet.org/assets/docs/shelter-standards-pdf (accessed 17 July 2019).

Newbury, S., Moriello, K.A., Kwochka, K.W. et al. (2011). Use of itraconazole and either lime sulphur or Malaseb Concentrate Rinse® to treat shelter cats naturally infected with microsporum canis: an open field trial. *Veterinary Dermatology* 22 (1): 75–79.

Patronek, G.P. and Bradley, J. (2016). No better than flipping a coin: reconsidering canine behavior evaluations in animal shelters. *Journal of Veterinary Behavior* 15: 66–77.

Spehar, D.D. and Wolf, P.J. (2019). Integrated return-to-field and targeted trap-neuter-vaccinate-return programs result in reductions of feline intake and euthanasia at six municipal animal shelters. *Frontiers in Veterinary Science* 6: 1–13.

Swanson, D. (2015). What's your magic number? Analyzing shelter capacity can increase live releases. *Animal Sheltering* (May/June), pp. 20–24.

Wagner, D.C., Kass, P.H., and Hurley, K.F. (2018). Cage size, movement in and out of housing during daily care, and other environmental and population health risk factors for feline upper respiratory disease in nine North American animal shelters. *PLoS One* 13 (1): e0190140.

Weiss, E. and Gramman, S. (2009). A comparison of attachment levels of adopters of cats: fee-based adoptions versus free adoptions. *Journal of Applied Animal Welfare Science* 12 (4): 360–370.

Weiss, E., Gramann, S., Dolan, E.D. et al. (2014). Do policy based adoptions increase the care a pet receives? An exploration of a shift to conversation based adoptions at one shelter. *Open Journal of Animal Sciences* 04 (05): 313–322.

2

Wellness

Brenda Griffin

College of Veterinary Medicine, University of Florida, Gainesville, FL, USA

2.1 Introduction: Wellness Defined

Simply stated, the primary goal of any animal shelter (no matter what resources, philosophy, or mission it possesses) must be for animals to be as physically and behaviorally healthy as possible during their stays. The protection of public health and safety must also be central goals. In this way, shelters also achieve the goal of public education, leading by example as they display good animal care practices.

Wellness is defined as the maintenance of good health. Both physical health and behavioral (or emotional) health comprise wellness. For example, a dog may be physically fit, free from infectious or other physical diseases, but suffering from severe anxiety. This animal cannot be assessed as truly healthy; his behavioral disorder must be addressed to ensure his well-being. A wellness program to optimize animal health in the shelter must therefore address both physical and behavioral health. In addition to addressing the animals themselves, addressing the shelter environment is also critically important when developing a wellness program for an animal shelter. Even the best-designed facilities cannot manage or prevent infectious disease and problem behaviors without thoughtful implementation of environmental wellness protocols. In small animal practice, environmental wellness is frequently not emphasized simply because many owners are accustomed to providing a reasonably healthy environment for their pets. In contrast, a structured program to address environmental wellness is essential in the context of an animal shelter regardless of the actual physical design of the facility. Proactive measures to maintain clean, sanitary environments that are not overcrowded, where animals are segregated (by species, health and behavior status), shielded from stressful stimuli, and provided with regular daily schedules of care by well-trained, dedicated staff are essential.

2.2 The Critical Importance of Wellness Protocols for Shelters

Infectious diseases, stress, and problem behaviors are common in cats and dogs housed in animal shelters. Pets entering shelters are highly stressed and at significant risk of acquiring infections and developing disease. The stress of even short-term confinement in a shelter can compromise both physical and behavioral health, negatively affect animal welfare and make cats and dogs less desirable

Infectious Disease Management in Animal Shelters, Second Edition.
Edited by Lila Miller, Stephanie Janeczko, and Kate F. Hurley.

to potential adopters. Though considerable progress has been made in recent years to increase the live release rate of animals in shelters, individual animals with compromised physical or behavioral health are still less likely to be adopted and more likely to be euthanized. Furthermore, when animals experience stress chronically, the attendant physiological and behavioral manifestations may persist even after adoption, compromising behavioral health and welfare in the long term.

The maintenance of good health or wellness of animals in shelters presents challenges for several reasons. Risk factors for the development of infectious disease include the frequent introduction of new animals often with unknown histories to the facility, high-density housing, housing animals of different ages and susceptibility levels in close proximity, induction of stress, and lack of adequate vaccination or insufficient time to respond to vaccination. All these risk factors, and others, exist in the shelter setting; therefore, a certain risk of infectious disease is inherent. In addition, certain diseases become endemic in facilities where populations of animals are housed, especially if wellness and disease control protocols are inadequate, or if staff lack training or if facility design and sanitation are poor.

Confinement of companion animals in a shelter can result in the display of a wide variety of behavioral indicators of stress, fear, anxiety, and/or frustration, including activity depression, hyperactivity, stereotypic behavior (such as pacing or circling), and barrier aggression, among others. Programs that reduce stress and related negative emotional states also serve to minimize the morbidity of endemic infectious diseases because stress has a profound influence on disease transmission as well as behavior. Shelter environments must be enriched to minimize stress, fear, anxiety, and frustration.

It is neither acceptable nor humane to house animals under conditions likely to induce illness and poor welfare. In addition, if animal shelters are to compete with other sources of animals for adoption, they must be able to present healthy animals in a healthy environment. Though very few regulations and mechanisms for oversight of animal shelters exist, shelters have an ethical obligation (and are increasingly expected by the public) to provide humane care for the well-being of every animal being handled. In order to meet this obligation, there is a critical need for a wellness program in every shelter.

2.2.1 Goals of a Shelter Wellness Program

The goals of a shelter wellness program are to minimize infectious disease and problem behaviors while optimizing the physical and behavioral health of the animals. Shelter wellness programs should not be based on control of a single disease or problem but should offer broad-based preventive strategies (a holistic approach). When shelters meet these goals, both public relations and adoption rates may be positively impacted. Further, shelter wellness programs must address both the health of individual animals and the health of the population. Shelter medicine has been compared to herd health (Hurley 2004). Indeed, much like a herd-health approach, population medicine in the shelter utilizes a systematic approach for optimizing animal health in the group. Unlike a herd-health program for large animals, where production (i.e. meat, milk, eggs, etc.) is the ultimate goal, ensuring the welfare of cats and dogs is the ultimate goal in the animal shelter. In order to implement a comprehensive wellness program for the shelter, establishing goals for and methods of monitoring the population is critical to ensuring animal health and welfare. Medical decisions must be weighed in the context of the population as well as the individual, while also considering animal welfare and the availability of resources. Finally, assessment and follow-up must be performed on a population as well as an individual level.

Wellness programs will vary depending on the shelter's mission, philosophy, and resources, and may even vary within shelters depending on such factors as intake rate and time of year. However, under no circumstances should a shelter engage in any practice or omission that would result in animals being allowed to suffer unnecessarily or unjustifiably. Inadequate or delayed veterinary care constitutes neglect, which is illegal according to some state laws. When situations arise in which animal welfare cannot be managed, whether due to physical or behavioral disease or environmental conditions such as overcrowding, euthanasia must be considered if no other remedies exist or it is beyond the shelter's ability to relieve animal suffering. Euthanasia, however, should not be used as a substitute for providing animals with proper care. Shelters should implement earnest programs to decrease the euthanasia of adoptable animals and community cats and seek alternatives to admitting an animal if it is beyond the shelter's capacity to provide appropriate care. For example, intake diversion programs may help provide alternative means of providing care for animals that do not need to enter the shelter system, such as food banks, low-cost veterinary clinics, or neuter-return programs for community cats. Comprehensive shelter wellness programs that include the delivery of efficient care, thoughtful and timely planning, evaluation, and follow-up are the foundations of shelter animal healthcare. These programs support the essential goals of animal sheltering: maximizing live release and animal welfare while minimizing euthanasia and suffering. Research is helping to better define protocols for limiting and treating physical and behavioral diseases common to shelter animal populations and to better assess their welfare or quality of life.

2.2.2 Quality of Life

Every attempt must be made to sustain quality of life for shelter animals. Like "happiness," quality of life remains difficult to define. Both physical and emotional factors contribute to quality of life, well-being, or welfare. These factors are broad, complex, and very individual. According to McMillan (2000), quality of life "is comprised of an array of affective states, broadly classified as comfort-discomfort and pleasure states. In general, the greater the pleasant and the lesser the unpleasant effects, the higher the quality of life."

Criteria are lacking for the objective measurement of the quality of life for cats and dogs; however, subjective assessments utilizing the most information possible can and should be made by medical and behavioral personnel at regular intervals (weekly or daily as indicated). Researchers are giving increased attention to validating quality-of-life measurements, which could help ensure humane endpoints for healthcare, define minimum housing standards, and be used for welfare audits in animal shelters as well as other settings where populations of animals are housed (Barnard et al. 2016). The Farm Animal Welfare Council's (FAWC) Five Freedoms represent a benchmark for measuring quality of life or assessing animal welfare (see Table 2.1). Since their introduction by council chair Dr. Roger Brambell in 1965, the Five Freedoms have been applied broadly as key animal welfare principles in numerous animal care settings.

Whereas the Five Freedoms emphasize freedoms from unpleasant experiences (hunger/thirst; discomfort; pain/injury/disease; fear/

Table 2.1 The Five Freedoms.

1) **Freedom from hunger and thirst** by ready access to fresh water and a diet to maintain full health and vigor.
2) **Freedom from discomfort** by providing an appropriate environment, including shelter and a comfortable resting area.
3) **Freedom from pain, injury, or disease** by prevention or rapid diagnosis and treatment.
4) **Freedom to express normal behavior** by providing sufficient space, proper facilities, and company of the animal's own kind.
5) **Freedom from fear and distress** by ensuring conditions and treatment that avoid mental suffering.

distress), it is recognized that good quality of life or good welfare is not merely the absence of negative experiences, but also the presence of positive ones. To this end, the FAWC continues to work to better define quality of life for animals across a spectrum of conditions that represent "a good life" to "a life not worth living." In the case of a life not worth living, defining the minimal acceptable treatment of animals is key. As such, FAWC supports "Banner's principles", which first and foremost state that "harms of a certain degree and kind ought under no circumstances to be inflicted on an animal."

According to the FAWC (2009), "achievement of a life worth living requires provision for an animal's needs and certain wants, and care by all involved. Wants are those resources that an animal may not need to survive or to avoid developing abnormal behavior, but nevertheless improve its quality of life. They may well stem from learned behaviors, so that once an animal has become accustomed to their provision, then withdrawal may lead to an adverse mental experience. They may also be innate such as space to play, to groom or engage in other normal behaviors." These tenets purported by the FAWC expand and enhance the principles of the Five Freedoms and can be used to help better define requirements for humane care that promote an acceptable quality of life for animals in a variety of settings, including shelters.

2.2.3 Guidelines for Standards of Care in Animal Shelters

In order to address the absence of professional guidelines for animal care in shelters, the Association of Shelter Veterinarians (ASV) published "Guidelines for Standard of Care in Animal Shelters" in 2010. The first of its kind, this groundbreaking document provides scientific and humane recommendations specifically for shelter animal care. It was written with the Five Freedoms as its basis to ensure all aspects of shelter practices support animal welfare. It identifies ideal, best and unacceptable practices as well as minimum standards of care for shelter animals. The document has been broadly supported by organizations including the National Federation of Humane Societies and the Society of Animal Welfare Administrators (now the Association for Animal Welfare Advancement), the National Animal Control Association, the American Society for the Prevention of Cruelty to Animals (ASPCA), and the Humane Society of the United States as a valuable aid to organizations for ongoing self-assessment and improvement of animal care regardless of the organization's mission or resources. The guidelines strongly support the importance of wellness programs for animal shelters and are an important source of information for any organization that cares for animals. They are available as a free download from the ASV website at http://www.sheltervet.org. The ASPCA offers a checklist for implementation of the guidelines at http://www.aspcapro.org. Compliance with the guidelines can be expected to improve animal care and welfare, however, it is currently voluntary.

2.2.4 Considerations Regarding Infectious Disease Transmission

Despite the fact that infectious agents are always present in the environment, under normal conditions, health is maintained. It is well recognized that the development of infectious disease is determined by a complex interaction of many factors surrounding the host, infectious agent, and the environment. The species, age, sex, general health, and immune status, as well as stress level and genetic predispositions of the host are all known to be factors that influence animal health (Greene 2012).

Infectious agents vary in virulence and modes of transmission. In many cases, they persist in the environment because they are resistant to disinfection, and many produce carrier states that contribute to continued environmental contamination or direct exposure of other animals. The amount and duration of exposure to an infectious agent, as well as methods of spread, routes of inoculation, carrier states, and mutation rates will all affect the likelihood that disease will spread in the shelter environment. Disease may be spread by direct contact with infected animals or carriers, via inhalation, ingestion, and contact with feces, urine, other bodily secretions, fomites, or even vectors such as fleas, ticks, flies and mosquitoes. Environmental factors also contribute substantially to disease, including housing density, ease of cleaning/disinfection, extremes or fluctuations of temperature, and air quality, among others. Environmental stressors such as loud or unfamiliar noises, unfamiliar stimuli, and unpredictable events are additional contributors. Thus, no single factor results in disease; rather, disease results from a combination of factors.

The importance of adhering to traditional general principles of infectious disease control must never be overlooked in an animal shelter. These include:

1) Vigilant surveillance and early recognition of disease.
2) Removal of infected animals (through isolation, transfer to foster care or other veterinary or rescue partners with adequate facilities, or euthanasia).
3) Mass vaccination and/or mass treatment.
4) Good husbandry and wellness practices (animals and environment).
5) Continual education and training of personnel.

Ultimately, disease control is best addressed proactively by establishing and implementing wellness protocols. Please see the Introduction in Chapter 1 for more information on the principles of infectious disease control in a shelter.

2.2.4.1 Population Management and Capacity for Care

In the field of shelter medicine, the term population management is used to refer to an active daily process of planning involving ongoing evaluation and efficient response as an organization cares for multiple animals (Newbury and Hurley 2013). Providing efficient evaluation and care of animals is the key to minimizing each animal's length of stay (LOS) in the shelter, and therefore reducing their risk for the development of disease and problem behaviors. When populations are efficiently managed, wellness care is effectively delivered to support the physical and behavioral health of animals and their environment, increasing the animals' resistance to disease as well as their emotional resilience. In order to be effective, population management must take into consideration an organization's ability and resources to provide care.

The maximum daily population in an animal shelter that allows for maintenance of recommended standards of care has been defined by the Association of Shelter Veterinarians' Guidelines for Standards of Care in Animal Shelters (2010) as "capacity for care." Many factors impact a shelter's capacity for care including the availability of housing, staffing, and all other resources necessary to provide humane care. When sheltering organizations operate without sufficient resources to provide proper animal care, animal health and welfare are compromised. Increases in the prevalence of infectious diseases are common, and likewise, increases in displays of fear, anxiety, stress and frustration-related behaviors by resident animals can be expected. The delivery of effective population management and operating within an organization's capacity for care are both key requirements for the successful implementation of a shelter wellness program. Please see the Introduction in Chapter 1 for more information about population management.

2.2.4.2 Components of a Shelter Wellness Program

Wellness starts with the prevention of both disease and problem behaviors. Prevention is more time and cost-efficient than treatment. In addition, it reduces suffering and is kinder to the animals as well as to the staff that must care for them. Table 2.2 contains the recommended components of a wellness protocol for

Table 2.2 Recommended components of a wellness protocol for shelter cats and dogs.

Animal Wellness = Physical Health + Behavioral Health	
Physical Health	Behavioral (Emotional) Health
History and physical examination	History and behavioral examination/observation
Vaccination	Proper housing
Parasite control/prevention	Enrichment including:
Spay-neuter	• Social companionship
Animal Identification (ID)	• Physical stimulation/exercise
Proper nutrition and physical exercise	• Mental stimulation
Grooming	• Positive training
Periodontal/oral disease prevention	Positive emotional environment
Individual-specific care	

Table 2.3 Recommended components of a wellness protocol for the shelter environment.

Environmental Wellness = Physical Environment + Emotional Environment	
Physical Environment	Emotional Environment
Population density	Mitigation of stressors and factors that elicit fear, including noise and unfamiliar stimuli
Segregation of animals and traffic patterns	Consistent daily routines
Cleaning and sanitation	Positive predictable interactions and events
Other facility operations:	
Heating, ventilation, and air conditioning (HVAC)	
Noise control	
Regular light/dark cycles	
Facility maintenance, etc.	
Staff training	

shelter cats and dogs, and Table 2.3 shows the recommended components of a wellness protocol for the shelter environment.

2.3 The Problem-Oriented Approach to Shelter Medicine

In animal shelters, it is important to have efficient systems that allow for the assessment of individual animals while affording consideration to the population itself. Indeed, shelter medicine represents a unique blend of both individual patient and population medicine. A useful system for patient evaluation is known as the "problem-oriented approach," which is widely accepted as the gold standard for small animal patient care and assessment.

A problem is defined as "any abnormality requiring medical or surgical management or one that interferes with quality of life" (Lorenz 1993). Thus, problems include both physical and behavioral conditions that require management or treatment and/or that affect welfare. In an animal shelter, problems are also defined as conditions that affect public health and safety (such as potentially zoonotic diseases or severe or unpredictable aggression).

The problem-oriented approach is used to systematically identify and address an animal's problems. With this approach, the clinical reasoning process is based on four steps: (i) database collection, (ii) problem identification, (iii) plan formulation, and (iv) assessment and follow-up. This approach enables the clinician to logically approach each patient to ensure thorough and accurate assessment so that appropriate and timely actions can be taken. A thorough, written or computerized medical record that includes all elements of the animal's assessment and care must be maintained for each patient. See the section later in this chapter on medical record keeping and data collection for more information.

2.3.1 Step 1: Database Collection

An initial minimum database should be obtained on every patient. Though the size of the database is often debated, there is no disagreement that it must include a complete history and a complete physical examination, including observation of behavior whenever possible. From the perspective of a shelter, resources and philosophy must be considered when deciding what to include in the minimum database for each patient. The author's recommendations may be found in Table 2.4.

The author recommends the addition of the tests in Table 2.4 to the minimum database for geriatric animals that will be offered for adoption: These procedures broadly screen many body systems and are very cost-effective. These should be viewed as extensions of the physical examination for the geriatric animal. Whenever time and resources allow, the veterinarian should also consider fine-needle aspiration for in-house cytologic evaluation of all cutaneous and subcutaneous masses. This simple and inexpensive practice of evaluating "lumps and bumps" may identify potential malignancies that would otherwise go unchecked and provide reassurance that any growths present should not be cause for undue concern by potential adopters.

2.3.1.1 History

Next to physical examination, history is the most important aspect of medical problem-solving. The history alerts the clinician to the presence of potential physical and behavioral problems; it can be especially helpful for identifying problems that might not be detected on a physical examination. When available, a history can provide valuable information that

Table 2.4 Recommended minimum database for cats and dogs in the shelter.

At Intake	Prior to Adoption
History	Ongoing physical and behavioral observations/monitoring
Physical examination (including scanning for a microchip)	Feline leukemia virus (FeLV)/Feline immunodeficiency virus (FIV) testing (cats)
Behavioral observations (including a determination as to whether the animal is safe to handle)	Heartworm (HW) testing of dogs (in HW endemic areas)
	Fecal exam (if diarrhea is present)
	Geriatric patients[a]:
	Packed cell volume (PCV)/Total solids (TS), urine specific gravity and dipstick

[a] Geriatric: Small dogs (under 20 pounds) 10 years; medium and large dogs (21 to 90 pounds) 7–8 years; giant dogs (over 90 pounds) 6 years; cats 9–10 years.

may save time, money, and stress on the animal and staff. In many cases, historical information may be used to expedite the disposition of the pet. However, in the shelter setting, it may not always be possible to obtain an accurate history. Stray animals are often brought in by animal control officers or good Samaritans who have little, if any, information about the animal. Some shelters provide a location (e.g. drop-off cages or runs) where animals can be relinquished after business hours. When this is provided, every effort should be made to obtain the history through questionnaires that the relinquisher can fill out when the animal is dropped off. That said, the use of unattended drop boxes is strongly discouraged because of the risks associated with leaving animals unattended at intake and for indefinite periods of time until staff return to work (ASV 2010). The presence of staff to directly accept the animal and obtain the owner's name and a history at the time of relinquishment is greatly preferred. Even so, surrendering owners may not provide thorough or accurate information because of fears that if they are honest about a pet's problems, the pet may be euthanized; to allay those fears, they should be encouraged that providing accurate information will help improve the care of the animal while in the shelter and will also help facilitate a better adoption match.

Intake procedures should be in place to capture basic patient information, including both physical and behavioral data such as vaccination history, known or suspected medical problems, regular diet and food preferences, elimination habits, handling preferences (e.g. likes to be petted, pulls on the leash, etc.), known fears, etc. It should also include the reasons for relinquishment as well as a bite history that provides details about any incident in which a bite has occurred. Please see Chapter 21 on Zoonosis for a comprehensive sample bite history form. The importance of obtaining accurate historical information cannot be overemphasized.

2.3.1.2 Physical and Behavioral Examination

Physical and behavioral examination and observation are the most important aspects of the minimum database. Every animal (that is deemed safe to handle) should receive a physical examination at or as close to the time of admission to the shelter as possible. Utilizing a physical examination form will ensure a complete and systematic review of all body systems. In addition to physical examination, behavioral examination or observation should also begin upon admission. Likewise, implementing a standardized system for recording behavior observations beginning at intake will ensure that the animals' emotional health receives equal consideration.

It is imperative that behavior is always described objectively and in context. This will provide the most accurate picture of the animal. For example, "the dog cowered when a staff member reached towards her with her hand" is an objective contextual observation and is much more informative than recording "the dog is afraid of people." The latter is subjective information without context, which is generally at least partly based on personal opinion and emotions and can be easily misinterpreted. Someone who reads that a dog is afraid of people will not know whether she cowered, ran away, or bit someone, nor will they know in what context the behavior occurred. Shelters should always focus on collecting and recording objective information and context to ensure that each animal's record reflects their behavior as accurately as possible.

Formal behavior testing or evaluation is not recommended as a routine practice for every animal. These tests lack validation and do not reliably predict future behavior in the home (Patronek and Bradley 2016). It is imperative to recognize that behavioral responses are profoundly influenced by stress. Nonetheless, to the extent possible, it is crucial to observe initial behavior and to continue monitoring behavior in order to recognize and mitigate stress and other negative emotional states that animals may be experiencing in the shelter. It is also necessary to learn as much as possible about each individual animal to aid in optimizing shelter behavioral care, outcome assessment, and adoption matching and counseling. Criteria to identify dangerous animals, such as history and/or displays of severe or injurious aggression, combined with risk assessment, should be in place to protect staff and public safety. Assessment of behavior should include history as well as information gleaned from every human and animal interaction with the animal. Information gleaned from interacting with animals during routine intake and husbandry procedures as well as enrichment, play, and training activities can be used to provide for each individual animals' emotional needs, ensure their welfare in the shelter, and make the best possible decisions about safety, placement, and matching.

Of particular importance in the shelter physical examination is an accurate physical description of the animal and careful inspection for the presence of identification, both of which may aid in pet–owner reunification. Photographing animals is a very useful adjunct to written descriptions, and microchip scanning should be systematically and correctly performed on every animal at the time of intake and prior to the animal being made available for adoption or being euthanized.

An additional critical aspect of the intake exam for shelter animals is the identification of conditions that require special housing considerations. Common examples include:

- animals suspected of being infected with contagious diseases that would require isolation,
- pregnant animals that appear near term,
- nursing mothers with litters,
- very young animals,
- injured or debilitated animals,
- other animals with special physical or behavioral needs who would benefit from additional bedding and care.

Animals that are very fearful or withdrawn should ideally be housed in quiet areas, and care should be provided by staff with experience assessing behavior. Animals exhibiting feral-like behavior or deemed unsafe to handle on entry should be identified so that they can be housed appropriately in enclosures that are especially secure and designed to minimize animal handling and stress, such as those that contain guillotine doors for dogs, or cat dens for cats. See Figure 2.1a and 2.1b.

2.3.2 Step 2: Problem Identification

The second step in medical problem solving is problem identification. Problems are identified based on the information gleaned from the animal's minimum database. These include historical, physical and behavioral problems as well as quality-of-life/welfare, public health, and/or safety concerns. Problems should be stated at their current level of understanding, and historical problems should be verified whenever possible.

2.3.3 Steps 3: Plan Formulation

If problems are identified, a plan can be formulated to address them within the mission, philosophy, and resources of the shelter, and with respect to state and local laws that stipulate legal holding periods that allow owners the opportunity to find and claim their pets. Plan formulation ideally involves outlining the clinical reasoning process to rule in/out potential causes or differential diagnoses for each problem identified. The plan should take into consideration three elements, including any necessary (i) diagnostic testing, (ii) initial therapy, and (iii) relevant staff and/or adopter education.

2.3.4 Step 4: Assessment and Follow-Up

The final step in medical problem solving is assessment and follow-up. This involves making calculated clinical appraisals based on available patient data and outcome options

(a)

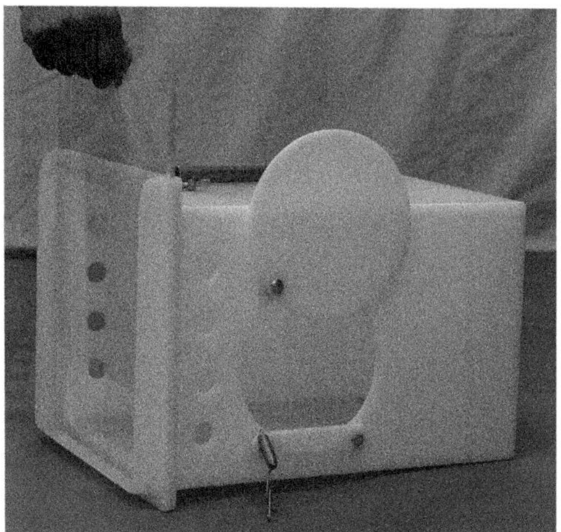

(b)

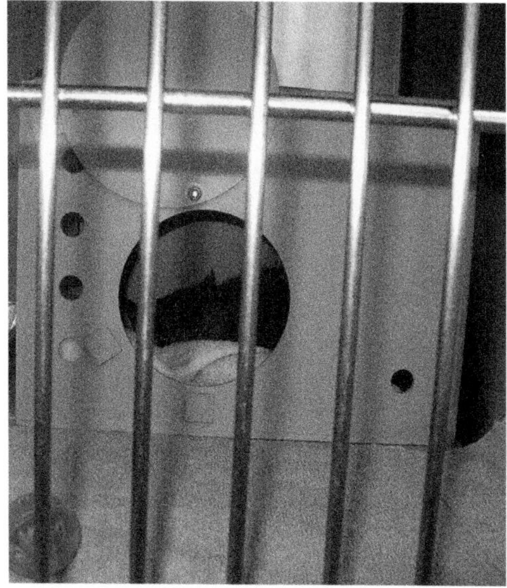

Figure 2.1 (a and b). A commercially available "cat den" serves as a secure hiding place for a fearful cat. The den's circular portal door can be closed from a safe and nonthreatening distance while the cage is spot cleaned as needed. The cat can also be securely transported in the den and the guillotine door provides a means of safe transfer to or from another box style enclosure, such as a trap or squeeze cage, if needed.

and documenting case progression over time. Timely action is essential in the shelter where animals may be triaged to adoption, foster care, rescue groups, isolation, or euthanasia. Plans and outcomes must be continuously moved forward through the shelter system with efficient ongoing assessments as needed. Regular reassessment is imperative, especially for animals that undergo long-term stays in shelters, to update known problems and to identify any new problems that may develop. In this way, all problems can be addressed in a timely fashion to ensure the wellbeing and safety of the individual animal as well as that of the population and the shelter staff.

A very useful initial assessment that facilitates triage of individuals and efficient population management involves designating animals as either "fast" or "slow track" based on the findings in their initial minimum database. Fast-track animals are those that enter the shelter in good physical and behavioral health and thus may be rapidly processed for immediate placement in adoption, foster care, or with rescue groups, serving to minimize the LOS of these animals. This, in turn, can be expected to free up more time and resources for slow-track animals that may require special medical and/or behavioral care. Identifying and triaging fast- and slow-track animals at intake facilitates efficient care, which helps reduce LOS, and ultimately promotes both individual animal and population health (Newbury and Hurley 2013). Please see the Introduction in Chapter 1 for more detailed information about fast- and slow-track management.

Many shelters elect to house animals with existing medical or behavioral problems that may be designated as slow-track animals. When special needs animals are housed in the shelter, it is imperative that an efficient and humane plan for diagnosis, treatment/management, monitoring, and housing is implemented. Special needs animals should not be kept in the shelter unless appropriate medical and behavioral care can be provided for them, including adequate pain control. When determining if animals with special needs can be humanely cared for in the shelter, the following goals and considerations should be addressed:

- Will the care provided to the animal result in a cure or adequate management of the disease or problem behavior?
- Will the animal be adoptable?
- What steps can be taken to minimize the holding time required for treatment?
- What measures must be implemented to prevent transmission of disease to other animals or people?
- Can the shelter afford the cost of and time for care?
- How will holding the animal impact resources available for other animals?
- Can adequate care realistically be delivered in the shelter or in foster care?
- What factors will be used to assess if the treatment plan is working or should be modified?
- If the animal is adopted, what can be done to decrease/eliminate the return of the animal for their special needs?
- If the pet is not adopted, what welfare assessments will be used to measure their quality of life in the shelter?
- Do humane long-term care options exist in the shelter?

A regular system of physical and behavioral health surveillance should be in place for the follow-up of all animals. At a minimum, walk-through rounds should be conducted twice daily by medically trained staff or volunteers to observe each individual animal as well as the environment for signs of problems. Early recognition and timely action are critical for effective control of infectious diseases and mitigation of emotional distress. According to the ASV Guidelines for Standards of Care in Animal Shelters (ASV 2010), "Just as a severe or rapid decline in an animal's physical health constitutes an emergency situation and requires an urgent response, so do such changes in the behavioral or mental health of an animal." Post-adoption follow-up should also be provided (especially for special needs animals); it may help increase adopter satisfaction and reduce shelter returns.

2.3.5 Medical Record Keeping and Data Collection

Medical records are essential in order to assure quality and timely medical care is provided. Record-keeping procedures must comply with state and local practice acts and federal drug laws (i.e. Drug Enforcement Act [DEA]) and should follow guidelines provided by state and national veterinary medical associations. Animal shelters commonly use commercially available software such as PetPoint (http://www.petpoint.com), Chameleon (https://chameleonbeach.com) or others to maintain, facilitate, and manage individual animal medical records as well as population data.

A medical record should be prepared for each animal that includes the intake date; an individual animal ID number; signalment; physical description; historical, physical, and behavioral findings and observations; results of microchip scanning; body weight and body condition score; names and dosages of all drugs administered or prescribed and routes of administration including vaccines, parasite control products, other treatments, and anesthetic agents; results of any diagnostic tests performed; surgical procedure(s) performed; any presumptive or confirmed diagnoses, abnormalities or problems that are identified; and any other pertinent information regarding the animal's condition. Standardized examination and operative/surgical reports may be used to document both normal and abnormal findings but should allow for additions or updates when necessary and as appropriate. The medical record should also document assessment and follow-up, including an assessment of the animal's adoptability or other outcomes. Copies of the patient's medical record should be made available to adopters so appropriate ongoing care can be provided.

In addition to the obvious need for medical record-keeping for individual animals, populations also benefit from thoughtful record keeping and data collection. For example, several goals of the shelter wellness program might include decreasing the incidence and prevalence of infectious diseases in the shelter and following adoption, decreasing the incidence of problem behaviors in the shelter, decreasing the rate of return of animals to the shelter for problem behaviors, increasing the adoption rate, decreasing the euthanasia rate due to disease, and so forth. By identifying and tracking measurable factors (often called performance targets in large animal medicine), it is possible to measure progress toward these goals. In shelter medicine, such factors may be more appropriately termed "welfare targets." Once baseline data (such as disease rates) are established, it may be possible to measure the impact of protocol changes on population health by evaluating individual welfare targets. A system for regular reporting will make it easier to identify both positive and negative trends in animal health.

Finally, record-keeping can be used to facilitate tracking of national and regional trends in animal sheltering. In the United States, Shelter Animals Count (https://shelteranimalscount.org) is an independent, not-for-profit organization that maintains a national database that promotes standardized data collection and sharing. Launched in 2015, this national initiative with "broad collaboration from the animal welfare community" seeks to enroll all U.S. shelters in order to generate evidence to elucidate the best sheltering practices for promoting and saving companion animals' lives and preventing homelessness.

2.4 Policy and Protocol Development

Shelters should have written policies and protocols in place that detail how medical and behavioral problems will be handled (Hurley 2004). Policies and protocols should be based on research and facts as well as the individual organization's mission, philosophy, and the availability of resources (including facilities, staff, and veterinary care). Policies and protocols are best established by a committee that is responsible for shelter health issues, including the shelter director or manager, medical and behavior staff, and other key individuals. The goals of the committee should be to establish definitions or descriptions of the disease or problem behavior in question, a description of the methods that will be used to diagnose or recognize the condition and a general policy regarding the disposition of animals affected by the condition. In addition, protocols should include details on who should be notified, housing guidelines, sanitation procedures, treatment, and documentation in each case. These written protocols should serve as guidelines for systematic triage and care of animals in the shelter.

In addition to establishing policies and protocols for commonly encountered diseases and problem behaviors of shelter animals, protocols should also be developed to ensure prompt recognition and treatment of pain and emotional distress in animals. Protocols should include provisions for conditions that cause both acute and chronic pain and/or distress. Many shelters receive animals that are victims of cruelty, neglect, and/or trauma; protocols should include provisions for recognition and triage, with the provision of adequate pain control and nursing care as a priority, or emergency euthanasia if necessary when animal suffering cannot be eased, including those in their stray holding period. For shelters that do not have a veterinarian on staff, protocols should contain information for obtaining emergency veterinary care and assistance with cruelty cases.

2.5 Wellness: Physical Health

The basic physical health of cats and dogs should be systematically addressed in the wellness program protocols. Protocols should include provisions for vaccination, parasite control, spay-neuter, identification, proper nutrition and physical exercise, grooming, periodontal/oral disease prevention, and individual-specific care (see Table 2.2). Protocols should be reviewed and updated periodically as needed.

2.5.1 Vaccination

The high likelihood of exposure to disease and stress and the potentially life-threatening consequences of illness in shelters make vaccination against certain diseases essential. There is no doubt that proper shelter vaccination protocols substantially reduce disease in the shelter and improve animal health. It is important for staff to be educated about the role and limitations of vaccines as part of wellness program training. Though they represent an essential component of a comprehensive wellness program for an animal shelter, vaccines are not "magic bullets" that can prevent disease altogether. Instead, vaccines are health products that trigger immune responses in animals and prepare them to fight future infections from disease-causing agents; they do not treat disease or provide instant immunity. In many instances, they provide only partial protection, lessening the severity of future diseases but not preventing them. For example, canine and feline upper respiratory disease (URI) cannot be prevented by vaccination, whereas canine distemper (CDV) and canine and feline parvovirus (CPV and FPV, respectively) can be effectively prevented when vaccines are used correctly. But even so, there may be sporadic cases of CPV, FPV, and CDV in shelters, especially in young puppies and kittens due to waning maternal antibodies and the window of susceptibility to these diseases. It must also be remembered that even the best vaccines take some time to provide protection, and vaccine failure may occur when animals enter the shelter already incubating disease. Finally, it is important to recognize that vaccine failure will occur in some individuals, regardless of the protocol used, and that vaccines are not available for all diseases seen in shelters.

Guidelines developed specifically for the vaccination of cats and dogs in animal shelters have been well described by the American Association of Feline Practitioners (AAFP) (Stone et al. 2020) and the American Animal Hospital Association (AAHA) (Ford et al. 2017). Certain "core vaccines" are recommended to be administered on intake whenever possible to all cats and dogs that enter shelters. Core vaccine recommendations for shelter animals vary from the guidelines for vaccination of privately owned pets. Shelter core vaccines target diseases that represent significant morbidity and mortality, are widely distributed in shelters, and for which vaccination has been demonstrated to provide relatively good protection against disease. Core vaccines for shelter cats include parenteral feline parvovirus (FPV or panleukopenia), FHV-1 (feline herpesvirus type 1 or feline rhinotracheitis virus), and feline calicivirus (FCV). Core vaccines for shelter dogs include parenteral vaccines against canine parvovirus (CPV), canine distemper virus (CDV), and canine adenovirus (CAV-2, hepatitis), as well as intranasal vaccines against *Bordetella bronchiseptica* (Bb) and canine parainfluenza virus (CPiV). Some vaccines are not generally recommended for use in animal shelters either because of undemonstrated efficacy in the shelter setting, low risk of disease transmission within shelters, and/or delayed onset of immunity following vaccination, rendering them impractical and of limited use in a shelter setting. In addition, when the use of unnecessary vaccines is avoided, costs and potential vaccination reactions are reduced. However, veterinarians should use their professional judgment when administering vaccines; general shelter vaccination guidelines may need to be adjusted for individual shelters due to the changing prevalence of a disease in the region, increased efficacy or safety of a vaccine, development of a new vaccine, etc.

Rabies vaccination is recommended in both cats and dogs prior to adoption when a licensed veterinarian is available to administer the vaccine (or by shelter staff in accordance with state laws). New owners should be advised that rabies vaccination for dogs is mandatory in most jurisdictions, and proof of vaccination may be required for dog licensing. Rabies vaccination is also warranted when animals are housed long term in shelter facilities. Animals being held for rabies bite quarantines should be vaccinated against rabies by a licensed veterinarian in accordance with state law and the guidelines provided by the current *Compendium of Animal Rabies Prevention and Control*. Though the Compendium is not law, it forms the basis for many state laws regarding the management of rabies and can be accessed at http://nasphv.org/Documents/NASPHVRabiesCompendium.pdf.

For more detailed information about vaccination, please refer to Chapter 9 on Vaccinations and Immunology, Chapter 22 on Rabies, and the individual disease chapters.

2.5.2 Parasite Control and Prevention

Parasite control and prevention represent essential components of shelter wellness programs. Wellness protocols for parasite control should be tailored to the given population, taking into account parasite prevalence, zoonotic potential, pathogenicity, cost, practicality, and safety. Both internal and external parasites are common in cats and dogs. Roundworms and hookworms are common intestinal parasites that possess zoonotic potential. Adult animals are often asymptomatic, whereas young puppies and kittens are most likely to exhibit clinical signs of infection, including diarrhea, anemia, and unthriftiness. The Centers for Disease Control and Prevention (CDC, www.cdc.gov) and the Companion Animal Parasite Council (CAPC, www.capcvet.org) strongly advise routine administration of broad-spectrum anthelmintics to all cats and dogs to control these potential zoonoses. Pyrantel pamoate is one of the safest, most cost-effective and efficacious anthelmintics for treatment of roundworms and hookworms. The author recommends the administration of pyrantel pamoate at a dosage of 10 mg/kg on entry to all adoptable cats and dogs with re-treatment in two weeks and then at monthly intervals. Kittens and puppies should be treated at two-week intervals until four months of age. For cats and dogs with diarrhea, a fecal flotation, direct fecal smear, and stained fecal cytology should be performed with treatment according to results. Even if results are negative, the administration of broad-spectrum anthelmintics should be strongly considered unless definitive enzyme-linked immunosorbent assay (ELISA) testing has confirmed the negative results. Ectoparasites, including fleas, ticks, lice, and mites (Otodectes, Notoedres, Sarcoptes, and Cheyletiella), are also common in cats and dogs entering shelters, and they require routine diagnosis and control measures. In addition to causing disease and discomfort in animals, some ectoparasites are responsible for transmitting zoonotic disease.

Heartworm disease is a serious vector-borne disease that is caused by the mosquito-borne filarial nematode *Dirofilaria immitis*. The testing of adoptable dogs over the age of six months is highly recommended in areas where canine heartworm disease is prevalent or dogs have been transported from areas with a high prevalence of heartworms, and when dogs exhibit clinical signs of the disease. Though cats can also be infected, heartworm testing is not recommended for cats due to the difficulty of interpreting the results. Shelters have adopted many strategies for testing, preventing and treating heartworm disease. Mosquito control is an essential component of any shelter heartworm prevention plan since *D. immitis* can be transmitted by over 70 species of mosquitoes. The ASV and the American Heartworm Society (AHS) worked together on a Heartworm Disease Resource Task Force to create a series of educational brochures that provide information to adopters about the disease (http://www.heartwormsociety.org 2017; http://www.sheltervet.org 2017). Downloadable, printable brochures help explain the shelter policy with regards to testing for and treating heartworms (i.e. whether a facility tests or treats the disease and which modalities are used) and recommendations for follow-up with a local veterinarian. These brochures offer shelter staff a concise and accurate tool to facilitate communicating about this complex disease. Please see Chapter 18 for more information about heartworm disease.

The CAPC maintains excellent online resources (www.capcvet.org) including numerous detailed parasite guidelines, parasite prevalence maps, and product tables that are very useful for informing wellness protocols for shelters. Chapters 17 and 19 contain more information about internal and external parasites respectively.

2.5.3 Spay-Neuter

Another essential component of a shelter wellness program is ensuring that cats and dogs are spayed or neutered prior to adoption. Surgical sterilization remains the most reliable and effective means of preventing unwanted reproduction of cats and dogs. In shelters where animals awaiting adoption may be held for long periods, reproductive stress from estrous cycling in queens and bitches and sex drive in tomcats and dogs can decrease appetite, increase urine spraying/marking and intermale fighting, and profoundly increase social and emotional stress. Spaying and neutering animals awaiting adoption is essential in shelters where cats and dogs will be housed for periods of longer than two to four weeks. These procedures decrease spraying, marking, and fighting; eliminate heat behavior and pregnancy; and greatly mitigate stress. This facilitates group housing and participation in supervised playgroups for exercise and emotional enrichment. In addition, the medical benefits of spay-neuter have been well described, including the elimination of pyometra and ovarian and testicular cancers, and decreased risk of mammary cancer, benign prostatic hyperplasia, prostatitis, and perianal hernias (Johnston et al. 2001).

2.5.4 Identification (Collar/Tag, Microchip)

In all animal care settings, a reliable means of animal identification is another crucial aspect of preventive healthcare or wellness. Identification of animals in the shelter in the form of a collar and tag or other types of neckband is essential for accurate surveillance of individuals, especially where litters or groups of animals are communally housed. Though the use of collars and tags as visually obvious forms of identification is extremely valuable, the provision of permanent identification in the form of a microchip is also very beneficial as a means of back-up identification and has been demonstrated to improve pet–owner reunification since collars and tags may be easily lost (AVMA 2013; Griffin 2016; Lord et al. 2007a, b, 2009; Slater et al. 2012; Weiss et al. 2011). Improving pet recovery following adoption is another important goal or welfare target for animal shelters to strive for; thus, applying collars and tags and implanting and scanning for microchips is another way for shelters to be proactive and to model excellent standards of pet care for the public.

2.5.5 Proper Nutrition and Physical Exercise

Proper nutrition and exercise have profound implications for wellness. Not only are they essential for the management of healthy body weight and condition, good nutrition also supports immune function and regular physical exercise is closely associated with behavioral health and well-being. A regular diet of good-quality, palatable commercial food consistent with life stage and health status should be offered, and appetite should be monitored to ensure the maintenance of an adequate nutritional plane. Animals that do not eat for more than one to two days should be evaluated for medical problems and stress, and appropriate action should be taken based upon the findings. In addition, fresh water must always be available. Finally, animals should be weighed at intake and at routine intervals throughout their shelter stay. This is especially important for undernourished animals, including those involved in starvation cruelty cases and for cats because significant or even dramatic weight loss may be associated with stress and/or feline upper respiratory infection (URI) during the first few weeks of confinement (Tanaka et al. 2012). On the other hand, excessive weight gain may occur in some individual animals housed long term. Ideally, bodyweight should be recorded weekly during the initial month of shelter care and then once a month or more often if indicated. Protocols must be in place to identify and manage unhealthy trends in body weight that can potentially compromise an animal's health, well-being, or adoption.

2.5.6 Grooming

Attention must also be given to proper grooming of animals in the shelter, including bathing, brushing and removal of matted hair, nail trimming, and ear cleaning. This is more than just a matter of cosmetics or appearance. Many animals enter shelters in urgent need of grooming, especially long-haired dogs and cats, with heavily matted hair coats and/or overgrown nails, which can be painful and/or associated with skin infections. In some cases, severe matting on extremities can compromise the blood supply and result in dangerous, gangrenous lesions. When animals are held in the shelter for long-term stays, a system of regular grooming must be implemented to prevent the accumulation of painful mats and overgrown nails. Care must also be taken to keep animals clean and dry. Being housed in soiled, damp, and/or wet environments is not only potentially stressful for animals, but such conditions predispose them to matting, pungent body odor, pyoderma, and pododermatitis, and therefore must be avoided. According to the ASV Guidelines for Standards of Care in Animal Shelters (2010), "Spraying down kennels or cages while animals are inside them is an unacceptable practice."

Some animals will require more grooming than others, depending on their type of hair coat and conformation. In addition to supporting a healthy hair coat and skin, regular grooming also provides an excellent opportunity to monitor health and body condition while checking for skin problems and lumps. Also, many animals enjoy contact and attention, and well-groomed animals are often more attractive to potential adopters.

2.5.7 Periodontal/Oral Disease Prevention

Dental or oral health is another component of addressing wellness; it extends far beyond bad breath. Plaque and tartar buildup are known to contribute to serious health concerns ranging from oral pain to chronic, intermittent bacteremia and organ failure. Some animals with dental disease may refuse to eat because of the discomfort and pain. In dogs, periodontal disease is one of the most common health problems, affecting an estimated 80% of canine patients over the age of five years. It is especially common in small breed dogs (Debowes 1998). Periodontal disease is very common in adult cats as well, and some cats also develop resorptive lesions, which are frequently very painful (Reiter 2012).

Stomatitis (inflammation of the mouth) is another painful oral condition that predominantly affects cats, although it is occasionally seen in dogs as well. Importantly, stomatitis may be more commonly seen in cats that are housed intensively such as cats originating from hoarding situations and those housed in large group settings long term (Merck 2016). Affected cats experience wide-spread oral inflammation around the teeth, which often extends into the back of the mouth (pharynx) and along the sides of the tongue. The exact cause is unknown; however, the vast majority of affected cats are chronic carriers of calicivirus, thus this virus may play a role in this chronic inflammatory process (Harley et al. 2011; Poulet et al. 2000). In a study of cats from large scale hoarding investigations, FCV was the most common viral respiratory pathogen detected, infecting 78% of the cats from the populations studied (Polak et al. 2014).

In an animal shelter, periodontal and oral disease prevention may be low on the list of priorities for wellness; however, it should be an important consideration for individual wellness care. When painful dental and/or oral disease is present and animals are kept for adoption or long-term stays, a plan for timely treatment must be implemented. Adopters of animals with dental disease should be advised to seek follow-up veterinary care as soon as possible.

In terms of simple and practical means of prevention, the use of products aimed at encouraging canine chewing activity is well recognized to be beneficial by maximizing self-cleansing and physiological stimulation of salivary flow. Furthermore, chewing is a normal behavior for puppies and dogs, and when dogs are confined, isolated, anxious, or otherwise stressed, they may engage in chewing as a coping strategy. For these reasons, as well as to help maintain oral hygiene, dogs of all ages should be provided with a variety of safe chew toys appropriate for their size and age. For cats, preventive efforts should focus on the reduction of stress and URI since FCV has been implicated as a likely contributing cause of oral inflammation, particularly in housed cats.

2.5.8 Individual-Specific Care

Wellness protocols may also be dictated by the specific needs of individual animals. In some cases, the needs of individuals may be anticipated based on particular physical or behavioral traits, or breed, if known, since many breed predispositions have been well documented. For example, caution must be taken with brachycephalic dogs to ensure they do not experience heat exhaustion, to which they are extremely sensitive given the conformation of their airways. This may affect the selection of holding/housing areas and exercise routines for these individuals. Poor airway conformation also predisposes brachycephalic dogs and cats to more severe URIs than other breeds. For these reasons, care should be taken to house brachycephalic animals in well-ventilated areas away from sick animals, and they should be prioritized for removal to foster care or rescue. In the author's experience, even intranasal vaccination of these breeds is best avoided because it can result in severe clinical signs of respiratory disease.

Similarly, certain other breeds require special care in the shelter depending on their medical or behavioral genetic predispositions. The pit bull is another example: Many of these dogs require extra attention regarding housing conditions in a kennel setting so that a propensity to learn or exhibit dog-dog aggression is not exacerbated through exposure to high levels of arousal and stimulation from other dogs. This type of behavior may be exhibited by other breeds and individual dogs as well and similar precautions should be taken regarding their care and housing.

2.6 Wellness: Behavioral Health

Just as a primary goal of animal care in the shelter is to maintain the physical health of animals, the behavioral or emotional health of animals likewise deserves careful attention and consideration. Good emotional or mental health implies a state of psychological or behavioral wellbeing. When animals possess good emotional health, they experience an array of positive emotional states (contentment, playfulness, relaxation) and can effectively function, learn, and adapt to everyday life. If faced with a stressful situation, they are able to cope and do not experience significant or prolonged stress, fear, anxiety, or frustration. In short, emotionally healthy animals are content, resilient and enjoy their lives, which should be the goal for any animal residing in a shelter.

When considering emotional health in the shelter, it must be recognized that animal shelters are not normal or natural environments in which to house cats and dogs. They are meant to serve as temporary housing for animals waiting to be reclaimed, rehomed, or returned to the field, and, in some cases, as temporary housing for animals that will be euthanized. Over the past several years, there has been a growing trend in animal sheltering to provide pets awaiting adoption with longer-term stays. If not chosen by an adopter, an animal may stay in the shelter for weeks, months, or even years. Long-term housing (i.e. greater than two weeks), however, predisposes animals to compromised behavioral health and welfare. In fact, maintaining the behavioral health and welfare of animals residing in shelters long term is extremely difficult because the risk of emotional distress and behavioral deterioration increases dramatically over time.

Cats and dogs experience many stressors in animal shelters, beginning at the time of admission to the facility. Even under the best possible conditions, animal shelters are stressful by their very nature: Incoming animals are confined and exposed to varying intensities of new and novel stimuli as well as to a variety of infectious disease agents. When confined long term, they often suffer from anxiety, social isolation, inadequate mental stimulation, and lack of exercise, all of which can adversely affect their physical and behavioral health and decrease their adoptability. This may increase their LOS in some shelters or result in euthanasia in others. Over time, the animal's emotional and/or physical well-being is compromised even further.

When addressing behavioral health in the shelter, just as with disease control, prevention is crucial. A behavioral wellness program starts with proactive strategies to decrease stress and promote a positive emotional environment from the moment animals arrive at the shelter until the moment their stay ends. As previously described, a thorough behavioral history and examination are essential and will provide an important baseline for action and follow-up. Also, ongoing examination and observation of behavior during all interactions are crucial in order to ascertain as much information as possible about an animal's emotional state, welfare, and personality. Careful attention must be given to housing and enrichment, and concurrent population management strategies must be employed to minimize LOS and maximize the best outcomes for animals.

2.6.1 The Role of Stress

Stress involves outcomes secondary to increased secretion of catecholamines and cortisol. The harmful effects of chronic activation of these hormones have been well described and include adverse metabolic responses that promote dehydration, mental depression, insulin resistance, peptic ulcer formation and increased susceptibility to infection (Greco 1991; Moberg 1985). Chronic stress can also alter metabolism sufficiently to cause weight loss, prevent normal growth, and result in persistent abnormal behavior deleterious to the animal. Stress responses and immunity are also intimately related; stress compromises the immune response, lowering resistance to infection (Griffin 1989). In fact, stress can trigger the shedding of certain viral pathogens, including reactivation of latent viral rhinotracheitis (feline herpesvirus) infections in cats (Gaskell and Povey 1977). In an animal shelter, minimizing stress has the potential to greatly improve animal welfare, decrease infection rates and disease transmission, and enhance adoptability.

A stressor represents any stress-producing factor or stimulus. Housing cats and dogs in animal shelters presents enormous opportunities for introducing stressors. Stressors may include illness; captivity; transport; crowding; isolation; changes in diet, environmental temperature, light patterns, and/or ventilation;

strange smells; noises; other animals; handling and restraint; irregular caregiving schedules; unpredictable daily manipulations; the absence of familiar human contact; and the presence of unfamiliar human contact. In fact, anything unfamiliar to a cat or dog can trigger apprehension and activate the stress response. The severity, chronicity, novelty, predictability, and duration of the stressor, as well as the individual's perception, influence the response to a stressor (McMillan 2002; Moberg 1985). An individual animal's perception of a stressor is influenced by its genetic makeup, personality, and prior socialization and experience.

If allowed, animals employ coping strategies in order to lessen the negative impacts of a stressor (Carlstead et al. 1993; McMillan 2002). There is marked variability among individuals regarding their ability to cope. Some examples of behavioral coping strategies include hiding, seeking social companionship, and acquiring mental stimulation. Those that are successfully able to cope will suffer less from the physical and mental impacts of stress and will adjust better to life in an animal shelter. That being said, it is rare to find an animal that thrives when housed long term in a shelter.

When animals are housed in shelters, stress frequently originates from the loss of control over conditions and lack of opportunities for engaging in active behavioral responses that would serve as a means of coping. When stress is perceived as inescapable or uncontrollable, the resulting stress response is most severe (Carlstead et al. 1993; McMillan 2002). This is an extremely important consideration when designing housing and husbandry protocols for cats and dogs in shelters.

2.6.2 Behavioral Needs of Cats and Dogs

In addition to basic physical needs (such as proper nutrition and shelter), certain behavioral needs are also fundamentally important for cat and dog wellness. First and foremost, they require freedom from fear and distress, as well as the freedom to express normal behavior. Most cats and dogs do not thrive in isolation; indeed, they are social animals, and thus the opportunity for social interactions represents a basic behavioral need. They also require the ability to create different functional areas in their living environments for elimination, resting, and eating. They require consistent routines or daily patterns of care, including consistent periods of light and darkness. Other important behavioral needs include the ability to find a hiding place, to sleep without being disturbed, and to be free of chronic harassment from humans, other animals, or environmental stressors. Cats and dogs also require mental stimulation and the ability to play and exercise at will. Finally, cats need to scratch, and dogs need to chew. For cats, scratching is a normal behavior that conditions the claws, serves as a visual and scent marker, and is a means of stretching. For dogs, chewing is a normal behavior that conditions the teeth, serves as a method of investigating their environment, and can be a healthy coping strategy because it provides a ready outlet to express a normal behavior.

Most animals experience at least some degree of fear and stress at the time of admission to a shelter. The "four F's" are often used to describe common types of behaviors associated with these emotional states: they include fight, flight, fret/fidget, and freeze behaviors. When fearful and stressed, some animals will display "fight" behaviors, such as struggling, growling, snarling, hissing, biting, or lunging, in an attempt to drive away a perceived threat. Others may display "flight behaviors" such as cowering, looking away, or moving away to escape, hide, or otherwise avoid contact. Still others will display "fret or fidget" behaviors: for example, they might move restlessly, nervously lick their lips, pace or shift about. And, some will display "freeze" behaviors: they may appear tense or frozen in a helpless state. Many stressed and fearful animals display a mixture of these fight, flight, fret/fidget, and freeze behaviors.

Manifestations of normal and abnormal behavior can indicate how successfully an animal is coping with its environment. In animal shelters, behavioral expressions of fear, anxiety, stress and/or frustration commonly manifest via inhibited or withdrawal, defensive, disruptive, and/or stereotypic behavior (Hubrecht 1993; Overall 1997). Inhibited or withdrawal behavior refers to activity depression or the absence of normal behaviors (such as grooming, eating, sleeping, eliminating, stretching, greeting people, etc.). Defensive behavior involves characteristic postural and/or vocal responses (e.g. barking, growling, lunging, hissing, swatting). Disruptive behavior involves the destruction of cage contents and/or the creation of a hiding place. Repetitive pacing, pawing, jumping and spinning are examples of stereotypic behaviors. Behavioral signs of stress and related negative emotional states may manifest as active communication signals or passive behaviors. Active signals may be subtle or obvious and include vocalization (growling, hissing), visual cues (facial expression, posturing of the body, ears, and tail), scent marking (urine, feces, various glands of the skin), and overt aggression among others. Passive signs include the inability to rest or sleep, feigned sleep, poor appetite, constant hiding, the absence of grooming, activity depression (decreased play and exploratory behavior) and social withdrawal (Griffin 2006; Rochlitz et al. 1998; Wemelsfelder 2005). High-density housing exacerbates these signs.

When cats and dogs are well adjusted and their housing and husbandry meet their behavioral needs, they display a wide variety of normal behaviors. Indeed, the best measures of emotional wellbeing and health in shelter cats and dogs are regular displays of species typical behaviors – in other words, cats should be "acting like cats" and dogs should be "acting like dogs": sleeping comfortably, but not all the time; exploring and playing at will; eating and eliminating normally; scratching or chewing; stretching and grooming; relaxing; seeking and receiving social contact – behaviors that, when displayed regularly and appropriately, indicate positive emotional states and good health.

Proper housing and enrichment, including social companionship, physical exercise, mental stimulation, and positive training, combined with a positive emotional environment are essential components of a comprehensive behavioral wellness program (see Table 2.2). Understanding the importance of minimizing stress and other negative emotional states and recognizing and responding to them are keys to maintaining proper behavioral welfare. Active daily monitoring by staff who are trained to recognize indicators of stress, fear, anxiety, and frustration is required to detect and respond to the needs of animals that are displaying these indicators. Some indicators that an animal needs additional attention include persistent hiding, agonistic behavior with conspecifics, activity withdrawal, or other markers as previously described. Staff should record their findings daily to ensure timely and appropriate steps are taken to decrease stress and enhance the animal's ability to cope in the shelter environment. Though subjective, staff should also attempt to estimate the severity of stress and note trends: What is the animal's emotional state? Is the animal acclimating to the environment? Assessment of the incidence and prevalence of stress and other negative emotional states among the population serves to measure the effects of the shelter's animal care protocols and establish important baselines to help measure the impact of changes in housing and stress reduction programs. In order to help shelters succeed at reducing stress and bolstering the emotional health of shelter animals, the Fear Free Shelter Program (https://fearfreeshelters.com) offers no-cost, high-quality, online course training and resources for shelter staff and volunteers on recognizing signs of fear, anxiety, stress and frustration in shelter animals and creating a positive emotional environment, including recommendations for Fear Free handling, housing, behavioral care, monitoring, and more.

2.7 Proper Housing

Housing design and its proper management can literally make or break the health of a population. Housing used for isolation, quarantine and other special needs should be appropriately separated at a distance away from the general population and designed for enhanced biosecurity and stress reduction to facilitate care and speed recovery. It is not enough for the design to only address an animal's physical needs (e.g. shelter, warmth); properly designed housing should also meet the behavioral needs of the animal while minimizing stress and other negative emotional states. Behavioral needs will vary depending upon such factors as life stage, personality, and prior socialization and experience. Regardless of the species in question, housing should always include a comfortable resting area and allow animals to engage in species-typical behaviors while ensuring freedom from fear and distress. Both the structural and social environment are key considerations for housing arrangements. Further, the environment must provide opportunities for both physical and mental stimulation, which become increasingly important as the LOS increases. Therefore, shelters should maintain a variety of housing styles to meet the individual needs of different animals in the population. Managing housing arrangements for populations of varying species, ages, sexes, personality types, social experiences, and stress levels requires knowledge of normal species behavior and communication, including social behavior. Staff training in behavior and communication are crucial to success.

A sense of control over conditions is well recognized as one of the most critical needs for behavioral health (McMillan 2002). Thus, housing design must provide a variety of satisfying behavioral options. The design of short-term housing should include provisions for housing individuals, litters or compatible pairs for intake evaluation and triage. Housing should be easy to clean and sanitize, well ventilated, and be safe for animals and caregivers. Even short-term housing should provide for the minimal behavioral needs of animals, affording animals with sufficient space to stand and walk several steps, sit or lie down at full body length, and separate elimination, feeding, and resting areas. This is often best accomplished with double compartment housing, in which a door or portal separates the resting and feeding area from the area for elimination. This is important for both dogs and cats. Resting areas should include comfortable surfaces and, if needed, extra bedding that can be disinfected or disposed of. To provide a refuge, a secure hiding place (such as a box, crate, or cat den, or a visual barrier placed over a portion of the front of the enclosure) should be provided for cats and dogs. See Figure 2.1a and 2.1b.

2.7.1 Long-Term Housing

The design of long-term housing (i.e. for confinement in the shelter for more than two weeks) should provide space that is mentally and physically stimulating and preferably esthetically pleasing (an important consideration to facilitate adoption). Alternatives to traditional cage housing (such as large runs) should be provided; enriched single or group housing is indicated. Though not always easy to accomplish in busy shelters, at an absolute minimum, healthy cats that are cage housed should be allowed a daily opportunity to exercise and explore in a secure enriched setting that can be easily disinfected. Biosecurity measures must be adhered to when providing enrichment opportunities for cats with an infectious disease such as URI or dermatophytosis. In some situations, outdoor enclosures may also be suitable for cats. Benefits include ample exposure to natural light and mental stimulation. Galvanized wire chain link panels (including a top panel) or specially designed fencing for cat enclosures (e.g. Purrfect Fence, http://www.purrfectfence.com) may be used (Griffin 2006).

Likewise, dogs should be provided with regular daily out-of-kennel time for physical exercise and appropriate social interactions. Outdoor enclosures provide opportunities for fresh air and exercise, as well as mental and social stimulation. If outdoor play enclosures are not available, dogs should be walked outside at least twice a day by experienced staff or volunteers who can ensure the dogs will not escape, transmit disease, bite or fight with other dogs they may encounter.

Co-housing affords animals with opportunities for healthy social contact with conspecifics, and when properly managed can help to meet their social needs, enhancing welfare. In fact, many animals can benefit from being housed with a compatible animal, provided there is sufficient space to distance themselves from each other, ready access to feeding, resting and elimination areas, and an adequate number of comfortable resting and hiding places. Family groups and previously bonded housemates are natural choices for co-housing, but unfamiliar animals who are compatible with one another may also be carefully selected for co-housing. Daily behavioral monitoring by staff trained to detect signs of social stress, bullying and incompatibilities is essential for success. Housing compatible animals in pairs or small groups (e.g. 3–4 animals) affords them the opportunity for healthy interactions and to build social relationships. Pair housing or small groupings facilitate effective monitoring and reduce the risk of conflict and infectious disease transmission. Grouping animals randomly or that are poorly compatible, fight with one another, or that bully others are unacceptable practices. Larger groups increase the odds of social conflict among animals. Similarly, the constant introduction of new animals and crowding induce stress and therefore should be minimized to ensure proper welfare.

Finally, "real life" rooms (e.g. rooms with a homelike environment) away from the kennel or cattery are useful, especially for those animals that remain in the shelter long-term.

2.7.2 Housing Design Considerations

The ASV Guidelines state "poor cat housing is one of the greatest shortcomings observed in shelters and has a substantially negative impact on both health and well-being." (ASV 2010). Several recommendations have been made for the appropriate dimensions and configuration of housing for cats in catteries and laboratories, but only a few existed specifically for cats housed in shelters until recently. Some websites that contain guidelines for appropriate housing for cats in shelters, as well as instructions for modifying existing housing, are listed in Table 2.5.

Table 2.5 Resources for cat housing.

Resource	Website
University of Florida	https://sheltermedicine.vetmed.ufl.edu
University of California- Davis	https://www.sheltermedicine.com
University of Wisconsin- Madison	https://www.uwsheltermedicine.com
Cornell University	https://www.vet.cornell.edu/hospitals/maddies-shelter-medicine-program)
Association of Shelter Veterinarians	https://www.sheltervet.org/assets/docs/shelter-standards.
American Society for the Prevention of Cruelty to Animals (ASPCA)	https://www.aspcapro.org
Humane Society of the United States (HSUS)	http://www.humanepro.org

Enclosures for cats should be large enough to allow them to stretch, groom, and move about while maintaining separate functional areas, at least 2 ft apart, for sleeping, eating and elimination. Unfortunately, many animal shelter facilities in the United States are equipped with small cages (e.g. 1.5–2.5 ft wide) that are inadequate for proper housing of cats. Double-sided enclosures (e.g. cat condos) generally afford more adequate space and have the benefit of easily allowing cats to remain securely in one side of the enclosure while the opposite side is cleaned. Traditional cages can be modified into condo-style enclosures by creating portals to adjoin two or three smaller cages. See Figure 2.2a and b. Runs can also be used to house cats and are especially useful for co-housing cats, as well as for stays that exceed two weeks. Larger enclosures allow for better air circulation, which is also an important consideration for control of feline URIs. Regardless of the housing dimensions and arrangement, a variety of elevated resting perches and hiding boxes should be provided to increase the size and complexity of the living space, and to separate it into different functional areas, allowing a variety of behavioral options. The physical environment should always include opportunities for hiding, playing, scratching, climbing, resting, feeding, and eliminating.

(a)

(b)

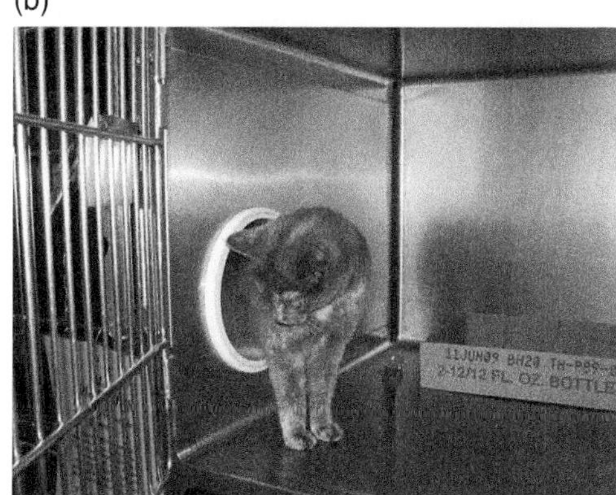

Figure 2.2 (a and b). Conversion of existing cages into condo-style units can be accomplished via the installation of a portal between cages by cutting a hole through the walls of adjacent cages and installing a section of PVC pipe with corresponding rims.

For dogs, indoor-outdoor access is generally preferred, but whatever the arrangement, dogs should be able to see out to observe their environment. While it is important for dogs to see out of their enclosures, enclosures that are arranged side by side should have solid sides to prevent direct contact with dogs in adjacent enclosures, and visual barriers should be provided on the front and back ends of enclosures as needed to shield occupants from stressful stimuli. Outside areas should provide protection from excessive sun, rain and wind. See Figure 2.3. Runs must be large enough to allow a dog to move about freely, and a clean, comfortable bed should be available for resting in a secure location. Double-sided enclosures are always preferred because they allow dogs to eliminate away from resting and feeding areas. (Though shelters often place dogs on both sides of the enclosure, this practice should be discouraged whenever possible because it defeats the goal of double-sided housing to provide an easily cleaned, enriched environment.) The addition of three-dimensional space (such as platforms, steps, or ramps) may be beneficial when space permits (Hubrecht 1993; Loveridge 1998; Overall 2005).

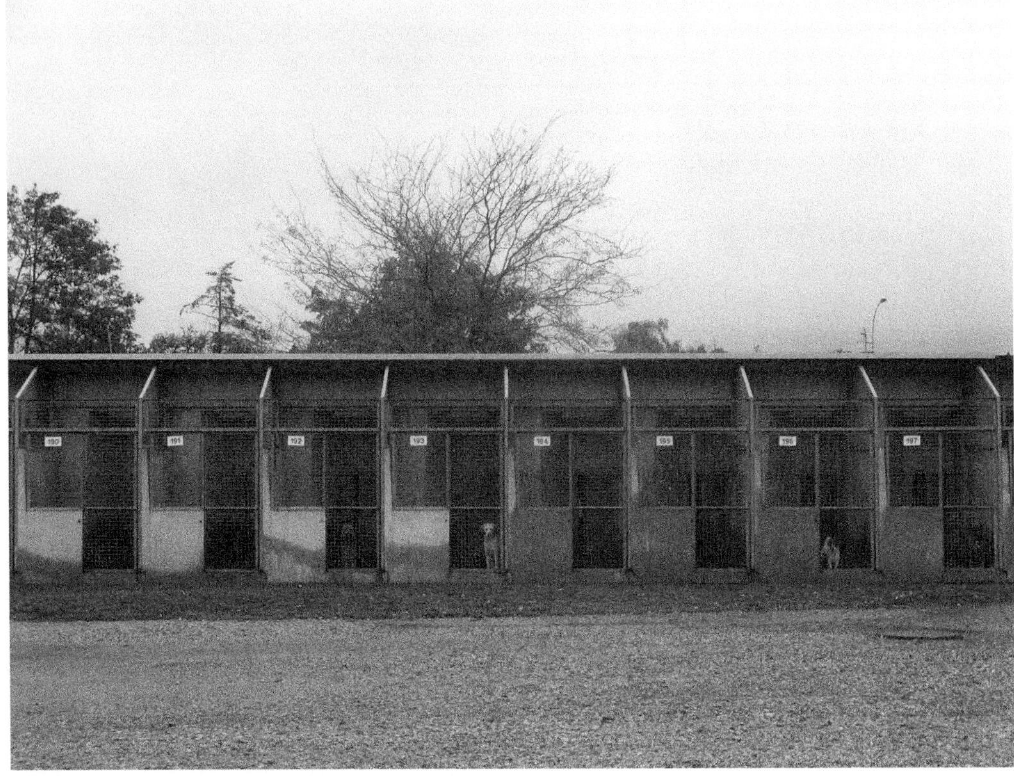

Figure 2.3 Outdoor section of a row of double-sided kennel runs. Indoor-outdoor kennel runs afford dogs with separate areas for resting and elimination. Note that solid sides prevent direct contact among dogs in adjacent runs, while the ends of the runs are partially unobscured to allow occupants to safely look out at their surroundings if they choose to do so.

The success of the adaptation of cats and dogs to novel environments depends on both the quality of the environment and the adaptive capacity of the animal. With proper behavioral wellness protocols in place, most animals will adapt and successfully cope with shelter life in the short term. However, some will never adjust and will remain stressed indefinitely, resulting in the decline of physical as well as emotional health. Novel environments tend to be especially stressful for poorly socialized and geriatric cats and dogs. Geriatric animals generally benefit from placement in foster care. The housing of feral cats should be avoided whenever possible; healthy feral and free-roaming cats can benefit from appropriately managed neuter and return programs in which healthy cats are vaccinated, surgically sterilized, and returned to their original site of capture (e.g. their home base).

The importance of proper staff training to recognize and prevent stress is critical for animal welfare and cannot be overemphasized. Long-term behavioral coping is extremely difficult for most animals, thus behavioral deterioration can be expected as LOS increases. This further underscores the importance of employing management strategies that minimize each animal's time in the shelter while maximizing the best outcomes.

2.8 Enrichment

Enrichment refers to a process for improving the environment and behavioral care of confined animals within the context of their behavioral needs. The purpose of enrichment is to reduce stress and improve wellbeing by providing physical and mental stimulation, encouraging species-typical behaviors, and allowing animals more control over their environment. Successful enrichment programs prevent the development and display of abnormal behavior and provide for the psychological wellbeing of the animals.

The ASV Guidelines state that "enrichment should be given the same significance as other components of animal care and should not be considered optional." It is not a task that can be neglected on busy days; instead, it bears repeating that it is a fundamentally important, core component of daily routine animal care that should be a part of every shelter's wellness protocol. Enrichment can be therapeutic and should be tailored to meet the needs of individual animals and improve behavioral health and emotional wellbeing. Enrichment opportunities for animals being treated for infectious disease are just as important as for healthy animals but must be tailored to meet their individual conditions and utilize appropriate biosecurity measures to minimize the risk of disease transmission. Ultimately, enrichment reduces stress and promotes positive emotional states.

Perhaps the most effective enrichment in a shelter is a trained animal care staff that enjoy working with animals and that are willing and able to spend ample quality time interacting with them daily to ensure social contact and tractability. Cats and dogs become accustomed to daily routines and generally respond strongly to their human caregivers. Whenever possible, caregivers should be assigned to care for the same animals on a regular basis and preferably at the same time each day so that they become aware of the habits and personality of each animal. This familiarity is necessary for better detection of physical or behavioral problems and enables staff to make better adoption matches. Caregivers should schedule time each day to interact with "their" animals in addition to the activities of feeding and cleaning. Some cats and dogs may prefer to be petted and handled while others will prefer to interact via a toy (e.g. cats chasing dangling feathers or dogs fetching a ball). Regular aerobic exercise is essential for dogs; the intensity and duration are defined by the individual's needs. Many dogs benefit greatly from participation in play-groups. Health, age, gender and reproductive status, personality and play-style should be used to guide the selection of groups. Play should be monitored to ensure that participants are comfortable with the types of play that are taking place and that they take natural breaks in their play.

Other forms of stimulation that engage the mind, body, and senses are important to enrich the environment and promote healthy mental and physical activities – dogs and cats need a variety of pleasant things to look at and listen to, good things to smell, and satisfying things to scratch or chew and taste as well as activities that provide exercise and social contact. They should be provided with sanitizable or disposable toys to stimulate normal behaviors and activities. Providing treats and novel sources of food is an important source of stimulation for both cats and dogs, and importantly provides dogs with opportunities for healthy chewing. It is easily accomplished by hiding food in commercially available food puzzle toys or cardboard tubes or boxes, empty plastic bottles, sections of PVC pipe, or similar items. The provision of scratching boards is especially important for cats. Empty cardboard boxes and paper bags are inexpensive and disposable, and they stimulate exploration and play behavior in addition to scratching.

Positive training (including clicker training) with food or play rewards can provide additional stimulation, activity and social contact for both dogs and cats. In addition to providing mental stimulation, teaching animals to engage with people and display good manners makes them more appealing to adopters and sets another example of good pet care. Commercially available synthetic cat pheromones (cheek gland- F3, and appeasing- F4) or a dog-appeasing pheromone may be beneficial to cats and dogs, respectively, as these products have been shown to help reduce anxiety in some animals. For singly housed animals and long-term residents, appropriate levels of additional enrichment should be provided daily. Cats and dogs need variety, control and choice, and individuals possess different preferences for environmental conditions, levels of activity, and social interactions with other animals and humans. The best enrichment program will provide for all these choices.

2.9 Environmental Wellness

The shelter environment has a profound influence on animal health and well-being; thus, systematic wellness protocols to address both the emotional and physical environment must be established. Environmental wellness protocols should include comprehensive practices to mitigate animal stress and fear; consistent daily routines; positive predictable interactions and events; provisions to ensure the maintenance of proper population density; animal segregation and traffic patterns; regular cleaning and sanitation; other facility operations; and staff training (See Table 2.3).

2.9.1 Emotional Environment

A healthy emotional environment provides regular and predictable caregiving by compassionate, well-trained staff members and actively reduces potential stressors and fear-inducing stimuli such as loud noises, other intense or overwhelming stimuli, haphazard schedules, and frequent interruptions. Positive predictable handling is crucial. Staff members should be well trained to recognize signs of stress and fear in patients and to mitigate them through environmental management and positive, calming interactions. Minimal, gentle restraint should be used to handle tractable patients since research indicates that gentle human contact can attenuate the adverse effects of unpleasant stimuli, eliminate fear responses, and alleviate signs of pain in animals (McMillan 2002). Animals quickly become accustomed to schedules of care (e.g. feeding, cleaning, enrichment activities), and rapidly learn to adapt to new and novel stimuli if fear responses are not overwhelming or sensitizing. For these reasons, from the moment an animal enters the shelter, steps should be taken to reduce stress and fear.

Housing design and soundproofing can help to control noises. Loud noise must be avoided (e.g. slamming the cage door while the animal is in the cage, loud equipment or loud music, etc.). In addition, white-noise recordings (such as the sounds of a fan blowing or rain falling) can be used to drown out other noises; the goal is to hide other sounds that might be distressing or disturbing. For example, many shelters might benefit from using white noise in cat areas to drown out the sounds of barking dogs. Also, for barking dogs, an evaluation of the motivation of the barker may help to solve the problem and alleviate the individual's distress as well as the impact on the environment. A solution for the problem may be as simple as moving a dog away from a door where there is constant provocative activity.

For cats, special care should be taken not to place them within spatial, visual or auditory range of other species, especially dogs. Creature comforts should be provided for all animals, including comfortable bedding and a hiding place or secure refuge. Soft bedding also allows animals to establish a familiar scent that aids in acclimation to a new environment. Importantly, cats instinctively feel more secure when they can perch at a high point; studies indicate that feline stress responses are significantly reduced when cats are housed in elevated cages compared to floor-level cages (McCobb et al. 2005). For these reasons, carriers containing cats should never be placed on the floor and cats should be preferentially transferred to elevated holding cages whenever possible.

Individuals that are exhibiting marked fear and stress at the time of entry should be housed in specially designated quiet areas away from other animals and foot traffic within the shelter. Whenever possible, animals should be housed in their same enclosure, and whenever appropriate, spot cleaning instead of complete sanitation should be performed to preserve their scent, which is necessary for stress reduction. Spot cleaning is also often preferred because daily removal of a cat from the cage for complete sanitation may be unnecessary for disease control and may create enough stress to reactivate latent viral rhinotracheitis (herpes) as mentioned previously (Gaskell and Povey 1977). Care should be taken during cleaning procedures to minimize stress and noise, and cats should be allowed to retreat to their hiding spot if they choose while their cage is quietly tidied and replenished around them as needed. Commercially available "cat dens" are ideal for this purpose. See Figures 2.1a and b. In most instances, dogs should be removed from their enclosures during cleaning procedures or allowed to move side to side of a double-sided enclosure to prevent undue stress. See Chapter 8 for more information about sanitation protocols.

The way in which animals are handled in the shelter has a profound impact on their behavior, health and wellbeing and impacts their ability to adapt to a new environment. When animals are provided with regular, consistent, predictable positive interactions and pleasant activities, they learn what to expect and can adapt and adjust to the routine. Even stressful events are less stressful if they are on a schedule. When aversive stimuli are unpredictable, chronic fear and anxiety may result. Conversely, if events that are perceived as stressful (such as cleaning) occur on a predictable schedule, animals learn that a predicable period of calm and comfort will always occur in between or afterwards. In other words, animals quickly learn consistent routines – and they will acclimate to a new environment much more quickly if they know who will be caring for them and when, and that the experience can then be a positive one. The importance of regular schedules of feeding, cleaning, exercise, and play cannot be overemphasized. Animals also respond to positive experiences in their daily routines. For example, feeding and playtime may be greatly anticipated; thus, scheduling positive daily events (e.g. a treat at 3:00 p.m. every day) should also be a priority.

Thus, a good emotional environment, combined with behavioral wellness care, promotes adaptation to the shelter environment because animals can learn to what to expect, have the ability to shield themselves from unpleasant stimuli, and are afforded the provision of basic essential creature comforts, as well as some control, variety, and choice.

2.9.2 Physical Environment

2.9.2.1 Population Density

Overcrowding is one of the most potent emotional and physical stressors recognized in housed animals (Griffin and Baker 2002; McMillan 2002). It increases both the number of susceptible animals and asymptomatic carriers in a given group, thus increasing the likelihood of disease transmission between group members through both direct contact and contaminated fomites. Overcrowding also increases the magnitude of many stressors in the shelter environment including noise, air contaminants and infectious agents, and compromises animal husbandry, inflating the risk for serious outbreaks of disease in the population. With too many animals to care for, shelter staffs' ability to provide proper care to animals and good customer service to the public becomes overwhelmed. In turn, this can negatively affect adoption rates since potential adopters often find an overcrowded and dirty shelter to be an overwhelming and uninviting environment, further compounding the shelter's crowding problem.

For all these reasons, shelters must limit the number of animals they house to the number for which they can provide reasonable care. A shelter's capacity for care is not simply a matter of space available for animals, but also of the shelter's ability to provide proper care to meet their physical and emotional needs. Though there is no single, simple formula available to determine the number of animals that a given facility should house, an assessment of housing capacity in relation to an organization's staffing, resources and population statistics can be used to estimate its capacity for care. At times, unexpected intake may result in temporary conditions of overcrowding, but a good wellness program dictates that protocols must be in place to alleviate overcrowding and maintain a modestly populated environment for the health and protection of the animals and staff within the organization's capacity for care. The ASV Guidelines for Standards of Care caution that "Every sheltering organization has a maximum capacity for care, and the population in their care must not exceed that level" (ASV 2010).

First and foremost, employing sound population management strategies and operating within the organization's capacity for care are crucial to prevent crowding, reduce euthanasia, and optimize positive outcomes. As a part of daily walk-through rounds for routine animal surveillance, thoughtful consideration should always be given as to why each individual animal remains in the shelter and what could be done to optimize or hasten a successful outcome for that animal (Hurley 2004). Ideally, overcrowding is prevented or reduced by decreasing the average length of time animals remain in the shelter, combined with limiting or diverting intake. Programs to increase and speed up adoption, redemption, transfer (to rescue or foster care) as well as return to field programs for neuter-return of community cats help to minimize euthanasia for space in open-admission shelters and maximize intake in limited admission shelters.

In some instances, when all other options have been exhausted, euthanasia may need to be performed in consideration of the population in order to alleviate overcrowding or prevent disease outbreaks from spreading out of control. Fortunately, as managed admissions have been embraced by many municipal or public shelters, this has become increasingly less common. However, when necessary, thoughtful euthanasia decisions, though always difficult, are a crucial part of the responsibility of every shelter. Euthanasia may be necessary at times for individual animals that are suffering from irremediable physical or behavioral disease or that pose a risk to public health or safety. Once a carefully thought-out decision is made to euthanize an animal, the procedure should be performed without delay. For example, aggressive dogs that cannot be safely rehabilitated within the resources of the organization or safely rehomed should not be held beyond their legal holding periods. Instead, they should be humanely euthanized as soon as possible to prevent undue stress and anxiety on the dog and risk for the shelter staff, public, and other animals. No matter what the underlying circumstances are surrounding the euthanasia of an animal, these decisions are always challenging. Delays in action, however, often prolong the suffering of sick or emotionally troubled animals, contribute negatively to population health and prolong the stress of individual animals in the shelter.

2.9.2.2 Segregation of Animals and Traffic Patterns

The segregation of animals entering shelters is essential for proper welfare, infectious disease control, staff safety, and compliance with animal control procedures. Different species should be housed separately from one another. Depending on a particular shelter's mission and functions, animals should be segregated into wards according to their physical, behavioral, adoption availability and legal holding status. For example, common ward designations include one or more areas for "healthy holding," adoption, and isolation. Proper traffic patterns throughout the shelter that direct people and animals from areas housing healthy and vulnerable animals first to areas housing sick animals last are important to minimize disease transmission and maintain health. Other considerations for animal segregation include the following:

- Kittens and puppies younger than four to five months are particularly susceptible to infectious disease, and extra care must be taken to limit their exposure – these holding areas should be easy to disinfect and have extra attention paid to close monitoring and appropriate biosecurity. However, biosecurity should not be emphasized to the extent that it becomes a barrier to socialization or adoption, as minimizing the LOS is particularly key to ensuring the proper social and emotional development of very young animals.
- Geriatric animals require comfortable, quiet quarters with secure footing and extra careful attention to stress reduction.
- Separate, quiet and low-stress housing areas are essential for fearful and reactive cats and dogs.
- A variety of separate flexible areas or wards can be used to meet the needs of those animals with special needs such as nursing mothers, neonatal orphans, animals awaiting foster care, those with non-infectious illness, etc.
- Isolation areas are used to segregate sick animals from the general population. Immediate isolation of sick animals is critical for effective disease control. Isolation should be targeted by species, age, and disease.
- Quarantine areas are used to segregate animals that appear healthy for observation for signs of disease. The routine use of conventional quarantines is more detrimental than beneficial in most animal shelters, but they can be of considerable value in specific instances, for example, observing animals involved in transport programs or during disease outbreaks, A plan should be in place for establishing quarantine areas if the need arises.

Thus, a variety of holding, adoption, and isolation areas is necessary for proper segregation of the population. Please see the Introduction in Chapter 1 and Chapter 6 on Outbreak Management for more information about population management, isolation and quarantine protocols.

2.9.2.3 Sanitation (Cleaning and Disinfection)

For wellness programs to be effective, a clean and sanitary environment must be maintained. Not only does this promote animal health, but it also promotes staff pride and public support. In addition to protocols for routine sanitation procedures, protocols should be in place for periodic deep cleaning and disinfection as well as procedures to be used in the event of disease outbreaks. Care should always be taken to avoid facilitating disease transmission during the sanitation process. Chapter 8 on Sanitation and Chapter 6 on Outbreak Management provide detailed information about cleaning and sanitation practices.

2.9.2.4 Other Facility Operations

The success or failure of virtually every aspect of a wellness program depends on facility operations. The adoption of clearly defined and well-designed management protocols, thorough training, and supervision of personnel with oversight by a knowledgeable professional are required for success. In addition to proper housing design, animal segregation, and sanitation procedures, there are several other very important aspects of facility operations to consider when designing a wellness program for the shelter environment.

Animal health can be compromised by inadequate ventilation or by ill-considered air pressure gradients that recirculate or cause the exchange of air between rooms. Poor ventilation and high humidity contribute to disease by promoting the accumulation of infectious agents as well as dust and fumes that may be irritating to the respiratory tract. Thoughtful consideration must be given to strategies to maintain good air quality (Hurley 2005). Good practices include improving ventilation, regular maintenance of filters, routine or as-needed vacuuming to control dust and dander, periodic deep cleaning, and the use of dust-free litter (or simply dumping dusty litter boxes outside). The best-case scenario, and what is typical in laboratory animal settings, is for the heating, ventilation, and air conditioning (HVAC) system to allow for 100% fresh (e.g. nonrecycled) air in each room so that the air entering a given room is exhausted out of the building and not recirculated to another room. The standard recommendation for an animal room is 10 to 15 air changes per hour, but more or less airflow may be acceptable or necessary depending upon the species housed and the anticipated housing density (ILAR 2011). Even when ventilation systems provide 10 to 15 room air changes per hour, this may not occur at the level of the cages or other animal enclosures.

Ventilation may be improved by housing design; for example, the use of flow-through condo-style cages, runs (especially the indoor-outdoor type), or room style housing may help. Cat cages that were designed with plexiglass fronts to minimize fomite disease transmission via contact with staff and adopters have been found to compromise ventilation and should probably be avoided whenever possible unless they are individually actively ventilated. Another reason to limit their use is that they also limit enrichment opportunities by restricting contact with staff, volunteers and potential adopters.

Another standard recommendation has always been to have separate ventilation systems for the various functional areas of the shelter to prevent the exchange of air among them. However, some shelter experts have called this recommendation into question because few diseases in shelters are truly transmitted via aerosolization, but instead are primarily spread via fomites. Though this recommendation seems prudent to consider whenever possible, it is very expensive to install and operate this type of ventilation system. If air quality remains good and the shelter maintains effective, comprehensive wellness protocols, this recommendation may not be necessary for maintaining animal health. More research in shelters is needed on this subject but in the meantime, the author recommends consulting with an HVAC specialist to analyze the shelter's needs and maximize the potential of the shelter's system.

Temperature and humidity should be controlled to keep animals comfortable. Drafts should be avoided. The recommended temperature range for cats and dogs is between 64 °F (17 °C) and 84 °F (28 °C) with a temperature setting in the low to mid-70s °F (20s °C) being typical (ILAR 2011). However, the temperature setting should match the animals' needs. For instance, sick animals, puppies, kittens, and animals recovering from surgery are more susceptible to lower temperatures than healthy animals. The location of the animal should be considered since cages located closer to the floor are always a few degrees colder than the ones above the floor level. In addition, it is important to consider the shelter's situation, finances, and climate conditions. Regarding humidity, the laboratory standards for cats and dogs state 30–70% humidity is desired (ILAR 2011). Higher humidity (70%) may be advantageous in treatment areas housing animals with URI, whereas less humidity (40–50%) in other areas may help with disease control by curtailing airborne transmission. Though the range considered acceptable is large, a given room should have a fairly constant humidity and avoid large fluctuations. It is recognized that hosing or even mopping a room will cause humidity spikes, but they should be short-lived with a well-ventilated room.

Regular light and dark cycles are important, and staff should be trained to ensure that lights are on during the day and turned off at night so animals may sleep; timers may be used to ensure control. The light should be sufficient to facilitate observation of all animals, especially in isolation and quarantine areas where close scrutiny of animals is required. Noisy or flickering lights are annoying and should be repaired as quickly as possible. Exposure to natural sunlight offers the advantage of diminishing disease transmission.

Regular pest control, via means that are safe for use around both humans and animals, as well as all aspects of building maintenance, are also important considerations for the maintenance of a healthy environment. Developing and following written standard operating procedures and daily, weekly, monthly, and quarterly checklists will ensure that systematic schedules of maintenance are carried out.

2.9.2.5 Staff Training

Regular staff training is essential to implement effective wellness programs. Staff knowledge, attitude, and skill will largely determine the success or failure of every aspect of the shelter's wellness program. Staff must be taught how to gather the essential historical information at the time of intake; to attend to all aspects of animal care including handling, feeding, cleaning, disease recognition, and behavioral care; and to offer adoption counseling that will help ensure a successful match. Adopters should receive written records and instructions for follow-up care with their veterinarian. In addition, post-adoption counseling and follow-up should be offered. The importance of regular staff training and assessment, and effective staff management and leadership cannot be overemphasized. The best-run shelters are ones with competent, compassionate, well-trained staff that work cooperatively in efforts to provide excellent animal care and public service.

2.10 Conclusion

Today more than ever, society expects high-quality care for animals in shelters. Indeed, shelters have a moral obligation to provide for the health and welfare of animals entrusted to them. Shelter animal health is dependent on the implementation of comprehensive wellness protocols, systematic surveillance, and excellent management. Shelters must establish solid goals for animal health and measure welfare targets. Wellness protocols and management practices must be regularly evaluated and revised to meet these targets. The bulk of the effort must focus on preventive strategies that minimize stress and ensure both the physical and behavioral health of animals. Indeed, the single most important means of managing disease in shelters is through prevention, which entails implementing excellent population management practices together with comprehensive population wellness protocols tailored for the shelter animals and environment. Staff training and education are critical since a dedicated and well-trained staff is essential for success. In addition, the shelter environment must support opportunities for animals that promote pleasurable feelings and experiences whenever possible. "Healthy and happy" cats and dogs are highly desirable pets; thus, appropriately designed wellness programs help shelters meet their ultimate goal of ensuring the welfare of animals in their care, which is essential for successful adoptions.

References

American Veterinary Medical Association (AVMA). Microchipping of Animals. (2013). Available at: https://www.avma.org/KB/Resources/Reference/Pages/Microchipping-of-Animals-Backgrounder.aspx (Accessed June 30, 2017).

Association of Shelter Veterinarians (ASV) (2010). Guidelines for Standards of Care in Animal Shelters (2010), available at http://www.sheltervet.org/assets/docs/shelter-standards-oct2011-wforward.pdf. (Accessed June 28, 2017).

Barnard, S., Pedernera, C., Candeloro, L. et al. (2016). Development of a new welfare assessment protocol for practical application in long-term dog shelters. *Veterinary Record* 178 (1): 18.

Carlstead, K., Brown, J.L., and Strawn, W. (1993). Behavioral and physiological correlates of stress in laboratory cats. *Applied Animal Behaviour Science* 38: 143.

Debowes, L.J. (1998). The effects of dental disease on systemic disease. In: The Veterinary Clinics of North America: Canine Dentistry, vol. 28 (ed. S.E. Holmstrom), 1057–1062. Philadelphia: WB Saunders.

Farm Animal Welfare Council (2009). Farm Animal Welfare in Great Britain: Past, Present and Future (Report). Oct. 2009, available at http://www.fao.org/fileadmin/user_upload/animalwelfare/ppf-report091012.pdf, (Accessed June 27, 2017).

Ford, R.B., Larson, L.J., Wellborn, L. et al. (2017). American Animal Hospital Association Canine Vaccination Guidelines. https://www.aaha.org/guidelines/canine_vaccination_guidelines.aspx (Accessed 9/8/2019).

Gaskell, R.M. and Povey, R.C. (1977). Experimental induction of feline viral rhinotracheitis in FVR-recovered cats. *Veterinary Record* 100: 128.

Greco, D.S. (1991). The effect of stress on the evaluation of feline patients. In: Consultations in Feline Internal Medicine (ed. J.R. August), 1991–1999. Philadelphia: W.B. Saunders.

Greene, C.E. (2012). Environmental factors in infectious disease. In: Infectious Diseases of the Dog and Cat, 4th (ed. C.E. Greene), 1078–1100. Philadelphia: W.B. Saunders.

Griffin, J.F.T. (1989). Stress and immunity: a unifying concept. *Veterinary Immunology and Immunopathology* 20: 263.

Griffin, B. (2006). Recognition and management of stress in housed cats. In: Consultations in Feline Internal Medicine (ed. J.R. August), 717–734. Philadelphia: W.B. Saunders.

Griffin, B. (2016). The epidemiology of lost cats: best practices for identification and recovery. In: Consultations in Feline Internal Medicine, vol. VII (ed. S. Little), 649–662. St. Louis: Elsevier.

Griffin, B. and Baker, H.J. (2002). Domestic cats as laboratory animals. In: Laboratory Animal Medicine (ed. J.G. Fox), 459–482. San Diego: Harcourt Academic.

Harley, R., Gruffydd-Jones, T.J., and Day, M.J. (2011). Immunohistochemical characterization of oral mucosal lesions in cats with chronic gingivostomatitis. *Journal of Comparative Pathology* 144 (4): 239–250.

Hubrecht, R.C. (1993). A comparison of social and environmental enrichment methods for laboratory housed dogs. *Applied Animal Behavior Science* 37: 345–361.

Hurley, K.F. (2004). Implementing a population health plan in an animal shelter: goal setting, data collection and monitoring, and policy development. In: Shelter Medicine for Veterinarians and Staff (eds. L. Miller and S. Zawistowski), 211–234. Ames: Blackwell Publishing.

Hurley, K.F. (2005). Feline infectious disease control in shelters. *Veterinary Clinics of North America: Small Animal Practice* 35 (1): 21–37.

Institute of Laboratory Animal Research (ILAR) (2011). Commission on Life Sciences, National Research Council. Guide for Care and Use of Laboratory Animals. Washington, D.C.: National Academies Press.

Johnston, S.D., Kustritz, M.R., and Olson, P.S. (2001). Canine and Feline Theriogenology. Philadelphia: W.B. Saunders.

Lord, L.K., Wittum, T.E., Ferketich, A.K. et al. (2007a). Search and identification methods that owners use to find a lost dog. *Journal of the American Veterinary Medical Association* 230: 211–216.

Lord, L.K., Wittum, T.E., Ferketich, A.K. et al. (2007b). Search methods that people use to find owners of lost pets. *Journal of the American Veterinary Medical Association* 230: 1835–1840.

Lord, L.K., Ingwersen, W., Gray, J.L. et al. (2009). Characterization of animals with microchips entering animal shelters. *Journal of the American Veterinary Medical Association* 235: 160–167.

Lorenz, M.D. (1993). The problem-oriented approach. In: Small Animal Medical Diagnosis (ed. M.D. Lorenz), 1–12. Philadelphia: Lippincott, Williams and Wilkins.

Loveridge, G.G. (1998). Environmentally enriched dog housing. *Applied Animal Behaviour Science* 59 (1): 101–113.

McCobb, E.C., Patronek, G.J., Marder, A. et al. (2005). Assessment of stress levels among cats in four shelters. *Journal of the American Veterinary Medical Association* 226: 548.

McMillan, F.D. (2000). Quality of life in animals. *Journal of the American Veterinary Medical Association* 216 (12): 1904–1910.

McMillan, F.D. (2002). Development of a mental wellness program for animals. *Journal of the American Veterinary Medical Association* 220 (7): 965.

Merck, M. (2016). Clinical management of large -scale cruelty cases. In: Consultations in Feline Internal Medicine, vol. VII (ed. S. Little), 663–673. St. Louis: Elsevier.

Moberg, G.P. (1985). Biological responses to stress: key to assessment of animal well-being? In: Animal Stress (ed. G.P. Moberg), 27–49. Bethesda: Waverly Press.

Newbury, S. and Hurley, K. (2013). Population management. In: Shelter Medicine for Veterinarians and Staff, 2e (eds. L. Miller and S. Zawistowski), 93–114. Ames: Blackwell.

Overall, K.L. (1997). Recognizing and managing problem behavior in breeding catteries. In: Consultations in Feline Internal Medicine, vol. 3 (ed. J.R. August), 634–646. Philadelphia: W.B. Saunders.

Overall, K.L. (2005). Environmental enrichment strategies for laboratory animals from the viewpoint of clinical veterinary behavioral medicine; emphasis on cats and dogs. *Institute of Laboratory Animal Research (ILAR)* 46 (2): 202–215.

Patronek, G.J. and Bradley, J. (2016). No better than flipping a coin: reconsidering canine behavior evaluations in animal shelters. *Journal of Veterinary Behavior* 15: 66–77.

Polak, K.C., Levy, J.K., Crawford, P.C. et al. (2014). Infectious diseases in large-scale cat hoarding investigations. *Veterinary Journal* 2: 189–195.

Poulet, H., Brunet, S. et al. (2000). Comparison between acute/respiratory and chronic stomatitis/gingivitis isolates of feline calicivirus: pathogenicity, antigenic profile and cross-neutralization studies. *Archives of Virology* 145: 243–261.

Reiter, A.M. (2012). Dental and oral diseases. In: The Cat: Clinical Medicine and Management (ed. S.E. Little), 329–370. St. Louis: Elsevier.

Rochlitz, I., Podberscek, A.L., and Broom, D.M. (1998). Welfare of cats in a quarantine cattery. *Veterinary Record* 143: 35.

Slater, M., Weiss, E., and Lord, L. (2012). Current use of and attitudes towards identification in cats and dogs in veterinary clinics in Oklahoma City, USA. *Animal Welfare* 21: 51–57.

Stone, A.E., Brummet, G.O. Carozza, E.M. et al. (2020) 2020 AAFP/AAHA Feline Vaccination Guidelines. *Journal of the American Animal Hospital Association* 56: 249–265.

Tanaka, A., Wagner, D.C., Kass, P.H. et al. (2012). Associations among weight loss, stress, and upper respiratory tract infection in shelter cats. *Journal of the American Veterinary Medical Association* 240 (5): 570–576.

Weiss, E., Slater, M.R., and Lord, L.K. (2011). Retention of provided identification for dogs and cats seen in veterinary clinics and adopted from shelters in Oklahoma City, OK, USA. *Preventive Veterinary Medicine* 101: 265–269.

Wemelsfelder, F. (2005). Animal boredom: understanding the tedium of confined lives. In: Mental Health and Wellbeing in Animals (ed. F.D. McMillan), 79–91. Ames: Blackwell.

3

Data Surveillance

Janet Scarlett

Cornell University College of Veterinary Medicine, Ithaca, NY, USA

The availability of scientifically and statistically reliable information is essential to improving the health of animal populations.

L.J. King

3.1 Introduction

The management of the health of shelter animals has improved dramatically over the past two decades. The development of shelter medicine training programs and the shelter medicine specialty has driven this progress. Many shelters have proactive healthcare plans for their populations with specific goals to improve population health. Population health-related protocols such as those designed to improve animal flow, standardize intake exams, and manage risk during outbreaks are now common. However, another component of population healthcare management, routine monitoring of disease-related summary data (metrics), has not been as widely adopted. This may be partially explained by the traditional emphasis on individual patient care for companion animals provided in veterinary training programs and private practices. Additionally, the widespread use of disease-related metrics has also been hampered by shelter software that has been slow to facilitate entry and retrieval of the necessary data.

Summary metrics relating to disease surveillance, animal flow and capacity (housing and staffing) are discussed in this chapter to encourage shelter veterinarians to incorporate the use of these metrics into their population healthcare plans. As these metrics are used more extensively, other influential measures can be added.

3.2 Disease Surveillance

Disease surveillance is an integral component of managing and minimizing disease in public health and preventive medicine programs for livestock (Anderson 1982; Horstmann 1974; King 1985; Langmuir 1963). William Farr is credited with formalizing the principles of human disease surveillance beginning in the mid-1800s in England. In the 1950s (during the height of polio outbreaks) in the United States, the Centers for Disease Control and Prevention (CDC) began formal surveillance programs for human communicable diseases (Langmuir 1963). It was not until the mid-1980s that the Animal and Plant Health Inspection Service (APHIS) took the lead in developing a national surveillance program for diseases of U.S. livestock species (King 1985).

Routine disease surveillance requires quantification of disease frequency, descriptions of disease distribution among subgroups of animals,

Infectious Disease Management in Animal Shelters, Second Edition.
Edited by Lila Miller, Stephanie Janeczko, and Kate F. Hurley.

analysis and interpretation of data. Formally, disease surveillance is defined as (i) the ongoing systematic collection, orderly consolidation, analysis and interpretation of health-related data in populations, and (ii) the prompt dissemination of this information to the people who are in a position to act on that data (Nelson and Williams 2007). Disease surveillance plans can include non-infectious disease, but this chapter will focus on infectious disease.

3.2.1 Importance of Disease Surveillance

Knowing the nature and extent of disease occurrence in shelter populations enables veterinarians to:

- assess population health in quantitative terms
- set objective and measurable disease-related priorities
- identify outbreaks
- plan and monitor the effectiveness of preventive and control measures
- rapidly identify "new" diseases/conditions
- justify grant proposals, and
- clearly communicate the health of their populations to interested constituencies (e.g. Boards of Directors, funding agencies, community).

The basic metrics of interest in disease surveillance in shelters are measures of morbidity (frequency of illness such as incidence), and mortality (frequency of death). Recommended definitions of these metrics for use in animal shelters have been discussed (Scarlett et al. 2017a). An incidence rate is defined as the number of newly diagnosed cases of a particular disease divided by the number of animals that could develop that disease in a specified period. This fraction is usually multiplied by 100 and expressed as a percentage. By comparison, prevalence refers to the percentage of cases of a particular disease that are present in a particular population at a given time. In this chapter, the terminology "frequency of disease" is used to encompass the disease incidence or prevalence, as well as death resulting from or euthanasia that occurs because of a particular disease. One of these terms (e.g. incidence) is used when the discussion pertains to that metric alone.

If disease incidence is increasing, it is important to ascertain why and to intervene to reduce its occurrence. An increase in disease is usually associated with a breakdown somewhere in the shelter's health-management protocols or signals the need for additional ones. Quickly identifying the possible causes of increased incidence is essential to maintaining population health. Even when the disease incidence is stable, quantifying the endemic level of diseases facilitates discussions of which diseases have priority for special attention (e.g. prevention, additional funding).

When discrepancies in the frequency of disease occur by host (e.g. kittens vs. adults), location (e.g. holding wards vs. adoption wards) or time of year (e.g. spring vs. fall) factors, these differences are often clues to underlying causes and/or additional steps that may need to be taken. They can indicate the need for new protocols, highlight breakdowns in current protocols, or suggest where and how a "new" disease agent entered the shelter and spread. The clues should lead to the development of hypotheses explaining the cause of the increased frequency, the precipitating event(s), and any factors supporting transmission in the shelter (if applicable). This knowledge then becomes the basis for preventive and control measures. If these measures are effective, disease rates decline, and recommendations can be made to prevent future increases in disease incidence. If rates fail to decrease, then protocols/initiatives are revised, and new approaches are instituted and evaluated.

Comparing the frequency of disease over time in a shelter or among shelters should be done thoughtfully. Interpretation of the differences in rates (or lack thereof) must always consider other explanations for what was observed. For example, comparisons of incidence rates before and after implementation of control measures can be a powerful means to assess the success and magnitude of the measures' effectiveness. However, changes in season affecting the age of entering animals or overcrowding due to an unanticipated seizure, for example, may explain the absence of an effect on disease rates, and not represent the failure of control measures. It is often necessary to consider ancillary information when interpreting any comparison. Similarly, demonstrating low incidence rates achieved in some shelters against those whose disease rates are high can be motivating. If done without thought, however, comparisons can also be discouraging (and unfair) if circumstances that can't be changed (e.g. characteristics of entering animals) between shelters are quite different.

Effective surveillance programs require good individual animal identification, a medical records system, a clear understanding of why surveillance is important, agreement on which diseases to include, clear definitions of those diseases, prompt disease reporting, incentives to report, and a management plan for affected animals. Regular timely analyses, clear surveillance reports, the ability to interpret and utilize those reports, and the dissemination of data to pertinent parties are essential. Protocols should be developed (e.g. documenting what to enter, when and by whom) to enhance the likelihood that diseases are identified, and pertinent data are entered consistently and completely.

3.2.2 Clear Objectives

Before initiating a disease surveillance program, clear objectives for the program should be outlined. The objectives must reflect the priorities of a shelter, be realistic, and be widely understood. Objectives could include, for example, quantifying the incidence of feline upper respiratory disease by host (e.g. age group, source) and time (season) factors, implementing appropriate control measures, and assessing the effectiveness of those measures.

3.2.3 Diseases/Signs to Surveil

One of the first steps in establishing a disease surveillance program is to create a list of the infectious diseases/signs that the medical staff believes are important to monitor. The focus should be on diseases/signs that are common (but could be reduced), particularly problematic (e.g. ringworm), or that are related to other medical goals (e.g. reducing time to recovery) of the shelter. The list should be short and manageable, with a focus on monitoring data that are likely to influence thinking and actions. Attempting to monitor too many diseases can overwhelm staff and lead to incomplete, inaccurate, or inconsistent data. It is better to collect and monitor data well for a few important diseases than to attempt to monitor many diseases and do it poorly; other diseases can always be added later. Once the list is established, the usual frequencies (endemic level) of those diseases should be calculated. (Note that some shelters develop an initial list and calculate the frequency of each disease, and then use the list to help decide which diseases to ultimately include in their surveillance program).

An annual medical profile is helpful in summarizing the yearly occurrence of disease for the shelter staff, the board of directors and other constituencies. The medical profile should be a part of the shelter's reported annual statistics. (An example is provided in Table 3.1). The shelter whose data appear in the table included the incidence and prevalence of major infectious diseases in its facility, mortality due to natural causes, and the number and percentage of euthanasias for medical reasons. This type of table provides a snapshot of the status of disease in the shelter, provides data to justify allocating funds for medical-related goals, and summarizes progress toward improving the population's health on an annual basis. The medical staff should monitor common diseases or those associated with particular goals more frequently for timely identification of concerning trends (see the section on frequency of review, interpretation and communication).

Table 3.1 Annual medical profile in an adoption guarantee shelter.

Disease	Number in Cats	Prevalence (%) in Cats	Number in Dogs	Prevalence (%) in Dogs
Coccidiosis[a]	106	24.7 (106/429)	81	15.2 (81/533)
Giardiasis[a]	36	8.4 (36/429)	51	9.8 (51/533)
Sarcoptic Mange[a]	–	–	37	8.6 (37/435)
Heartworms[b]	–	–	162	9.3 (162/1746)
FeLV[b]	30	0.91 (30/3310)	–	–
FIV[b]	112	3.4 (112/3310)	–	–
Disease	**Number in Cats**	**Incidence (%) in Cats**	**Number in Dogs**	**Incidence (%) in Dogs**
URTD/CIRD[c]	637	18.3 (637/3484)	106	4.8 (106/2227)
Mortality (all causes)	55	1.6 (55/3484)	18	0.81 (18/2227)
Euthanasias for medical reasons	216	6.2 (216/3484)	31	1.4 (31/2227)
• Treatable[d]	0	–	–	–
• Non-treatable	216	6.2 (216/3484)	31	1.4 (31/2227)

[a] Animals positive for this organism among those tested with signs possibly associated with this disease.
[b] Animals positive for this organism among those tested during the intake examination.
FeLV, feline leukemia virus.
FIV, feline immunodeficiency virus.
[c] Disease that developed among the shelter animals while they were in residence in the shelter.
URTD, feline upper respiratory tract disease.
CIRD, canine infectious respiratory disease, also known as kennel cough.
[d] Could be treated in the future with additional resources.
Source: L.J. King, National Animal Health Monitoring System in the USA: a model information system for international animal health, Rev. Sci. Tech. Off. Int. Epiz., 1988, 7 (3), 583–588.

One issue complicating the collection of surveillance data is the failure to reach a diagnosis. For this reason, some software programs enable shelters to retrieve both "diagnoses" and "clinical signs" (check your software). From a disease-surveillance standpoint, a diagnosis is preferable, but since a specific diagnosis is often not possible in shelters, recording and monitoring important clinical signs can be helpful. An unusual frequency of diarrhea might prompt the collection and submission of samples for diagnostic testing and identify, for example, an outbreak of giardiasis. Sometimes, the level of uncertainty of diagnosis is incorporated into disease data. For example, some studies incorporate case descriptors such as "possible," "probable" or "confirmed" or "presumptive" vs. "confirmed" for diagnoses and incorporate these levels into their analyses. It can be helpful to have data regarding both diagnoses and signs, particularly when diagnoses are suspect, or the shelter wishes to monitor disease severity. If both signs and diagnoses are collected, they should be in separate data fields to avoid double counting.

To achieve consistency of data recording among staff over time, shelters need written descriptions of each of the diseases they include in the surveillance system. Staff members require training regarding those definitions and the importance of adhering to them. For some diseases, this is relatively easy. A diagnosis of feline leukemia virus (FeLV), for example, is based on a positive result on a commercially available, validated test; for other diseases, such as canine infectious respiratory disease (also known as kennel cough or CIRD), defining cases is more difficult, as respiratory signs alone rarely establish a definitive diagnosis. In these instances, a "working definition" of the disease can be used (as is often true during outbreak investigations) or the incidence of certain clinical signs may be monitored. Despite the difficulty, if no attempt is made to standardize the grounds for a diagnosis or create a working definition, it is hard (if not impossible) to interpret changes in disease frequency. The key is to standardize *as much as possible* what staff diagnose as a particular disease or identify as a clinical sign. The definitions need not be perfect, only consistently applied.

The collection of the date of the *first* diagnosis is essential to mark the onset of each new case so that incidence measures can be calculated for specific time periods. For diseases that can occur more than once in an individual animal (e.g. upper respiratory tract infections), **only the first episode** during a particular timeframe is counted as a new or incident case. If the medical team has an interest in reoccurring illnesses, the rate of second occurrences can be calculated and reported separately. If second (or other) occurrences are monitored during a time period of interest, the denominator includes only animals with a first occurrence in that timeframe. Fortunately, since most animals do not reside in most shelters long enough to experience second infections of most diseases, the rate of second infections is usually ignored. An exception may be in sanctuaries.

3.2.4 Data Collection, Analysis, Interpretation, and Communication

Disease surveillance takes time and resources to do well. An effective surveillance program must be valued, planned, and well-executed. Written protocols governing what, where, when, and by whom each component will be performed are essential.

Several staff members are usually involved in data *collection* during an animal's passage through the shelter system. For infectious disease surveillance, shelter intake (for denominators) and medical data (for numerators) are obviously needed, but data related to movement, outcomes, daily observations and other events could also be important to address questions that arise from surveillance. Quality and completeness of all relevant data are key components. Everyone involved with data collection must be trained and held accountable for providing good data. Without explicit protocols, staff may be unsure of how, what, when, and where to collect specific pieces of information.

How and by whom the data will be routinely *analyzed* should be clear. This includes the metrics (e.g. incidence, mortality) and subgroups of animals to monitor, the trends to track, and any other metrics that are important to the shelter's medical-related goals.

Since disease risk frequently varies by age group, source (e.g. stray), and over time, separate incidence rates should be calculated for each of these factors. Data can contradict common beliefs. For example, after reviewing Figure 3.1, medical staff members were surprised that the incidence (or risk) of feline upper respiratory tract disease (URTD) was actually higher in the fall and winter months than in the spring and summer. Further analyses demonstrated that this was true among both kittens and adult cats. The staff did see more sick cats in the spring and summer, but the cat intake was also much higher. With these results, the shelter heightened its adherence to its preventive protocols in the fall and winter. Similarly, surveillance data can confirm suspicions and provide evidence to change behavior and shelter protocols. A veterinarian had the clinical impression that the survival rate among fostered un-weaned kittens could be improved by making changes to their management in foster homes; foster care providers were resistant to change. The data (see Figure 3.2) demonstrated a survival rate of only 71%. The providers were unaware of this rate, and they also found it unacceptable. The veterinarian updated protocols and made presentations to explain the basis for the changes. Over the next several years, survival rates increased to over 90%.

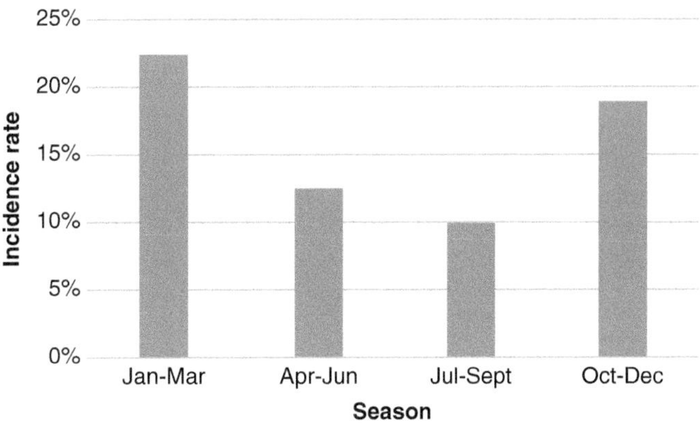

Figure 3.1 Incidence rate of URTD among cats by season.

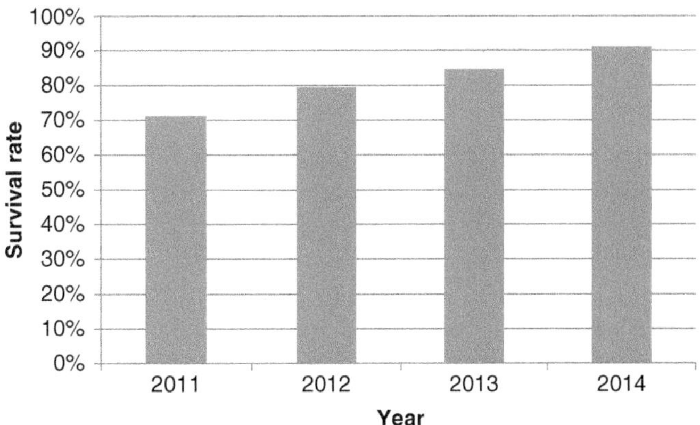

Figure 3.2 Annual survival rates of un-weaned kittens in foster care 2011–2014.

Routine monitoring and analysis of data augment the daily observations of the medical staff, adding to their understanding of the state of the health of the population. When routinely incorporated into population care, data surveillance can improve the health and welfare of shelter animals.

3.2.5 Frequency of Review, Interpretation and Communication

A key component of disease surveillance is regular data review and communication (Anderson 1982; Nelson and Williams 2007). Regular *review* by medical staff facilitates prompt recognition of changes in disease frequency and heightens responsiveness to these changes. This facilitates the timely achievement of disease-related goals and enables the medical staff to inform the administration and other shelter staff of health changes in a timely manner. No less than monthly reviews of the frequency of some diseases (e.g. upper respiratory tract infections) at regular staff meetings are warranted. Monthly reviews have the added benefit of maintaining interest in disease surveillance and attention to the collection of quality data. It is powerfully motivating for staff to realize that their adherence to protocols was responsible for falling disease rates and the achievement of other goals.

The timing of some analyses can be prespecified, but other analyses may need to occur as the data suggests new questions. Frequency of monitoring is usually related to the incidence and severity of the disease, and whether the shelter has specific goals related to that disease. Generally speaking, high-incidence diseases (e.g. feline URTD) will be monitored more frequently (e.g. monthly) than those of lower frequency. Disease outbreaks also trigger more frequent monitoring.

Interpretation of the results should include staff that may have insight into a particular analysis. The medical staff should obviously be involved but, in many instances, the shelter manager, kennel personnel or volunteers may also have important insights into why disease is manifesting as it is. For example, the interpretation of data relating to a rise in the mortality of fostered kittens might involve the shelter manager, veterinarian, executive leadership, foster-care providers and others empowered to make protocol changes based on that data.

The ability to interpret and *communicate* findings based on the data is heavily influenced by the data presentation; the presentation can obscure or enhance the message it contains. It is beyond the scope of this chapter to make recommendations for effective data presentation, but references are provided (Knaflic 2015; Tufte 2001). A consistent recommendation in these references is to keep presentations simple and focused on the message that needs to be conveyed; it is important to avoid ostentatious presentations that obscure that message.

3.2.6 Data Quality and Administrative Buy-In

Since disease surveillance requires the commitment of staff throughout a shelter, members of the shelter administration and management staff must believe in and support surveillance efforts. Staff training and incentives enhance the collection of quality data. When staff members understand the rationale for, and the importance of, complete and accurate collection of information, data quality rises. Resources are wasted in the collection of poor-quality data, and analyses of that data can be misleading. Summary reports should be shared with staff on a regular basis. A review of the analyses facilitates discussions aimed at reducing disease and provides an opportunity to celebrate staff contributions to declining disease rates!

3.2.7 Recording Changes Affecting the Surveillance Program

Changes that can have an impact on disease frequency occur routinely in shelters. For example, turnover in foster-care providers or staff, shifting shelter priorities, or changes to the economy of the community can impact the magnitude of disease rates and their interpretation. For example, in one community, the 2008 economic downturn resulted in the surrender of an increased number of animals requiring veterinary care because owners could not afford treatment. If the nature and timing of those changes are not recorded, people forget, and incorrect conclusions may be drawn from the data. One strategy for capturing these changes is a "Log of Events and Protocol Changes" that is updated as changes occur. An example of a log is provided in Table 3.2.

Table 3.2 Log of events and protocol changes for 2015.

Date	Relevant Events
1-Jan	Animal control contracts from Sunny and Marlow towns discontinued. Owner surrenders will continue to be accepted.
20-Feb	A seizure of 60 dogs from Mary Smith is undertaken. The number of dogs exceeds the housing capacity of the shelter. Crates are set up and dogs are housed in staff offices.
25-Apr	Grant (~$20,000) received to increase Trap Neuter Return (TNR) efforts.
30-Apr	The shelter eliminated the part-time veterinarian position due to financial concerns.
9-Jul	The intake policy changed. Nuisance feral cats managed by providing traps and spay-neuter services. Animal Control officers trained to vaccinate stray animals before bringing them to the shelter.
10-Sept	Shelter eliminated two full-time staff positions due to budget crisis; shelter is understaffed.
23-Oct	Funding restored, and two staff members rehired.
15–23-Dec	Mega adoption event.

3.3 Length of Stay (LOS) in Shelters

The length of time animals spend in a shelter affects their likelihood of exposure to infectious agents; it also affects their stress levels (which impacts susceptibility to infection). Several studies have linked increased length of stay (LOS) with enhanced risk of feline and canine URTD in shelters (Dinnage et al. 2009; Edinboro and Glickman 2004; Edinboro et al. 1999; Gourkow et al. 2013). The average length of stay (ALOS) is a measure of the average speed with which animals are moved or flow through a shelter. When animal movement is slow (i.e. the ALOS is high), not only does the risk of disease and stress increase, but fewer animals are processed in the same time period compared to when the flow is fast. If intake remains constant or increases, slow movement (or high ALOS) often leads to overcrowding, another important risk factor for many infectious diseases.

The ALOS is calculated by summing the LOS of all animals of interest and dividing that sum by the total number of animals contributing to LOS values during a specified time period. Time periods of greatest interest are usually by month, season, and year. Monitoring graphs of these averages over time can identify patterns, suggest goals, gauge progress toward minimizing ALOS, and reveal associations between ALOS and disease risks. Many commercially available shelter software systems can calculate ALOS for specific populations and over specific time periods.

A common initial objective of shelters is to reduce the overall ALOS. Progress can often be accelerated by using data to identify the subgroups, procedures, or areas in the shelter that contribute disproportionately to slowing transit times through the shelter. By evaluating the ALOS of various subgroups, e.g. time spent waiting for common procedures to be performed (e.g. behavior evaluations, spay-neuter, dentistry), and time spent in specific areas (e.g. holding, adoptions), a shelter can identify and focus its efforts on specific impediments that cause delays in animal transit through the facility. Common subgroups to monitor are those of age group, source (e.g. seized, stray), general health status (e.g. healthy, sick) and in some shelters, breed-type. Since time-related factors (e.g. seasonal intake, volunteer availability) often affect flow, regular assessments of ALOS by these factors may highlight opportunities for preemptive interventions.

The ALOS of senior cats was much longer than staff anticipated in the shelter associated with Figure 3.3. After reviewing this graph, the shelter gave the highest priority to reducing the ALOS of its oldest cats. Also, monthly and seasonal differences in ALOS often become apparent when graphed, raising questions as to why. Evaluating these discrepancies can suggest strategies that will minimize or eliminate them.

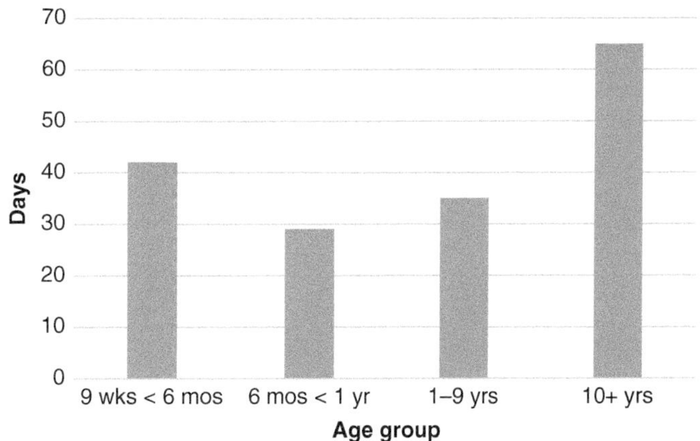

Figure 3.3 Average LOS of cats by age group.

Increases in LOS not only enhance risks for disease, but disease also increases the LOS, animal suffering and costs to the shelter. Data such as those in Figure 3.4 are useful in explaining requests for funding to enhance disease control measures, in this case, for controlling feline URTD. The data demonstrated that this disease significantly increased ALOS and the associated costs of care in this shelter.

A few words of caution are in order regarding ALOS calculations. There are at least three approaches to calculating the ALOS for shelter animals during particular periods of time (Scarlett et al. 2017b). It is beyond the scope of this chapter to describe the differences, but when using ALOS values supplied by shelter software, it is important to understand the method of calculation and the strengths and limitations of the method used.

In addition, current shelter software only provides ALOS values. In many shelters, the frequency distributions of LOS values do not display a Gaussian or Normal (bell-shaped) distribution. Instead, data are skewed to the right with a few animals having unusually long LOS. These highest LOS values pull the average upwards, away from the center of the data; this results in more than half of the animals having LOS less than the average. If this is true, the average may not be the optimal metric to monitor, depending on the purpose for which the ALOS is being monitored. Instead, the median, by definition, reflects the true middle of the distribution of age data and may provide a more accurate picture of the true situation for most animals in the shelter. One example of this exists for shelters with a few animals residing in the shelter for very long periods. The overall ALOS is especially problematic in such a scenario and it may appear high, even though the majority of animals have a lower (and more acceptable) LOS. Similarly, since some groups (e.g. those in foster care or awaiting court proceedings) may have LOS dictated by their circumstances, they should be monitored separately from other animals.

3.4 Capacity for Care

The ability of shelters to meet the needs of their animals is called a shelter's capacity for care (C4C) (http://www.millioncatchallenge.org/resources/capacity-for-care). When shelters have more animals than they can house humanely or too few staff members to provide basic care, conditions adverse to animal well-being can result (e.g. high disease rates, numerous animals housed in small spaces or in

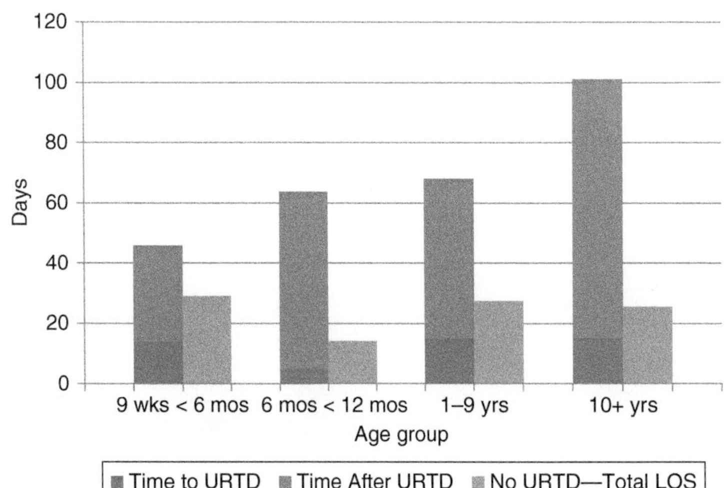

Figure 3.4 Average LOS of cats with and without URTD by age group.

carrying crates, dirty cages). It is often easy to recognize when a shelter is overcapacity or understaffed; quantitatively measuring overcrowding or deficits in staffing may be more difficult depending on the type and quality of data available but is worth the extra effort.

3.4.1 Housing Capacity

Why use metrics for monitoring housing capacity? This can be a valuable tool to reduce or avoid overcrowding. Common strategies for reducing overcrowding include increasing the number of housing units (either through construction or finding alternative housing sites), managing intake, and reducing the LOS. Building new housing is usually impractical and even when possible, will not resolve overcrowding if intake chronically exceeds the outflow of animals. The use of offsite adoption venues is also helpful but is rarely effective as the only approach to eliminating overcrowding; reducing the ALOS and/or managing the number of animals admitted over time are also approaches used by many shelters. The success of efforts to reduce ALOS at the population level is monitored as discussed previously. Similarly, efforts to reduce the number of incoming animals can be monitored over time using intake data.

The relationships between ALOS, intake, and the available housing space can be used to predict the effect of changing any one of these factors on the others over time (See the formula below). These predictions help set goals and motivate staff to achieve them.

During a specified period of time:

$$\text{Intake (\# of new animals that can be housed)} = \frac{\text{Number of humane housing spaces} \times \text{Number of days}}{\text{ALOS (days)}}$$

It is important to note that using this formula assumes that all humane housing spaces are occupied in the shelter at the beginning of a time period; it is used to calculate how many additional animals the shelter can expect to be able to provide humane housing for based on the number of spaces and the average length of stay.

To use the formula, a shelter must start by estimating the number of animals by species that can be humanely housed at any given time. The *Guidelines for Standards of Care in Animal Shelters* (Newbury et al. 2010) provide recommendations that may be used to determine which housing is humane. If the shelter experiences wide fluctuations in the number and/or age groups of animals entering by season, then the number that can be housed at any given time should be estimated by species, age group and by season. Counting the number of housing spaces is done making assumptions (e.g. two kittens or one adult cat per humane housing unit). (These numbers should be as accurate as possible but need not be perfect as they are used to generate estimates.

After estimating the number of available housing units, the shelter can acquire the ALOS for animals from its software system (by season and age group, if appropriate) and use those values to determine how many additional animals they can admit to the facility in that period of time while remaining within their humane housing capacity. Alternatively, the shelter can specify target ALOS values, depending on the intent of the calculations. The usefulness of the formula is illustrated in the following example. (Age group is ignored to simplify the calculations).

Shelter A historically receives an average of 260 cats during the months July–September (92 days), which results in some cats being euthanized and others being temporarily housed in stacked portable wire cages. The shelter has 40 humane housing spaces for cats and historically has had an ALOS during this period of 22 days per cat. The formula suggests that the shelter should only accept approximately 167 cats to avoid overpopulating during this period.

$$\underset{(\text{July–September})}{167\,\text{additional cats}} = \frac{40\,\text{housing units} \times 92\,\text{days}}{22\,\text{days}}$$

What would happen if the shelter reduced its ALOS? Looking at Table 3.3, if the shelter could reduce its ALOS to 14 days, it could successfully house an estimated 262 cats (enabling it to avoid overcrowding during the period). The shelter can make this ALOS a goal to work toward.

If the shelter also wished to manage its intake, it could modify the formula to estimate the number of cats (on average) that should be admitted daily during the period with a given ALOS. If both sides of the formula are divided by the number of days in the period, the average number of cats to be admitted daily can be estimated according to the modified formula below.

$$\text{Animals to admit daily} = \frac{\text{Number of humane housing units}}{\text{ALOS}\,(\text{days})}$$

If the ALOS remained at 22 days, the shelter would need to reduce its weekly intake to approximately 12 (1.8 cats/day × 7 days) cats to avoid overpopulating (Column 4, Table 3.3). If the shelter were to reduce its ALOS to 18, they could comfortably accept 15 cats/week (2.9 cats/day × 7 days).

To summarize, the formula can be used to estimate the:

1) ALOS of animals needed to avoid overcrowding with a given intake and number of housing units;
2) number of animals to admit in a specified period based on the number of available housing units and ALOS;
3) predicted effect of reducing the ALOS on the number of animals that should be admitted to avoid overcrowding.

The formula can be used to estimate any one of its component parts (if the other values are known or target values are inserted). Thus, a shelter could also calculate the number of housing units needed to comfortably house animals with a specific ALOS and rate of intake. Additionally, this formula can be used to determine the number of animals to have on the adoption floor based on a specific ALOS in the adoption area and adoption rate (see the Adoption Driven Capacity calculator on the Koret Shelter Medicine website http://www.sheltermedicine.com/library/resources/capacity-for-care-c4c-magic-number-calculator). These uses, assumptions associated with the use of the formula, and the calculations are explained in more detail in other sources (Koret Shelter Medicine 2015; Newbury and Hurley 2013a; Scarlett et al. 2017c).

Other metrics can also be used to manage population numbers. For example, a shelter could compare the number of animals actually housed in the building (daily in-shelter inventory) to the estimated number of available

Table 3.3 The effect of lowering ALOS on the estimated number of cats that can be admitted during July–September without overcrowding in Shelter A.

Number of housing units	Average LOS (days)	Cats that could be housed in the period	Approximate number of cats to accept
40	22	167	1.8/day 12/week
40	18	204	2.2/day 15/week
40	14	262	2.9/day 20/week

housing units. If the number of animals housed in the building exceeds the number of humane housing units available, the number of "excess animals" and the percent overcapacity could be monitored over time and strategies implemented to reduce it.

The use of the formula produces estimates because the component parts are estimated. Nonetheless, these estimates are tools that have helped manage the populations of a growing number of shelters, in combination with reducing ALOS, managing intake, improving the quality of housing and other approaches (Karsten et al. 2017).

3.4.2 Staffing Capacity

Inadequate staffing to provide basic care (cleaning and feeding) often leads to breaches in shelter biosecurity. When this happens, exposure to infectious agents and disease frequency increases. Therefore, monitoring staff numbers is an important component of a comprehensive disease control program. The National Animal Control Association (NACA) recommends that staff spend a minimum of 15 minutes per animal providing basic care (NACA 2014). Using these recommendations, a shelter's capacity to provide basic care can be assessed by (i) estimating the amount of time that staff should be engaged in basic animal care daily; (ii) calculating the number of hours staff actually is engaged in basic care daily; and (iii) comparing the two estimates. Calculations are described in more detail in other sources (Newbury and Hurley 2013b; Scarlett et al. 2017d).

If staff time for basic care is insufficient or less than that which is suggested in the guidelines, the shelter should consider an investment in additional staff positions, cross-training of non-animal care staff, or a reduction in the numbers of animals in the shelter. If a shelter meets the guidelines, it should be noted that the recommended daily time per animal is a *minimum* estimate solely for feeding and cleaning. Other staffing-related recommendations are also available (Newbury and Hurley 2013b). Shelters should strive to increase the available staff time per animal to maximize the welfare of the animals in their care. Since staffing needs can vary widely (e.g. by season, after a seizure of several animals, and with the changing physical and behavioral needs of the animals), shelters should evaluate the adequacy of staffing on a regular basis and as animal care needs change. Some shelters routinely utilize trained volunteers to assist staff in providing animal care and enrichment; when these volunteers are adequately trained and reliable and available to help with daily care, they may be counted toward the total amount of available animal care time for the shelter.

3.5 Other Disease-Related Metrics

Disease surveillance, the ALOS, and C4C metrics are not the only ones that can be useful to shelters. Once data monitoring becomes routine, other disease-related metrics such as the average time to disease recovery, percentage occupancy of isolation wards, ratio of sick-to-healthy animals, or average sick-days can be monitored to enhance insight into disease control and understanding and management of population health.

3.6 Software Needs

Many shelters already have protocols outlining the active identification and reporting of animals with infectious diseases. Much of that data is entered into software programs but retrieving disease rates in a useful format is challenging. Shelter software companies have generally been slow to provide disease rates or facilitate flexible, efficient retrieval of much of the data needed to calculate these rates. Fortunately, the ALOS and daily census metrics are now routinely provided.

Medical staff need the ability to obtain overall morbidity, mortality, and medically related euthanasia rates, as well as the ability to classify these rates by age group, source, and over various time periods. Since trends and group comparisons are usually best understood when graphed, an easy means to produce visual presentations is also essential. Inevitably, regular monitoring of basic data leads to new questions and additional analyses. As these new questions arise, software also needs the flexibility of data retrieval that helps veterinarians and shelter staff address such questions.

Software providers should facilitate retrieval and graphing of disease surveillance and related data. They should understand that, without a clear understanding of the incidence of disease, veterinarians cannot assess whether and to what degree their disease-management recommendations are effective. Similarly, their efforts to set health priorities and communicate the importance of their health-related goals are hampered by words like “a lot, some or very little disease” because they cannot quantify disease at the population level.

3.7 Shelters Without Shelter-Specific Software

For veterinarians working for shelters without software or with unwieldy software, the frequency of diseases of interest to the shelter can be monitored by hand or in a spreadsheet. Most shelters have staff or volunteers who could tally numbers or work with the data in spreadsheets. Spreadsheets should:

- Identify diseases in each species that are important to monitor.
- Record each affected animal’s unique identifier along with the diagnosis (e.g. URTD) and its first date of recognition.
- Capture these data in a notebook, spreadsheet or by some other means.;
- Count all newly diagnosed diseases for various periods (e.g. month of August).
- Include data regarding other factors that may affect disease risk, such as those related to the host (e.g. age group), place (e.g. off-site location) or time (e.g. season) to enhance the usefulness of surveillance data.

3.8 The Future

Disease surveillance in shelters today is predominantly active (not passive or sentinel) surveillance. That is, medical personnel have protocols to actively identify common infectious diseases, report them internally and ensure that affected animals receive appropriate care as soon as possible. In the future, once individual shelters enhance their disease surveillance by using their data more extensively, reporting across communities, regions and at the national level becomes possible. Shelter Animals Count is a collaborative initiative of sheltering organizations that currently focuses on the national collection of basic animal entry and outcome data, but it could expand its data collection to include disease-related and other data in the future (http://shelteranimalscount.org). Such data could lead to surveillance efforts at regional and national levels, similar to those of CDC and APHIS; this would enhance understanding of regional variations in disease incidence and enhance disease management.

3.9 Summary

Shelter medicine has improved the care of shelter animals dramatically over the past two decades. Veterinarians can now find full- and part-time job opportunities in animal shelters, and veterinarians with a background and training in shelter medicine can bring specific knowledge as well as an arsenal of tools to improve animal health and welfare in animal welfare organizations. Monitoring disease-related metrics is an additional tool that will enhance the care of shelter populations, as it has for human and livestock populations. For this to occur, veterinarians must embrace the importance of data, enhance their skills at their interpretation, and insist that software companies facilitate the entry, retrieval and visualization of relevant data.

References

Anderson, R.K. (1982). Surveillance: criteria for evaluation and design of epidemiologic surveillance systems for animal health and productivity. *Proceedings of the 86th Annual Meeting of the U.S. Animal Health Association*, Nashville, TN (7–12 November 1982). Richmond, VA, US: Carter Printing Company.

Dinnage, J.D., Scarlett, J.M., and Richards, J.R. (2009). Descriptive epidemiology of feline upper respiratory tract diseases in an animal shelter. *Journal of Feline Medicine and Surgery* 11: 816–825.

Edinboro, C.H. and Glickman, L. (2004). A placebo-controlled trial of two intranasal vaccines to prevent tracheobronchitis (kennel cough) in dogs entering a humane shelter. *Preventive Veterinary Medicine* 62: 89–99.

Edinboro, C.H., Janowitz, L.K., Guptill-Yoran, L., and Glickman, L. (1999). A clinical trial of intranasal and subcutaneous vaccines to prevent upper respiratory infection in cats at an animal shelter. *Feline Practice* 27: 7–13.

Gourkow, N., Larson, J.H., Hamon, S.C., and Phillips, C.J.C. (2013). Descriptive epidemiology of upper respiratory disease and associated factors in cats in an animal shelter in coastal western Canada. *Canadian Veterinary Journal* 54: 132–138.

Horstmann, D.M. (1974). Importance of disease surveillance. *Preventive Medicine* 3: 436–442.

Karsten, C.L., Wagner, D.C., Kass, P.H., and Hurley, K.F. (2017). An observational study of the relationship between Capacity for Care as an animal shelter management model and cat health, adoption and death in three animal shelters. *Veterinary Journal* 227: 15–22.

King, L.J. (1985). Unique characteristics of the National Animal Disease Surveillance System. *Journal of the American Veterinary Medical Association* 186: 35–39.

Knaflic, C.N. (2015). Storytelling with Data, 1e. Hoboken: Wiley.

Koret Shelter Medicine (2015). Calculating shelter capacity information sheet. http://www.sheltermedicine.com/library/resources/calculating-shelter-capacity. (accessed 12 April 2017).

Langmuir, A.D. (1963). The surveillance of communicable diseases of national importance. *New England Journal of Medicine* 268: 182–192.

National Animal Care and Control Association (NACA) (2014). Determining kennel staffing levels resource sheet. https://www.nacanet.org/determining-kennel-staffing-needs/ (accessed 12 April 2017).

Nelson, K.E. and Williams, C.F. (2007). Infectious Disease Epidemiology, 25–42. Boston: Jones and Bartlett Publishers.

Newbury, S. and Hurley, K. (2013a). Population management. In: Shelter Medicine for Veterinarians and Staff, 2e (eds. L. Miller and S. Zawistowski), 106–110. Ames: Wiley Blackwell.

Newbury, S. and Hurley, K. (2013b). Population management. In: Shelter Medicine for Veterinarians and Staff, 2e (eds. L. Miller and S. Zawistowski), 109–110. Ames: Wiley Blackwell.

Newbury, S., Blinn, M.K., Bushby, P.A. et al. (2010). Guidelines for Standards of Care in Animal Shelters. https://www.sheltervet.org/assets/docs/shelter-standards-oct2011-wforward.pdf (accessed 17 December 2017).

Scarlett, J.M., Greenberg, M., and Hoshizaki, T. (2017a). Every Nose Counts Using Metrics in Animal Shelters. A Maddie's Guide, 1e, 147–149. CreateSpace.

Scarlett, J.M., Greenberg, M., and Hoshizaki, T. (2017b). Every Nose Counts Using Metrics in Animal Shelters. A Maddie's Guide, 1e, 92–96. CreateSpace.

Scarlett, J.M., Greenberg, M., and Hoshizaki, T. (2017c). Every Nose Counts Using Metrics in Animal Shelters. A Maddie's Guide, 1e, 98–106. CreateSpace.

Scarlett, J.M., Greenberg, M., and Hoshizaki, T. (2017d). Every Nose Counts Using Metrics in Animal Shelters. A Maddie's Guide, 1e, 106–109. CreateSpace.

Tufte, E.D. (2001). The Visual Display of Quantitative Information. Cheshire, CT: Graphics Press.

4

Diagnostic Testing

Brian A. DiGangi

American Society for the Prevention of Cruelty to Animals (ASPCA), New York, NY, USA

For most diagnoses all that is needed is an ounce of knowledge, an ounce of intelligence, and a pound of thoroughness.
– Anonymous

4.1 Introduction

A diagnostic test can be defined as any tool used to obtain information that enables the practitioner to identify a disease or condition. In veterinary medicine, diagnostic tests typically include physical examination findings, information gleaned from interviewing an owner or caretaker, history of the patient and its relatives or cohorts (i.e. anamnesis), and paraclinical findings reported by laboratory tests and imaging studies (Blood and Studdert 1999). Determining the cause of disease enables the veterinarian to prescribe appropriate treatment and render a prognosis. In the face of an infectious disease outbreak, obtaining a diagnosis can guide management decisions to mitigate the impact of the outbreak. Of particular importance in the shelter setting, obtaining a diagnosis also ensures efficient resource allocation and maximizes the quality of life for shelter animals.

In addition to identifying the cause of an acute or chronic disease, diagnostic testing may also be utilized to identify both animals with subclinical infection and those that are free from infection (Evermann et al. 2012). Such distinctions allow the shelter veterinarian to determine the risk of co-housing individual animals and to develop rational biosecurity protocols to prevent the introduction and spread of disease within the shelter environment.

Diagnostic tests for infectious diseases can be broadly categorized as direct or indirect. Direct testing methodologies rely on detection of the pathogen itself (e.g. culture, polymerase chain reaction [PCR]), while indirect testing methodologies focus on detecting the body's response to the pathogen or disease process (e.g. antibody testing, biochemical profile). It is important for the practitioner to understand the testing modality that is being used, as well as its limitations. For example, direct testing methods do not necessarily indicate whether the pathogen identified is dead or alive, nor can they always quantify the severity of the disease. Similarly, indirect testing methods often cannot distinguish between current or previous exposure to a pathogen or active disease.

In the face of resource limitations common in many shelter organizations (i.e. time, money, training, expertise), the utility of a comprehensive diagnostic testing strategy is often overlooked or considered unattainable; however, such limitations are not a reason to ignore best practices. For many practitioners,

Infectious Disease Management in Animal Shelters, Second Edition.
Edited by Lila Miller, Stephanie Janeczko, and Kate F. Hurley.

the joys and challenges of shelter practice lie within creatively meeting the spirit of those practices in the face of limited resources. Thoughtfully employed diagnostics can lead to cost-effective protection of animal health and welfare—a goal that is shared by everyone.

4.2 Obtaining Diagnostic Samples

Every organization with a medical program should strive to maintain some minimum diagnostic testing supplies and equipment for an in-house laboratory. See Box 4.1. Such items are commonly available through veterinary and medical supply distributors at minimal cost (<$500 for disposable supplies listed in Box 4.1). Inexpensive, gently used diagnostic equipment can often be found online or through local human hospitals. Maintaining an in-house laboratory will allow the practitioner to establish a presumptive or definitive diagnosis in the majority of infectious diseases common in animal shelters. An in-house laboratory also supports the ability to perform all the diagnostic procedures described in the sections on core diagnostic tools and primary diagnostic testing, and many of the procedures in the section on secondary diagnostic testing. Additional supplies and equipment can be obtained when expanding the scope of an in-house laboratory or as needed for the routine collection of samples for submission to diagnostic laboratories. In many cases, diagnostic laboratories will provide sample or test-specific collection equipment at no charge. Care should be taken to ensure that the type and number of samples, the manner of collection (i.e. sterility), along with the collection container (including preservatives or additives) are appropriate for

Box 4.1 Minimum Recommended Diagnostic Testing Supplies and Equipment

Supplies

Syringes (1 cc, 3 cc)
Needles (21–25 gauge (g) x 1″)
Blood collection tubes (Sterile "red top," EDTA "purple top")
Microhematocrit capillary tubes and tube sealant pad
Microscope slides
Romanowsky-type stain (e.g. Diff-Quik, Siemens Healthcare Diagnostics Ltd., Deerfield, IL)
Sodium nitrate solution (e.g. Fecasol, Vetoquinol, Fort Worth, TX)
Mineral oil
Coverslips
Cotton swabs
Scalpel blades
Small containers with 10% formalin

Equipment

Stethoscope
Scale
Thermometer
Microscope (10×, 40×)
Microhematocrit centrifuge
Refractometer
Portable blood glucose monitor or glucose reagent strips
Wood's Lamp (ultraviolet light, 365 nm wavelength)
Refrigerator

Test Kits

Urine chemical reagent strips
Blood urea nitrogen test strips (e.g. Azostix®, Shelby Scientific, Macomb, MI)
Commercial diagnostic test kits (e.g. heartworm antigen, canine parvovirus antigen, feline leukemia virus, feline immunodeficiency virus)

both the type of diagnostic test to be conducted and the interpretation of its results.

Many diagnostic tests rely on the collection of a sample of tissue, blood, urine, feces, or other bodily fluid (versus those that rely on contemporary historical, physical, or clinical findings). For such specimens, the diagnostic utility of the sample is often only as good as the collection technique and specimen handling. With careful planning and staff training, many diagnostic samples can be collected cage-side or even in a foster-home environment. Test kit manufacturers and diagnostic laboratories often have instructions and consultative services readily available to provide such direction when needed. Though veterinarians should direct the process, many individuals comfortable with basic animal handling can be trained to perform the actual sample collection for the most common diagnostic tests where permissible under applicable laws and regulations.

Once collected, diagnostic samples should be handled with care, particularly when being prepared for shipment to an outside laboratory. In general, cytologic samples should be rapidly air-dried and stored at room temperature; care should be taken not to crush or smear slide preparations. If not evaluated within 4 hours of collection, samples of blood, bodily fluids, or those intended for culture should be stored under refrigeration and processing should occur within 24 hours. See Chapter 5 for information on the collection and handling of necropsy specimens.

4.3 Types of Diagnostic Tests

Common diagnostic tests described in this chapter have been divided into core, primary, secondary, and diagnostic laboratory tests based on their resource requirements, knowledge and skill needed to conduct the tests and interpret the results, and their feasibility for being conducted within the resource limitations of most animal shelters.

Core diagnostic tools include a case history, physical examination findings, and response to treatment. These tools require minimal to no equipment, can be performed and interpreted by trained non-veterinary personnel and, with the exception of diagnosis by the response to treatment, should be performed on every animal that enters the shelter system.

Primary diagnostic testing in the animal shelter encompasses routine use of enzyme-linked immunosorbent assay (ELISA) test kits, diagnostic cytology, fecal examination and urinalysis. In most cases, these tests can be performed and interpreted by trained non-veterinary personnel within the shelter itself and are commonly used as both screening tests and first-line diagnostic tests for animals exhibiting specific clinical signs.

Secondary diagnostic testing includes complete blood count and blood chemistry analysis, diagnostic imaging, culture, and necropsy. These are utilized in specific clinical scenarios and when core and primary diagnostic tests are unable to provide a definitive diagnosis or direct the management plan. Many of the secondary tests can be conducted by in-house laboratories but results require interpretation and application by a veterinarian.

Diagnostic laboratory tests should be conducted by trained personnel in a diagnostic laboratory, and these results also require interpretation and application by a veterinarian. These tests are often reserved for select cases requiring a definitive diagnosis. Though all these tools (and many more not covered here) can provide a wide variety of clinical diagnostic information, this chapter will focus on those tools most likely to be applicable to the diagnosis and management of infectious diseases encountered in the shelter environment.

4.3.1 Core Diagnostic Tools

4.3.1.1 Case History

Often overlooked, but perhaps the most critical and readily available diagnostic tools include a case history, physical examination findings, and response to treatment for a presumptive diagnosis. It is tempting to dismiss the utility of a good case history in the shelter setting where many animals may not have an owner available for questioning, however, an attempt should always be made to collect such information. It is quite possible that an animal control officer, good Samaritan, pet owner, community volunteer, or other individual obtained some information on the animal's origin, has interacted with the animal, and has observed the animal prior to a clinical examination. Even if such information does not reveal clues about specific medical or behavioral care that may be indicated, it may direct housing of the animal in the shelter, prioritize the animal for veterinary evaluation, initiate an investigation into animal cruelty, or provide other information critical to protecting the health and welfare of that animal in the shelter system. Typical case-history questions used in private practice can be adjusted to address similar points relevant to the care of shelter animals. See Table 4.1.

4.3.1.2 Physical Examination

A thorough physical examination is an essential diagnostic modality that may be underutilized in a busy shelter. A complete description of physical examination techniques is beyond the scope of this chapter, but a few key points relevant to utilizing the physical examination as a diagnostic modality should be emphasized. Ideally, every animal will receive a physical examination by a veterinarian on intake or, at some point, before its release from the shelter; this is legally required whenever a medical diagnosis is made, a treatment plan is prescribed, or a surgical procedure is being performed. However, laypersons operating under the guidance of a veterinary-designed protocol can conduct a purposeful and accurate physical examination in most circumstances on shelter animals. (Shelters should ensure compliance with their state veterinary practice act and any other federal, state, and local regulations.) Physical examination generally includes the collection of both subjective and objective data points that can be assessed together to determine the most appropriate next steps in meeting that patient's individual needs. See Table 4.2.

The patient examination should progress from pure observation and least invasive measures and, as safety and comfort of both the examiner and the patient increase, proceed to an evaluation of areas that require a hands-on approach or may include manipulation of painful or diseased body parts. Unless an urgent medical need is apparent, an in-depth evaluation of a presenting complaint or existing condition is generally left until the end of the procedure. This allows the practitioner to have completed the entire physical examination in case a patient's pain or sensitivity to a diseased or injured area limits further evaluation.

Subjective patient assessment typically includes details about the presenting complaint, evaluation of the animal's mental state, food and water consumption, and any obvious signs of pain or discomfort. Assessment of respiratory rate and character should also occur at this time to avoid over-interpretation of abnormal findings that may be attributed to the stress and/or discomfort of animal handling. This portion of the examination can often be conducted without removing the animal from its primary enclosure. In addition, evaluation for obvious signs of infectious disease and behavioral characteristics should occur prior to handling. This information will alert the handler of any special precautions that may need to be taken to minimize contamination, limit disease transmission, ensure safe handling, and minimize stress.

An objective evaluation includes the systematic evaluation of body parts and organ systems to identify abnormalities and should begin with an assessment of the animal's signalment (e.g. age, sex and neuter status, breed or breed-type). The body weight should be recorded along with a body condition score

Table 4.1 Clinical case history questions for private and shelter practice.

Category	Private Practice Questions	Shelter Practice Questions
Environment	What percentage of the time does the animal spend inside versus outside? Is there exposure to fields, woods, bodies of water?	Is the pet known to live indoors or outdoors? If outdoors, is there access to shelter that can provide protection from the elements?
Diet	What kind of food is fed? How often? How much? Any changes in appetite?	Is there evidence the animal has regular access to clean, species-appropriate food? Is there evidence of regular access to a clean water source?
Medical history	What previous medical conditions have been diagnosed, treated, or managed?	Is there evidence of chronic illness or ongoing medical treatment?
Behavioral history	What previous behavioral conditions have been diagnosed, treated, or managed?	Is there a history or evidence of fear, anxiety, or aggression?
Reproductive history	Is the animal neutered or intact? Is there a history of breeding, lactation, and/or successful parturition?	Is there evidence the animal has been neutered (e.g., tattoo, ear tip)? Is there evidence of breeding, lactation, and/or successful parturition?
Vaccination status	Which vaccinations has the animal received? When were vaccinations administered?	Is there history or evidence (i.e., vaccination tag) of prior vaccination?
Current medications	What medications, nutraceuticals, or supplements are given?	Is there a history or evidence of medication administration?
Current condition	What is the presenting complaint?	Are there any injuries or illnesses noted on or prior to presentation?

and an indication of the scoring system being used (i.e. nine-point or five-point scale).

Generally, one of two methods of conducting the hands-on portion of the physical examination is employed: the practitioner can utilize a systems-based approach (i.e. gastrointestinal (GI) system, cardiovascular system, etc.) or a directional approach (i.e. start at the nose and work one's way to the tail). The examiner should develop a method that is comfortable to them and that they can perform consistently so as not to inadvertently omit a particular body part or system. Assessment of hydration status and recording of heart rate, respiratory rate, and body temperature may also be conducted during this phase of examination and should take into account species, breed, age, and environmental considerations. For example, the normal heart rate in puppies and kittens can be considerably higher than that of adults; that of cats is typically higher than that of dogs. Similarly, excitement, stress, and high ambient temperatures can cause temporary increases in body temperature. Finally, if the animal has an obvious wound, injury or disease, or the animal is presented for evaluation of a particular condition, additional examination of those items should be conducted (e.g. wound assessment, orthopedic examination, neurologic examination, etc.). If the physical examination is not conducted by a veterinarian, the findings thus far can be utilized to

Table 4.2 Physical examination approach, normal findings and common abnormalities.

Examination Phase	Normal Findings	Common Abnormalities
Subjective		
Mental state	Alert and responsive Friendly, approachable	Depressed, obtunded, comatose Withdrawn, stereotypic behavior, aggression, hiding, feigning sleep (cats)
Food and water consumption	Empty food and water bowls Evidence of urination and defecation seen or reported	Consistently full food and water bowls, no interest in treats Urination or defecation not seen or reported
Pain/discomfort	Non-painful	Vocalization, aggression, limping/difficulty walking, intense scratching, shaking of the head, difficulty breathing, panting, licking or guarding
Objective		
Injuries/wounds/ existing conditions	None	Puncture wounds, lacerations, abrasions, swollen limbs, broken legs
Signs of infectious disease	None	Coughing, sneezing, ocular discharge, nasal discharge, vomiting, diarrhea, hair loss
Body condition score (9-point scale)	4–5	1–3 (too thin), 6–9 (too heavy)
Hydration	Well-hydrated	<5% History or evidence of vomiting or diarrhea 5–7% Dry or tacky mucous membranes, delayed capillary refill 8–10% Skin tenting >10% Mental depression, sunken eyes, weak or rapid pulse
Temperature[a]	99–102 °F (Canine) 99–101.5 °F (Feline)	<98 °F Canine, Feline >103 °F Canine, >102 °F Feline
Heart rate[a]	70–120 bpm (Canine) 120–140 bpm (Feline)	<70, >120 bpm (Canine) <120, >140 bpm (Feline)
Respiratory rate[a]	18–34 bpm (Canine) 16–40 bpm (Feline)	<12, >40 bpm (Canine, Feline)
Organ systems	No abnormalities found	Examples included but not limited to: • Ocular, nasal, aural discharge; • Heart murmur or arrhythmia; • Coughing, sneezing, difficulty breathing; • Painful abdomen, vomiting, diarrhea; • Hair loss, flaking, crusting, redness of skin

[a] Normal heart rate (beats per minute or bpm) and respiratory rate (breaths per minute or bpm) will vary considerably based on age, species, and breed and may exceed the parameters listed. In general, puppies and kittens have higher rates than adult animals and large breed dogs will have lower rates than smaller breeds. Environmental influences such as stress and ambient temperature can also temporarily impact heart rate, respiratory rate and body temperature.

identify animals in need of veterinary evaluation and treatment. Initial physical examination in the shelter setting typically focuses on the identification of conditions requiring urgent care (e.g. wounds, injuries) and those with signs of infectious disease that could pose a risk to other animals in the population (e.g. respiratory, GI, dermatologic disease).

It is important that shelters have detailed standard operating procedures (SOPs) to outline what steps should be taken to ensure appropriate care and further assessment if there is evidence of an infectious disease or condition requiring further veterinary care.

4.3.1.3 Response to Treatment

A final core diagnostic tool with which the shelter practitioner should be proficient is the appropriate use of response to treatment to make a presumptive diagnosis. Response to treatment refers to the empirical prescribing of medications or courses of treatment without confirmation of a diagnosis. Rather, a presumptive diagnosis and treatment are based on historical information and physical examination findings, and the diagnosis is presumed to be correct based on the resolution of the clinical problem. Careful utilization of this technique can provide benefits of immediately addressing existing conditions, minimizing opportunities for infectious disease transmission, and, when the presumptive diagnosis is correct, reducing the time and costs associated with obtaining a definitive diagnosis before initiating treatment. However, there are significant downsides to relying on this technique on a routine basis. When used indiscriminately, reliance on response to treatment can result in misdiagnosis; misuse of pharmaceuticals; prolonged time to diagnosis, treatment, and disease resolution; and an overall ineffective use of resources. Utilizing response to treatment as a basic diagnostic tool may be considered in the following circumstances:

- An urgent threat to animal health or welfare
- Severe medical resource limitations
- Diagnostic testing options are limited in accuracy, availability, or practical turnaround time
- Inability to obtain veterinary care (e.g. after-hours or irregular access to veterinary support)
- Treatment is likely to provide substantial benefit but unlikely to cause harm.

In each case, a response to treatment protocol should be developed under the direction of a veterinarian familiar with the shelter population, community resources, and limitations. Model protocols include the following components:

- Re-evaluation of patient status after starting treatment and regularly thereafter
- The appropriate use of first-line antimicrobials (e.g. amoxicillin vs. amoxicillin and clavulanic acid) (See Chapter 7 for more information.)
- Defined end-points after which definitive diagnostics or a revised treatment plan will be pursued
- Periodic review of SOPs including evaluation of antimicrobial choices based on definitively diagnosed conditions.

Common shelter scenarios in which response to treatment may be beneficial include mild upper respiratory infections (URIs), mild enteritis, first-time urinary tract infections (UTIs), minor wounds, and superficial pyoderma.

4.3.2 Primary Diagnostic Testing

4.3.2.1 ELISA

The ELISA is perhaps the most readily available and widely utilized diagnostic test in veterinary medicine. In general, ELISAs provide immediate results, are easy to use, cost-effective, able to be conducted outside of a laboratory setting, highly accurate, and adaptable for the detection of a wide variety of analytes. In the shelter setting, ELISAs are commonly utilized for the detection of both antigen and antibodies to common pathogens (e.g. *Dirofilaria immitis, Giardia* spp., and feline leukemia virus [FeLV] antigen; *Ehrlichia* spp., *Anaplasma* spp., *Borrelia burgdorferi, Leptospirosis* spp., and feline immunodeficiency virus [FIV] antibody), assessment of antibody titers against common pathogens (e.g. canine distemper virus, canine parvovirus, canine adenovirus-2, feline panleukopenia, feline herpesvirus-1, feline calicivirus), and the detection of hormone levels for example, relaxin and luteinizing hormone (see Table 4.3). Test kits for the detection of metabolic biomarkers are also available. Anticoagulated whole blood, serum, or plasma can typically be utilized in point-of-care ELISA test kits depending on manufacturer instructions. Particularly

Table 4.3 Common diagnostic tests, indications, and collection and handling techniques for in-house laboratories (Belford and Lumsden 1998; Bowman 2014; Rosenfeld and Dial 2010a, b; Zajac and Conboy 2012).

Diagnostic Test	Indications	Collection and Handling Techniques
Cytology		
Fine needle aspirate	Evaluate mass lesions in the skin, subcutaneous tissue, thorax, and abdomen	1) (A) Insert a 21–25 g needle attached to a ≥5 ml syringe into the lesion; apply 3–5 ml of vacuum; move the needle forward and back while altering direction; release the vacuum and withdraw needle; (B) Insert a 21–25 g needle directly into the lesion; move the needle forward and back while altering direction; withdraw the needle. 2) Remove needle (A) and aspirate 3–5 ml of air into the syringe; (A, B) attach the needle to the syringe and depress the plunger to deposit a drop of aspirated material onto the slide.
Impression smears, imprints, or swabs	Superficial lesions, otic cytology, surgical biopsy specimens	1) Ensure the sample site is clean and dry. 2) Gently press clean glass slide on or rub cotton swab across the surface of the tissue. 3) Roll cotton swab across a clean microscope slide.
Scrapings	Diagnosis of external parasites (e.g., *Demodex* spp.), pyoderma, cutaneous lesions, surgical biopsy specimens	• Hold a sterile scalpel blade at a 90° angle to the surface of the tissue; scrape vigorously across the surface • The edge of a glass slide can also be utilized to obtain superficial surface samples • For diagnosis of demodicosis, utilize a scalpel blade and scrape until capillary bleeding occurs • For cutaneous lesions and surgical biopsy specimens, ensure the tissue is clean and dry prior to scraping
Immunoenzyme assays		
ELISA	Antigen or antibody detection: infection or exposure (e.g., *Anaplasma* spp., *Borrelia burgdorferi*, canine parvovirus, *Dirofilaria immitis*, *Ehrlichia* spp., feline panleukopenia, feline leukemia, *Giardia*), antibody titer assessment (canine parvovirus, canine distemper, feline panleukopenia) Hormonal assays: luteinizing hormone, relaxin	• Vary by assay; see individual techniques below and refer to test manufacturer guidelines

(Continued)

Table 4.3 (Continued)

Diagnostic Test	Indications	Collection and Handling Techniques
Multi-well test kits (e.g. ASSURE®/FeLV, DiroCHEK®, TiterCHEK® CDV/CPV [Zoetis, Parsippany-Troy Hills, NJ])		• Anticoagulated whole blood, serum or plasma samples[a] • Samples can be fresh, refrigerated for up to 7 days, or frozen and thawed[a] • Store test kits under refrigeration until the expiration date • Allow samples and test kits to reach room temperature before testing
Single-well test devices (e.g. SNAP tests [IDEXX Laboratories, Westbrook, ME])		• Anticoagulated whole blood, serum, plasma, or fecal samples[a] • Samples can be fresh, refrigerated up to 1 week, or frozen and thawed[a] • Allow samples and test kits to reach room temperature before testing • Store test kits under refrigeration until expiration date OR at room temperature for 90 days (or until expired) • Test kits removed from refrigeration for more than 24 hours should be used within 90 days or until expired
Lateral flow assays (e.g., Solo Step® tests [Heska Corporation, Loveland, CO], VetScan® [Abaxis, Union City, CA], WITNESS® tests [Zoetis, Parsippany-Troy Hills, NJ])		• Anticoagulated whole blood, serum, plasma, or fecal samples[a] • Samples can be fresh, refrigerated for 3–7 days (up to two weeks for feces), or frozen and thawed[a] • Run within 10 minutes of opening test pouch[a] • Store test kits at room temperature until the expiration date
Fecal Examination		
Direct fecal smear	Nematode larvae, protozoan trophozoites, heavy eggs, motile organisms	• Refrigerate if not examined within 1–2 hours of collection • Examine within 30 minutes if evaluating for protozoan trophozoites • Break up a small piece of feces in a drop of saline on a glass slide; use a coverslip • Feces remaining on rectal thermometer after use is sufficient • Use of water instead of saline can result in lysis of fragile organisms • Dried fecal smears may be stained though motility will be lost

Fecal flotation	Nematode eggs, cestode eggs, protozoan cysts	• Approximately 1 teaspoon (4 grams) of fresh feces should be analyzed • Centrifugation methods will recover more eggs, species with fewer eggs, and dense eggs; eggs will float in less time but additional steps are required • Gravitational methods are suitable for screening • Sodium nitrate solution will float eggs in 10 minutes; immediate evaluation is necessary to reduce distortion • Saturated sucrose solution will float eggs in 15–20 minutes
Hematology		
Complete blood count	Minimum metabolic database	• Use largest bore needle available to minimize hemolysis • Collect directly in anticoagulant (e.g. EDTA) and promptly mix • Ensure proper anticoagulant to sample ratio to minimize dilution of cell counts
Chemistry	Minimum metabolic database	• Use largest bore needle available to minimize hemolysis • Collect without anticoagulant; allow to clot for 15–20 minutes (serum) • For small volume samples (e.g. puppies, kittens, exotics), collect with lithium heparin and centrifuge immediately (plasma)
Blood glucose	Hypo or hyperglycemia	• Process whole blood sample within 30 minutes or separate serum and refrigerate until analysis • Stress, meals, anemia, sample handling and instrument variation can all lead to erroneous results • Portable monitors are likely to slightly underestimate the concentration
Urinalysis		
Specific gravity	Minimum metabolic database, dehydration, evidence of urinary tract disease	• Use refractometer, reagent strip stick readings inaccurate

(*Continued*)

Table 4.3 (Continued)

Diagnostic Test	Indications	Collection and Handling Techniques
Reagent strips	Minimum metabolic database, dehydration, evidence of urinary tract disease	• Note collection method; cystocentesis and catheterization preferred; midstream voided sample acceptable • Use refractometer to measure specific gravity, strip readings inaccurate • Drop urine onto each pad, do not dip the strip in the sample • Analyze immediately or refrigerate for up to 6 hours • Allow refrigerated samples to reach room temperature prior to analysis • Leukocyte, nitrite, and specific gravity readings unreliable • Protect strips from air, light and moisture; mind expiration dates
Sediment analysis	Minimum metabolic database, dehydration, evidence of urinary tract disease	• Note collection method; cystocentesis and catheterization preferred; midstream voided sample acceptable • Collect 2–6 ml of urine • Allow refrigerated samples to reach room temperature prior to analysis • Analyze within 4 hours or store under refrigeration up to 24 hours • Centrifuge sample for 5 minutes at 1,500 RPM, decant supernatant, resuspend sediment prior to analysis • Examine stained and unstained sediment • Examine at 10x for crystals, casts, and epithelial cells • Examine at 40x for microorganisms, red blood cells, white blood cells
Culture	Evidence of urinary tract disease	• Note collection method; cystocentesis and catheterization preferred; midstream voided sample acceptable • Use a sterile collection method and storage container • Aerobic culture is indicated in most circumstances • Store under refrigeration and transport to the diagnostic laboratory within 12 hours

[a] Vary widely based on specific tests and kit manufacturer, follow manufacturer's product insert guidelines.

as pertains to feline retrovirus (FeLV and FIV) testing, samples of saliva or tears have also been used in such test kits and while historically have resulted in an unacceptably low sensitivity, newer devices may be more accurate (Westman et al. 2016, 2017).

As the name implies, ELISAs are testing methods that rely on the detection of an enzyme-linked protein within a variety of test samples to indicate either a qualitative or semi-quantitative result. ELISAs can be direct or indirect, though the former are not routinely used outside of diagnostic laboratories. The basic operational principles of indirect ELISAs for antibody detection are as follows:

1) Test substrates are pre-coated with the antigen by the manufacturer.
2) A biological sample containing the antibody to be detected is exposed to the substrate.
3) Antibody in the sample binds to the pre-coated antigen creating an antigen–antibody complex. Unbound antibody is washed away.
4) An enzyme-labeled antibody (i.e. conjugate) binds to the antigen–antibody complex. Unbound labeled antibody is washed away.
5) An enzyme-substrate reacts with the enzyme-labeled antigen–antibody complex, resulting in a color change indicating the test result.

In such tests, the intensity of color change is proportional to the amount of antibody present in the sample. Detection of antigen can be accomplished similarly, however, the well is pre-coated with antibody allowing for binding and identification of antigen in the test sample.

A sandwich ELISA is a variation on the indirect ELISA commonly used to detect specific antigens. Many of the commercially-available point-of-care test kits utilize this methodology in the form of manually activated bi-directional flow devices (SNAP® tests [IDEXX Laboratories, Westbrook, ME]) or lateral flow devices (also known as rapid immunochromatography). The former devices are largely automated and self-contained; the benefits of which include minimization of background coloration, reduced washing time, and an increased opportunity for binding of the test sample to indicators (O'Connor 2015). Lateral flow assays generally offer more rapid analysis with fewer steps, lower operational costs, and greater environmental stability, however, they may be subject to decreased sensitivity and greater difficulty with interpretation of results, particularly in hemolyzed samples (O'Connor 2015; Sajid et al. 2015). Additional variations on the indirect ELISA include the labeled antigen ELISA and the competitive ELISA, see Table 4.4.

4.3.2.2 Diagnostic Cytology

Examination and interpretation of cellular samples is a rapid, inexpensive, and minimally-invasive tool that shelter practitioners can use to help establish a definitive diagnosis, establish a morphological diagnosis (e.g. mixed septic inflammation), or rule out differential diagnoses (Belford and Lumsden 1998). Cytologic samples can be obtained through a variety of techniques depending on the location or type of lesion and the preliminary or differential diagnosis, most commonly including fine needle aspiration (FNA); impression smears, imprints, or swabs; and skin scrapings. Diagnostic cytology can also be used as a component of the evaluation of fecal samples or bodily fluids such as urine, blood, effusions and secretions (Table 4.3). Once a sample is obtained, it is prepared for evaluation under a microscope. In general, for fine needle aspirates, impression smears, imprints, and swabs, identification and description of cellular characteristics or microbial agents are needed, and samples should be stained prior to evaluation. Identification of external parasites, such as *Demodex* spp., is usually performed on unstained preparations while evaluation of bodily fluids is often performed on both stained and unstained preparations. Romanowsky stains, such as modified Wright-Giemsa and Diff-Quik® (Siemens Healthcare Diagnostics Ltd., Deerfield, IL), can be utilized

Table 4.4 ELISA technique variations (Tizard 2013).

Technique	Methodology	Detects	Examples
Indirect	Pre-coated Ag + Test sample Ab + Enzyme-linked Ab + Enzyme substrate	Ab in sample	TiterCHEK CDV/CPV (Zoetis, Parsippany-Troy Hills, NJ) Canine VacciCheck® (Biogal Galed Labs, Kibbutz Galed, Israel) Feline VacciCheck (Biogal Galed Labs, Kibbutz Galed, Israel)
Sandwich	Pre-coated Ab + Test sample Ag + Detection Ab + Enzyme-linked Ab + Enzyme substrate	Bound Ag	DiroCHEK (Zoetis, Parsippany-Troy Hills, NJ) SNAP tests (IDEXX Laboratories, Westbrook, ME) Solo Step tests[a] (Heska Corporation, Loveland, CO) VetScan[a] (Abaxis, Union City, CA) WITNESS HEARTWORM[a] (Zoetis, Parsippany-Troy Hills, NJ)
Labeled antigen	Pre-coated Ag + Test sample Ab + Enzyme-linked Ag + Enzyme substrate	Bound Ab	Not commonly used outside diagnostic laboratories in companion animals
Competitive	Pre-coated Ab + Test sample Ag with Enzyme-linked Ag + Enzyme substrate	Bound Ag/Inverse of Ag in sample	Not commonly used outside diagnostic laboratories in companion animals

Ag, antigen; Ab, antibody.
[a] lateral flow assays.

for most cytologic preparations. Such stains contain both an acid and basic dye that bind to basic and acidic cellular structures respectively, allowing for visualization and recognition under the microscope (Rosenfeld and Dial 2010a). New methylene blue stain may be useful for preparations with heavy blood contamination, visualization of fungal agents, and analysis of urine sediment.

Though detailed descriptions and definitive diagnoses may require the expertise of a cytopathologist, shelter practitioners should be able to classify cytologic preparations in order to obtain a preliminary diagnosis and establish the next steps in a diagnostic or treatment plan. Three general categories of lesions with distinct cellular characteristics have been described:

- Inflammatory: the presence of white blood cells greater than that expected from blood contamination
- Non-inflammatory: non-neoplastic lesion; cyst, sialocele, seroma, hematoma
- Neoplasia: homogenous cell population, characterized as benign or malignant.

Table 4.5 Inflammatory lesions and infectious differential diagnoses (Rakich and Latimer 2011; Rosenfeld and Dial 2010a).

Type	Cell Population	Infectious Differential Diagnoses
Purulent	Neutrophils (>85%)	Bacterial infection, typically Gram +
Pyogranulomatous	Neutrophils (>50%) Macrophages (<50%)	Fungal infections Foreign bodies Mycobacteria Protozoa
Granulomatous	Macrophages (>85%)	Fungal infections Foreign bodies Mycobacteria Protozoa
Eosinophilic	Eosinophils (>50%)	Parasites *Pythium* spp.
Lymphocytic	Lymphocytes (>85%)	Chronic bacterial infections Acute viral infections Protozoa

Most lesions of an infectious nature will be classified as inflammatory and can be further described as purulent, pyogranulomatous, granulomatous, eosinophilic, or lymphocytic depending on the predominant inflammatory cell type present. Such descriptions can narrow the list of potential causative agents (Table 4.5). Identification of an inflammatory cytologic lesion, particularly those with signs of degeneration, should prompt careful observation for microbial agents. Among those agents typically identified through direct microscopy are: bacteria, mycobacteria, superficial yeasts (*Malassezia* spp., *Candida* spp.), fungal organisms (*Blastomyces, Cryptococcus, Histoplasma, Coccidioides, Sporothrix*), fungal hyphae (*Zygomycetes*), parasitic oomycetes (*Pythium* spp.), protozoa (coccidia, *Trichomonas* spp., *Leishmania* spp.), and algae (*Prototheca* spp.) (Rakich and Latimer 2011).

4.3.2.3 Fecal Examination

A fecal examination is a primary tool for the diagnosis of endoparasitism in companion animals and typically consists of both direct fecal smears and flotation concentration techniques. (Note that fecal antigen detection for select pathogens is also commercially available as discussed in the section on ELISA testing found under primary diagnostic testing.) The direct fecal smear—microscopic evaluation of a small particle of feces mixed with saline—is ideal for the evaluation of delicate nematode larvae (e.g. *Aelurostrongylus* spp., *Ancylostoma* spp., *Filaroides* spp., *Strongyloides* spp.) and protozoan trophozoites (e.g. *Giardia* spp., *Tritrichomonas* spp.) (Bowman 2014) (Table 4.3). Direct smears also allow for the evaluation of organism motility and identification of organisms that are easily distorted by flotation solutions. Due to the small sample size evaluated, direct fecal smears have low sensitivity. That is, while a positive fecal smear can confirm endoparasitism, a negative fecal smear does not rule out infection. Fecal smears can also be stained for more detailed examination and parasite identification, though motility will be lost with such preparation (Zajac and Conboy 2012).

In most cases, direct fecal smears should be performed in tandem with fecal flotation techniques. Such techniques allow for the separation of fecal and food material, fats and dissolved pigments, and parasite eggs and cysts based on the density of the suspension liquid. Flotation techniques that involve centrifugation of the sample will result in higher sensitivity than those that rely on passive gravitational suspension of eggs. This is most important when low numbers of parasites are expected (e.g. *Giardia* spp., *Trichuris* spp.). If a passive flotation method is pursued, sodium nitrate (e.g. Fecasol®, Vetoquinol, Fort Worth, TX) or saturated salt solutions should be used. Though they are ideal for centrifugation techniques, the high viscosity of sugar solutions and the lower specific gravity of zinc sulfate solutions can impede the passive flotation process (Zajac and Conboy 2012). In the absence of centrifugation or proper flotation solutions, the likelihood of inaccurate test results warrants consideration of additional diagnostic testing or empirical treatment of patients exhibiting clinical signs consistent with parasitic infection.

Once the sample is prepared and the surface layer transferred to a coverslip, the sample should be scanned under the 10× objective lens of a microscope. To maximize the contrast between parasites and background debris, the microscope condenser should be lowered and the light intensity and diaphragm should be reduced. Samples prepared in sodium nitrate solution should be evaluated immediately to avoid distortion of any parasites and crystallization of the preparation (Bowman 2014; Zajac and Conboy 2012).

4.3.2.4 Urinalysis

Urinalysis is useful for the evaluation of renal function, assessment of urinary tract diseases, and the analysis of systemic disease processes that impact the urinary system. There are four main diagnostic tests utilized to evaluate the urinary system: urine specific gravity, urine chemical analysis (i.e. use of reagent strips or "dipstick"), urine sediment analysis, and urine culture (Table 4.3). Urine sediment analysis and urine culture are of the most utility regarding the diagnosis of infectious diseases, though direct testing may be warranted under certain circumstances (e.g. canine distemper virus, leptospirosis).

Analysis of urine sediment can aid in the diagnosis of bacterial, fungal, algal, and parasitic diseases of the urinary tract. The sample should be obtained through cystocentesis or catheterization in order to confirm that any pathogens identified originate in the kidneys or bladder. If that is not feasible, a midstream voided urine sample can be utilized to minimize contamination from the urethra and external environment. After obtaining the specific gravity and urine chemical analysis, the sediment can be prepared for microscopic evaluation through low-speed centrifugation (1,500–2,000 RPM for 5 minutes), decanting of the supernatant, resuspension, and preparation on a glass slide. Both unstained and stained drops of urine should be evaluated for cells, casts, crystals, and infectious organisms. Fat droplets, spermatozoa, mucous, and other contaminants may also be identified. Preparations can be stained with a Romanowsky stain after drying for detailed identification of cellular elements and examination under oil immersion; however, crystals will be dissolved by the fixative component. Supravital stain (e.g. Sedi-Stain) or new methylene blue can be applied to a wet-mounted sample if preservation of crystals is desired; however, cellular detail is lost, examination under oil immersion is not possible, and accumulation of bacteria and stain precipitate resulting in sediment artifacts are common (Anthony 2014). The presence of more than five white blood cells per high-power field indicates urogenital tract inflammation and the sample should be carefully evaluated for the presence of bacteria (Tripathi et al. 2011). Bacteria in the absence of white blood cells could indicate contamination of the sample during collection or processing. Both rod and coccoid bacteria can be found, with progressively motile rods being the most common. Yeast are the most common fungal organisms identified and are usually contaminates from the lower urinary tract (Rosenfeld and Dial 2010c).

A large number of bacterial organisms in the presence of red and/or white blood cells along with clinical signs of urinary tract disease are an indication for bacterial culture with antimicrobial sensitivity. Alternatively, a rapid immunoassay has been evaluated for point-of-care diagnosis of urinary tract infections (UTIs) in dogs and found to be highly accurate (Jacob et al. 2016). The most common organisms identified in bacterial cultures of dogs and cats include *Escherichia coli, Klebsiella* spp., *Staphylococcus* spp., *Enterococcus* spp., *Proteus* spp., and *Pseudomonas* spp. with *E. coli* accounting for up to 55% of isolates (Thompson et al. 2011). The International Society for Companion Animal Infectious Diseases recommends the use of amoxicillin or trimethoprim-sulfonamide for first-line antimicrobial treatment of uncomplicated UTIs and only when such infections are deemed to be clinically significant, as defined by the presence of clinical signs such as dysuria and pollakiuria, along with the identification of bacteria in the urine (Weese et al. 2011). Antimicrobial resistance to fluoroquinolones, third-generation cephalosporins, and clavulanic acid-potentiated β-lactams are increasingly reported, so their use should be limited to those cases in which resistance to first-line antimicrobials has been documented (Thompson et al. 2011; Weese et al. 2011). Animals that have been empirically treated for a UTI that has not resolved should have a urine culture performed at a diagnostic laboratory.

4.3.3 Secondary Diagnostic Testing

4.3.3.1 Complete Blood Count and Blood Chemistry Analysis

Along with a urinalysis, a complete blood count and blood chemistry analysis are typically considered part of the minimum metabolic database allowing the practitioner to gain an overall assessment of a patient's ability to oxygenate the body, respond to infection or inflammation, and perform the most basic organ functions (Table 4.3). Complete blood counts should include both a quantitative analysis (i.e. a count of the number of cells of a particular type) as well as a qualitative analysis (i.e. microscopic evaluation of cellular morphology in a blood smear). Quantitative analysis is typically performed by automated hematology analyzers, though manual counts can be obtained through the use of a hemocytometer. If neither automated nor manual counts are feasible, assessment of packed cell volume (PCV) is a readily available means of assessing the degree of anemia and the oxygen-carrying capacity of the blood and can be combined with a simple blood smear for a more thorough assessment. The PCV represents the percent of the patient's total blood volume comprised of red blood cells and is directly measured after centrifugation of a sample. Though a measure of the same parameter, a patient's hematocrit (Hct) is calculated based on the red blood cell count and cell volume. Agglutination of red blood cells or inclusion of platelets in the count will, therefore, impact the Hct but not the PCV. Normal PCV values are 37–55% for dogs and 26–45% cats. An additional benefit of obtaining a PCV is the ability to subjectively assess plasma and measure protein concentrations (see below). Qualitative analysis of red and white blood cells can be assessed by microscopic examination of the long or "feathered" edge of a blood smear. Examination after air-drying and staining with a Romanowsky stain can enhance the diagnostic value. Cells should ultimately be examined under the 100× objective with oil immersion and should be assessed for color, size, shape, inclusions in red blood cells (e.g. Howell-Jolly bodies, Heinz bodies, basophilic stippling) and signs of toxicity in white blood cells (e.g. basophilia, vacuolation, Döhle bodies). A variety of infectious agents may also be identified in both red blood cells (e.g. *Mycoplasma* spp., *Babesia* spp., and *Cytauxzoon*) and white blood cells (e.g. intracellular bacteria, *Ehrlichia* spp., *Anaplasma* spp., *Hepatozoon* spp.). Viral inclusion bodies of canine distemper virus can also occasionally be seen within red blood cells and within the cytoplasm of white blood cells (Rosenfeld and Dial 2010d; Webb and Latimer 2011). Finally, particularly when subjected to centrifugation methods, microfilaria of *D. immitis* may also be identified on blood smear analysis.

Blood chemistry analysis may include a variety of parameters to assess the function of major organ systems (e.g. renal, hepatic), total proteins, electrolytes, and metabolism of carbohydrates and lipids. These assessments are most thoroughly and accurately performed through the use of calibrated, automated biochemical analyzers either in-house or at a diagnostic laboratory. If complete biochemical profiling is not available, crude assessments of total proteins, blood urea nitrogen (BUN), and blood glucose can be conducted in almost any setting.

As mentioned above, after obtaining a PCV, an analysis of the remaining plasma can easily be undertaken. Plasma color and transparency should first be visually assessed. For both dogs and cats, plasma is normally clear and colorless; yellow plasma indicates icterus, pink or red indicates hemoglobinemia, and white to pink opaque plasma indicates lipemia. Finally, the plasma sample can be used to assess plasma protein concentration with a refractometer. Normal protein concentrations range from 5.5–7.5 g/dl in dogs and 6.5–8.5 g/dl in cats. Refractometric protein readings can be falsely elevated in samples that are lipemic, hemolyzed, or when there are high concentrations of glucose, urea, sodium, or chloride in the sample (Evans 2011). Complimentary analysis of the PCV and plasma protein can provide useful information to narrow the list of differential diagnoses:

- Low PCV, Normal protein: anemia
- Low PCV, Low protein: chronic blood loss
- High PCV, Normal protein: increased red blood cell production, hemorrhagic gastroenteritis, endocrinopathy
- Normal PCV, Decreased protein: protein-losing disease, acute blood loss, liver failure
- Normal PCV, High protein: dehydration, increased immune response.

Urea is a waste product of dietary protein digestion formed in the hepatocytes and excreted through the kidneys. As such, assessment of the BUN concentration can be a useful indicator of decreased glomerular filtration and, when interpreted in light of the animal's hydration status and urine specific gravity, a crude screening test of renal function. Outside of a concentration reported from a biochemical analyzer, BUN levels are commonly assessed through the application of a whole blood sample on semi-quantitative colorimetric reagent test strips. Such strips have been correlated with serum urea concentrations as measured with an automated analyzer in both dogs and cats. Dogs with BUN concentration estimates >15 mg/dl and cats with estimates >50 mg/dl were accurately categorized as azotemic in 98% of samples evaluated (Berent et al. 2005).

A final point-of-care quick assessment test is the measurement of blood glucose concentration. Glucose is the primary cellular energy source and is obtained from dietary carbohydrates, the breakdown of glycogen in the liver (glycogenolysis) and the synthesis of glucose from amino acids and fats (gluconeogenesis). Alterations in blood glucose concentration can indicate dysfunction in a wide variety of organ systems including the renal, hepatic, and endocrine systems. In addition, sepsis and congenital metabolic diseases are important causes of hypoglycemia while analysis immediately or shortly after a meal or a stressful event (particularly in cats) are noteworthy explanations for hyperglycemia (Duncan 1998). Normal fasting blood glucose concentrations range from 60 to 125 mg/dl in dogs and 70 to 150 mg/dl in cats.

Care must be taken when obtaining a blood sample for the measurement of glucose concentration. Acute stress, such as that due to aggressive handling or restraint, and a recent (<12 hours) meal are likely to result in falsely elevated measurements. Additionally, blood glucose concentration decreases ~10% per hour at room temperature, so samples should be processed within 30 minutes or the serum should be separated and refrigerated until testing (Evans 2011).

Glucose concentrations in whole blood can be measured by using colorimetric reagent strips or portable blood glucose meters. Reagent strips are not reliable for the detection of hypoglycemia, and the presence of anemia may result in falsely elevated concentrations. Excessive washing and incomplete coverage of the reagent pad can also result in erroneous results. Elevated blood glucose concentrations above the renal threshold can also be detected in urine samples through the use of urine chemical reagent test strips (Evans 2011). Portable blood glucose meters can provide measurements that are comparable to those obtained with reagent strips and biochemical analyzers; however, there is substantial variation between models (Cohen et al. 2009, 2000). In general, such meters tend to underestimate blood glucose concentrations and have greater divergence from reference measurements when samples are hyperglycemic. Meters that are designed and calibrated specifically for use in companion animals are preferred and thought to be less likely to report falsely decreased blood glucose concentrations (Kang et al. 2016). As with reagent strips, anemia can result in an overestimation of the blood glucose concentration. Despite these pitfalls, imprecise results from portable blood glucose meters are not likely to lead to alterations in clinical decision-making (Cohn et al. 2000; Wess and Reusch 2000a, b).

4.3.3.2 Additional Secondary Tests

Several additional diagnostic tests can be conducted in-house depending on both facility and veterinary resources. Common examples of such tests include diagnostic imaging and necropsy. Many shelters have the capability to perform diagnostic imaging in the form of radiographs (X-rays) and/or ultrasounds. Such tools can be rapid and useful methods of establishing diagnoses and identifying emergent conditions. In order to ensure that images are of diagnostic quality and, in the case of radiographs, that staff and patient exposure to radiation are minimized, these tools should only be used by appropriately trained personnel; in some jurisdictions, specific licensing requirements may restrict which staff members can take radiographs. Diagnostic images require interpretation by a veterinarian.

Finally, in the event of an unexplained patient death, a gross necropsy should be conducted. Frequently overlooked as a diagnostic tool, a necropsy can help establish a diagnosis and alert the practitioner to any conditions that may impact both the human and the remaining animal population within the shelter. The collection of tissue samples for histopathologic examination and ancillary diagnostic testing (bacteriology, virology, cytology) should also be considered based on gross necropsy findings. Samples can always be collected and held for submission pending initial results, but failure to collect appropriate samples at the time of necropsy may preclude obtaining a definitive diagnosis and significantly limit the information that can be obtained from the necropsy. See Chapter 5 for more information on this topic.

4.3.4 Diagnostic Laboratory Tests

4.3.4.1 Serology

Serology is the measurement of antigen–antibody interactions for diagnostic purposes and is commonly used for the diagnosis of infectious disease as well as risk management during a disease outbreak. In some cases, serology is used to determine whether an animal has been previously exposed to an infectious agent, vaccinated, or actively infected. Primary binding tests are those that directly measure the binding of antigen to antibody, usually in a qualitative form (i.e. positive or negative). Examples of these include ELISAs and lateral flow assays, immunofluorescent antibody (IFA) tests, Western blotting, and immunohistochemistry. Secondary binding tests measure the results of antigen–antibody interaction *in vitro* and typically provide a quantitative result in the form of a titer; examples include hemagglutination inhibition (HI) and complement fixation (CF).

Tertiary testing methods, such as serum neutralization, measure the protective effect of antibodies in live organisms and also provide results in the form of titers. A final category of serologic tests is the molecular assay that detects nucleic acids. These tests, which can be both qualitative and quantitative, include PCR, reverse transcriptase PCR, and real-time PCR (Tizard 2013).

4.3.4.1.1 Primary Binding Tests *(Note that ELISAs including lateral flow assays are common primary binding tests; these have been discussed earlier in the text.)*

IFA tests can be either direct or indirect. Direct fluorescent antibody tests can detect the presence of specific antigens within a tissue sample. With IFA, antibody labeled with a fluorescent marker is applied to a tissue sample that has been treated with antibody specific to the antigen of interest. The fluorescent marker binds to the antibody, revealing the presence of antigen when examined under a dark-field microscope with an ultraviolet light source. This method is commonly used for the detection of rabies virus in brain tissue and FeLV in white blood cells. Indirect fluorescent antibody tests can be used to detect the presence of either tissue antigen or, more commonly, serum antibody. This technique is similar to direct fluorescent antibody testing, however, the sample to be tested is treated with antibodies against the molecule of interest prior to fluorescent labeling. This allows for amplification of the fluorescent signaling, determination of specific classes of antibody in the sample (i.e. IgG, IgM, IgA, etc.), and a quantitative estimation of the amount of antibody in the sample (Tizard 2013). Indirect fluorescent antibody tests are commonly used for the detection of brucellosis and rickettsial organisms.

Western blotting is a method of antigen or antibody detection primarily used for complex proteins including microorganisms and parasites. With this technique, protein antigens are separated via electrophoresis and immobilized on a nitrocellulose membrane. The antigens are then visualized through the use of an enzyme or radioimmunoassay (Tizard 2013). Western blotting is commonly used for the detection of antibodies against FIV, *Borrelia* spp., *Ehrlichia* spp., *Leishmania*, and *Neorickettsia* spp.

Immunohistochemistry can be utilized to identify specific antigens within histopathological tissue specimens. Prepared tissue sections are treated with an enzyme-labeled antibody that binds to the antigen of interest. When exposed to an enzyme substrate, the labeled complexes produce a distinct brown color which can be identified by the pathologist. Immunohistochemistry has a wide variety of applications but is most commonly used for the diagnosis of viral diseases such as feline infectious peritonitis, canine distemper virus, and canine parvovirus and is frequently performed on postmortem tissue samples.

4.3.4.1.2 Secondary Binding Tests Serum antibody levels are typically quantified and reported as "titers." In practice, test serum is diluted in a series of tubes and a known amount of antigen is added to each dilution. The most diluted sample in which a reaction occurs provides an estimate of the amount of antibody within the serum sample. The reciprocal of this dilution is reported as the titer (e.g. a sample in which the 1:32 dilution of serum was the highest sample dilution to display a reaction, has a titer of 32) (Figure 4.1). There are several caveats to the use and interpretation of antibody titers that should be understood:

- A titer from one laboratory may not be the equivalent of a titer at another laboratory.
- A titer determined by one method may not be the equivalent of a titer determined by another method.

Figure 4.1 Antibody titration.

Serial dilutions of test sample are made.

Undiluted 1/2 1/4 1/8 1/16 1/32

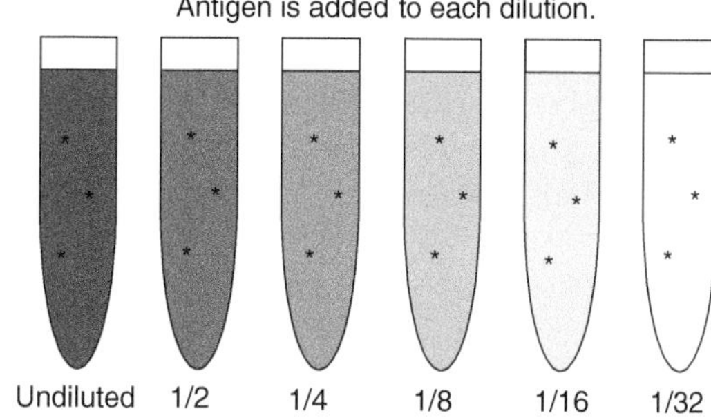

Sample titer equals reciprocal of greatest dilution in which desired reaction is observed.

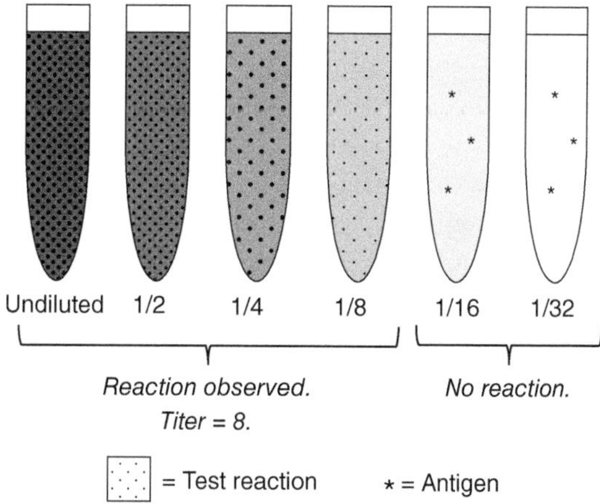

- What constitutes a "protective" titer differs for various pathogens and may vary between laboratories.
- The method in which a titer was determined to be "protective" may vary between laboratories.
- Lack of a "protective" titer may not indicate susceptibility.
- In most cases, a single titer measurement cannot distinguish between previous exposure and current infection.
- Titer detection alone cannot establish the cause of existing disease.
- In puppies and kittens, titers cannot distinguish between maternal antibodies and those derived from vaccination or previous exposure.

In-house ELISA test kits can be used to measure antibody titers against canine distemper, canine adenovirus, canine parvovirus, and feline panleukopenia (see the discussion in the section on primary diagnostic testing) (Gray et al. 2012; Mazar et al. 2009; Mende et al. 2014); however, laboratory testing methods are considered the gold standard. Practitioners should be aware of the particular method utilized when interpreting clinical results, making case management decisions, and comparing literature references.

Agglutination, or clumping, of red blood cells in a serum sample occurs when antibodies cross-link large particles of antigen (i.e. one antibody binds to two antigens). In the presence of excess antibody, the antigenic particles become saturated and further agglutination is inhibited. This reaction is the basis for antibody titration through HI. In these tests, a serial dilution of the test serum is exposed to soluble antigen (e.g. viral particles) cross-linked to red blood cells. Antibodies within the test serum bind to the soluble antigen causing agglutination of the cross-linked red blood cells—hemagglutination—until the antibodies are exhausted and further hemagglutination is inhibited. The reciprocal of the highest serum dilution that completely inhibited hemagglutination represents the HI titer for that sample. In addition to its use for measuring antibodies, HI can also be used to identify specific viruses (Tizard 2013). HI is commonly employed to measure antibodies against adenoviruses, coronaviruses, herpesviruses, influenza, and parainfluenza. HI is considered the gold standard titer testing method for canine and feline parvoviruses (Ford 2013).

CF testing relies on the classical complement pathway resulting in the binding of antibodies to red blood cells and their subsequent rupture and hemolysis. After the disruption of existing antigen–antibody complexes, test serum is mixed with a known amount of a new complement source, allowed to form new antigen–antibody complexes, and an indicator in the form of antibody-linked red blood cells is added. If antibody is present in the sample, the complement is consumed and the red blood cells remain intact. In the absence of antibody, the complement binds to the antibody-linked red blood cells and is lysed. Conducting the reaction within serial dilutions of test serum allows quantification of antibodies. The reciprocal of the highest dilution of serum in which no more than 50% of the red blood cells are lysed represents the CF titer for that sample (Tizard 2013). CF is commonly employed to measure antibodies against adenoviruses, parvoviruses, mycobacterial infections, and coccidioidomycosis.

4.3.4.1.3 Tertiary Tests Serum neutralization testing or, when in reference to viruses, virus neutralization (VN) is used to estimate the ability of antibodies within a test sample to disrupt (i.e. neutralize) the biological activity of an antigen. Such activity can include hemolysis of red blood cells, lysis of nucleated cells, and disease or death in animals. In these tests, serial dilution of the test serum is exposed to a constant amount of antigen (i.e. live virus). Antibodies within the test serum bind to the antigen, blocking critical attachment sites thus preventing them from infecting live cells. The reciprocal of the highest serum dilution that prevents lysis of 50% of cells, infection in 50% of tissue cultures or infection in 50% of live animals represents the VN titer for that sample. In addition to its use for measuring antibodies, VN can also be used to identify specific viruses (Tizard 2013). VN typically has higher sensitivity compared to secondary binding tests such as HI and CF and is commonly employed to measure antibodies against adenoviruses, caliciviruses, herpesviruses, and parvoviruses. VN is considered the gold standard titer testing method for canine distemper virus (Ford 2013).

4.3.4.1.4 Molecular Assays The detection of the nucleic acid of an infectious agent can be accomplished through the use of molecular assays such as PCR, reverse-transcriptase PCR (RT-PCR), and real-time PCR. The ability of such assays to detect minute quantities of nucleic acid makes them among the most sensitive diagnostic testing methods available (Tizard 2013). Another important benefit of molecular assays is their ability to detect organisms in animals that are subclinical carriers or latently infected (Evermann et al. 2012), allowing for quicker identification of animals that may present an infectious disease risk to the population. This benefit may be particularly useful during the response to a disease outbreak when quantitative results are available to distinguish between vaccinates and infectious animals. However, as with antibody titer analysis and other methods of antigen detection discussed above, molecular detection of an organism merely indicates its presence. It does not indicate whether the detected organism is alive or dead or whether it is the cause of active disease. For these reasons, interpretation of results should take into account clinical signs and the possibility of latent stages of infection (e.g. herpesviruses, feline retroviruses). The high sensitivity of these assays makes careful sample collection and handling, as well as submission to a reliable laboratory with high-quality control standards, of the utmost priority as sample contaminants will readily be detected. Molecular methods can be used to detect pathogens in samples of blood and tissue or, increasingly, in culturettes or swabs containing trace amounts of respiratory secretions or feces.

Molecular assays rely on the PCR to detect trace amounts of pathogen DNA. For RNA viruses (e.g. feline calicivirus, canine distemper virus), RT-PCR may be performed. In this assay, reverse transcriptase is used to convert the viral RNA to DNA prior to the PCR process. Real-time PCR allows for the quantification of DNA through the use of fluorescent labeling of the DNA (or a DNA probe), which can be tracked and quantified as the PCR progresses, allowing for the determination of initial DNA quantity, less susceptibility to contamination, and greater sensitivity of detection. Standard PCR techniques analyze DNA bands at the completion of a variable number of amplification cycles and rely on size discrimination for identification, which can result in comparatively lower precision and sensitivity of detection (Applied Biosystems n.d.; Tizard 2013). Real-time PCR can also be completed on RNA viruses through reverse transcriptase real-time PCR.

For the detection of common causes of both respiratory and GI disease, diagnostic laboratories offer real-time PCR analysis of a variety of pathogens common to either dogs or cats. Such services carry the benefit of screening for a variety of pathogens with a single sample (and single fee), fast turnaround time (one to three days), and ready identification of potential co-infections. Pathogen detection may be inhibited in aged samples or those from patients receiving antimicrobial therapy and, in the case of respiratory PCR panels, recent modified live-virus vaccination can interfere with the interpretation of results. Samples for respiratory PCR analysis should include a conjunctival and deep pharyngeal swab collected on a sterile, plastic-stemmed swab and placed in a sterile tube. Samples obtained via trans-tracheal wash or bronchoalveolar lavage may also be accepted and would be most appropriate to collect from animals with suspected lower airway disease. Samples for GI PCR analysis should include fresh feces (minimum 1 gram) placed in a sterile container. Both respiratory and GI samples can be refrigerated for up to 10 days (IDEXX Laboratories 2017).

4.3.4.2 Microbiological Tests

Microbiological culture is a commonly used test that, with the exception of dermatophytosis cultures, generally requires the use of diagnostic laboratory services (see Chapter 20 on Dermatophytosis for more information about the performance and interpretation of ringworm cultures). Almost any bodily fluid, excretion, or tissue can be submitted for culture to determine whether or not infectious organisms are present (most commonly bacterial or fungal agents). In contrast to molecular assays, a culture can identify live pathogens, the species of organism(s) present and, when antimicrobial sensitivity is evaluated, which pharmaceutical treatments are likely to be effective and at what dosages. Repeat cultures can be used to evaluate a patient's response to a treatment course and to determine when an infection has been resolved. Unless sampling from a contaminated area such as a wound or a sample of skin or hair (e.g. ringworm cultures), samples must be collected and handled using aseptic techniques in order to provide meaningful results. Fecal samples submitted for culture should include specific differential diagnoses to direct the microbiologist. Similarly, when fastidious microorganisms not easily cultured on standard media are suspected (e.g. *Mycoplasma* spp., anaerobes, spirochetes, *Mycobacterium* spp.), the laboratory should be consulted for recommendations on sample collection, preparation, storage, and transportation. Additionally, if the animal is receiving antimicrobial therapy at the time of sample collection, this must be taken into account for proper interpretation of results. Common indications for culturing include UTIs, non-healing or contaminated wounds, and severe, chronic, or non-responsive diseases of the respiratory, GI, and dermatologic systems.

Virus isolation is a specialized type of microbiological culture that relies on the need for viruses to replicate in living tissue. Most commonly, laboratory cell cultures are inoculated with test samples, incubated, and evaluated for structural changes due to viral infection (i.e. cytopathic effect). Once an active virus is cultivated, identification can be confirmed through the use of the serological methods described above. Common samples for virus isolation include tissue (belonging to viral target organs), anticoagulated whole blood, respiratory secretions, and urine. Samples should be kept in sterile containers, refrigerated, and arrive at the diagnostic laboratory within 24 hours. In addition to its utility for the identification of novel organisms and to monitor the microevolution of certain viruses (e.g. influenza), virus isolation is commonly used for confirmation of infection with adenoviruses, FeLV, and parvoviruses. Virus isolation of these pathogens may take between one and 4 weeks, limiting the usefulness of this modality in urgent clinical cases.

4.4 Indications for Diagnostic Testing

In the animal shelter setting, diagnostic testing can be employed on both an individual animal and population level basis. Before developing a testing strategy for either of these scenarios, the shelter practitioner should consider the costs and benefits of diagnostic testing as it relates to shelter operations, testing methodology, animal and human health, and the specific disease of interest (Box 4.2). Performing diagnostic tests is generally indicated when the disease in question is common in the shelter population, is likely to be acquired or transmitted in the shelter, presents a risk for spread into the community, requires immediate treatment and/or could be life-threatening, or poses a zoonotic risk (Hurley and Pesavento 2013).

4.4.1 Individual Animal Testing

There are two high-level indications for diagnostic testing of individual animals, including (i) screening for common diseases found in a population and (ii) diagnosis of existing disease states. Screening tests are those that are conducted on all members of a defined population for the detection of diseases that are commonly present but have not yet become clinical. Screening tests provide for early detection of disease, thus allowing for earlier management and, in most cases, an improved prognosis for the individual animal while also having potentially (widespread) implications for the health and well-being of the larger population in the case of contagious diseases. For these reasons, they are a key component of a comprehensive preventive care strategy. Such testing

Box 4.2 Diagnostic Testing Considerations

Shelter Operations

Does testing fall within the shelter's operational mission?
Are there enough resources to devote to testing?
Will test results alter current or future operations?
Do the costs of testing impact other services?

Testing Methodology

What tests are available for the disease in question?
How does disease prevalence impact test accuracy?
Can samples be collected, handled, prepared, and stored appropriately?
Do staff have the time, knowledge, skill, and training to conduct point-of-care tests accurately?

Animal and Human Health

Will test results alter the management of animals?
Will test results impact human health?

Disease Characteristics

Is the disease common?
Is infection or transmission within the shelter or community likely?
Is immediate treatment required?
Is the disease life-threatening?
Is there a zoonotic risk?

is most useful for diseases that have a long preclinical phase and for which the benefits of early treatment outweigh the expense of conducting the test, the cost of disease progression in the individual (both in terms of money and welfare), and the cost of disease transmission within the shelter population. In most cases, if performed, screening should be conducted at the time of shelter intake to realize these benefits; however, screening at other times may be considered for diseases that do not pose immediate threats in order to improve animal flow through the shelter system and promote more efficient utilization of resources. Diseases for which screening tests are commonly conducted include canine heartworm disease, feline retroviruses, and dermatophytosis.

Diagnosis of existing disease states can also protect the health and welfare of individual animals and, in the case of transmissible or zoonotic diseases, the health of the entire shelter population, both animal and human. In addition to those indications described for screening tests, when it comes to disease diagnosis, practitioners should also consider how the results of a particular diagnostic test will alter the treatment or management plan for the individual animal or the shelter population at large.

4.4.2 Population Level Testing

There are two high-level indications for diagnostic testing on a population level, including (i) disease surveillance and (ii) diagnosis and management of a disease outbreak. Surveillance has been defined as "the use of data to monitor health problems to facilitate their prevention or control" (United States Department of Health and Human Services 2012). It involves the active collection of data, such as clinical signs and diagnostic test results, within an at-risk population and is used to set priorities, plan and conduct disease control programs, and assess the effectiveness of control efforts (United States Department of Health and Human Services 2012). In the animal shelter, disease surveillance can help identify and document common conditions in incoming animals, detect disease trends within the shelter, and identify emerging diseases (Hurley and Pesavento 2013).

Though disease surveillance often occurs informally, such as monitoring for general trends during daily rounds, scheduled and formalized surveillance can provide more objective, actionable data. One example of this might be a periodic evaluation of fecal samples from dogs admitted within one week to assess concordance with prophylactic deworming protocols. The mathematical goal of surveillance testing is to detect at least one animal with the infection or disease of interest and not to determine prevalence in the shelter population; therefore, the ideal number of animals to test should be calculated based on the lowest assumed rate of infection and the desired confidence limits. Sampling enough animals to ensure at least 90% probability of detection is recommended (Table 4.6).

In addition to testing clinically healthy animals, it is useful to perform disease surveillance in cohorts of animals with specific clinical syndromes. For example, collecting oropharyngeal swabs from cats with clinical signs of upper respiratory disease may help guide empirical treatments and direct husbandry practices in order to minimize disease transmission once particular pathogens are identified. This type of surveillance may help inform preventive care practices and be helpful in understanding baseline disease characteristics should frequency or severity of clinical syndromes increase or animals fail to respond to treatment as expected.

Table 4.6 Surveillance testing sample sizes for ≥90% probability of detection (National Research Council 1991).

Assumed Infection Rate (%)	Number of Animals to Test
2	120
3	80
4	60
5	45
10	25
15–20	15
25–30	10
≥40	5

The frequency of surveillance is dependent upon the importance of the specific disease to the management of the population, historical trends, and resource availability; typical intervals include monthly, quarterly, biannual, or annual testing (National Research Council 1991). Results should be interpreted in terms of time (e.g. seasonal disease trends), location (e.g. building, ward, housing unit), and the individuals affected (e.g. species, age, sex, clinical signs) (United States Department of Health and Human Services 2012).

Diagnostic testing plays a key role in individual animal risk assessment during a disease outbreak response. Definitive identification of the cause of an infectious disease outbreak is a critical step in its mitigation and control (O'Quin 2013). In such circumstances, consideration should be given to testing of animals that are presumed to be infected; exposed and at risk of infection; exposed but not at risk of infection; and those not yet exposed (Hurley and Pesavento 2013). Testing every animal is generally not necessary and may not yield more actionable results. Though the precise number of patients to test will depend on the stage of infection, diagnostic test accuracy, and disease prevalence, a minimum of three to six samples for both GI and respiratory diseases have been recommended in human outbreak investigations (British Columbia Provincial Infection Control Network 2011; Plantenga et al. 2011). See Chapter 6 for more information on this topic.

4.5 Accuracy and Testing Strategy

The accuracy of diagnostic test results is commonly assessed through calculation of sensitivity, specificity, and predictive value reported as percentages. Sensitivity refers to a test's ability to report a positive test result in an animal that is actually infected. It can be calculated by dividing the number of true positive test results by the total number of cases that are actually positive (true positives + false negatives). A test with high sensitivity will report few false negative results. Specificity refers to a test's ability to report a negative test result in an animal that is not infected. It can be calculated by dividing the number of true negative test results by the total number of cases that are actually negative (false positives + true negatives). A test with high specificity will report few false positive results. Sensitivity and specificity refer to the characteristics of a specific diagnostic test, clinical sign, or disease syndrome, and remain constant regardless of the population being evaluated (Rothman 2012).

Predictive value refers to the usefulness of a particular test, sign, or syndrome in classifying animals with the infection or disease of interest. As such, predictive value is highly dependent on the prevalence of disease within the population being evaluated (Rothman 2012). Whereas sensitivity and specificity report the percentage of accurate test results, predictive value reports the percentage of patients that are likely to have accurate results. Positive predictive value can be calculated by dividing the number of true positive test results by the total number of positive test results (true positives + false positives). A test will have a high positive predictive value when the disease is common in the population and the diagnostic test utilized has high specificity. Negative predictive value can be calculated by dividing the number of true negative test results by the total number of negative test results (true negatives + false negatives). A test will have a high negative predictive value when the disease is not common in the population and the diagnostic test utilized has high sensitivity. See Figure 4.2.

Understanding these measures of accuracy is critical to designing rational diagnostic testing strategies for both individual animals and the shelter population as a whole. With each diagnostic test employed, there comes a risk of either false positive or false negative test results that may have a far-reaching impact. Therefore, such decisions should only be made after an assess-

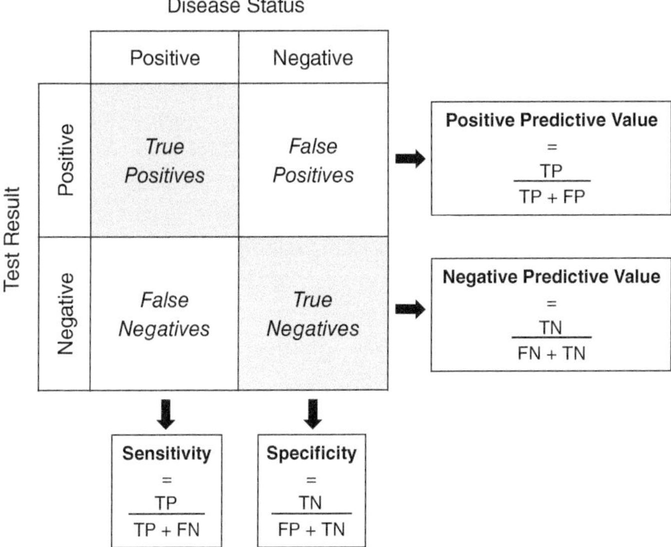

Figure 4.2 Sensitivity, specificity and predictive value. TP, true positives; TN, true negatives; FP, false positives; TN, true negatives.

ment of the cost–benefit ratio for the individual animal or shelter population and the acceptance of the risk posed by erroneous results. The following questions should be considered:

- Could an inaccurate test result lead to euthanasia?
- How would an inaccurate test result impact other animals in the shelter or community?
- Could treatment for a disease not present or lack of treatment for a disease that is present negatively affect the animal's well-being in the shelter or its disposition? How might that treatment impact other animals in the shelter or community?
- How could an inaccurate test result burden an adopter? Might it discourage adoption altogether?
- What are the costs of both accurate and inaccurate test results (e.g. money, time)?

Once it has been decided to perform diagnostic testing and the consequences of both positive and negative test results have been considered, a strategy can be developed. When there is a substantial risk for negative consequences from a false negative result, then a strategy that results in a high negative predictive value should be developed. An example of this can be seen with canine parvovirus testing in a dog with vomiting and diarrhea. Obtaining a false negative test result would allow the disease to progress and allow for continued transmission to other dogs in the shelter or community. If a negative antigen test result is obtained, repeating the original diagnostic test or using additional diagnostics such as a complete blood count or blood smear evaluation to acquire evidence in support of the original negative test result will increase the sensitivity of the testing strategy, minimize the risk of a false negative, and increase the negative predictive value of the result. When there is a substantial risk for negative consequences from a false positive result, then a strategy that results in a high positive predictive value should be developed. An example of this can be seen with canine parvovirus testing in a shelter for which treatment is not possible and infected puppies are euthanized. In this case, the consequences of a false positive result are extreme, so limiting testing to dogs with clinical signs of GI disease will limit testing to a population in which the disease is more common, minimizing the risk of false positives and increasing the positive predictive value of test results.

4.6 Standard Operating Procedures

4.6.1 Protocol Development and Staff Training

The definitive diagnosis of a disease is legally defined as the practice of veterinary medicine in many jurisdictions and should be performed only by veterinarians or under direct veterinary supervision. However, the establishment of SOPs, including diagnostic testing protocols, is not only a best practice for animal shelters but is also an essential component of meeting industry guidelines for shelter animal care. Such protocols must be written, detailed, current, accessible to staff and volunteers and should be developed with veterinary input. Protocols should define common illnesses, offer initial management steps, and detail the expected course of disease and response to treatment (Newbury et al. 2010). Protocols that pertain to disease diagnosis should describe the indications for diagnostic testing, the performance of common diagnostic tests, recognition and response to adverse treatment effects, and discuss the documentation of testing procedures (Association of Shelter Veterinarians 2014). Though diagnostic testing protocols should be veterinary-directed, it is important that staff and volunteers are included in their development to ensure understanding and assess feasibility (Steneroden 2004).

Once protocols are established and written, staff must be trained on their implementation.

Training techniques should be targeted toward the desired outcome which, in the case of diagnostic testing, is typically the performance of new skills. Therefore, performance and competency-based strategies should be utilized and generally include: a verbal and written description of the skill to be acquired, demonstration of the target skill, practice of the target skill, performance feedback, and repetition until mastery. Mastery of the skill in a simulated learning environment should be followed by training in an actual work scenario (Parsons et al. 2012). Training should be continuous to ensure the maintenance of skills, account for the turnover of shelter staff and volunteers as well as changes in standard procedures and should involve periodic observation of staff to ensure adherence to established protocols (Steneroden 2004).

4.6.2 Diagnostic Algorithms

The use of medical diagnostic algorithms is popular in both human and animal healthcare. Such an approach is thought to minimize unnecessary testing, control costs, and provide uniform quality care (Mushlin and Greene 2010). It is important to remember that such tools should be used with caution, particularly in complex cases, and should not be used as the sole means of disease diagnosis. However, in routine clinical scenarios, they have demonstrated enhancements in diagnostic accuracy when used in combination with clinical assessment (Riches et al. 2016). The following diagnostic algorithms are provided to help the shelter medicine practitioner obtain a diagnosis in common clinical scenarios in which infectious diseases are likely to be involved. See Figures 4.3–4.5.

4.7 Conclusion

A thoughtfully employed diagnostic testing strategy can ensure cost-effective protection of animal health and welfare in the shelter environment. Practitioners need not dismiss diagnostic testing as unattainable or unrealistic simply due to resource limitations. In fact, many of the most clinically useful diagnostic tools require minimal financial investment and thoughtful use of timely, targeted testing can often be a more cost-efficient strategy when all operational costs are considered. Careful use of the core diagnostic modalities—case history, physical examination, and response to treatment—will establish a sound treatment plan in many, if not the majority of shelter patients. With a modest budget, basic diagnostic supplies and equipment can be obtained allowing for a great spectrum of diagnostic capabilities through both primary and secondary diagnostic tests at a minimal cost. Such information can adequately guide the short- and long-term care of a variety of medical conditions in the shelter environment. Resources should also be reserved for advanced diagnostic laboratory testing and disease outbreak response when indicated.

Shelter practitioners should have a keen understanding of the benefits and drawbacks of each testing modality in order to select the most appropriate test for a given clinical situation and accurately interpret the results. Diagnostic testing protocols should be developed for both individual- and population-level health maintenance; they should be written and accessible. Such protocols should be designed by a veterinarian with knowledge of the animal population as well as familiarity with shelter medicine principles and take into account the risks and benefits of testing as well as those of obtaining erroneous results. Consideration of each of these factors in the development of sound diagnostic protocols can lead to efficient and effective disease treatment and, better yet, disease prevention—the ultimate rewards for all of us working to improve animal health and welfare.

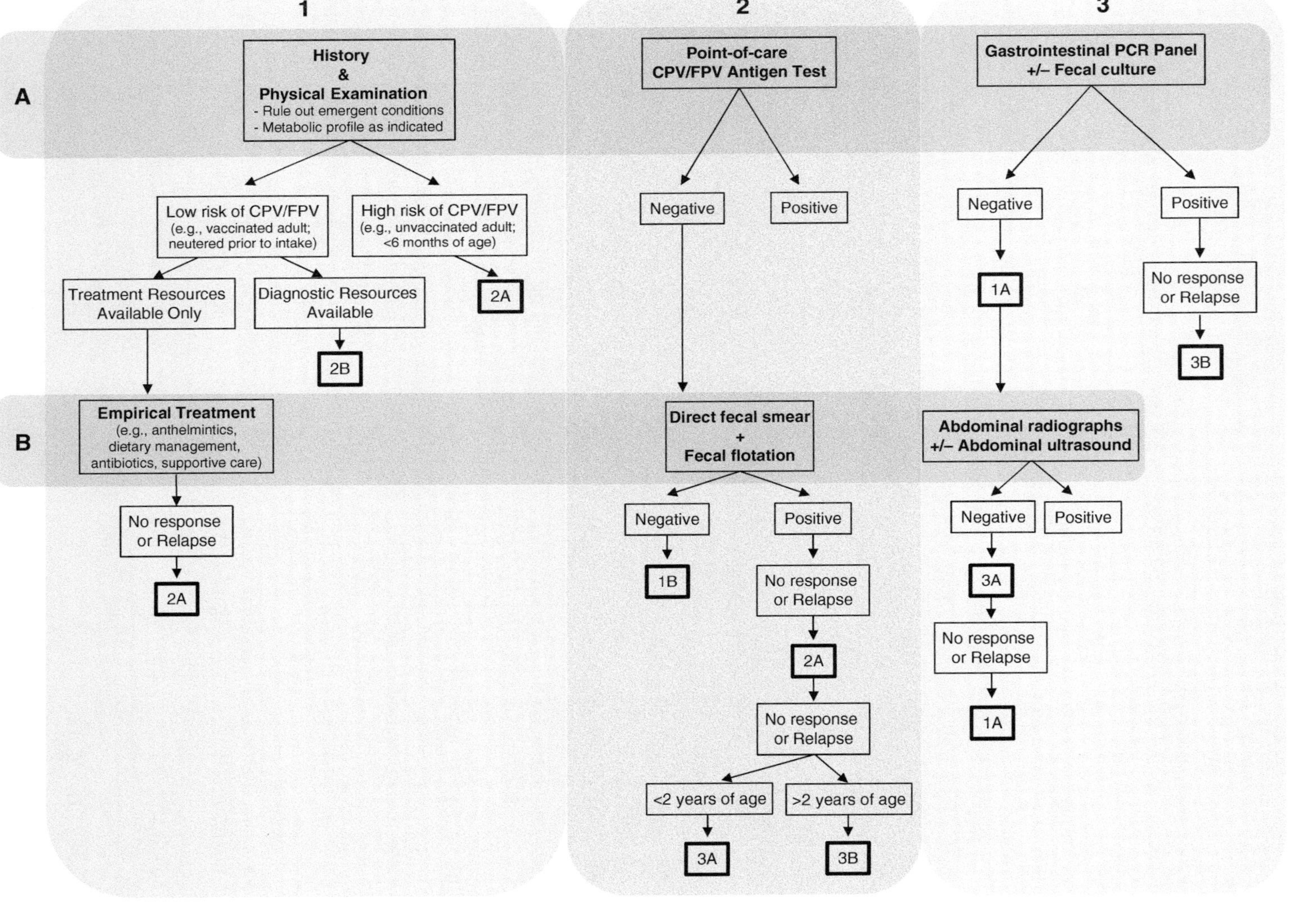

Figure 4.3 Infectious disease diagnostic algorithm for clinical signs of common infectious GI diseases including vomiting, diarrhea, anorexia, and weight loss. CPV, canine parvovirus; FPV, feline parvovirus.

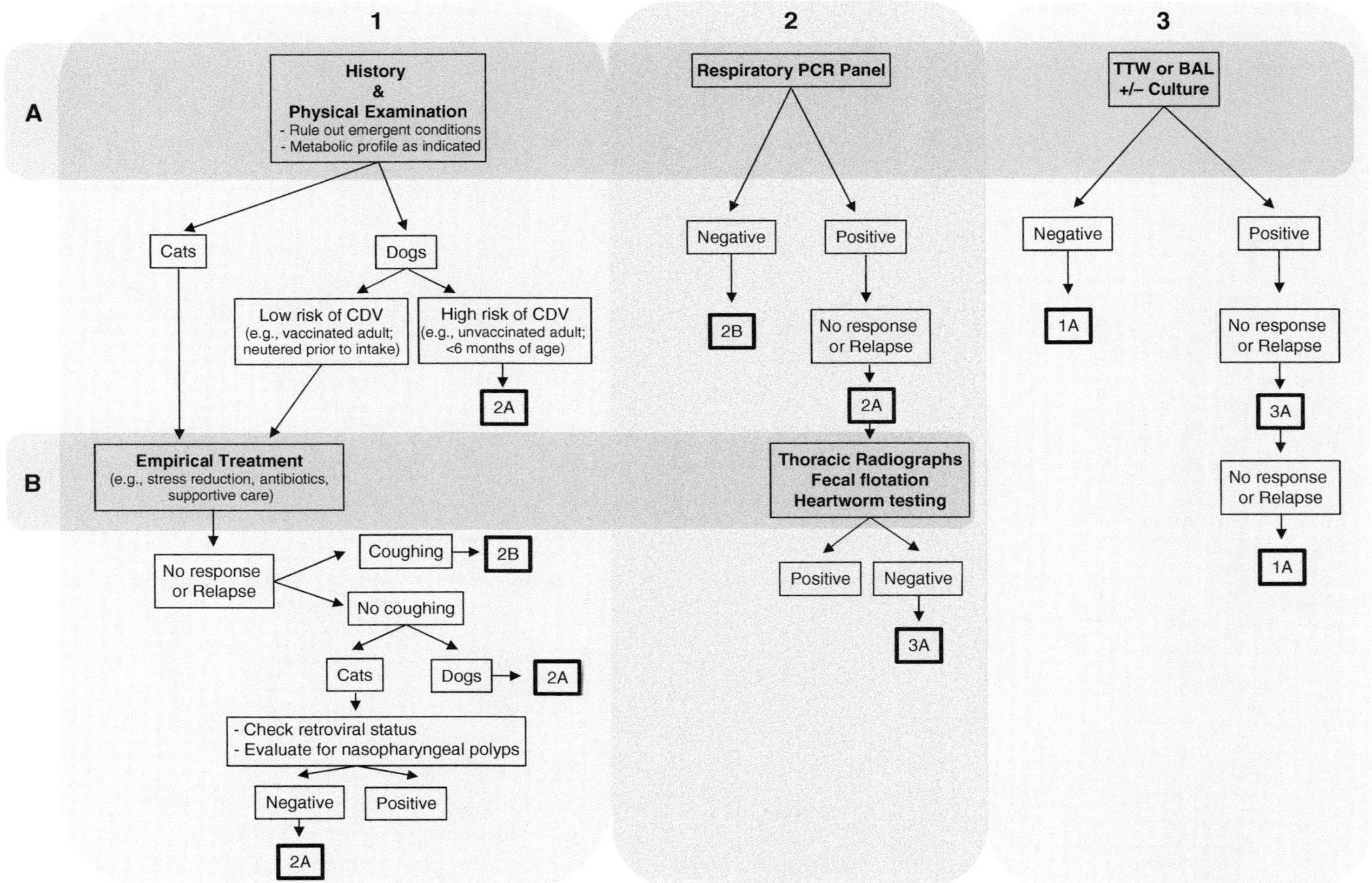

Figure 4.4 Infectious disease diagnostic algorithm for clinical signs of common infectious respiratory diseases including sneezing, coughing conjunctivitis, and oculo-nasal discharge. CDV, canine distemper virus; TTW, trans-tracheal wash; BAL, bronchoalveolar lavage.

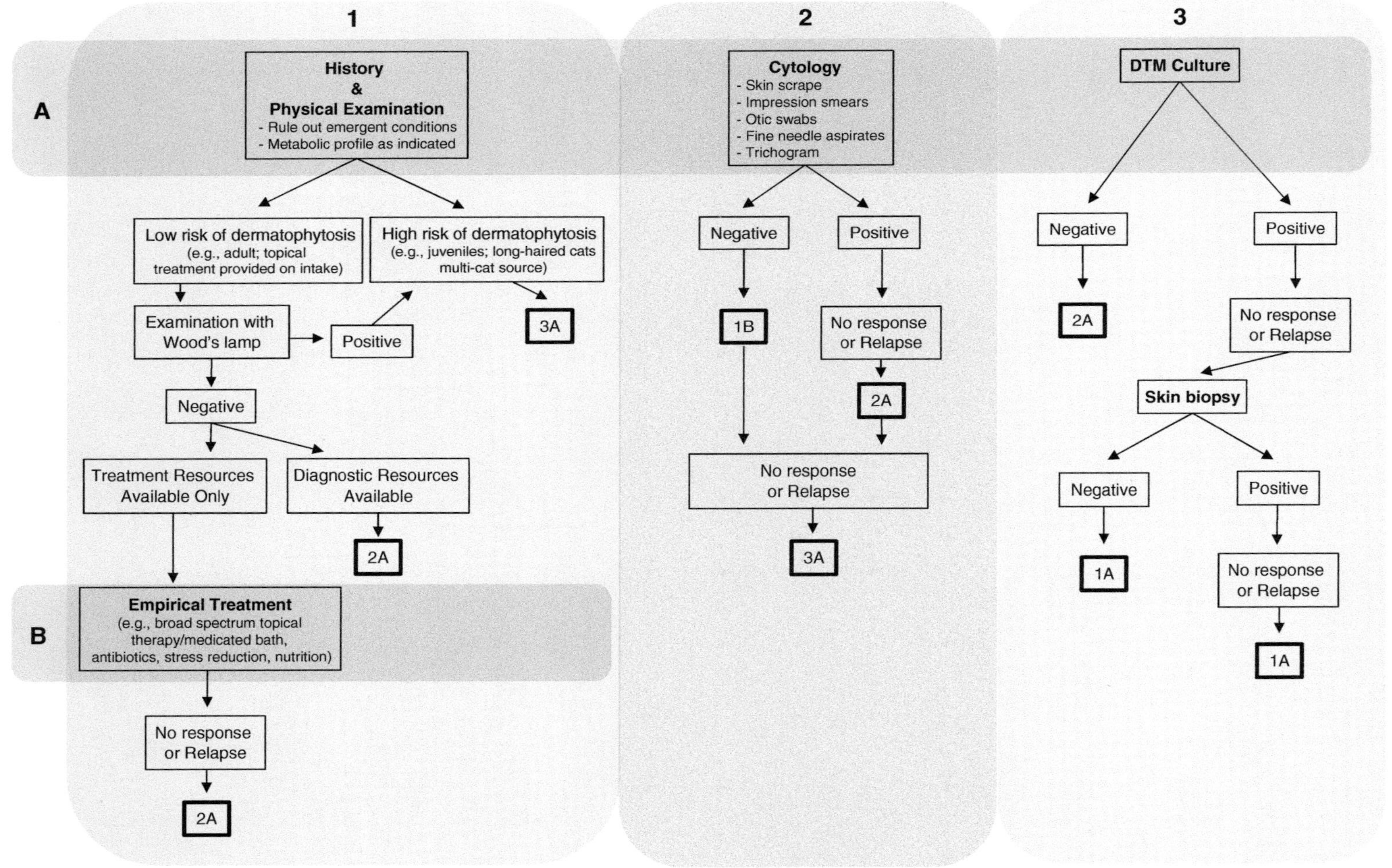

Figure 4.5 Infectious disease diagnostic algorithm for clinical signs of common infectious dermatologic diseases including alopecia, pruritus, papules, pustules, scaling, crusting, erythema, and nodules. DTM, dermatophyte test medium.

References

Anthony, E. (2014). Urine-Titled to Know: Urine Sediment Evaluation. *Veterinary Team Brief* (April), pp. 10–12.

Applied Biosystems. (n.d.) Real-Time PCR vs. Traditional PCR. Applied Biosystems. https://www.gene-quantification.de/abi-rtpcr-pcr.pdf (accessed 21 February 2018).

Association of Shelter Veterinarians (2014). Position Statement: Veterinary Supervision in Animal Shelters. Association of Shelter Veterinarians. http://www.sheltervet.org/assets/docs/position-statements/veterinarysupervisioninanimalshelters.pdf (accessed 17 February 2017).

Belford, C. and Lumsden, J.H. (1998). Cytopathology. In: BSAVA Manual of Small Animal Clinical Pathology (ed. M.G. Davidson), 121–140. Cheltenham: British Small Animal Veterinary Association Shurdington.

Berent, A.C., Murakami, T., Scroggin, R.D. et al. (2005). Reliability of using reagent test strips to estimate blood urea nitrogen concentration in dogs and cats. *Journal of the American Veterinary Medical Association* 227: 1253–1256.

Blood, D.C. and Studdert, V.P. (eds.) (1999). Saunders Comprehensive Veterinary Dictionary, 2e, 334. London: Harcourt Publishers Limited.

Bowman, D.D. (2014). Diagnostic parasitology. In: Georgis' Parasitology for Veterinarians, 10e (ed. D.D. Bowman), 326–398. St. Louis: Elsevier Saunders.

British Columbia Provincial Infection Control Network (2011). Collection of specimens. In: Respiratory Infection Outbreak Guidelines for Healthcare Facilities, 11–12. British Columbia: British Columbia Provincial Infection Control Network.

Cohen, T.A., Nelson, R.W., Kass, P.H. et al. (2009). Evaluation of six portable blood glucose meters for measuring blood glucose concentration in dogs. *Journal of the American Veterinary Medical Association* 235: 276–280.

Cohn, L.A., McCaw, D.L., Tate, D.J. et al. (2000). Assessment of five portable blood glucose meters, a point-of-care analyzer, and color test strips for measuring blood glucose concentration in dogs. *Journal of the American Veterinary Medical Association* 216: 198–202.

Duncan, J. (1998). Clinical biochemistry. In: BSAVA Manual of Small Animal Clinical Pathology (ed. M.G. Davidson), 61–86. Cheltenham: British Small Animal Veterinary Association Shurdington.

Evans, E.W. (2011). Proteins, lipids, and carbohydrates. In: Duncan and Prasse's Veterinary Laboratory Medicine: Clinical Pathology, 5e (ed. K.S. Latimer), 173–209. Ames: Wiley Blackwell.

Evermann, J.F., Sellon, R.K., and Sykes, J.E. (2012). Laboratory Diagnosis of Viral and Rickettsial Infections and Clinical Epidemiology of Infectious Disease. In: Infectious Diseases of the Dog and Cat, 4e (ed. C.E. Greene), 1–9. St. Louis: Elsevier Saunders.

Ford, R.B. (2013). Vital vaccination antibody titers versus vaccination. *Today's Veterinary Practice* 3: 35–38.

Gray, L.K., Crawford, C.C., Levy, J.K. et al. (2012). Comparison of two assays for detection of antibodies against canine parvovirus and canine distemper virus in dogs admitted to a Florida animal shelter. *Journal of the American Veterinary Medical Association* 240: 1084–1087.

Hurley, K. and Pesavento, P. (2013). Disease recognition and diagnostic testing. In: Shelter Medicine for Veterinarians and Staff, 2e (eds. L. Miller and S. Zawistowski), 329–341. Ames: Blackwell.

IDEXX Laboratories Inc. (2017) IDEXX Laboratory Test Directory 2017. IDEXX Laboratories Inc. https://www.idexx.com/

small-animal-health/directory-tests-services.html (accessed 9 April 2017).

Jacob, M.E., Crowell, M.D., Fauls, M.B. et al. (2016). Diagnostic accuracy of a rapid immunoassay for point-of-care detection of urinary tract infection in dogs. *American Journal of Veterinary Research* 77: 162–166.

Kang, M.H., Kim, D.H., Jeong, I.S. et al. (2016). Evaluation of four portable blood glucose meters in diabetic and non-diabetic dogs and cats. *The Veterinary Quarterly* 36: 2–9.

Mazar, S., Larson, L. and Lavi, Y. (2009). Sensitivity, specificity, accuracy and difference between positive and negative mean results of the ImmunoComb® Canine VacciCheck Antibody Test Kit for Canine Distemper. Parvo and AdenoVirus, Spectrum Labs. http://vaccicheck.com/wp-content/uploads/2014/02/VacciCheck-Performance-Wisconsin.pdf (accessed 20 February 2018).

Mende, K., Stuetzer, B., Truyen, B. et al. (2014). Evaluation of an in-house dot-enzyme-linked immunosorbent assay to detect antibodies against feline panleukopenia virus. *Journal of Feline Medicine and Surgery* 16 (10): 805–811.

Mushlin, S.B. and Greene, H.L. (2010). Preface. In: Decision Making in Medicine: An Algorithmic Approach, 3e (eds. S.B. Mushlin and H.L. Greene), xvii. Philadelphia: Mosby, Inc.

National Research Council Committee on Infectious Diseases of Mice and Rats (1991). Principles of rodent disease prevention. In: Companion Guide to Infectious Diseases of Mice and Rats, 1–8. Washington: National Academy Press.

Newbury, S., Blinn, M.K., Bushby, P.A. et al. (2010). Guidelines for Standards of Care in Animal Shelters: The Association of Shelter Veterinarians. https://www.sheltervet.org/assets/docs/shelter-standards-oct2011-wforward.pdf (accessed 1 June 2020).

O'Connor, T.P. (2015). SNAP assay technology. *Topics in Companion Animal Medicine* 30: 132–138.

O'Quin, J. (2013). Outbreak management. In: Shelter Medicine for Veterinarians and Staff, 2e (eds. L. Miller and S. Zawistowski), 349–370. Blackwell Publishing, Ltd.

Parsons, M.B., Rollyson, J.H., and Reid, D.H. (2012). Evidence-based staff training: a guide for practitioners. *Behavior Analysis in Practice* 5: 2–11.

Plantenga, M.S., Shiferaw, B., Keene, W.E. et al. (2011). Specimen collection and confirmation of norovirus outbreaks. *Emerging Infectious Diseases* 17: 1553–1555.

Rakich, P.M. and Latimer, K.S. (2011). Cytology. In: Duncan and Prasse's Veterinary Laboratory Medicine: Clinical Pathology, 5e (ed. K.S. Latimer), 331–364. Ames: Wiley Blackwell.

Riches, N., Panagioti, M., Alam, R. et al. (2016). The effectiveness of electronic differential diagnoses (DDX) generators: a systematic review and meta-analysis. *PLoS One* 11: 1–26.

Rosenfeld, A.J. and Dial, S.M. (2010a). Obtaining samples from different body systems and evaluating cytology. In: Clinical Pathology for the Veterinary Team (eds. A.J. Rosenfeld and S.M. Dial), 193–206. Ames: Blackwell Publishing, Ltd.

Rosenfeld, A.J. and Dial, S.M. (2010b). Sample handling and laboratory standardization – developing standard operating procedures. In: Clinical Pathology for the Veterinary Team (eds. A.J. Rosenfeld and S.M. Dial), 1–18. Ames: Blackwell Publishing, Ltd.

Rosenfeld, A.J. and Dial, S.M. (2010c). Components of the urinalysis. In: Clinical Pathology for the Veterinary Team (eds. A.J. Rosenfeld and S.M. Dial), 129–138. Ames: Blackwell Publishing, Ltd.

Rosenfeld, A.J. and Dial, S.M. (2010d). Abnormalities in the red and white cell populations. In: Clinical Pathology for the Veterinary Team (eds. A.J. Rosenfeld and S.M. Dial), 45–74. Ames: Blackwell Publishing, Ltd.

Rothman, K.J. (2012). Epidemiology in clinical settings. In: Epidemiology: An Introduction, 2e, 198–217. New York;: Oxford University Press.

Sajid, M., Kawde, A.N., and Daud, M. (2015). Designs, formats and applications of lateral flow assay: a literature review. *Journal of Saudi Chemical Society* 19: 689–705.

Steneroden, K. (2004). Sanitation. In: Shelter Medicine for Veterinarians and Staff, 2e (eds.

L. Miller and S. Zawistowski), 37–48. Ames: Blackwell Publishing, Ltd.

Thompson, M.F., Litster, A.L., Platell, J.L. et al. (2011). Canine bacterial urinary tract infections: new developments in old pathogens. *Veterinary Journal* 190: 22–27.

Tizard, I. (2013). Immunodiagnostic techniques. In: Veterinary Immunology (ed. I. Tizard), 494–514. St. Louis: Elsevier Saunders.

Tripathi, N.K., Gregory, C.R., and Latimer, K.S. (2011). Urinary system. In: Duncan and Prasse's Veterinary Laboratory Medicine: Clinical Pathology, 5e (ed. K.S. Latimer), 253–282. Ames: Wiley Blackwell.

United States Department of Health and Human Services (2012). Public health surveillance. In: Principles of Epidemiology in Public Health Practice, 3e, 5-1–5-73. Atlanta: Centers for Disease Control and Prevention.

Webb, J.L. and Latimer, K.S. (2011). Leukocytes. In: Duncan and Prasse's Veterinary Laboratory Medicine: Clinical Pathology, 5e (ed. K.S. Latimer), 45–82. Ames: Wiley Blackwell.

Weese, J.S., Blondeau, J.M., Boothe, D. et al. (2011). Antimicrobial use guidelines for treatment of urinary tract disease in dogs and cats; antimicrobial guidelines working group of the international society for companion animal infectious diseases. *Veterinary Medicine International* 2011: 1–9.

Wess, G. and Reusch, C. (2000a). Evaluation of five portable blood glucose meters for use in dogs. *Journal of the American Veterinary Medical Association* 216: 203–209.

Wess, G. and Reusch, C. (2000b). Assessment of five portable blood glucose meters for use in cats. *American Journal of Veterinary Research* 61: 1587–1592.

Westman, M.E., Malik, R., Hall, E. et al. (2016). Diagnosing feline immunodeficiency virus (FIV) infection in FIV-vaccinated and FIV-unvaccinated cats using saliva. *Comparative Immunology, Microbiology and Infectious Diseases* 46: 66–72.

Westman, M.E., Malik, R., Hall, E. et al. (2017). Comparison of three feline leukaemia virus (FeLV) point-of-care antigen test kits using blood and saliva. *Comparative Immunology, Microbiology and Infectious Diseases* 50: 88–96.

Zajac, A.M. and Conboy, G.A. (2012). Fecal examination for the diagnosis of parasitism. In: Veterinary Clinical Parasitology, 8e (eds. A.M. Zajac and G.A. Conboy), 3–170. Ames: Wiley Blackwell.

5

Necropsy Techniques

Patricia A. Pesavento

Department of Pathology, Microbiology, and Immunology, School of Veterinary Medicine, UC Davis, Davis, CA, USA

5.1 Introduction

The loss of an animal is always discouraging, but it is a valuable and accurate way to establish a cause of death; so, it is especially useful if other animals are at risk. In this chapter, the focus is on the necropsy techniques that help to identify sample collection in the case of infectious or toxic problems. How to collect excellent and useful tissue samples that accurately identify problem pathogens is the goal and can be very time efficient compared to the performance of a full or forensic-type necropsy. Consider an outbreak of respiratory disease in a kennel run where one affected dog either dies or is euthanized: Extensive testing, whether by culture or polymerase chain reaction (PCR) on oral swabs of in-contact animals can be expensive and nonetheless confounding, since potentially causative bacteria or viruses will circulate in the population due to either recent vaccination or simply because pathogens can be present but not clinically important. It would require a small, time- and money-consuming epidemiologic study to be confident of the cause in this way. Yet a single sample of lung tissue, taken from the affected dead animal, in a measured combination of culture, histologic review, and/or viral testing, will reveal the problem—and any pathogen in that sample should not be present, and IS significant. It is respectful to both the individual and the population to obtain as much useful information as possible from any animal that dies.

Necropsy can provide an opportunity to gain valuable insight into diseases, treatment, and husbandry practices in a single shelter. In the bigger picture, well-performed diagnostics provide the power to understand whether, and when, shelter animals are more susceptible to disease. They can also help identify new, or unexpected pathogens.

Consider, for example, the situation faced by this shelter:

Linda is a technician at Metro City All-Paws Rescue. She has noticed that, over the last few months, the mortality rate in the feral cat room seems high. She checks the records and confirms that, in the past month, 8/40 cats have died and in the previous month, 5 cats died. Averaging over the year prior, the monthly mortality was 1 death/~40 cats total. After consulting with the team, they recognized that many of the recent deaths have been associated with both upper respiratory (URI) signs and skin abscesses. Limited diagnostics had been performed on affected cats and both herpesvirus and calicivirus were found by oropharyngeal swab samples.

In the case of contagious disease, toxins, or husbandry problems, a necropsy performed on affected or sentinel cases could potentially save

Infectious Disease Management in Animal Shelters, Second Edition.
Edited by Lila Miller, Stephanie Janeczko, and Kate F. Hurley.

the lives of many more cats. In the example above, pre-mortem diagnostic tests had been performed on some of the cats with upper respiratory tract problems that had died, but the agents detected were common in the shelter environment and were therefore not convincingly the cause of death. Moreover, it was unclear to the shelter staff whether the URI or the abscesses were related to the animals' deaths, to each other, or just coincidental findings. An unexplained increase in mortality is one of the most compelling reasons for a shelter to perform a necropsy. See Table 5.1 for a partial list of reasons to perform a necropsy, with specific attention to those significant to a shelter.

An estimated 6.5 million companion animals entered US animal shelters in 2016 according to the American Society for the Prevention of Cruelty to Animals (ASPCA 2017). Shelters are intensive housing situations where transmission, exposure, and susceptibility to infectious disease are heightened. If compared to the dairy industry, with 9 million cows in the United States in 2017 (https://www.ers.usda.gov/data-products/dairy-data), necropsy is not just warranted but state and federally mandated (and funded) for large animal herd health clinicians to track infectious disease. There are hundreds of clinicians and pathologists employed to perform large animal diagnostics in the US and Canada. In contrast, and despite the real and intimate interface with the human population, few states provide funding for necropsy or diagnostics of shelter animals. There is a need for more methodical scrutiny for emerging diseases, infectious diseases, and zoonoses, and necropsy is the most accurate method to collect effective diagnostic samples, assess diagnostic accuracy, and to predict disease emergence. The purpose of this chapter is to provide practical guidelines for necropsy and for collecting, storing, and shipping samples for diagnostic testing.

For ideal infectious disease surveillance, a board-certified or accredited pathologist would examine all deaths at a given shelter. If that is an option, animals that die should be turned in immediately, without freezing of the carcass, for the most accurate results. However, state-subsidized diagnostics are not an option for most shelters. Full necropsy services at state diagnostic laboratories or veterinary schools are available, and although costs vary, they can be quite high for small animals. In contrast, performing a necropsy/sampling at a shelter and testing, or at least storing samples (for possible future examination) is relatively inexpensive and both biopsy services ("necropsy in a bottle") and microbiology services are readily available. Shelter personnel need to be trained to recognize lesions, and to perform a necropsy as part of the overall healthcare plan for their shelter population.

Table 5.1 Reasons to perform a necropsy in a shelter.

1) When there is unexplained death, or deaths, in the population
2) When there is the possibility that contagious disease could affect other shelter animals (including to limit future losses)
3) When zoonoses are suspected (when contagious disease from an animal could affect human workers or visitors)
4) To evaluate the effects of treatment, especially when a new treatment is involved or if a reaction to a drug or disinfectant is suspected
5) To document the accuracy of a clinical diagnosis
6) To document a legal case (e.g. suspected poisoning or cruelty)
7) To enhance discussion of husbandry and health maintenance programs with animal shelter specialists.

5.2 Why Sample Tissues at Necropsy?

Expedient pathogen identification can help minimize deaths and maximize successful outcomes from infectious illnesses. Appropriate

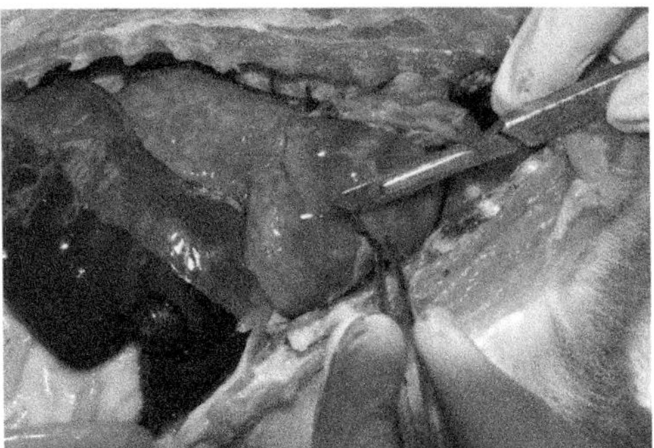

Figure 5.1 The prosector takes a sample of lung. Samples taken for microbiological analysis (culture or PCR) should be taken first during a necropsy. Use a sterile scalpel blade or scissors to take a section, and/or use a sterile swab to sample.

and adequate sample collection can help with such identification and is one of the most important reasons for a shelter to perform a necropsy. See Figure 5.1.

Necropsy has its limitations, and necropsy findings can be inconclusive as to the actual cause of death. Some conditions are simply not characterized by lesions that can be detected either grossly or microscopically. However, it is a very useful method to rule in (or out) infectious/inflammatory vs. OTHER causes of death. It is the intention of this chapter to put clinicians in a confident position to collect samples correctly so that the best material is available for analysis and diagnosis. Samples collected at necropsy can be used for culture, cytology (impression smears), molecular diagnostics (polymerase chain reaction or PCR), serology (antibodies are generally stable in postmortem blood for serology tests), histological analyses (of target tissues or all tissues collected) or other tests.

5.3 The Necropsy

5.3.1 General Considerations

To complete an effective necropsy, specific and consistent protocols (procedure, sampling, documentation) should be followed. The optimal time to perform a necropsy is as soon as possible after the animal's death. Depending on environmental conditions, changes in tissues occur in minutes after an animal has expired. It is important, for an accurate diagnosis, to take appropriate tissue samples for culture and/or microscopic examination in a timely fashion. If a necropsy cannot be performed immediately, the animal should be placed in a cooler (for up to two days post-death). Tissue integrity and most pathogens and toxins are stable during that time, although overgrowth of postmortem bacteria becomes a problem. For any longer time window, freezing the carcass is warranted.

Any animal that dies should be examined to the best of one's time and ability; however, a necropsy performed specifically for sample collection can be much shorter (for example, collecting gastrointestinal (GI) samples in a dog with diarrhea to confirm or exclude parvovirus). Here are a few important considerations before performing a necropsy:

1) **Zoonoses**: It is important to be aware that animals in the shelter may have a disease that is transmissible to humans (zoonosis) and, even more likely, a disease transmissible to other animals. The situation postmortem is no different than when the animal was alive, however, exposure to some agents is higher when a necropsy is performed (e.g. blood-borne pathogens, anthrax, rabies, and some fecal pathogens). The necropsy should be performed in a quiet, isolated, well-ventilated space. Precautions should be taken consistently (protective clothing, gloves, mask) during a necropsy, and any unfixed tissues should be placed in leak-proof containers or disposed of as medical waste according to the protocols specified by the state or institution.
2) **Handling cadavers**: If the necropsy cannot be carried out immediately, cadavers should be stored in a refrigerator (+2 °C to +4 °C) as soon as possible after death until the necropsy can be performed. A cadaver

should be frozen only if necessary; while still present in the tissue, some microbes will not be viable after freezing.

3) **Euthanasia:** Euthanasia policy and strategy is widely variable among shelters. The method of euthanasia should always be documented. There are both gross and histologic sequelae to any form of euthanasia, and it is important to understand whether a lesion is "real" or simply related to the method of euthanasia. For example, intra-abdominal administration of pentobarbital can result in puncture trauma, a layer of chemically induced necrosis on the surfaces of abdominal organs, or in peri-mortem intra-abdominal hemorrhage (See Figure 5.2).

Also, because euthanasia solution is caustic, intra-abdominal administration of euthanasia solution is not the best route of administration if an animal has an enteric (gastrointestinal) disease and histopathological analysis is anticipated.

The clinical history (including duration) and knowledge about any therapy are both vital to the appropriate interpretation of findings. In a shelter with the capacity to provide medical resources, necropsy may be limited to animals that have received medical care, such as antibiotics, which can compromise postmortem culture results. It is always beneficial to perform a necropsy on a more recently affected or moribund animal, rather than one that had recovered but might be weakened and subject to a secondary disease process.

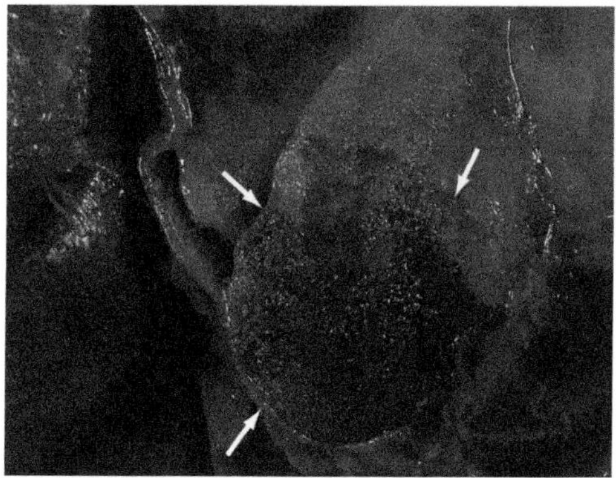

Figure 5.2 Euthanasia can cause artifactual changes to tissues. Here the granular, dull texture of the region of lung defined by the arrows is caused by intrathoracic contact with beuthanol during intracardiac euthanasia.

5.3.2 Documentation

5.3.2.1 Written Data

Pre-mortem information: Historical and clinical information are equally as important in the investigation as transcribing observations at the necropsy. Pre-mortem information includes clinical signs, date of intake and onset of illness, location held in the shelter, and all treatments received. Especially in a shelter, this information is necessary to identify patterns of susceptibility to disease over time, whether geographical, age-related, treatment-associated, time of year, etc. This information is also essential to interpret the necropsy and histological lesions, and/or to compare future or past cases. Pre-mortem and historical information can be written on a separate form or can be included on the necropsy form itself.

Necropsy results: There are several well-organized necropsy templates available (see resources below) and a shelter should have copies of one of these on hand. Which directions, forms, and/or templates are used are not important; they are designed to remind the prosector (the person doing the dissection) to be methodical, thorough, and consistent. It is important to try to be as objective as possible in reporting observations; specifically, to describe abnormalities without presuming cause (without adding interpretation). For example, if the liver appears large, the organ should be weighed or, if there is no scale, describe how this interpretation was made: "The edges of the liver lobes were rounded and the caudal aspect of the liver extended to. . .." The features (shape, position, color, consistency) should also be noted if the liver is abnormal. In this same example, the objective gross diagnosis is "hepatomegaly," or large liver. Knowing if a liver is too big or too small is useful, as the differential causes are entirely different, but the interpretation of organ size based on weight relies on its comparison (ratio) with the bodyweight of the animal.

If an organ or system was not examined, this should also be noted (e.g. if only the abdominal cavity and gastrointestinal system were examined and sampled, there should be a note on the report saying that organs within the thoracic cavity were NOT examined).

5.3.2.2 Photographic Data

Visual data can have great importance in the communication of necropsy findings, and with digital hegemony, most shelters own or have access to a digital camera. Photographic data is complementary to the written description of a lesion and can be even more persuasive than a written report in the legal documentation of findings. A photograph should never be substituted for a written record since two-dimensional photographs can only rarely fully represent the texture, cut surface, depth, and extent of any single lesion or systemic process.

5.4 Steps in Performing a Necropsy

5.4.1 The Materials Needed for a Necropsy

Not all the listed equipment will be needed to perform each necropsy, but Table 5.2 is a good starting list of the things that should be on hand for any given situation. Maintaining a devoted "necropsy kit" can save time.

5.4.2 General Information

There is no single CORRECT method to perform a necropsy, but consistency is important. If a cadaver is opened in the same way for each necropsy, one is more likely to recognize/discriminate abnormalities of any sort (e.g. size, position, color). Even in the case where the animal's disease appears to be limited to, for example, the respiratory system, the author recommends that the animal's body be opened in the same way so that both body cavities are examined visually. Respiratory distress can arise from abnormalities in organs not present within the thoracic cavity. In addition, concurrent diseases, if present, can be very important to disease progression. The most common example of this seen in shelters is immunosuppression caused by viral diseases like canine distemper virus, which can predispose a dog to a "secondary" infection such as bacterial pneumonia, or parvovirus (panleukopenia) in a dog

Table 5.2 Necropsy kit.

1) Camera
2) Notebook or Pathology Form
3) Protective clothing
    - Gloves (latex, nitrile, or rubber)
    - Boots
    - Mask (to cover mouth and nose)
    - Eyewear or goggles
4) Instruments
    - Sharp knife (and/or scalpel)
    - Knife sharpener
    - Scissors
    - Forceps
    - Small shears
    - Ruler
5) Collection gear
    - Specimen container (plastic) with a tight-fitting lid for fixed samples (plastic tubs, Rubbermaid, specimen cups, Tupperware type)
    - 10% buffered formalin (for fixed specimens/histology)
    - Plastic bags with closure (whirl-pack, zip-lock) for unfixed samples (fresh or frozen)
    - Tags (to identify specimens)
    - Collection vials (can be used for urine, blood, joint fluid, etc.)
6) Transport/shipping containers
    - Ice packs
    - Heavy-duty bags, or leak-proof containers
    - Packing material (preferably absorptive)
7) Cleaning and disinfecting materials

or cat, which can predispose the infected animal to other enteric pathogens.

Step by step instructions on how to perform a necropsy are available from several books and web-based sources. Five sources are listed below. While not all these protocols specifically use dogs and cats as models, the general approach to a necropsy is similar in all domestic species. The 5th listed resource by Severidt, for example, although specifically addressing cattle, has an excellent section on sample handling and submission.

5.4.2.1 Resources for Performing a Complete Necropsy

1) The Veterinary Necropsy Report Checklist and Guidelines form (DD Form 1626) was created by the Armed Forces Institute for Pathology (AFIP), Division of Veterinary Pathology. It can be found at https://www.esd.whs.mil/Portals/54/Documents/DD/forms/dd/dd1626.pdf (or search veterinary pathology, Form 1626).

   It is a comprehensive, 12-page document with sections for data and interpretation (pages 1-2), gross necropsy findings (pp. 3–8) and a detailed necropsy protocol (pages 9-12). Included is a tissue checklist (page 7) to record tissues collected during the necropsy.
2) *The Necropsy Book* by Drs. John M. King, Lois Roth-Johnson, David C. Dodd and Marion E. Newsom. This succinct, small book guide is available from the Charles Louis Davis-Thompson Foundation, which is a non-profit organization for the advancement of comparative pathology education. It is widely used by veterinary schools to teach basic necropsy techniques to veterinary students. It is an inexpensive manual and contains an organ-based approach to a necropsy, including many drawings. The information on patterns is particularly useful for making the best decisions during the gross necropsy for sample collection. It is available at http://store.cldavis.org/thenecropsybookfifthedition.aspx
3) Necropsy Guide for Dogs, Cats, and Small Mammals, 1st Edition by Sean P. McDonough and Teresa Southard (editors). This book has "how-to" guides, but also has many very useful photos of common diseases, common artifacts, and methods of fixation and sampling.
4) *Necropsy of Wild Animals* by Linda Munson DVM, Ph.D. This is a PDF document available on the web, composed by Dr. Linda Munson, and maintained by the University of California's Wildlife Health Services. It can be found at http://www.cldavis.org/ghpn/tools/Necropsy%20of%20Wild%20Animals.pdf. It is an excellent reference for the steps in a complete necropsy, including drawings, and the "models" are felines and canids. The site includes a comprehensive tissue checklist for the collection of samples during a necropsy.
5) *Dairy Cattle Necropsy Manual* by Julie Severidt, Dennis Madden, Gary Mason, Frank Garry, and Dan Gould. This is a web-based set of directions, with color photographs, for a necropsy of a ruminant. It is available from Colorado State at http://csu-cvmbs.colostate.edu/Documents/ilm-dairy-cow-necropsy-manual.pdf. It has a well thought out discussion of considerations for sample shipping. See Table 5.3

5.4.2.2 Opening the Animal for Analysis and Sampling

It is important to think about the samples that should be collected PRIOR to the necropsy and have materials at hand that are necessary for collection. Samples destined for microbiology or other infectious disease diagnostics should be taken first, with sterile instruments if possible, and with minimal handling. If a sample needs to be refrigerated or frozen, do so as soon as possible after collection. While many premortem tests can be performed postmortem, tissues collected postmortem, if collected properly, can be more accurate for establishing the cause of disease. For example, a culture of lung

Table 5.3 Resources for performing a complete necropsy.

Resource	Author
Veterinary Necropsy Report Checklist and Guidelines form (DD Form 1626)	Armed Forces Institute for Pathology (AFIP), Division of Veterinary Pathology. https://www.esd.whs.mil/Portals/54/Documents/DD/forms/dd/dd1626.pdf
The Necropsy Book	John M. King, Lois Roth-Johnson, David C. Dodd and Marion E. Newsom. http://store.cldavis.org/thenecropsybookfifthedition.aspx
Necropsy Guide for Dogs, Cats, and Small Mammals, 1st Edition	Sean P. McDonough and Teresa Southard, editors
Necropsy of Wild Animals	Linda Munson http://www.cldavis.org/ghpn/tools/Necropsy%20of%20Wild%20Animals.pdf
Dairy Cattle Necropsy Manual	Julie Severidt, Dennis Madden, Gary Mason, Frank Garry, and Dan Gould. http://csu-cvmbs.colostate.edu/Documents/ilm-dairy-cow-necropsy-manual.pdf.

tissue to diagnose a bacterial cause of pneumonia is more accurate than a culture from an oropharyngeal swab that would contain several potential commensal bacteria.

5.4.2.3 Necropsy Analysis and Sampling, a Beginning

1) Place the carcass on its left side.
2) Assess the general condition.

   Determine the nutritional state of the animal. This can be done using a body condition scoring system but should also include looking for external (subcutaneous) and internal fat stores. In most animals, stores of fat surrounding the kidney and the heart are the longest retained, so these should be specifically examined if emaciation is suspected. Note the muscle mass of the animal.
3) Oral exam

   Note the condition of the teeth, look for masses or ulcers on the lingual, buccal and/or gingival mucosa.
4) Cut the skin along the ventral midline from the chin to the tail.
5) Reflect the right limbs by cutting through the muscles to the hip and shoulder joints.

   Reflect the skin to the level of the backbone (See Figure 5.3).
6) Open the two body cavities (abdomen, chest):
   a) Open the abdominal cavity by cutting through the body wall musculature along the caudal border of the ribcage and extend the cut to the pelvic region. Open the right side of the chest cavity by cutting the ribs along the sternum and adjacent to the backbone (see Figure 5.3).
   b) Record any abnormal locations or sizes of organs.

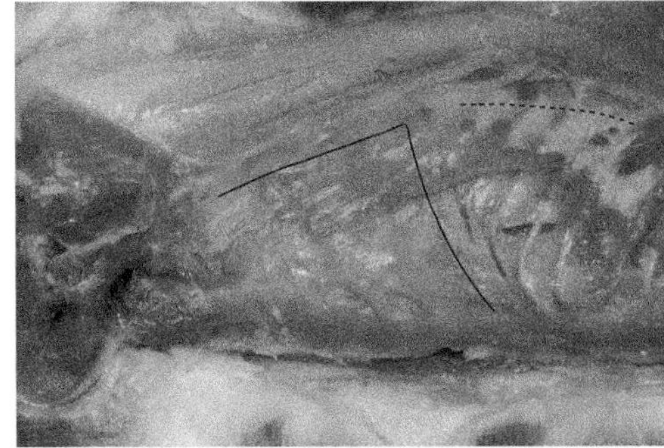

Figure 5.3 Prepare to open the animal by reflecting the skin. A cut along the thin, black solid line will reveal the abdominal cavity; continue the incision across the pelvic region and along the ventral midline. Open the thoracic cavity by cutting the ribs along the dotted line to the thoracic inlet and finish the opening by cutting each rib just dorsal to the vertebrae.

c) Record the quantity, color, and contents of any fluids in the body cavities.
d) Note the amount and quality of food in the digestive tract.
e) If samples of organs are to be taken for culture or microbe analysis of any type, do so early, before they have been removed and handled. A description of the best samples to take for common shelter problems is provided in the next section.

7) The organ systems should be examined in a methodical manner, which can be guided by any of the resource sites listed in the previous section. A tissue checklist should be on hand. For samples destined for histopathology, a sharp knife or scalpel should be used, the tissues held at the edges only and quickly placed in formalin. If a complete necropsy is desired (e.g. if there is a sudden death) samples should be taken from all listed organs (refer to the tissue checklist), including normal and abnormal regions. Samples that include both abnormal areas and surrounding normal areas are best. Do not scrape surfaces of tissues. Histopathology samples from any organ should be no thicker than 1 cm so that formalin penetration of the tissue is adequate, but multiple samples should be taken so that they represent the range of lesions (See Figure 5.4)

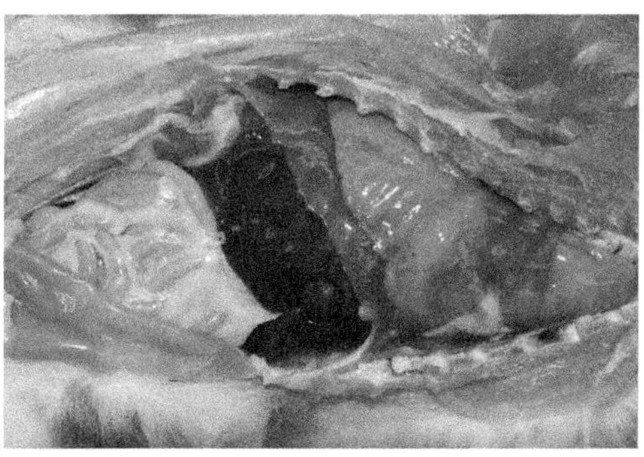

Figure 5.4 A properly opened body ready for diagnostic sampling.

8) Specific tissues to sample in the case of gastrointestinal or respiratory disease are listed separately later in the chapter. For shipping, if the appropriate ratio for fixation has been used (10 formalin:1 tissue), and there has been an appropriate time of fixation, most of the formalin can be removed once the specimen is fixed. It is important to leave just enough formalin so the sample does not dry during shipment. Proper fixation depends on the sample size and the density of the tissue. For properly cut samples of most visceral organs, 24 hours is usually sufficient. Waste formalin is considered hazardous waste and must be handled following current state and federal regulations, as well as U.S. Environmental Protection Agency guidelines. Similarly, the size and quantity of formalin containers that can be shipped may be limited, which may be of particular importance when multiple samples are collected.

For shipping samples, four layers of packaging are generally required to include a primary watertight inner receptacle, absorbent material, a secondary watertight inner receptacle, and sturdy outer packaging. The second receptacle should contain any required clinical history and request forms. Both the shipping company and the receiving laboratory should be consulted to ensure proper packaging prior to sample submission. Remaining samples can be placed and stored in a large plastic container of formalin in case additional samples are needed.

5.4.2.4 Tissue Checklist for Necropsy

The following tissues should be preserved in 10% buffered formalin at a ratio of 1 part tissue to 10 parts formalin. Tissues should be no thicker than 1 cm.

1) Liver – sections from each lobe, including gall bladder
2) Kidney – sections should extend from cortex to medulla and be collected from each kidney (see Figure 5.5)

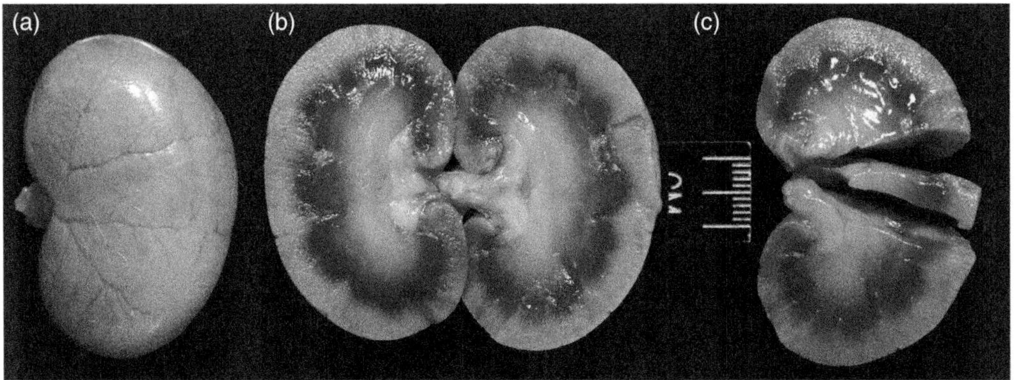

Figure 5.5 Sections to be submitted for histological analysis need to be thin enough to properly fix in formalin. In this example, the (a) kidney has been cut along a (b) mid-sagittal plane. (c) A properly cut section for fixation in 10% buffered formalin is pictured.

3) Stomach – sections from fundus (body) and pylorus
4) Gastrointestinal (GI) Tract
   a) Oral/pharyngeal mucosa and tonsil – plus any areas with erosions or ulcerations
   b) Tongue – cross section near tip including both mucosal surfaces

   Segmental (up to 5 cm long) sections of:

   c) Esophagus
   d) Small intestines – duodenum, jejunum, ileum
   e) Large intestines – cecum, colon
5) Spleen
6) Pancreas
7) Adrenal gland
8) Heart – longitudinal sections including atrium, ventricle and valves from both left and right sides
9) Lung – regional samples including cranioventral, caudodorsal, and hilar with major bronchus included
10) Lymph nodes – possibilities include iliac, mesenteric, hilar, mandibular, retropharyngeal
11) Thymus (if young animal)

Other possible tissue sections to consider (case dependent):

12) Skin – any affected regions
13) Brain – if there are neurologic signs, the entire brain should be submitted, cut longitudinally along the midline
14) Reproductive tract – entire uterus and ovaries with longitudinal cuts into the lumen of uterine horns, or both testes (transversely cut) with epididymis
15) Salivary gland
16) Trachea
17) Nasal turbinates
18) Thyroid/parathyroids – leave intact
19) Urinary bladder, ureters, urethra- cross-section of the bladder and 2 cm sections of ureter and urethra
20) Eye – intact
21) Spinal cord (if neurologic disease)- sections from cervical, thoracic and lumbar cord
22) Skeletal muscle – diaphragm, cross-section of thigh muscles
23) Bone marrow – Opened rib or longitudinally sectioned ½ femur; marrow must be exposed for proper fixation

5.5 The Diagnostic Shelter Necropsy

Consider the following case history:

There is an outbreak of diarrhea, with a concurrent increase in mortality, in cats and kittens in a large, municipal shelter. Several cats and kittens have been found dead within the past few weeks. The bodies were disposed of and the cages cleaned thoroughly but even with isolation procedures in place, the number of affected animals appears to be increasing. The shelter manager and part-time veterinarian at the shelter both suspect that the feline panleukopenia virus is the culprit. Animals are vaccinated at intake and every two weeks during their stay, but the disease presentation seems more aggressive than they have seen in the past, and several older cats have been affected. A fecal antigen test was performed on two affected animals, but the result was negative for viral antigen on the first and weakly positive on the second animal. Although apparently well yesterday, a cat and a three-month old kitten were found dead at morning rounds. They believe both animals are part of this outbreak, although diarrhea was seen in the cat's cage but not in the kitten's cage. What is the best way for staff to establish the cause of gastrointestinal disease in their feline population?

This scenario is not at all uncommon in shelters. If accurate (sensitive and specific) pre-mortem tests are available and results are consistent in affected animals, a cause for increased morbidity and mortality is comfortably determined. However, there are many reasons (e.g. less sensitive test, unusual presentation for a disease, unusual behavior of the disease in a population, non-responsive to treatment for that disease) a shelter might seek additional information about a disease. In this case, although feces from one cat was positive for the presence of feline panleukopenia virus, the disease seemed to be occurring in the face of vaccination and isolation and was occurring in animals less commonly associated with the suspected disease (older animals).

What should they do? Staff are understandably very busy and need to efficiently diagnose the problem. The tests have been somewhat equivocal and doing full necropsies on each of these animals would likely be very time-consuming; moreover, they are not sure the gross exam will be helpful since they are not exactly sure what they are seeing.

In a shelter (herd) situation, it is sometimes practical, sufficient, and time-efficient to ask a more specific (limited) question about disease or death of an animal. Gastrointestinal and respiratory diseases, in particular, are frequent problems in shelters. To ask a more limited question of a necropsy means that the necropsy itself can be simplified. Necropsy samples can be the best samples to definitively diagnose a cause of disease, and proper necropsy sampling in a sentinel case or an infectious outbreak will save other animals.

5.5.1 Sampling a Carcass, General Considerations

The success of infectious disease diagnosis depends largely on the quality of the specimen and the conditions under which the specimen is transported and stored before it is processed in the laboratory. It would be naive to generalize; depending on the suspected agent and the test, the optimum sample and optimum conditions for stabilization during transport are variable. For example, if a bacterial agent is suspected, freezing the specimen could compromise future culture; however, DNA would remain intact and a PCR test relying on extracted bacterial DNA would be unaffected. Some viruses, on the other hand, can withstand freezing, especially if samples are stored in the proper media. There are specific transport media that stabilize viruses and prevent bacterial overgrowth. What this means, of course, is that if the cause of the disease is completely open and multiple tests are going to be performed, multiple types of samples are necessary. Collection is simpler if a certain agent is highly suspect, or if a single agent needs to be ruled in or out.

Because gastrointestinal disease and respiratory disease are the most common infectious diseases associated with morbidity and mortality in the shelter environment, the following section is devoted to the sampling of a cadaver in these types of outbreaks.

5.5.2 Necropsy and Sampling for Gastrointestinal Disease

The following sample collection would be a good starting point for sampling any enteric disease (diarrhea and/or vomiting) of unknown origin in both dogs and cats. While causes of diarrhea can be remote from the gastrointestinal system (heat shock, for example), MOST contagious or toxin-associated GI disease results from a direct attack on the gastrointestinal system. Moreover, the distribution of lesions (grossly) is very helpful in determining the cause of disease. See Table 5.4

1) **Feces:**
   If abundant, feces collection can be made from the distal colon. Even if scant, feces can be scraped from the colonic mucosa or obtained by a swab. Postmortem feces are useful samples for multiple tests, including fecal antigen test (parvoviruses, see below). Pooling feces from the small intestine and colon has been noted to increase the sensitivity of the parvo antigen tests, which is sensible for a viral infection with a segmental distribution and episodic shedding. Also, the feces can be used for direct smear/fecal flotation/parasite analysis, or viral analyses. If collecting formalin-fixed tissue for histologic correlate analysis, tissue should be collected from an undisturbed (unsampled) region of the colon (mucosa is fragile and will slough easily with handling).
2) **Formalin-fixed tissues:**
   Histological samples should be taken in ALL CASES, no matter what supplementary diagnostic tests are chosen. Histology can provide a definitive diagnosis, it can direct to possible causes, or it will confirm or refute the results of other diagnostic tests. A general list for sampling an animal with enteric disease is found below. In nearly all cases, these samples would be sufficient to diagnose or exclude common shelter enteric pathogens. In cases where the agent or cause is unexpected, these samples would establish whether an enteric disease is inflammatory, infectious, toxic, or neoplastic.

Table 5.4 Necropsy and sampling for GI disease.

1) Feces
2) Formalin-fixed tissues
3) Microbiology
4) Molecular diagnostics
5) Toxicology
6) Serology

5.5.2.1 Tissue Checklist for Gastrointestinal Disease

Tissues should be no thicker than 1 cm. Tissues should be placed immediately in 10% buffered formalin at a ratio of 1 part tissue to 10 parts formalin.

a) Duodenum, two (up to 5 cm long) segments
b) Pancreas (1 cm section, can be left attached to the duodenum)
c) Jejunum (proximal, mid, distal), at least three (up to 5 cm long) segments
d) Ileo-ceco-colic junction (these regions can be sampled individually, or this region can be sampled in its entirety. If the latter is chosen, the sample should be opened enough so that formalin can perfuse the mucosa throughout the section, but do not scrape or touch the mucosa while handling.) See Figures 5.6 and 5.7.
e) Colon, distal, one sample (proximal is included in sample listed in d)
f) Liver, up to 1 cm wide sections (from all distinct lobes, including gall bladder)
g) Mesenteric lymph node
h) Any regions perceived to be abnormal

3) **Microbiology:**
   Screening for bacterial or fungal organisms of significance can be performed on feces, small intestinal contents, or a combination of both. Be aware that antibiotic therapy can skew or prevent the culture of many bacteria. Any pre-mortem therapy should

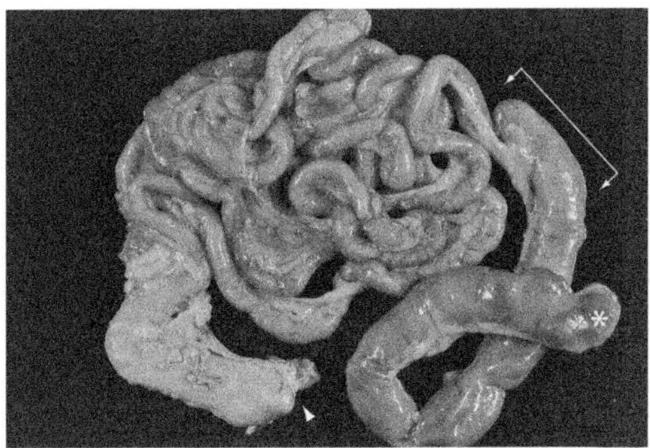

Figure 5.6 The intestines, extending from the gastroesophageal junction (arrowhead) to the distal colon (asterisk) have been removed. In the case of GI disease (or for any complete necropsy) the ileo-ceco-colic junction (bracketed by arrows) is one of the important sections for submission.

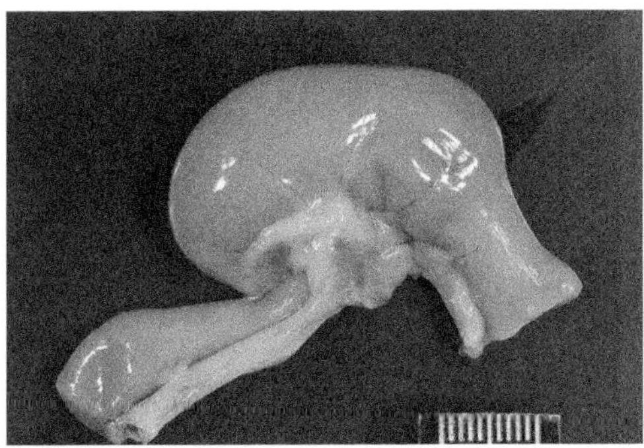

Figure 5.7 The ileo-ceco-colic junction is pictured. The intestine can be opened along a sagittal plane for greater penetration of the formalin fixative.

be noted in the submission form and on the necropsy report. Feces can be collected in any number of different sterile or clean containers, including bags, urine cups, or tubes. If feces are submitted, it should be specified on the request that *significant* enteric organisms (such as *Salmonella*, *Clostridia*, and *Campylobacter*) are of concern. Culture results need to be correlated with histologic findings; *Clostridia*, for example, can be cultured from normal intestines, so histologic correlates or toxin testing has to be performed concurrently with culture. *Salmonella*, although always significant for herd health and zoonotic reasons, can be shed asymptomatically in cats and dogs. Be aware also that so-called "commensal" (usually non-pathogenic) organisms can become virulent (e.g. some strains of *E. coli*). Diagnosis in these cases would require a combination of histologic and microbiologic results or specialized microbiologic analysis. Specimens destined for culture should be transported and processed as soon as possible; delays of more than 48 hours are undesirable. If processing is delayed, refrigeration is preferable to storage at ambient temperature; freezing will kill many types of bacteria (see adjunct diagnostics).

4) **Molecular diagnostics:**
Detection and characterization of pathogenic organisms increasingly rely on DNA or RNA amplification techniques (PCR). These samples need to be taken early in the postmortem from tissue minimally manipulated, but the tissue can be frozen immediately and used at a future date if warranted. DNA or RNA from the infectious agent will degrade at rates dependent on time, environmental factors (temperature, pH) and the organism itself. Ideally, samples from affected organs are fresh or fresh/frozen for molecular analysis. Most diagnostic laboratories or veterinary schools can offer guidance and a list of possible tests, the preferred or potentially useful tissue samples, and the preferred method of shipment. Whole blood (e.g. heart blood) or highly vascularized tissues (spleen, liver, lung) are reliable sources for circulating infectious agents (bacteria, viruses, or hemoparasites).

Individual PCR tests and enteric PCR "panels" are available in many commercial laboratories and veterinary schools. For enteric disease, feces are usually the sample of choice for DNA/RNA retrieval, but individual laboratories vary and should be consulted directly. There are important considerations for whether and when to use PCR for diagnostic analysis. (See Chapter 4 for more details.) For accurate assessment of causation, PCR results should be correlated by histopathologic analysis of formalin-fixed tissue. For example, if *Salmonella spp.* is detected by PCR, the correlative lesion of *Salmonella* associated GI disease is an acute and necrotizing enteritis. It is true that if many cases in a single outbreak are evaluated by a single test, correlation and causation can be established by epidemiologic findings (e.g. only and all cases of enteric disease are positive for *Salmonella*). However, this can be both unfeasible (depending on the incidence of disease) and expensive. Using histopathology, correlated with PCR (or a number of other diagnostic tests), can establish causation in an individual animal. While PCR is an excellent way to rule out KNOWN causes of disease, most diagnostic PCR assays are not designed to detect newly emergent disease. This is another reason to include histologic analysis of tissues in the diagnostic plan: by ruling out common diseases, a newly emergent cause for disease can be more quickly identified. The most difficult emergent diseases to recognize and identify are those that mimic known diseases. For retrospective analyses, DNA can also be extracted from tissue embedded in paraffin, however, this is offered by a more limited number of laboratories.

5) **Toxicology:**
   It is best to contact a toxicology laboratory, state laboratory, and/or a poison control center such as the ASPCA (http://www.aspca.org/apcc) for guidance. The appropriate sample for analysis is dependent on the type of toxin, among other variables. In the case of GI illness, source (food) and stomach contents should be saved. For heavy metal analysis, samples of liver and kidney should be collected, placed in separate plastic bags, and frozen until submitted. If a toxin is suspected but unknown, a necropsy should be performed and, in addition to histologic samples, liver, kidney, fat, stomach contents, and muscle samples should be frozen until submitted.
6) **Serology:**
   Serodiagnostic tests are tests performed on serum or plasma to detect either the presence of antibodies to a particular pathogen or the presence of circulating antigens from the pathogen itself. Both of these types of tests can be performed postmortem on serum obtained from a pooled blood source (e.g. heart, major veins). The significance of the result should be considered before this particular technique is used; few tests are validated for postmortem serum. Nonetheless, a positive titer is generally considered significant. See Chapter 4 for more details on serologic testing.

5.5.2.2 Parvovirus (Canine Parvovirus (CPV), Feline Panleukopenia Virus (FPV))

In the shelter, the most common causes of intestinal disease associated with mortality are the canine and feline parvoviruses. Suspicion and caution for this disease, therefore, is high; however, no clinical or gross finding is specific to parvoviral enteritis. This is a good reason to perform a necropsy on a dog or cat that is either suspicious for or known to be infected with parvovirus.

1) Establishing cause:
   a) Tissues for histology: Necropsy with histology can confirm the presence of parvovirus and would be important in ruling out parvovirus during an investigation of an unusual outbreak of GI disease. Acute cases of parvovirus are nearly pathognomonic by histologic analysis and chronic (historic) cases can also be detected by a pathologist; the architecture of the small intestine is not restored to normal for two to three weeks post-infection.
   b) Other tests: In dogs, although the parvovirus antigen tests on feces are highly sensitive during viral shedding in the early stages of infection, these peak viral titers are brief and occur at the same time as, or prior to, the onset of clinical

signs (Greene 2011). Subsequent viral shedding is known to fluctuate, and if the fecal antigen test is performed late after infection, virus in feces may be undetected. Testing of nearby, recently exposed animals is warranted, and in an animal that has died, feces should be retested at the time of necropsy with fecal material collected from pooled segments of the lower intestine (duodenum, jejunum, and colon). Numerous cases of dogs or cats have been seen whose feces were negative one to two days prior to death and submitted for evaluation of "non-parvoviral diarrhea." These same animals were often positive by fecal antigen tests at the time of necropsy and in these cases, there was concurrent histologic confirmation of parvoviral disease to establish etiology.

Tissue and fecal samples from dogs or cats collected at the time of necropsy are also useful for PCR amplification of virus. There is a higher sensitivity by using the PCR on infected tissues as compared with fecal antigen retrieval (Decaro and Elia 2005). In addition, many laboratories offer additional diagnostic methods on tissue samples such as immunofluorescence or immunohistochemistry.

2) Unusual presentation:

   The progression of any disease can vary greatly among affected animals. Among the factors that can alter the "normal" course of disease are co-infections, viral dose and virulence, and/or the animal's age, breed, and clinical presentation.

3) Concurrent disease(s):

   Parvoviral disease, even when suspected or confirmed clinically, may be exacerbated by concurrent infections with bacteria, *Giardia*, hookworms, or other enteric viruses such as coronavirus. Samples should be gathered that can potentially rule concurrent disease either in or out.

5.5.2.2.1 Gross Findings of Parvoviral Disease

The gross findings of parvoviral disease, although caused by a similar virus, manifest somewhat differently in the dog and cat. It would be unlikely that a puppy or adult dog would die suddenly of parvovirus in the absence of dehydration, diarrhea, and other well-documented clinical signs. On the other hand, kittens can die per-acutely of panleukopenia, with no preceding signs noted. On necropsy, dogs commonly have segmental to diffuse sub-serosal hemorrhage (reddening) that predominantly affects the small intestine (See Figure 5.8).

The small intestine can be flaccid and/or dilated. There will be scant ingesta within the intestinal system and no formed feces within the colon. On section of the small intestine, the mucosa is segmentally to multifocally discolored tan to dark red (necrosis, congestion, hemorrhage). Peyer's patches, which are more concentrated in the distal small intestine and ileum, can be dark red (lympholysis).

In cats, the findings can be similar but are usually subtle. The small intestine is flaccid or dilated, but not always reddened, and the GI contents, although typically watery or scarce, do not always contain blood. In both dogs and cats, the mesenteric lymph nodes are enlarged, congested and wet (edematous). Because the effect of panleukopenia on bone marrow and primary lymphoid tissues is quite predictable in the feline form of the disease, it is a good

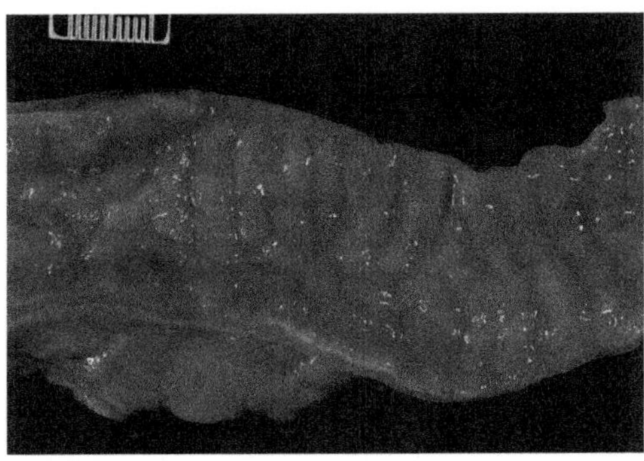

Figure 5.8 Canine parvovirus (CPV). The intestines are segmentally thick, edematous, and hemorrhagic, and the mucosal surface (pictured here) is dull and felt-like.

idea to include these tissues when performing a necropsy on either a dog or a cat.

5.5.3 Respiratory Disease, General

The following collection would be a good starting point for sampling any respiratory disease of unknown origin in dogs or cats. While causes for respiratory distress can be remote from the respiratory system, most cases of infectious pneumonia or upper respiratory infections (URI) result from a direct attack on the respiratory tissues. Gross lesions of the lung are difficult to interpret. This is, in no small part, because there are often peri-mortem lung changes, and such variability makes a baseline interpretation of "normal" very difficult. Histologic samples are of paramount importance when trying to discern factors contributing to lung disease. In cats, in particular, analyzing the upper respiratory tract as well as the lung is important; many common infections of the upper respiratory tract can contribute to fulminant respiratory disease, and severe URI is often interpreted as pneumonia (infection of the lower respiratory system).

1) Microbiology:

   In respiratory disease, depending on the lesions and clinical course, bacterial cultures can be taken from the nasal cavity, frontal sinus (swab immediately after opening) and/or lung. In general, because URI is so common in kittens and cats in a shelter, cultures should be taken from both the nasal cavity/sinus and the lungs. In dogs or cats with a clinical course clearly associated with the lower respiratory tract (pneumonia), lung tissue should be submitted. Accurate culture results require using sterile techniques. During a necropsy, these should be the first specimens taken, and the tissue should be minimally or not manipulated. This can be achieved by using sterile instruments and/or a swab stick, or by placing a piece of tissue directly into a sterile container. It is important to alert the microbiology laboratory that the specimen was taken at the time of necropsy. Antibiotic therapy can skew or prevent the culture of many bacteria. Any pre-mortem therapy should be noted in the submission form and on the necropsy report.

2) Molecular diagnostics:

   Fresh or fresh/frozen lung or upper respiratory tissue samples are necessary to diagnose agents contributing to pneumonia (former) or URI. These samples need to be taken early in the postmortem stage, using sterile technique, and from tissue minimally manipulated. DNA or RNA from the infectious agent will degrade at rates dependent on time, environmental factors (temperature, pH) and the organism itself. Ideally, samples from affected organs are fresh or fresh/frozen for molecular analysis. Most diagnostic laboratories or veterinary schools can offer guidance and a list of possible tests, the preferred or potentially useful tissue samples, and the preferred method of shipment.

3) Formalin-fixed tissues

   Histological samples should be taken in ALL CASES no matter what supplementary diagnostic tests are performed. Histology can provide a definitive diagnosis, identify possible causes, or confirm or refute the results of other diagnostic tests. The following is a general list for sampling an animal with respiratory disease. In nearly all cases, these samples would be sufficient to diagnose or exclude common shelter respiratory pathogens.

5.5.3.1 Tissue Checklist for Respiratory Disease

Tissues should be no thicker than 1 cm. Tissues should be placed immediately in 10% buffered formalin at a ratio of 1 part tissue to 10 parts formalin.

a) Nasal conchae, sinus
b) Trachea, 1-2 cartilage rings

c) Lung, multiple samples, including cranioventral portions of the cranial lobe(s), the caudal and dorsal regions of the caudal lobes and hilar region including major bronchus
d) Hilar lymph nodes, and/or lymph nodes from the thoracic inlet
e) Heart-longitudinal sections including atrium, ventricle and valves from both left and right sides.

5.5.3.2 Common Respiratory Diseases in the Shelter

5.5.3.2.1 Canine Distemper Virus (CDV)
Clinical impressions are rarely sufficient to differentiate canine distemper from other causes of infectious canine respiratory disease. Pre-mortem testing options are limited; serological tests are limited by viral immunosuppression and interference due to maternal or vaccine-induced antibodies and fluorescent antibody (FA) testing (cells from the conjunctiva, blood, respiratory tract epithelium, or urinary bladder) is very specific but has low sensitivity. Another pre-mortem test is PCR (on urine sediment, epithelial swabs, bronchoalveolar lavage, buffy coat preps, or CSF); however, PCR may also detect vaccine virus in recently vaccinated animals and for this reason the use quantitative reverse transcriptase PCR (RT-PCR) is recommended. If an animal dies of suspected distemper, or if the presentation of the disease is unusual and confirmation is necessary, distemper can be identified reliably on necropsy samples and histopathology by a qualified pathologist.

Gross findings: If the lungs are involved, canine distemper virus will be disseminated and affect all lobes. In most cases, oculo-nasal discharges are thick and mucopurulent. The lungs are generally edematous or consolidated (interstitial pneumonia). Thick, foamy to mucopurulent hemorrhagic exudates may be found in the airways. Secondary (bacterial) infection is common, both because of viral damage to the airways and because of lymphoid depletion. Therefore, a cranioventral distribution of lung consolidation (bronchopneumonia) does NOT rule out distemper. Lymphoreticular tissues are characteristically involved and are the primary site for viral replication. There can be enlargement of the tonsils and/or atrophy of the thymus. Hyperkeratosis ("hardpad disease") of the nose and/or footpads is sporadically present. There are no gross lesions of the central nervous system even when nervous signs are uniquely present. The heart should always be examined, opened, and sampled when investigating respiratory outbreaks; right heart failure (e.g. as a result of heartworm disease) often poses clinically as respiratory distress.

Histopathology: In addition to the list above for general respiratory disease, histopathologic samples useful in the diagnosis of CDV include the brain and bladder. Samples submitted for histology and paraffin-embedded are also used for immunohistochemistry, which is one of the definitive methods of identifying CDV induced respiratory and/or neurologic disease.

Molecular diagnostics: PCR can be used to detect virus in lung, CSF, feces, or urine. False positives are possible within one to three weeks of vaccination. The diagnostic laboratory should be consulted regarding testing details.

5.5.3.2.2 Canine Infectious Respiratory Disease (CIRD, "Kennel Cough," Multiple Agents) Canine infectious respiratory disease is caused by a combination of both viral and bacterial agents. The range of morbidity and mortality can be attributed to several problems, including husbandry, but in ANY case, knowing the spectrum of infectious agents that are contributing to the disease is helpful in identifying problems, developing isolation procedures and ongoing therapy. Many laboratories offer tests for common agents of CIRD, though new bacterial and viral agents continue to be identified. Confirmation of specific causative agent(s), whether novel or typical, requires a combination of histology, microbiology, and (for the viral component) PCR or virus isolation. Histology (including PCR or immunohistochemistry) is also necessary to rule in/out viruses as contributory or causative in an outbreak of respiratory disease.

Gross findings: The gross lesions of CIRD typically reflect the aerogenous introduction of bacteria into the pulmonary tissues. The lungs are congested and consolidated, most consistently within the cranial and ventral portions of the cranial lobes. There can be pleural mottling that may involve multiple lobes. Depending upon whether a viral component is acute or chronic, the bronchopneumonia could be superimposed on a more diffuse pattern of lung involvement (interstitial pneumonia). The thoracic cavity should be examined for excessive pericardial and thoracic fluid production (normal is less than 5 ml in both cavities), +/− concurrent pericarditis and pleuritis.

Histological, microbiological (lung), and molecular diagnostic (lung) samples should be taken according to the general respiratory disease protocol above.

5.5.3.2.3 Canine Influenza: (CIV) As with most viral diseases, it can be difficult to determine the role of a virus in a clinical event. Reliable diagnosis of many viral diseases by serology requires both acute and convalescent serum samples. Virus detection by PCR in respiratory secretions from acutely ill or recently exposed animals is possible, but false negatives are not uncommon. The Becton-Dickinson Flu-A ELISA test may also be used on nasal secretions from acutely affected animals. While the mortality rate of canine influenza is fairly low (5–8%), if an animal does die or is euthanized with respiratory disease, the most accurate test for the virus is a PCR test of respiratory tissue. This, combined with histological features of viral-induced pneumonia, would be the "gold-standard" for the presence, and effect, of the virus. In several identified cases of CIV, there was a concurrent and severe bacterial pneumonia, so samples for culture and antibiotic sensitivity should be concurrently submitted.

Gross findings: Influenza virus will be hematogenously disseminated (affect all lobes). The lungs can be hemorrhagic or consolidated (interstitial pneumonia). Again, lungs are among the most difficult of organs in which to detect gross changes; histological analysis is of paramount importance in evaluating the sequelae of the virus and/or co-infections in the lungs. The tissue collection protocol that was elaborated for respiratory disease sample collection should be followed.

PCR: Fresh, or fresh frozen respiratory tissue is always best, but RNA extracted from paraffin-embedded tissues has been used to detect the virus. Laboratories that offer this type of testing are limited but will accept samples by courier. Some specific instructions are listed below.

US:

https://www.idexx.com/en/veterinary/reference-laboratories/canine-feline-influenza

California:

https://pcrlab.vetmed.ucdavis.edu/veterinary-diagnostics

New York:

https://ahdc-portal.vet.cornell.edu/#!/test_fee/search

Wisconsin:

https://www.wvdl.wisc.edu/index.php/canine-influenza-information-for-veterinarians

5.5.3.2.4 Feline infectious respiratory disease (FIRD) (Upper respiratory infection (URI)) FIRD is typically multifactorial, and, like CIRD, recognition of the contributory infectious agents can be very helpful in organizing a response. Moreover, unusual agents, or unusually virulent agents have plagued some shelters. The most commonly recognized agents involved in infections limited to the upper respiratory tract are feline calicivirus (FCV), feline herpesvirus (FHV1), *Mycoplasma*, *Chlamydia*, and occasionally *B. bronchiseptica* (Pesavento and Murphy 2014). Other bacterial organisms such as *Streptococcus canis* have also and more recently been described in outbreak situations (Pesavento et al. 2007). Nasal swabs can be performed postmortem, and sampling in an outbreak of severe FIRD should include the histological samples described in the general section on respiratory disease. Many diagnostic laboratories now offer PCR panels for the most common organisms associated with FIRD. Nonetheless, the presence of the pathogen does not always imply causation, and concurrent culture and histology can be very helpful in identifying the cause. Gross assessment cannot distinguish among even the most common agents involved in FIRD, however, it is helpful to note the character of the nasal conchae, lungs, and whether or what type of fluid is present within the sinuses.

5.6 Other Shelter Necropsies

5.6.1 Necropsy on a Previously Healthy Animal Found Dead

5.6.1.1 Acute Death

Common causes of acute death, with special attention to possible shelter situations or submissions are anaphylaxis, physical trauma (with neurologic or hemorrhagic consequences), intestinal malpositions (volvulus, intussusception), cardiomyopathy, electrocution (lightning or chewing on electric cords), gunshot, drowning, septicemia, heatstroke, dehydration, or ingestion of toxins or poisons (plant or synthetic, including disinfectants). Note that the most common cause of acute death in incompletely vaccinated shelter cats is panleukopenia. While some of these conditions may be obvious on gross necropsy (physical trauma, intestinal malpositions, gunshot, cardiomyopathy), in others histopathology is useful (e.g. some toxins, septicemia); still others are unlikely to have either gross or histological lesions (e.g. anaphylaxis, dehydration, electrocution, some toxins, heat stroke). Even in this latter subset, a gross necropsy effectively rules out most possible causes of disease. In all cases, diagnosis requires a good history to arrive at the definitive diagnosis.

5.6.2 Feline Infectious Peritonitis (FIP)

There is no single, predictable target organ for feline infectious peritonitis (FIP). The virus widely (systemically) disseminates in macrophages, and the clinical outcome is dependent on both the host immunity and the specific organ affected. Histopathology on biopsy or necropsy specimens remains the gold standard for diagnosis. Many of the pre-mortem tests, and especially a cumulative amount of information, can be highly suggestive of the disease. If an animal dies or is euthanized with suspect FIP, a necropsy with histology would be diagnostic.

Gross findings: In the effusive form, there will be fluid within either or both the thoracic and abdominal cavities. The fluid is high in protein and may vary from slightly viscous to gelatinous. The surfaces of the viscera are covered with tiny (1–5 mm) friable, pale tan to white plaques (fibrin) that can give the surfaces a granular appearance (See Figure 5.9).

In the non-effusive (chronic) form, there will be nodules (granulomas) of variable size

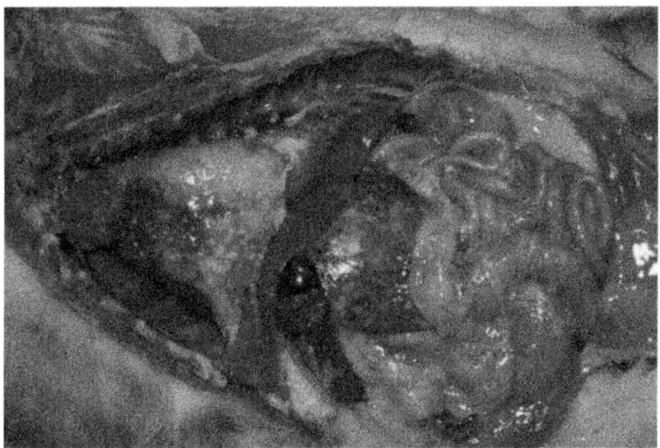

Figure 5.9 Feline infectious peritonitis (FIP) virus (feline coronavirus). In the effusive form of FIP, along with intracavitary fluid, the surfaces of abdominal and thoracic viscera are covered with small (1–2 mm) to coalescing pale tan plaques.

present in one or multiple organs. These can vary in color from off white to light tan, in texture from slightly firm to soft. The nodules are typically associated with capsular or serosal vessels, although when abundant this can be difficult to distinguish. Within organs, the granulomas can be scattered throughout the parenchyma. Lymph nodes are often enlarged.

Formalin-fixed tissues: Samples should be taken from affected organs (in the case of the non-effusive form, this would be any viscera with detectable granulomas). In the case of the effusive form, multiple samples should be taken from affected viscera (liver, GI, lung). If the clinical presentation is limited to the nervous system and FIP is suspected, it is imperative to submit the brain. Brain lesions are, however, rarely uniquely present.

5.7 Conclusion

It is impossible to provide necropsy guidelines for every infectious disease encountered in shelter animals—therefore a few characteristic diseases were selected. It is hoped that the information in this chapter will enable the shelter veterinarian to work more closely with pathologists and microbiologists to develop good shelter surveillance programs. This chapter should aid veterinarians in collecting samples so that the pathologist and the diagnostic laboratory can analyze and diagnose problems more accurately. Necropsy has multiple potential roles in shelter animal health: it is a method to detect disease, to establish the cause of death, to assess diagnostic suitability in a single animal, and as a source of knowledge to apply to future cases.

References

American Society for the Prevention of Cruelty to Animals (2017). Are Anmal Shelter Outcomes Improving? https://www.aspca.org/blog/are-animal-shelter-outcomes-improving (accessed 4 August 2020).

Decaro, N. and Elia, G. (2005). A real-time PCR assay for rapid detection and quantitation of canine parvovirus type 2 in the feces of dogs. *Veterinary Microbiology* 105 (1): 19–28. http://www.fedex.com/us/packaging/guides/Clinical_fxcom.pdf.

Greene, C.E. (ed.) (2011). Infectious Diseases of the Dog and Cat. St. Louis: Saunders-Elsevier.

Pesavento, P.A. and Murphy, B.G. (2014). *Common and emerging infectious diseases in the animal shelter. Veterinary Pathology* 51 (2): 478–479.

Pesavento, P.A., Bannasch, M.J. et al. (2007). Fatal Streptococcus canis infections in intensively housed shelter cats. *Veterinary Pathology* 44 (2): 218–221.

6

Outbreak Management

Jeanette O'Quin

The Ohio State University, Columbus, OH, USA

6.1 Introduction

By their very nature, animal shelters generate conditions that foster the transmission of infectious diseases and are therefore highly vulnerable to disease outbreaks. When outbreaks that begin or are amplified in the shelter spread outside of the shelter they can have far-reaching impacts on both animals and people (Schorr-Evans et al. 2003; Van Immerseel et al. 2004; Wright et al. 2005). Early disease detection and response can lessen the consequences when preventive measures fail.

Outbreaks of uncommon but serious pathogens such as *Streptococcus equi* subspecies zooepidemicus and virulent systemic feline calicivirus (VS-FVC) have resulted in both high morbidity and mortality with devastating consequences (Hurley 2004; Byun et al. 2009). Similarly, outbreaks of more common pathogens such as feline panleukopenia (FPV), canine parvovirus (CPV), and canine distemper (CDV) have led to widespread effects in both the shelter and the community (Lamm and Rezabek 2008; Goddard and Leisewitz 2010; Newbury et al. 2010).

Less obvious, yet equally damaging, are outbreaks of ubiquitous diseases such as feline infectious respiratory disease (FIRD) and canine infectious respiratory disease (CIRD) complex. Though rarely fatal, a higher than expected number of cases would constitute an outbreak, as would an expected number of cases with a greater percentage developing a more protracted or serious course of illness, such as pneumonia. If not handled properly, outbreaks can continue for weeks, months or even years, taxing a shelter's resources and threatening the public's confidence in the quality of care provided by the shelter.

The pathogens most likely to cause outbreaks in shelters are discussed elsewhere throughout this textbook along with disease-specific prevention and control strategies. Cases of infectious disease in a shelter can be introduced from the community through sporadic cases or as spillover from an outbreak. They can also occur through recrudescence (i.e. reactivation), or from exposures that occur in the shelter. Regardless of the source, it is the shelter's responsibility to prevent these cases from becoming an outbreak and to prevent them from spreading disease back into the community.

Infectious Disease Management in Animal Shelters, Second Edition.
Edited by Lila Miller, Stephanie Janeczko, and Kate F. Hurley.

This chapter will discuss the broader concepts of outbreak management and demonstrate their application to the recognition, investigation, and management of infectious disease outbreaks in animal shelters.

6.2 Infectious Disease Outbreaks

An outbreak is defined as a greater number of cases than would normally be expected at a given place and time and/or a marked increase in the severity or duration of signs. For a disease that is not endemic, (i.e. not normally found in that shelter) the identification of a single case may warrant an outbreak response in order to prevent additional spread. It is more challenging to recognize an outbreak of an endemic disease because some background level of infection is expected. Historic trends in that facility can be helpful for comparison; however, shelters should also check with industry guidelines and contact similar facilities to request their infection rates. Outbreaks that have continued unchecked for months to years should not be used to determine an acceptable level of a specific disease. See Chapter 3 for more information on data surveillance.

6.3 Infectious Disease and Outbreak Response Plan

Every shelter should have a written infectious disease and outbreak response plan, and all staff should be familiar with their specific role(s). Since housing options, disease risks, and available resources vary among shelters, there is no one-size-fits-all plan. What is effective for one shelter could be disastrous if implemented in another. Sample plans and templates (e.g. those available from university-based shelter medicine programs and national animal welfare organizations) are valuable planning aids provided they are customized with details specific to the shelter in which they will be used.

Comprehensive plans should include the shelter's infectious disease policy, outbreak management plan, and disease-specific protocols (Figure 6.1). An infectious disease policy outlines which diseases or conditions the shelter will treat and under what circumstances. These policies should be based in part on the shelter's mission, but also on the additional resources available including funding, suitable treatment space, and the skilled human resources needed to provide appropriate care (Hurley and Baldwin 2008).

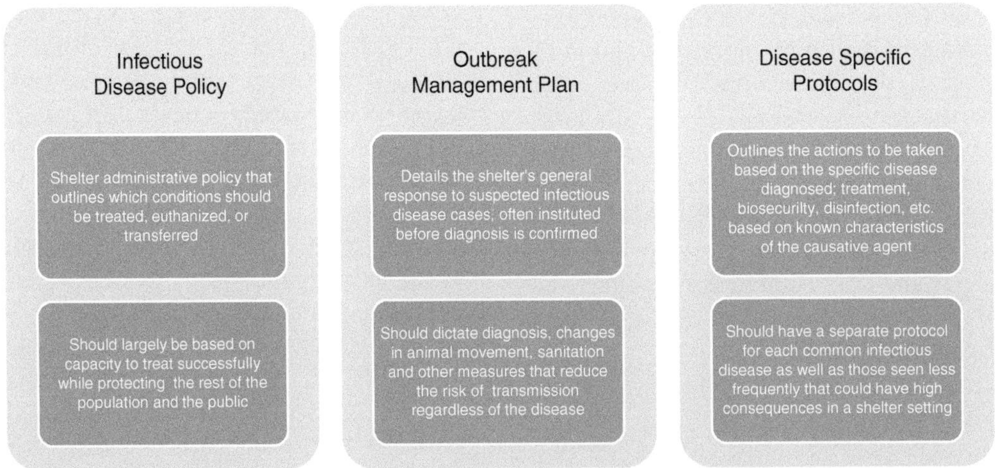

Figure 6.1 Components of an infectious disease and outbreak management plan.

These resources need to be made available without compromising care or services provided to the general population. For each disease, the shelter's policy should detail what animals will be treated, euthanized, transferred to another facility, or treated offsite (e.g. veterinary hospital, skilled foster care). Several other factors that may influence the shelter's approach to a specific disease should also be considered. These may include the number of animals affected, the severity of disease in an individual, and the presence of other health or behavioral concerns. For example, two cases of CPV may be within a shelter's capacity for care, but that same shelter may not be able to manage 20 cases or a single case that has developed pneumonia and requires oxygen therapy. The policy should describe circumstances that influence decisions to treat as well as how those decisions will be made. Considerations for developing an infectious disease policy can be found in Table 6.1. Because this information will guide the development of outbreak management plans and disease-specific protocols, this policy should be the first step toward completing an infectious disease and outbreak management plan.

When an adverse health event is recognized, the exact cause may not initially be known. For this reason, outbreak management plans should be broad-based and applicable to any potential infectious disease situation. With the primary goals of diagnosis and prevention of disease transmission, they should detail the specific actions to be taken by the shelter. It is recommended to consider the worst-case scenario with respect to the unknown pathogen's ability to spread, survive in the environment, and withstand disinfection. At a minimum, plans should include the identification and segregation of sick (and sometimes exposed) animals, control of fomite and staff movements, and enhancement of sanitation efforts. Ideally, specific staff positions should be identified as responsible for the implementation of the various components. Key considerations to help guide the development of an effective outbreak management plan can be found in Table 6.2.

Table 6.1 Considerations for infectious disease policies.

How contagious is this disease to other animals, including other species?
How contagious is this disease to people?
What percentage of the shelter population is susceptible to this disease?
How is this disease transmitted and can the shelter effectively prevent it?
How difficult is it to eliminate from the environment through cleaning and disinfection?
How severe is this disease, what are the welfare concerns during treatment?
What is the prognosis or likelihood for recovery?
How long is recovery expected to take?
Can the shelter effectively treat this disease with minimal risk to animals and people?
Does the shelter have the space, staffing, and funding to treat this disease without compromising basic care provided to the general population?
Is the shelter able to place the majority of similar animals that do not have this disease?
In what circumstances will cases of disease typically treated in the facility be euthanized or sent elsewhere for treatment (e.g. severity of signs, behavior concerns, over capacity, etc.)?
How many animals are affected; is this within your capacity for care for this disease?
What off-site options can be made available (veterinary hospital, foster care, etc.) for effective treatment of this disease?

Table 6.2 Considerations for outbreak management plans.

Describe what constitutes an unusual health event and how it should be reported for further medical evaluation
Designate persons to whom unusual health events should be reported, outline the chain of communication and the authority for decision making
Summarize diagnostic options and identify laboratories for testing, including specific test recommendations based on the clinical signs present
Increase frequency of medical walk-throughs to identify additional cases and separate them from the general population, if warranted
In some cases (e.g. specific signs or large numbers affected) it may be necessary to stop all movement of animals until diagnosis is made and/or exposures are identified
Designate separate areas for isolation of clinical animals and for quarantine of healthy but meaningfully exposed animals, and determine their capacity
Establish isolation and quarantine protocols (PPE, fomite reduction, etc.), restrict human and animal traffic in these areas to the minimum required to provide necessary care
Identify alternative options should isolation and quarantine capacity be exceeded (e.g. repurpose other areas in the facility, off-site treatment, transfer, foster care, euthanasia)
Increase frequency of cleaning and disinfection; base disinfection on an easily transmitted and difficult to kill pathogen (e.g. parvovirus) until the disease is identified
Adjust schedules to prevent staff from working with susceptible populations after working with animals that are exposed or sick
Plan for additional staff time that will be needed to provide proper medical care, ensure humane conditions, and perform additional cleaning and disinfection tasks
Develop a system to inform and educate staff and volunteers so that all understand the outbreak protocols that are being implemented
Outline data collection needed to monitor the health event and aid in decision making, identify responsible party for record keeping
Set parameters for determining when it may be necessary to suspend certain functions (e.g. services for owned animals, off-site events, intake, adoptions)
Establish MOUs with animal care partners (e.g. shelters, veterinary clinics, rescues) that could provide assistance if needed (e.g. divert intake, provide off-site care)
Determine when and how the public and/or other animal care partners in the community should be notified of an outbreak
Develop a media communication plan and designate a spokesperson for the shelter

PPE-Personal Protective Equipment
MOU-Memorandum of Understanding

Efforts should be made to obtain a timely diagnosis so that disease-specific protocols can be initiated. These protocols are more detailed and based on the known characteristics of the pathogen. Protocols should include prevention measures, recommended treatment, management of animals that were meaningfully exposed, and length of time after resolution of clinical signs before the animal can be made available for surgery or adoption. Disease-specific protocols may be comprehensive and separate from the outbreak management plan, or they can be addendums to the plan, describing just the additions or deviations from the plan that are needed based on the pathogen. Considerations for developing disease-specific protocols can be found in Table 6.3.

Shelters should develop disease-specific protocols for all of the common infectious diseases

Table 6.3 Considerations for disease specific protocols.

Description of clinical signs and typical progression of disease to aid in recognition
Susceptible species and zoonotic potential
Effectiveness of vaccine (if one is available), recommended type (killed, MLV, etc.) and duration to onset of immunity
Mode (direct contact, fomite/indirect contact, airborne, droplet, vector borne) and ease of transmission
Infectious dose (the amount of a pathogen needed to cause infection)
Incubation period (the time between exposure and the appearance of the clinical signs)
Shedding periods, the length of time an infected animal is contagious before clinical signs develop (preclinical) and following resolution of disease (post clinical)
Subclinical shedding, i.e. the likelihood that animals will be contagious without developing clinical signs
Durability and longevity of the pathogen in the environment, including kennels, foster homes, and outdoor walk areas if relevant
Sanitation practices specific to this pathogen, including recommendations for personal protective equipment (PPE) and disinfectant type, frequency, dilution and contact time
Where animals with signs should be held pending diagnosis, where they will be isolated after diagnosis and who is authorized to handle them
Recommended screening and confirmatory diagnostic tests
If (depends on the pathogen) and how to identify animals that were exposed (depends on mode of transmission, proximity to infected animal, and other management practices)
Assessment of exposed animals to determine meaningful risk (e.g. titer testing, species, vaccination status, etc.) and appropriate quarantine of those meaningfully exposed
Treatment options and expected recovery time
Circumstances, if any, which would warrant interruption of services (e.g. intake, adoption, direct service to the public, etc.)

in their shelter and community. Additionally, it is recommended to have protocols for high-consequence diseases that could be introduced to the shelter. Some diseases to consider include:

- Canine parvovirus (CPV)
- Canine distemper virus (CDV)
- Canine infectious respiratory disease (CIRD)
- Canine influenza virus (CIV)
- Rabies
- Ringworm
- Feline panleukopenia (FPV)
- Feline infectious respiratory disease (FIRD)
- Feline leukemia virus (FeLV)
- Feline immunodeficiency virus (FIV)
- Feline coronavirus (FECV/FIP)
- *Tritrichomonas fetus*
- *Giardia spp.*
- *Coccidia spp.*
- *Campylobacter spp.*
- *Salmonella spp.*
- *Streptococcus zooepidemicus*
- *Leptospira spp.*
- *Brucella canis*
- Sarcoptic mange
- Multidrug-resistant bacterial infections
- Other infectious diseases relevant to your shelter

Shelters should develop their infectious disease and outbreak management plans when they are not in the midst of an outbreak. During a crisis, time is not available to fully evaluate the options and decisions tend to be driven by emotions. Planning allows management to identify needs and find ways to increase the shelter's life-saving capacity. For example, a shelter that currently has no place to effectively isolate highly infectious animals could repurpose another space in the shelter, recruit skilled foster care providers willing and able to house and treat animals, or establish a memorandum of understanding (MOU) with another shelter or veterinary clinic to provide treatment.

Having detailed plans in place will facilitate decision making when saving time is of the utmost importance. These plans should be reviewed and revised regularly to ensure they remain relevant and reflect the best use of the shelter's available resources. Shelters should ensure that the infectious disease and outbreak management plan covers prevention, detection, investigation, and response activities.

6.4 Outbreak Prevention

Traditional herd biosecurity measures such as limiting the turnover of animals, acquiring new animals from a disease-free source, ensuring that all incoming animals have been tested and received appropriate preventive medical care prior to arrival, and limiting human traffic through the facility are not reasonable given the mission of most shelters (Hurley and Baldwin 2012). Outbreak prevention in shelters, therefore, relies heavily upon infection control strategies designed to strengthen individual resistance to disease and minimize exposure to pathogens. These strategies include vaccination and prophylactic deworming at (or before) intake; separation by species and health status, treatment of pre-existing conditions, provision of suitable nutrition, effective sanitation, adequate exercise and appropriate enriched housing, as well as other measures that alleviate stress and ensure both physical and mental well-being. Failure to meet these needs can elevate disease incidence and outbreak potential. (More information on these measures can be found in Chapters 1, 2, 8, and 9.)

Animals with signs of infectious disease on intake should be isolated immediately rather than placed in the general population. Timely recognition and segregation of potentially contagious animals will reduce the risk of disease spread. For this reason, it is recommended that medical staff member(s) walk through the shelter at least once a day to perform rounds to visually observe animals for signs of illness (Newbury et al. 2010). Training all staff to recognize the common clinical and behavioral signs of disease will increase the timely detection of sick animals, and disease reporting will be improved when staff fully understand why this is essential to the continued health and welfare of sheltered animals.

Quarantining healthy animals on intake to make sure they are not incubating an infection, has not been a successful method of disease reduction in shelters (Hurley and Baldwin 2012), and is not recommended as a general practice. A prolonged length of stay, for any reason, has been associated with increased risk of disease in shelters (Newbury and Hurley 2012). Some intake circumstances present a higher risk of disease transmission to shelter populations and may warrant a quarantine of those specific animals. For example, an outbreak of disease in the community animal population may result in a higher percentage of exposed and infected animals being admitted to the shelter. Similarly, animals entering from a known high-risk source, such as an animal hoarding or disaster response situation may present a greater risk to the general population. In situations where the risk is known to be higher, quarantine of animals from those specific locations may be warranted. At the same time, the risk associated with prolonged length of stay from routine quarantine must be balanced against the risk of disease in incoming animals.

Perhaps the most insidious and preventable risk factor for shelter disease outbreaks is overcrowding. The deleterious effects resulting in a higher disease burden are well known and cannot be overcome by even the most comprehensive healthcare program (Newbury and Hurley 2012). A shelter's capacity for care is not simply based upon the number of housing units in the facility. Among other factors, determinants of capacity include the number of animals admitted and their duration of stay, the size and condition of the housing, and staffing levels and training (Newbury et al. 2010). Methods for determining a shelter's capacity for care are further detailed in Chapter 1.

Although housing too many animals is often undertaken with the best of intentions to save more lives, this management decision compromises the health and welfare of the entire shelter population. Animals housed in overcrowded conditions are more stressed which reduces their immune system's ability to fight off infection. Additionally, the increase in animal density leads to more opportunities for contact between animals, an increase in pathogens shed into the environment, and a reduced ability to adequately clean and disinfect the environment. Overcrowding increases the likelihood of disease outbreaks and interferes with disease control strategies, ultimately negatively impacting lifesaving efforts.

In addition to causing animal suffering, an increase in disease can damage an organization's standing in the community, leading to fewer adoptions and further perpetuating the vicious cycle of overcrowding, stress, and disease. A heavy financial and emotional toll is also exacted on the shelter and its staff who are already at risk for compassion fatigue.

6.5 Outbreak Detection

Early identification and rapid implementation of planned interventions can reduce the duration and severity of a disease outbreak, thereby lessening its potential impact. Some outbreaks are so unexpected or severe that they are hard to miss. Others, however, may not be apparent without the benefit of ongoing disease surveillance.

Data collected over time on the incidence of various diseases in a shelter population can be used to determine whether the current caseloads represent a departure from expected levels or merely reflect a normal fluctuation in the background disease burden. Several methods of tracking these statistics are available and can be facilitated using commercially available shelter software programs as well as standard programs such as Microsoft Excel.

Unusual health events such as serious illness, uncommon signs, unexplained death, or an increase in the number of illnesses, should be reported and recorded. Clinical signs commonly associated with infectious disease (e.g. sneezing, ocular, and nasal discharges, fever, diarrhea, hair loss) should also be reported for follow-up management. Determining, in advance, exactly what needs to be reported and to whom is essential for effective, timely management and this information should be included in the infectious disease and outbreak management plan. An animal found dead in the cage, for example, should be a rare event that is required to be reported so that the cause of death can be determined. For endemic shelter diseases, it may be useful to establish a reporting threshold so that the occurrence of a specific number of cases in a given time period will trigger an investigation. This is a more objective assessment than relying on memory and the perception of what *seems* like more than the usual number of cases. Not every event will be an outbreak or even an infectious disease; however, vigilance will ensure timely outbreak detection that helps to maintain a healthy shelter population. (See Chapter 3.)

6.6 Outbreak Investigation

When an outbreak is suspected, the nature and cause of the illness should be determined in order to guide appropriate interventions. While the primary goals during an outbreak are to alleviate suffering and halt the spread of disease, properly conducted investigations can also provide information that assists in the prevention of future occurrences.

Many questions need to be answered during an outbreak investigation. These include:

- What is the cause of the disease?
- How is the disease transmitted?
- How many animals are affected?
- When and where were the current cases exposed?
- What are the risk factors for infection?

Both clinical and epidemiologic methods are employed during an outbreak investigation. Though some key components of an investigation are described here in a seemingly logical order, in practice, these often occur simultaneously rather than sequentially.

6.6.1 Define and Identify Cases

In order to connect a case to an outbreak under investigation, a standard set of criteria must first be defined. Identifying cases that are part of the outbreak is an essential investigatory step. There should also be some focus on the detection of earlier cases since the first case to be recognized may not have been the first to occur. Depending on the disease, canvassing community partners such as other shelters and veterinary clinics may be warranted to determine if shelter cases are part of a much larger outbreak.

A case definition should be developed based on specific clinical signs and diagnostic tests as well as epidemiologic criteria such as time and location. Counting all dogs with diarrhea, while an effective way to detect potential outbreaks by syndromic surveillance of diarrheal illness patterns, would be too inclusive to define cases in an outbreak of CPV. (Syndromic surveillance uses specific symptoms such as diarrhea or sneezing to help identify potential outbreaks and signal the need for additional diagnostics.)

A sample CPV case definition follows: all dogs housed in Shelter A between March 15, 2021 and August 31, 2021 with compatible clinical signs (e.g. lethargy, inappetence, ±vomiting, diarrhea ±blood), and a known exposure or a positive diagnostic finding (e.g. fecal antigen test, pronounced leukopenia or pathognomonic necropsy lesions). If a positive fecal antigen test had been required by this case definition, the dogs with false negative test results would have been excluded from the case count. Ideally, the case definition will be structured to include all cases related to the outbreak while excluding those that are unrelated.

No case definition is perfect, and revisions based on new findings or changing investigatory needs may be warranted. Revision of the initial definition may be indicated, for example, when the outbreak cause is confirmed or when investigators wish to differentiate between cases acquired in the community and those acquired in the shelter. As an investigation progresses, modifications may be made to expand or narrow the case definition as long as all cases in the outbreak are included based on the same criteria.

6.6.2 Diagnosis

Another critical step in an outbreak investigation is identifying the causative agent. An initial list of differential diagnoses or a tentative diagnosis may be based on the clinical presentation including the type and severity of signs, course of illness, morbidity, mortality, and other associated factors. This can be used to guide the selection of appropriate diagnostics and the implementation of initial control measures. Diseases most likely to be found in shelter animals should be considered before exploring those that are considered rare or unusual. Co-morbidity, or simultaneous infection by more than one pathogen, can complicate the situation, making both diagnosis and outbreak management more difficult.

Even if the diagnosis seems obvious based on clinical signs, verification is necessary. Atypical disease presentations are more common in a shelter environment (Hurley and Baldwin 2012) and some of the more virulent pathogens have nonspecific signs that can be easily confused with other more common diseases. For example, initial assumptions that an outbreak of unusually severe CIRD is canine influenza may be proven incorrect when diagnostic testing reveals other respiratory pathogen(s) at fault. Conversely, a sudden increase in cases of canine respiratory disease that is assumed to be an outbreak of endemic CIRD may be proven incorrect when testing confirms CDV. Without a proper diagnosis, these two situations could result in treatment and control measures that were unnecessary or inadequate.

In addition to identifying the causative agent of an outbreak, various diagnostic tools can be used to establish a link with seemingly unrelated cases, confirm new cases, identify a common source, detect at-risk animals, assess environmental contamination, and evaluate the effectiveness of treatment and prevention measures.

6.6.3 Data Collection

Systematic data collection and analysis are the foundation of an outbreak investigation and should include both time and location of disease occurrences, as well as descriptive information about each diseased animal. When coupled with a comparison of affected versus unaffected animals, factors associated with infection and populations at risk can be identified. While a diagnosis is being sought, this information can guide initial control measures and even assist in determining the cause of an outbreak. Ongoing monitoring can be used to evaluate the effectiveness of intervention strategies and keep decision-makers and community partners, including the media if needed, apprised of the status of an outbreak.

Data collection starts with complete shelter records that document an animal's history if available, health, medical care, and location in the shelter from intake to final disposition. Creating a table of cases associated with the outbreak that includes pertinent information about each case, commonly called a line list, facilitates investigation and will assist in the epidemiologic analysis of temporal and spatial distribution patterns. Each row represents a single case and each column represents an important variable. The information included in a line list may vary based on the disease being investigated but, in general, should include the animal's identification (ID) number, sexual status, age, intake date, vaccine type and date if relevant, date of disease onset, signs observed, method of diagnosis, location at the time of diagnosis, and the final outcome. Some shelters may also want to record the length of time to recovery in order to examine the impact of extended stays on housing capacity. An example of a disease outbreak tracking form can be found in Appendix 6.A.

6.7 Outbreak Epidemiology

Epidemiology is the study of the distribution and determinants of health-related events in a population, and the application of this study to the control of health problems (WHO 2010). It is largely based on the understanding that most diseases do not occur randomly but are related to complex interactions of environmental and individual host factors that vary by location, time, and the subgroup of a population.

While clinical assessment and diagnostics can identify the causative agent, epidemiology can be used to detect patterns and examine causal relationships between potential risk factors and outcomes. Some questions to be answered include who is affected, why them, and why not others? Even in the absence of a known cause, epidemiology can help identify variables that increase or decrease the individual risk of disease, and this information can be used to help prevent new cases.

Infectious disease data can be summarized in several ways. Descriptive epidemiology organizes the data with respect to the animal, place, and time in an effort to answer the questions *who*, *what*, *where*, and *when*. Animal data such as species, breed, age, sex, recent use of medications, and vaccination status at the time of exposure, may be used to describe the affected population.

Location is often related to disease exposure so stratifying cases by location or creating a spot map of case distribution within a facility or room may provide information on the geographic extent and origin of the outbreak. Graphs, such as epidemic curves described below, are commonly used to depict frequency trends over time and to compare disease incidence in subpopulations.

Statistics commonly used to describe and quantify disease frequency include morbidity, mortality, incidence, and prevalence. (See Chapter 3.) When investigating an outbreak, the importance of comparing unaffected to affected individuals should not be overlooked. Analytic epidemiology compares subgroups based on various outcomes and risk factors in an effort to answer the questions *why* and *how*. Measures of association such as relative risk and odds ratios, and measures of potential impact, such as risk ratio and attributable fraction, can be calculated to further characterize the relationship between disease determinants and illness. Since shelters are typically dealing with a defined population of animals, calculation of attack rates can be a useful way to analyze possible contributing factors.

6.7.1 Attack Rates

Comparisons made between affected and unaffected groups based on specific known exposure criteria can provide information vital to the identification of potential disease contributors. First, a table should be constructed with a row for each suspected source or contributing factor requiring analysis, and columns for ill, well, the sum of ill and well, and attack rate. The columns should be repeated under both exposed and unexposed headings (Table 6.4). Attack rates, which are actually proportions, can then be calculated by dividing the number of ill animals by the sum of ill and well for each column. The factors that have most likely played a role in the outbreak will have the greatest difference in attack rates between exposed and unexposed groups.

As an example, consider a shelter experiencing an outbreak of CPV. Eighty dogs were housed in the shelter's two wards, A and B; 40 of them met the outbreak case definition that included the onset of illness between November 1st and November 31st. In this example, 39 (49%) had been vaccinated with a modified live CPV vaccine prior to arrival; the other 51% were vaccinated between 16 and 36 hours following arrival. Based on available information, the investigators selected a few risk factors they believed might be contributing to the outbreak, and calculated attack rates to test their hypotheses. (Table 6.5)

Table 6.4 Parvovirus attack rates (AR) for 80 shelter dogs.

	Exposed				Unexposed			
	Ill	Well	Total	AR%	Ill	Well	Total	AR%
Risk Factor	a	b	a + b	a/(a + b)	c	d	c + d	c/(c + d)
Housed in Ward A	22	28	50	44%	18	12	30	60%
From zip 12345	36	20	56	64%	4	20	24	17%
Vaccinated prior to arrival	6	33	39	15%	34	7	41	83%
Arrived in control van	20	20	40	50%	20	20	40	50%

Table 6.5 Parvovirus attack rate (AR) for 41 shelter dogs not vaccinated prior to arrival.

	Exposed				Unexposed			
	Ill	Well	Total	AR%	Ill	Well	Total	AR%
Risk Factor	a	b	a+b	a/(a+b)	c	d	c+d	c/(c+d)
From zip 12345	33	3	36	92%	1	4	5	20%

As presented in Table 6.4, vaccination prior to arrival at the shelter shows a substantial difference in attack rates (15%, 83%), which supports what is known about the efficacy of vaccination against parvovirus. Being housed in Ward A shows a moderate difference in attack rates (44%, 60%) indicating a greater proportion of cases in Ward B. Arrival in an animal control van shows no difference (50%, 50%). Those from zip code 12345 demonstrate a marked difference (64%, 17%), not unlike that seen with vaccination prior to arrival.

As is often the case, multiple factors are interacting. The data summarized in Table 6.4 suggest that a community outbreak in zip code 12345 is the likely source of exposure; however, the difference in attack rates was likely tempered by the highly protective nature of vaccination. To look closer at this interaction, another attack rate was calculated for zip code 12345 exposure using only the subpopulation of dogs that were not vaccinated prior to arrival (Table 6.4). Without this confounder, the difference in attack rates is even more dramatic (92%, 20%). Several potential recommendations can follow from this epidemiologic analysis: Dogs being surrendered from zip code 12345 should be quarantined on arrival, nonclinical dogs from zip code 12345 should be titer tested to assess protective antibody titers (PAT), community awareness and/or free vaccination clinics could be offered in zip code 12345.

Additionally, the table shows that all but 4 of the 40 infected dogs came from zip code 12345. The cases that were not from zip code 12345 could represent community-acquired cases or, perhaps more worrisome, secondary transmission of parvovirus within the shelter. Secondary cases occur from exposure to primary cases, and tertiary cases from exposure to secondary cases. In this example, this would indicate that new cases were being acquired in the shelter. This is important to ascertain as it likely represents a failure in biosecurity and sanitation.

Examining the time interval between arrival at the shelter and the onset of disease may aid in differentiating community from shelter exposure sources. If this outbreak were to progress with secondary and tertiary cases, the link to zip code 12345 would likely not be as apparent in an analysis of the entire outbreak. For this reason, examining the onset of the outbreak separately may provide information that would otherwise be obscured by disease propagation within the shelter.

As a final note, attack rate comparisons can provide valuable information, but they do not always represent a causal relationship. Results must be interpreted within the context of the actual body of knowledge. A significant difference in attack rates, for example, may be found if patterned versus solid coat color were to be listed as a possible exposure.

6.7.2 Epidemic (Epi) Curves

One of the simplest tools for describing an outbreak is a simple plot of the number of cases in a population over time. This frequency distribution, commonly referred to as an epidemic curve (epi curve), is made by placing the time

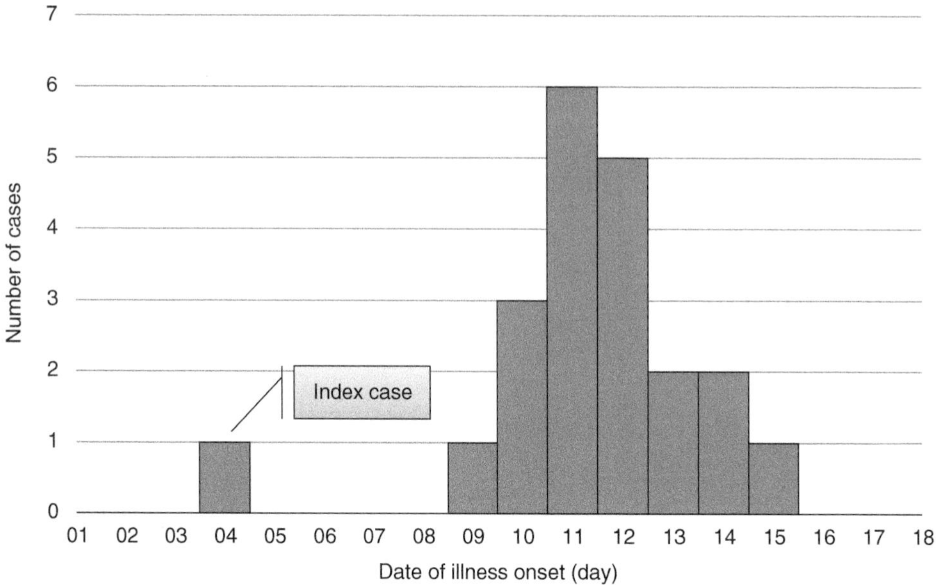

Figure 6.2 Point source outbreak.

interval (hour, day, month, year) on the x-axis and the number of new cases during each time interval on the y-axis. In Figure 6.2, each tick on the X-axis is a single day and the y-axis indicates the number of new cases that occurred on that day. Epi curves are useful for studying any disease outbreak. In addition to depicting the presence and magnitude of an outbreak, epi curves can be used to better understand the pattern of disease spread within a population, estimate the incubation period, characterize at-risk populations, and assess the effectiveness of control strategies. Typically, the patterns observed in epi curves fall into three different categories: point source, continuous, and propagated.

A point source pattern is observed when a cluster of cases occur following exposure to a common source for a brief period of time. The curve rises swiftly to a peak and gradually declines as shown in Figure 6.2, provided additional exposures are avoided. Cases typically occur within one incubation period, which can provide valuable information if the infectious agent is not yet known. An example of this pattern might be seen if a kitten was diagnosed with FPV; susceptible animals receiving an infective dose as a result of that exposure would develop illness approximately one incubation period from the index case. Ideally, the infected and exposed animals would be isolated from the general population and environmental decontamination would prevent additional cases.

A continuous pattern results from exposure to a common source that is present for an extended period of time. The curve rises sharply but instead of peaking and declining; it tends to plateau as shown in Figure 6.3. A classic example of this is exposure to a contaminated food or water source. The exposure would continue until the source was identified and removed. Play yards that are heavily contaminated with roundworm and hookworm eggs could provide a continuous source of exposure for parasitic infections in shelter animals.

A propagated pattern is more commonly seen in contagious disease outbreaks and indicates ongoing disease transmission within the shelter. Rather than being exposed to a common source, new secondary and tertiary cases

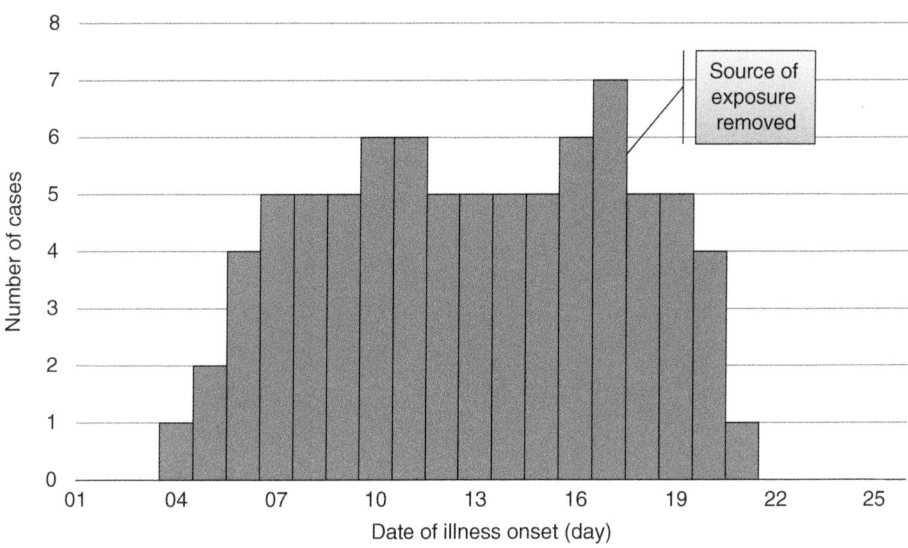

Figure 6.3 Continuous source outbreak.

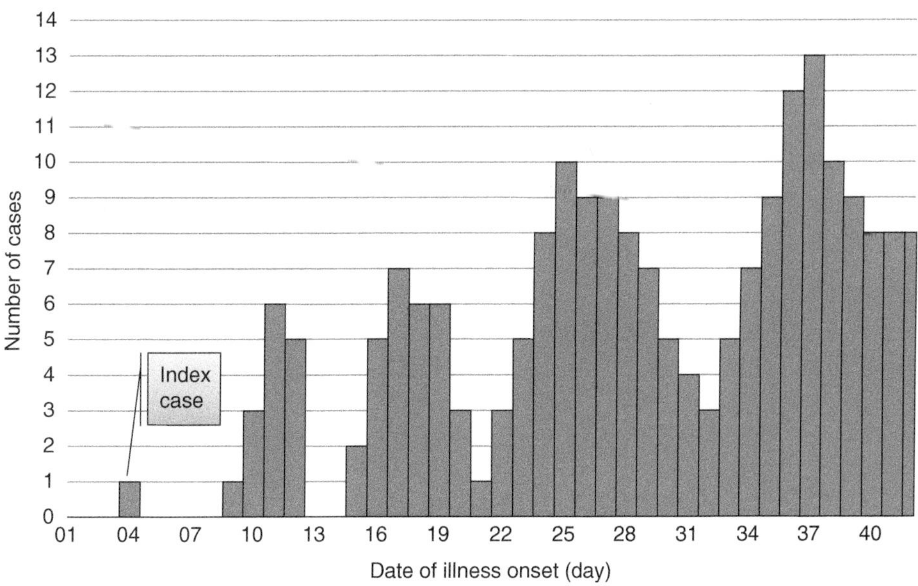

Figure 6.4 Propagated outbreak.

result from exposure to one or more animals actively shedding the pathogen. As shown in Figure 6.4, the curve rises rapidly and typically displays a series of successively higher peaks until adequate control measures are implemented, or until all susceptible animals have been exposed and develop immunity or die. A steady influx of susceptible animals into animal shelters; however, can perpetuate this outbreak pattern indefinitely.

In extended outbreaks, sometimes lasting months to years, the curve will reach a steady-state with periodic fluctuations reflecting the presence or absence of other contributors to

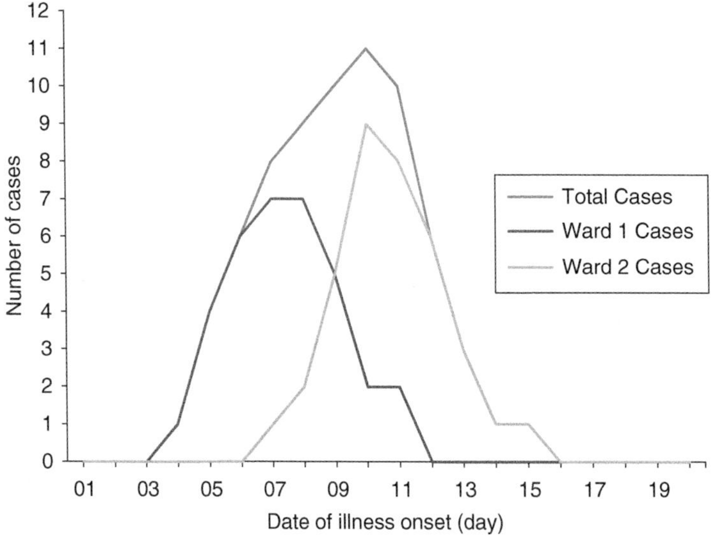

Figure 6.5 Epidemic curve stratified by location.

the disease burden. It is imperative that those reviewing disease trends in a shelter do not mistake this relatively flat part of the curve as a normal or expected background level of endemic disease. Consistently elevated levels of shelter-acquired diseases indicate a serious problem in shelter operations that compromises animal health and welfare.

Outbreak progression may change the pattern of an epi curve, providing additional information for investigators. If a diagnosed case of FPV, as mentioned above in the point source exposure, was isolated from the population but exposed cats were not quarantined, a secondary case could develop in the population that exposes a new group of cats. At low levels, these propagations can look like unrelated point sources when they actually stemmed from the same index case. If ongoing transmission was not prevented, the curve would take on a typical propagated pattern over time.

If the pattern becomes more sporadic with several peaks no longer separated by incubation period time intervals or if it forms a plateau, this could indicate that there is an ongoing source of exposure in the shelter, perhaps from insufficient cleaning and disinfection or, if cases are being treated in-house, from inadequate isolation protocols.

In addition to mapping frequency patterns, epi curves can be used to compare subpopulations within the shelter population. Case counts can be classified based on specific variables such as age, location or vaccination status to help determine which animals are most at-risk. As shown in Figure 6.5, the total outbreak curve demonstrates the magnitude and frequency of cases, while the location curves suggest that the outbreak started in Ward 1 and spread to Ward 2. Based on that information, animal movement within the shelter and sanitation procedures may need to be reviewed.

6.8 Control Measures

Outbreak control measures are intended to prevent transmission of disease to susceptible animals within the shelter and the community at large. When dealing with zoonotic disease, the focus must also be placed on protecting humans from infection. Ideally, control measures will be based on a presumptive or confirmed cause of disease but, in some cases, mitigation efforts are instituted while the search for an identifiable cause is ongoing.

Timely implementation of control measures is greatly facilitated when outbreak management and disease-specific protocols are detailed in a written infectious disease and outbreak management plan (Tables 6.1–6.3). In an outbreak, a situation report and refresher training for all staff should be provided as soon as possible to ensure that management, staff and volunteers know exactly what is expected of them.

The impact of specific control measures, like those detailed below, should be continuously evaluated during an outbreak and modified as needed. Collecting and analyzing epidemiologic data as described above can assist with this assessment and also provide useful information for avoiding similar outbreaks in the future.

6.8.1 Enhanced Disease Surveillance

When an outbreak is suspected, disease surveillance should be enhanced to quickly identify and respond to new cases. This can be accomplished by increasing the number of times trained staff perform rounds from the recommended once per day (Newbury et al. 2010) to two or more times per day. All staff should be encouraged to watch for and report signs of illness. These efforts can be facilitated by staff training on disease detection and having an established mechanism for reporting suspected health issues in the shelter to the appropriate managers so timely action can be taken.

Additional time should be taken to observe animals for clinical signs before handling them. This is especially important for staff who may otherwise transmit infection during routine cleaning activities. If illness is suspected, cleaning that enclosure should be delayed until the animal has been evaluated and moved out of the general population. For diseases with a high morbidity and/or a significant percentage of contagious animals that don't show clinical signs, temporarily treating all animals as if they were infected and changing personal protective equipment (PPE) (e.g. gloves, gown) between each animal may be justified.

6.8.2 Isolation, Quarantine, and Other Alternatives

Isolation refers to the physical separation of infected animals from the rest of the population. In addition to reducing the exposure of susceptible animals, trained staff working in isolation areas can improve the delivery of specialized care to those that are ill.

Quarantine refers to the physical separation and observation of animals that are currently disease-free but have been exposed to a pathogen and therefore may become ill or infectious themselves.

6.8.2.1 Isolation

Pathogen shedding is highest in animals that are displaying clinical signs of illness. Even for ubiquitous diseases, clinically ill animals should be separated from the general population and from animals that are being isolated for other unrelated diseases. When the diagnosis has not yet been determined or when reliable diagnostics for confirming disease in individuals are not readily available, it is best to assume that all animals displaying clinically compatible signs during an outbreak are infected and treat them accordingly, regardless of the extent of the illness. The severity of clinical signs is an ineffective and dangerous way to estimate the risk of disease transmission. With most diseases, mildly affected and recovering animals are still contagious. When the disease agent is known, the post-recovery shedding period can be used to help determine how long the animal should remain separate from the general population. Ideally, recovered animals should not remain in the same isolation area with acutely ill animals still receiving treatment.

6.8.2.2 Quarantine

When there are significant consequences associated with additional cases developing in the general population, animals that were potentially exposed should be identified and evaluated individually for their risk of developing an infection. Risk and exposure assessments are discussed later in the chapter.

Those at meaningful risk (exposed and at risk for infection as a result of that exposure) should be quarantined and observed for signs of illness (Newbury and Hurley 2012). They should also remain separated from other sick animals and from those who are quarantined for other reasons. For instance, puppies exposed to CPV should not be quarantined in the isolation area for CIRD. Doing so might maximize the use of limited space, but it presents a significant threat to the CIRD dogs who are already ill and may be at greater risk for infection.

Animals that have been meaningfully exposed should not be returned to the general population until the typical incubation period for that disease has passed with the animal showing no signs of infection. An animal that develops the disease during the quarantine period should be handled as a new case based on the shelter's infectious disease policy and disease-specific protocol. Any animals that were sharing quarantine with this case should undergo a new exposure risk assessment with the possible outcome of extending the quarantine. Depending on the pathogen and other circumstances such as the date of vaccination, the new risk assessment may find that the animal was unlikely to have been susceptible at the time of the most recent exposure, in which case, the original quarantine would be completed without the need for an extension. For example, an adult dog that was vaccinated two days prior to being exposed to CPV was considered meaningfully exposed and was quarantined with several other dogs. On day 11 of 14, one of the other dogs in quarantine was diagnosed with CPV. Though the adult was exposed again, enough days had passed following his vaccination that he was not considered susceptible at the time of his second exposure. He does not need to be quarantined for an additional 14 days, but he should complete the remaining 3 days of the original quarantine. A three-month-old puppy in the same situation would be considered meaningfully exposed because of his young age. Maternal antibodies may have interfered with his vaccination leaving him susceptible to disease. He should begin a new 14-day quarantine.

6.8.2.3 Isolation and Quarantine Parameters

Some shelters are designed with dedicated isolation and quarantine wards, which should ideally possess an independent air supply with negative pressure ventilation. Other shelters must create space for temporary or permanent use by repurposing areas originally intended for other functions, or by dividing a room into smaller partitioned areas. These areas should be constructed of non-porous materials that can be easily disinfected, and individual housing should be appropriately sized with solid barriers between animals. Whenever possible, areas selected for isolation and quarantine should be located outside of the main human and animal traffic patterns within the shelter.

Protocols for maintaining the integrity of isolation and quarantine wards should be standardized and enforced. Additional details on cleaning and disinfection, fomite control, dedicated animal care supplies, and protective outer garments are provided in Chapter 8 on sanitation and will not be covered in this chapter. Contact with the animals, while they are potentially contagious, should be limited to what is necessary to ensure adequate and humane care.

6.8.2.4 Alternatives to Isolation and Quarantine

Shelters that lack appropriate isolation/quarantine space or are unable to adequately protect the general population from the risk created by having contagious animals in the facility, should consider alternatives to isolation and quarantine. Shelters can cultivate options such as off-site treatment through foster-care programs, conditional adoption programs, treatment at local veterinary clinics, and transfer to other suitable sheltering facilities or rescue organizations. The preferred options will be largely dependent on the diagnosis. Factors such as pathogenicity, transmission modes, the severity of disease and zoonotic potential may eliminate some choices if they pose a significant threat to human or animal health.

Even shelters that have dedicated isolation and quarantine space should explore alternatives in case an outbreak surpasses their ability to provide necessary medical care while ensuring humane living conditions. Overcrowding can increase stress and delay recovery, thereby causing avoidable suffering. Additionally, overworked staff usually do not have enough time to clean and disinfect appropriately and are more likely to make biosecurity mistakes, increasing the chance that disease will spread to areas outside of isolation/quarantine. Exceeding the shelter's capacity for care can worsen an outbreak. Assessing available resources in advance and establishing realistic limits for in-house care with respect to specific disease conditions will minimize the need for euthanasia and maximize live outcomes.

When employing off-site housing options, preventing the spread of disease from the shelter into the community is a priority. Anyone receiving sick or quarantined animals from a shelter should be fully informed about the disease and its risks, be capable of preventing disease transmission and have a clear understanding of who is responsible for medical care costs, including those incurred by their own resident pets if they become infected. This information should be provided in writing, ideally with a signed consent form or MOU. Exposed animals do not always develop disease so giving them priority for foster or rescue placement over those who are already infected may have several advantages, both financial and emotional.

6.8.3 Risk and Exposure Assessment

Infection is dependent on both the level of exposure (dose) and the susceptibility of the animal. Rather than quarantining all animals that might have been exposed, which is generally not recommended, each animal should be evaluated to assess their risk of developing disease. Species is a common barrier to disease transmission. For some diseases, vaccines can provide near-sterilizing immunity (e.g. panleukopenia, parvovirus, distemper, rabies), which means that those who have mounted an appropriate immune response to the disease are extremely unlikely to become infected. Only those at meaningful risk need to be quarantined, thereby maximizing the use of resources, and minimizing disruption to other shelter functions. Many factors involving the pathogen, the environment and the animal's general health and immune status can impact whether or not an animal will develop an infection following exposure.

6.8.3.1 Pathogen Related Factors

Considerations for assessing exposure dose include the distance pathogens can travel, mode of transmission, infectious dose, durability of the infectious agent in the environment, and the frequency of carrier states in animals. For example, Giardiasis, a disease caused by a protozoan, only requires a very low number of oocysts to cause infection. These oocysts are also very durable, surviving typical shelter cleaning protocols and persisting in the environment for weeks. The combination of low infectious dose and durability in the environment make Giardia highly communicable.

It makes intuitive sense that those closest to a source of infection for the longest period of time will have the highest dose of exposure. Littermates, co-housed animals, and playgroup partners will have had the closest contact and should be assessed as having a high level of exposure. For many diseases, animals can be contagious before they develop clinical signs. This preclinical shedding period (usually a few days) should be determined for the specific disease and potential exposures during that timeframe should be identified and assessed.

The primary method of disease transmission helps determine the safe distance required to avoid infection from a source. Common feline respiratory pathogens are spread by airborne droplets with highest pathogen loads within 5 ft of the cat; while common canine respiratory pathogens are spread by aerosols that can travel much farther, sometimes more than 25 ft (Gaskell and Povey 1982). Physical barriers such as walls significantly reduce the risk of exposure. However, fomite transmission must also be considered; the movement of staff and shared animal care items play a significant role in disease transmission.

6.8.3.2 Environment-Related Factors

Room and housing size and layout, ventilation, housing, sanitation and husbandry practices all contribute to exposure levels. Walls present a barrier to a large extent, keeping pathogens in or out. Smaller rooms have the advantage of housing, and therefore exposing, fewer animals. Airflow patterns and the recycling of air should also be taken into consideration depending on the pathogen. It is less than ideal, for instance, to have airflow from a room with clinical cases of CDV into a room with susceptible puppies.

Housing design and cleaning processes can increase or decrease the risk of exposure. Stacked cages that allow feces and urine to enter the cages below or runs that receive *dirty* water from neighboring runs during the cleaning process are conducive to the spread of enteric parasites and other pathogens. The use of high-pressure hoses to remove animal waste can result in the discharge of tiny particles into the air. These particles may carry along several pathogens, effectively blanketing the room and its occupants. All waste should be removed before the use of sprayers when cleaning.

Allowing puppies or cats to play on the floor while their cages are being cleaned may provide them with some exercise, but it also creates greater opportunity to have direct contact with animals in other cages as well as any contaminants that are on the floor. Similarly, tying dogs to or near neighboring cages provides an opportunity for close contact between occupants. These actions can lead to significant exposures and should be considered when assessing at-risk status.

6.8.3.3 Host Related Factors

As previously mentioned, exposure does not always lead to disease. Animals possess both innate and acquired immunity that can reduce or eliminate their vulnerability. Other factors such as species, age, health status, and medication usage can influence susceptibility.

The species barrier is effective against diseases with a narrow host range. For example, cats do not need to be quarantined if exposed to CDV and dogs do not need to be quarantined during an outbreak of FPV. However, it should be noted that cats are susceptible to both FPV and CPV (Ikeda et al. 2002). Dogs, cats and humans are susceptible to *Bordetella bronchiseptica*.

Young animals under five months are at the highest risk, as they may not yet have developed active immunity to most infectious agents. Regardless of age, host-specific factors such as stress, malnutrition, and pre-existing disease conditions including those that attack the immune system (e.g. FeLV, FIV), are known to reduce resistance and should be taken into consideration when determining at-risk status.

Certain drugs are also known to reduce disease resistance. Chemotherapeutic agents and long-term use of steroids have been shown to compromise immunity. Antibiotics can increase susceptibility to some infections, such as Salmonella, because their use alters the normal balance of protective bacteria.

For some infectious diseases such as CDV, CPV, and FPV, vaccination is highly protective and properly vaccinated adults develop near-sterilizing immunity. When exposed, quarantine is rarely indicated for these animals. Positive serology (titer testing) results for those viruses are also suggestive of protection and may be worth the cost in the face of an outbreak, especially when prior vaccination history is not known (Lappin et al. 2000). (See the section on serology for CPV, FPV, and CDV, Chapter 4 and 9.)

For other diseases, such as canine influenza virus and most respiratory diseases, vaccines provide only partial immunity. This reduces the likelihood of disease and the severity of disease but may not prevent infection or subsequent shedding. For this reason, vaccinated dogs should be quarantined if exposed to canine influenza, which is known to cause severe outbreaks in dog populations, including those housed in shelters.

6.8.3.4 Serology for CPV, FPV and CDV

Serology can be performed to measure the number of antibodies present in the blood against a specific pathogen. In cats and dogs five months of age and older who are lacking clinical signs of illness, a positive titer test correlates very strongly with protection from infection with that disease even if exposure occurs (Larson et al. 2009; Burns and Ford 2016) This means that titer testing can be a very valuable tool to assess the risk of infection following a potential exposure. Blood should be drawn and tested at the first opportunity after an exposure to obtain the most reliable results. As the days after exposure pass, the chance that a positive result may represent infection rather than protection increases.

A positive titer test is not a guarantee that the animal was protected at the time of exposure, but the majority of the time that will be true (Schultz et al. 2010). These animals can be placed in a low-risk category and managed per the shelter's disease-specific protocols. For many shelters, this means that they can move through the process to adoption without a quarantine period (Newbury and Hurley 2012).

Positive titers in animals that have clinical signs of disease may represent protection, but the chance that they could be the result of infection is higher, making interpreting the results more difficult (Newbury and Hurley 2012). It is recommended that these animals have diagnostic tests run and be either isolated or quarantined accordingly. Positive titer results in juvenile cats and dogs under the age of five months also cannot be relied upon to accurately represent protection (Newbury et al. 2009). They may instead be the result of maternally derived antibodies passed in their mother's milk. These gradually decrease over the first four months of life and can interfere with vaccine efficacy. In general, puppies and clinically ill dogs are in a higher risk category due to difficulties interpreting their titer results.

Titer tests can be sent out for laboratory analysis with a typical turnaround time of two to four days. There are also two tests available at the time of publication that can be conducted in the shelter in under 30 minutes. No test is perfect and there is a chance of false positive results for all three of these diseases. Studies have found that it is far more likely to have a false negative result, especially with FPV, which means that the test indicated that there was not adequate protection when in fact there was (DiGangi et al. 2011; Litster et al. 2012).

The measurement of titers to assess the risk of infection in animals exposed to CDV, CPV, or FPV can save lives. These animals can get adopted more quickly, leaving more resources to quarantine the animals that are in a higher risk category. Compared to the cost of a quarantine period, titer testing can also be cost-effective. See Chapters 9 and 4 for more information on the use and interpretation of titers in disease exposure risk assessments.

6.8.3.5 Other Related Factors

Risk and exposure assessments are unavoidably subjective; the risk will never be zero even in the absence of an outbreak. Every animal intake has the potential to introduce infectious disease. The goal then becomes the identification of those who were exposed to an infectious dose *and* have a higher than normal risk of infection as a result of that exposure.

In addition to assessing meaningful risk, shelters must also consider the need for and expected length of quarantine, the number of animals needing quarantine, and the potential impact on the shelter and the community if outbreak control measures fail. Risk assessments will naturally be more conservative for some diseases than others based on the known ease of transmission, the severity of the disease, mortality rate and zoonotic potential.

6.8.4 Sanitation

Once infected and exposed animals have been moved from their enclosures, their housing and the surrounding environment can be thoroughly cleaned and disinfected. Sanitation products and usage protocols should be reviewed (see Chapter 8) and altered if needed to ensure they are effective against the current pathogen; this is especially important for pathogens that are difficult to inactivate (e.g. parvo and calici viruses, dermatophytes). It is also important to verify, ideally through first-hand observation, that all cleaning and disinfection procedures are being performed correctly and in a manner that will not inadvertently contribute to disease spread. Methods such as progressing from clean areas to contaminated areas, wearing protective outer garments, and reducing fomites are important outbreak control measures. The importance of staff biosecurity cannot be overstated, including the proper use of protective outer garments and frequent hand hygiene.

Stronger concentrations of cleaning agents are not beneficial during an outbreak (unless noted on the label for specific conditions); in fact, this common practice can cause harm. Attention should be given to proper cleaning to remove all liquid and solid wastes prior to the application of disinfectants, and to ensuring that the disinfectant is properly prepared and applied and remains wet for the full recommended contact time. Animals should never be returned to wet cages. Even when disinfecting chemicals are used appropriately, they are not a replacement for thorough mechanical cleaning, which remains a very effective method of reducing environmental contamination.

The frequency of sanitation may need to be increased in the face of an outbreak; for non-localized outbreaks, the entire facility should be cleaned and disinfected, including transport vehicles, areas where no animals are housed and the items that are not typically part of the daily sanitation routine (e.g. doors, ledges, cage tops).

Fomite control should be implemented, as this is one of the most common means of disease transmission. The use of items that cannot be adequately disinfected between uses should be avoided; the use of disposable equipment whenever possible is advised. It is also important to remember that cleaning tools and equipment (e.g. trash cans, scrub brushes, squeegees) can serve as fomites and aid in the spread of infectious agents. Ideally, each room or ward will have its own dedicated set of equipment.

6.8.5 Determine Additional Staffing Needs

The tasks and activities involved in mounting an outbreak response will require additional staff hours. This can be especially crippling for shelters that are often already chronically understaffed. Even shelters that are adequately staffed need to plan for the expanded staff requirements during an outbreak.

In addition to their normal duties, medical staff will be needed to identify, diagnose and treat sick animals. They will also be assessing risks and exposures, including running titers or other tests as needed. If the outbreak involves risk to recently adopted animals, they may also be evaluating them and addressing concerns from the owners. For some tasks, the staff hours needed can be estimated, similar to estimating the time needed for cleaning or surgery based on the anticipated number of animals. If a shelter plans to run diagnostics on 200 dogs that were exposed to distemper, they can determine the amount of time it takes to put on new PPE, restrain the dog to collect blood and swabs, prepare the samples, and dispose of the PPE. If this takes 15 minutes per dog, then the shelter should plan for 50 hours dedicated to this task for each of the two to three people that would be needed to perform this task together. In order to accomplish the sample collection of all of the dogs in a shorter period of time, additional staff teams will be needed.

Similarly, front office staff may be handling more calls and visits from the public while staff will likely be performing additional cage transfers, treatments, and sanitation tasks. Shelters are encouraged to plan ahead for increasing staff capacity. Employing some part-time staff when needed is one way to create staffing flexibility. Utilizing temporary services and *borrowing* volunteer staff from other shelters or veterinary clinics can also transiently bolster staffing levels.

6.8.6 Protect at-Risk Animals in the Shelter

When an outbreak is suspected, efforts to identify individual animals that may be susceptible to infection and provide them with additional protection can help reduce the spread of disease. These protections may include restricting their movements within the facility, avoiding potentially contaminated areas (e.g. outdoor areas, playrooms), and limiting the staff that have contact with them. Their exposure to fomites should be reduced by replacing shared or common use items such as litterboxes, kongs, toys, and food bowls with disposable items. For vaccine-preventable diseases, the administration of an appropriate vaccine, provided it has not been given within the last two weeks, may increase immunity, especially in those less than 18 weeks of age (Davis-Wurlzer 2006).

6.8.7 Protect at-Risk Humans

When dealing with zoonotic diseases, visitors, staff, and volunteers become part of the at-risk population. Access to animals being treated in the shelter should be controlled and restricted to essential trained staff only, and disease-specific protections should be put in place. When developing shelter policies and protocols for handling zoonotic diseases, careful consideration should be given to the shelter's ability to prevent human cases while also providing appropriate treatment, behavioral and environmental enrichment to the patients. The potential consequences if human cases occur in the shelter or the community could be disastrous. (See Chapter 21.)

Refresher training for staff on disease-specific prevention is warranted during an outbreak, as is a review of outbreak management procedures concerning how to notify supervisors and when to seek medical care. Federal Occupational Safety and Health Administration (OSHA) regulations require that employers make their employees aware of any health risks and provide all necessary PPE. The shelter should report suspected and confirmed cases of zoonotic disease in humans to the local public health officials. It is the shelter's responsibility to know which animal and zoonotic human diseases are subject to mandatory reporting; in some states, zoonotic disease outbreaks (typically defined as two or more related cases) must be reported.

In general, staff who have contracted a zoonotic disease should not report to work until they are no longer contagious. However, with some diseases such as ringworm, the spread of disease can be effectively prevented by mitigating the risk of exposure (e.g. covering ringworm lesions), using additional PPE, and restricting activities to reduce contact with susceptible animals and people. All medical decisions should be made between the patient and their licensed healthcare provider. Veterinarians must not diagnose or treat disease and injuries in humans; this activity is considered illegal and can result in severe penalties. First aid can be provided, including the washing of injuries, including bite wounds.

6.8.8 Protect Incoming Animals

Strict disease prevention measures should be in place to protect susceptible animals that enter a shelter during an outbreak. Consideration should be given to all animals regardless of the purpose or length of their stay. This includes surrenders, impoundments, visiting pets owned by staff and volunteers, foster appointments, and community pets brought to the shelter for services such as training classes, surgery or medical care.

Even if all of the outbreak cases are isolated, there is a benefit to providing housing that is separate from the resident animals in order to further reduce the potential for exposure via subclinical shedding from animals in the general population. If the shelter cannot provide a suitable, uncontaminated environment for incoming animals, then entry for those animals should temporarily be refused.

In addition to physical separation and vaccination, there are some treatments that may sometimes be employed to reduce individual susceptibility. For example, cats entering a shelter during a ringworm outbreak can be given a prophylactic lime sulfur dip (Newbury and Moriello 2014). This would provide some residual protection should exposure occur despite the biosecurity measures already being taken. However, prophylactic use of antibiotics for all animals entering a shelter is inappropriate and ill-advised. Most pathogens involved in FIRD are viral and antibiotics are not effective. Their use, even when indicated, can alter normal other protective flora and thus make animals more susceptible to some infections such as Salmonella. Additionally, indiscriminate use of antibiotics can lead to the development of resistance that poses a risk to both human and animal health.

6.9 Decision-Making

When an infectious disease outbreak is suspected, many decisions need to be made, and time is at a premium. Though preliminary information, including the cause, may be unavailable or incomplete, general outbreak control measures should begin immediately. Regardless of the disease, isolation of the sick, enhanced surveillance including identification of exposed animals, careful sanitation, and protection of at-risk and incoming animals as described above will reduce the risk of disease transmission. Veterinary direction of clinical assessment, diagnosis and treatment is essential; consultation with veterinary professionals should be sought if not readily available from a staff veterinarian.

6.9.1 Animals in the Community

A decision must be made whether or not services to privately owned animals (e.g. sterilization, outpatient medical care, daycare, obedience classes) can be safely provided during an outbreak, and what additional precautions may be needed to ensure their protection. Similar consideration should be given to programs that take shelter animals into the community (e.g. off-site adoption events, publicity spots, and humane education outreach). If disease transmission to the public or their pets cannot be prevented, that activity should be temporarily suspended or altered to mitigate the risk. Services such as outpatient medical care can usually be maintained if facility space and equipment are not shared with shelter animals. When dealing with airborne pathogens, the building's ventilation system and airflow pathways must be considered when making these decisions.

Alternatives to canceling activities or services can also be explored. Obedience classes can be moved to an off-site location and surgical space may be obtained from a nearby veterinary practice or mobile surgical clinic. Rather than taking a shelter animal to scheduled public relations activities, an animal that is in foster care and was unaffected by the outbreak may be taken instead.

Shelters engaged in animal transfer activities with rescues and other sheltering organizations should also carefully consider the risk of transferring disease. Animals should not be transferred without full disclosure of recent disease activity in the source shelter. Some receiving organizations may still be willing and able to offer appropriate care for infected and exposed animals, aiding affected shelters with their outbreak relief efforts. Discussions about these issues with transfer partners, in advance of need, are strongly encouraged.

6.9.1.1 Animals Entering the Shelter

Depending on the causative agent, disease severity, and magnitude of the outbreak, a temporary restriction of intake may be indicated, and should definitely occur if incoming animals cannot be adequately protected from exposure. The addition of susceptible animals merely propagates an outbreak, ultimately causing greater suffering and potential loss of life. That said, many measures can be taken to shorten the duration of intake restrictions, lessen the impact, or even prevent the need for them altogether.

Some shelters already have the necessary space and population management policies to adequately provide an uncontaminated environment to safely house incoming animals. Other shelters may need to create this space by relocating some resident animals and thoroughly disinfecting the newly available space. Intake restrictions, if necessary, may only need to be in place for the time it takes to assess the situation, isolate the sick animals, and disinfect a suitable area for receiving new arrivals. This process is often referred to as creating a "*clean break.*" (See Chapter 11 for more information about establishing a clean break.)

A risk assessment should be conducted for each animal presented for intake. Species, age, and vaccination status are important determinants with obvious implications in specific disease events. In most cases, animals that are assessed as low risk and not likely to become infected if exposed can be handled following usual protocols. Entry for at-risk animals can be refused, diverted, delayed, or allowed provided they can be housed in a manner sufficient to protect them from disease.

6.9.1.2 Suspending Intake

When the shelter cannot adequately protect incoming animals, it will be necessary to restrict or fully suspend intake. There are many approaches to accomplish this and shelters will need to customize the restrictions to best fit their situation.

It may be necessary to turn all animals (or all those who are determined to be at-risk) away with an explanation, leaving it up to the surrenderer to locate other available options. For highly vaccine-preventable diseases such as CDV, CPV and FPV, adult animals could be tested for protective antibody levels before deciding whether or not they should be admitted to a shelter experiencing an outbreak of one of these diseases. They could be housed with very low risk of contracting disease, provided they have no known history of exposure, no clinical signs and they possess an adequate titer. Those without protective titer levels could be diverted elsewhere or vaccinated and sent back to their home or into foster care for a period of time, thereby delaying intake until a sufficient immune response has occurred or until outbreak control measures are no longer needed.

For shelters (i.e. typically municipal or open admission) that receive or pick-up stray animals, there may be a legal obligation to receive them regardless of conditions at the shelter. However, municipalities are often willing to temporarily suspend a mandate to take in animals when fulfilling that mandate would put the animal's life in jeopardy. It is essential to discuss these issues in advance with municipal administrators and legal counsel in order to determine what options are available to the shelter under various outbreak situations.

Even if intake cannot be completely halted it can be drastically reduced. For example, owner surrenders could be diverted to another local shelter and/or all intake could be deferred except those that are suffering, are in harm's way, or represent an immediate threat to public health or safety. Additionally, if the disease risk warrants, those animals could be housed at an off-site location or be accepted by a partner shelter.

Suspending or restricting intake can be a challenge, especially for open admission facilities. Advanced planning can help reduce both the need to do so and the potential impact on the community. Relationships should be developed with other local shelters and rescue groups that may be willing to receive diverted animals, thus providing the time needed to effectively contain the outbreak. And it is important to make partner organizations aware as soon as possible when diversion to their facilities may be necessary.

6.9.2 Quarantining a Shelter

Though hopefully rare, there are times when an entire facility must be quarantined, with no animals entering or leaving. In some cases, shelter activities that involve unaffected species can continue, but in other cases, there is not enough separation of space to ensure that visitors would not inadvertently carry the infectious agent to pets outside the shelter.

A quarantine might be recommended during a widespread outbreak affecting large areas of a shelter to facilitate enhanced sanitation and allow more control of risk factors. There are frequent reports in the news of shelters closing to manage outbreaks of CPV, CDV or ringworm. Concurrent outbreaks of multiple pathogens are a strong indication that a shelter should be closed so the management and staff can evaluate its protocols and make necessary adjustments to contain and control the disease.

Shelter closure may be indicated when the disease is known to be severe and highly contagious, or when the disease presents a significant zoonotic risk. Reportable animal diseases may also lead to a shelter quarantine. For instance, shelters and pet stores in Rhode Island are required to report cases of CDV to the state veterinarian, who has the authority to investigate and quarantine the entire facility if indicated.

6.9.3 Requesting Assistance from Shelter Medicine Experts

Infectious disease management in animal populations can be quite complex. Outbreak management in animal shelter populations is even more of a challenge. Shelters developing protocols for outbreak management, actively managing outbreaks or considering wide-scale euthanasia or mass depopulation are strongly encouraged to consult with a shelter medicine expert before making decisions. Deciding when and who to call for assistance is an important step in outbreak planning and response. Reaching out to experts for guidance on planning and prevention measures will establish a professional relationship and may help avoid an outbreak altogether.

6.9.4 Requesting Assistance from Public Health Authorities

Many diseases affect humans as well as animals, and zoonotic disease outbreaks should be reported to the local health department, whether or not human cases are known to have occurred. Reporting may be mandatory for some diseases; shelters should include specific reporting requirements and contact information in their infectious disease and outbreak management plans. Health departments can also provide PPE recommendations, diagnostic services, and assistance with disease and exposure investigations, making them a valuable resource for shelters. On more than one occasion, a confirmed case of rabies in an animal shelter has sparked a public search for visitors and volunteers who may have been exposed (CDC 2011). Shelters are then flooded with calls and could easily be overwhelmed without the support of health officials to screen the dozens or perhaps hundreds of persons needing a risk assessment to determine the need for prophylactic anti-rabies treatment. Shelters should not hesitate to seek assistance to handle these types of cases.

6.9.5 Caring for the Caregivers

Managing an outbreak introduces many changes to the daily routine for shelter staff. The additional work created by outbreak response activities often translates into overtime for staff. This creates additional stress for those already dealing with the fact that the animals in their care are suffering from diseases they were unable to prevent. If euthanasia of affected or exposed animals is necessary, the feelings of sorrow and guilt can be almost unbearable, especially if the animals were healthy on intake and acquired disease in the shelter.

The staff and volunteers are an essential part of the shelter, and the impact that an outbreak will have on their mental and emotional health should be considered. It is important to ensure that all staff are kept updated on the response activities shelter-wide so they are aware of more than their specific role. This could be as simple as a daily email or posting announcements in a common work area. In addition to what has been accomplished and what will be happening, positive outcomes should be included as they occur (e.g. fewer cases were diagnosed, favorite dog Belle is responding to treatment).

The staff should be reminded of behavioral health employee benefits and encouraged to take advantage of them, both during and following an outbreak. Some shelters have brought counselors in during working hours, setting up an area where private conversations can occur. Shelters are encouraged to find ways to show appreciation to the staff and recognize their feelings and their contributions to the response efforts.

Following the outbreak, the staff should be provided with a summary and engaged in constructive discussion about how the outbreak occurred and how outbreak response and prevention efforts can be improved. This can be valuable information for preparing or revising an infectious disease and outbreak management plan, and it demonstrates an interest in both staff contributions and disease prevention.

6.10 Working with the Media

While the public and the press are not aware of most outbreaks, some may reach the attention of the media. This is most likely to occur when there are large numbers of sick animals being adopted, an increase in animal deaths, disease transmission to humans, or someone makes a complaint. It is recommended that shelters appoint a spokesperson to respond to media requests, thus ensuring the quality, accuracy and continuity of the information being shared with the public. When dealing with the press it is best to be honest and forthcoming. If it is too early to know exactly what the cause is, the available information should be provided along with the steps that are being taken to address the situation. Offering to provide regular updates to the media demonstrates transparency and may reduce the frequent requests for more information which can otherwise detract from response efforts.

Social media outlets, including Facebook and Twitter, can be utilized to share information and updates from the shelter. Ideally, all official communications from the shelter should go through the person who was selected to be the shelter's spokesperson to help ensure relevance, accuracy and consistency.

Social media is very participatory, however, and anyone can share his or her opinions on these public forums. Comments can be quite inflammatory. Response to negative posts is not necessary, and in many cases should be avoided. Even when attempting to correct misinformation, this can simply devolve into an online argument that does not clarify or improve the situation. Ignoring non-constructive comments is often best. Instead, shelters can post factual information about the disease and updates about what has occurred and what is being done. In some cases, temporarily closing public comments may be warranted.

While newspaper and television reports can at times be inaccurate, overall, they represent a powerful means of sharing information about an investigation with the public and other interested parties. An Idaho shelter outbreak of multidrug-resistant *Salmonella typhimurium* affected dozens of cats and sickened 49 people, resulting in 10 hospitalizations (Dunn et al. 2004). The shelter released joint statements with the department of health and kept the community apprised of outbreak status and response efforts. This was a significant investigation involving both state and federal health officials. Despite the well-publicized threat to public health, the executive director later reported that the adoption areas were busy as soon as the shelter reopened to the public (Hurley 2004).

Taking a proactive approach by reaching out to the media provides an opportunity to educate the public on the importance of relevant disease preventive measures. For example, announcing a confirmed case of rabies in the shelter provides an excellent opportunity to teach the public about the disease and discuss the importance of keeping pets current on their rabies vaccination, further demonstrating compassion and a commitment to serving as a community resource for animal health and welfare issues.

6.11 Community Considerations

Sheltered animals are not a separate population; instead, they represent a subgroup of the larger community population. A shelter is a place where various subgroups of animals (e.g. stray, feral, displaced, cruelty victims and owned) temporarily converge. Some shelters are expanding the borders of their source population by transferring animals from other communities, states, and countries. Just as the growth of travel and commerce has increased human disease risks, so too have animal disease risks been increased by the ease with which animals move across large distances (O'Shea 2010). Whether for disaster relief, animal rescue efforts or other reasons, the importation of surplus animals may introduce rare or foreign diseases not typically found in that area.

As previously discussed, sheltered animals can become a source of disease exposure to animals outside of the shelter. In addition to those that are clinically ill, consideration must be given to the introduction of subclinical and carrier animals into the community. These animals appear healthy and are more likely than sick animals to be taken to puppy or kitten classes, animal parks, or other public venues. Minimizing infectious disease levels in animal shelters not only reduces the risk of outbreaks, but it can also reduce the disease burden for the rest of the community as well.

Shelter animals are also an important sentinel for local disease trends. Intake often mirrors disease prevalence in the community, and the comparatively large numbers of animals received by a shelter make significant fluctuations more likely to be noticed. Shelters may also detect the emergence of new pathogens such as CIV, which was first confirmed to have spread from racing greyhounds to companion dog populations in a Florida shelter (Crawford et al. 2005).

Emerging pathogens may enter and spread through a shelter, or they may mutate within a shelter. Many factors, including concentrated populations of animals in various states of health, from a wide geographic area and in a transient state, make this environment highly conducive to the emergence and spread of novel disease agents. The potential development of antimicrobial drug-resistant organisms is of particular concern. Active disease surveillance and monitoring of population health provide for early event detection, protecting both the community and the shelter from disease outbreaks. For instance, reports of a sudden influx of dogs diagnosed with a vector-borne disease may prompt investigation and public health alerts that reduce the risk to both humans and animals through increased awareness and vector control. Shelters should strive to work with community partners involved in animal health and well-being. Maintaining good communications with veterinarians, local and state health officials, animal placement agencies, and other animal care professionals in the community can aid in detection and response to unusual disease events.

6.11.1 Zoonotic Disease Concerns

Approximately 75% of recently emerging infectious diseases affecting humans are of animal origin; approximately 60% of all human pathogens are zoonotic (Taylor and Woolhouse 2000). The majority of zoonotic diseases acquired from contact with shelter animals or their environs are not reported to public health agencies, so the frequency of their occurrence is unknown. Typically, only incidents with poor outcomes, lawsuits, or large numbers of exposures are documented. Despite the paucity of data from shelter reporting, the health risks to humans from companion animals are well documented.

Zoonotic disease transmission is relatively uncommon; however, millions of animals generating tens of millions of animal contact hours accumulated through the provision of care and rehoming efforts represent an occupational health risk for staff and volunteers. This risk parallels that of pet store workers who were the largest group affected by a recent outbreak of *Campylobacter jejuni* in humans, with over 100 cases associated with puppies at pet stores (Montgomery et al. 2018). Nearly half of those cases occurred in persons working in the pet stores.

Shelters have a responsibility to protect human health by implementing zoonotic disease prevention measures and providing education to staff and adopters as needed. It is important to note that a meaningful percentage of the population are immunocompromised, and many of them do not know this about themselves. Modern shelters owe their origins to animal control efforts aimed at protecting the public from animal bites and rabies. Shelters still play an important role in community health and have an obligation to protect both animals and humans. See Chapter 21 for more information.

6.12 Conclusion

Though developing an infectious disease and outbreak management plan can seem like a daunting task, the benefits of having one during an outbreak are innumerable. The development process itself can also lead to improvements in general disease prevention strategies. Ongoing surveillance and early detection methods provide the opportunity to minimize potential impacts on a shelter and the surrounding community when an outbreak cannot be avoided. A methodical, epidemiologic approach to outbreak investigation is very advantageous; providing input into both the selection of appropriate control measures and the evaluation of their efficacy. Preventing an outbreak altogether is clearly preferred; however, shelters that are prepared to implement a swift and effective response are better able to protect the health and wellness of the animals in their care.

6.A Sample Disease Outbreak Tracking Form

Animal ID	Sex	Age	Date entered shelter	Date/type of vaccine	Date of disease onset	Coughing	Sneezing	Fever	Location at time of diagnosis (room/cage #)	Method of diagnosis (clinical signs, culture, snap test, necropsy, etc.)	Outcome R = recovered D = died E = euthanized

Case Definition: ____

____.

References

Burns, K. and Ford, R. (2016). To titer or revaccinate. *Journal of the American Veterinary Medical Association*. https://www.avma.org/javma-news/2016-07-01/titer-or-revaccinate (accessed 4 August 2020).

Byun, J.W., Yoon, S.S., Woo, G.H. et al. (2009). An outbreak of fatal hemorrhagic pneumonia caused by *Streptococcus equi* subsp. *zooepidemicus* in shelter dogs. *Journal of Veterinary Science* 10: 269–271.

CDC (Centers for Disease Control) (2011). Public health response to a rabid dog in an animal shelter – North Dakota and Minnesota, 2010. *MMWR (Morbidity and Mortality Weekly Report)* 59: 1678–1680.

Crawford, P.C., Dubovi, E.J., Castleman, W.L. et al. (2005). Transmission of equine influenza virus to dogs. *Science* 310: 482–485.

Davis-Wurlzer, G.M. (2006). Current vaccination strategies in puppies and kittens. *Veterinary Clinics of North America Small Animal Practice* 36: 607–640.

DiGangi, B.A., Gray, L.K., Levy, J.K. et al. (2011). Detection of protective antibody titers against feline panleukopenia virus, feline herpesvirus-1, and feline calicivirus in shelter cats using a point-of-care ELISA. *Journal of Feline Medicine and Surgery* 13 (12): 912–918.

Dunn, J., Carter, K., Tengelsen, L. et al. (2004). Salmonella Typhimurium DT104 infections among persons adopting cats from an animal shelter. 42nd Annual Meeting of the Infectious Disease Society of America in Boston, MA (30 September–4 October 2004).

Gaskell, R.M. and Povey, R.C. (1982). Transmission of feline viral rhinotracheitis. *Veterinary Record* 111 (16): 359–362.

Goddard, A. and Leisewitz, A.L. (2010). Canine parvovirus. *Veterinary Clinics of North America Small Animal Practice* 40: 1041–1053.

Hurley, K.F. (2004). Outbreak of drug resistant Salmonella at an animal shelter. *Animal Sheltering* (November), pp.10–12.

Hurley, K.F. and Baldwin, C.J. (2008). Developing infectious disease policies and procedures in an animal shelter. In: *Maddie's Infection Control Manual for Animal Shelters* (eds. C.A. Petersen, G. Dvorak and A.R. Spickler), 66–79. Des Moines: Center for Food Security and Public Health, Iowa State University, College of Veterinary Medicine.

Hurley, K.F. and Baldwin, C.J. (2012). Prevention and management of infection in canine populations. In: *Infectious Diseases of the Dog and Cat* (ed. C.E. Greene), 1124–1130. St. Louis: Elsevier/Saunders.

Ikeda, Y., Nakamura, K., Miyazawa, T. et al. (2002). Feline host range of canine parvovirus: recent emergence of new antigenic types in cats. *Emerging Infectious Diseases* 8: 341–346.

Lamm, C.G. and Rezabek, G.B. (2008). Parvovirus infection in domestic companion animals. *Veterinary Clinics of North America Small Animal Practice* 38 (4): 837–850.

Lappin, M.R., Jensen, W., and Andrews, J. (2000). Prediction of resistance to panleukopenia, herpesvirus 1 and calicivirus utilizing serology. *Journal of Veterinary Internal Medicine* 14: 364.

Larson, L.J., Schultz, R.D., and Newbury, S. (2009). Canine and feline vaccinations and immunology. In: *Infectious Disease Management in Animal Shelters* (eds. L. Miller and K.F. Hurley), 61–82. Ames: Wiley-Blackwell.

Litster, A.L., Pressler, B., Volpe, A. et al. (2012). Accuracy of a point-of-care ELISA test kit for predicting the presence of protective canine parvovirus and canine distemper virus antibody concentrations in dogs. *The Veterinary Journal* 193 (2): 363–366.

Montgomery, M.P., Robertson, S., Koski, L. et al. (2018). Multidrug resistant *Campylobacter jejuni* outbreak linked to puppy exposure – United States, 2016-2018. *MMWR (Morbidity and Mortality Weekly) Report* 67: 1032–1035.

Newbury, S. and Hurley, K.H. (2012). Population management. In: *Shelter Medicine for Veterinarians and Staff*, 2e (eds. L. Miller and

S. Zawistowski), 93–114. Ames: Wiley Blackwell.

Newbury, S. and Moriello, K.A. (2014). Feline dermatophytosis: steps for investigation of a suspected shelter outbreak. *Journal of Feline Medicine and Surgery* 16 (5): 407–418.

Newbury, S., Larson, L.J., and Schultz, R.D. (2009). Canine distemper. In: *Infectious Disease Management in Animal Shelters* (eds. L. Miller and K.F. Hurley), 161–172. Ames: Wiley Blackwell.

Newbury, S.P., Blinn, M.K., Bushby, P.A. et al. (2010). Guidelines for Standards of Care in Animal Shelters. The Association of Shelter Veterinarians. https://www.sheltervet.org/assets/docs/shelter-standards-oct2011-wforward.pdf (accessed 5 June 2020).

O'Shea, P.L. (2010). Shelter-animal relocation raises infectious disease concerns. *DVM Newsmagazine*. Advanstar Communications Inc. https://www.dvm360.com/view/shelter-animal-relocation-raises-infectious-disease-concerns (accessed 5 August 2020).

Schorr-Evans, E.M., Poland, A., Johnson, W.E. et al. (2003). An epizootic of highly virulent feline calicivirus disease in a hospital setting in New England. *Journal of Feline Medicine and Surgery* 5: 217–226.

Schultz, R.D., Theil, B., Mukhtar, E. et al. (2010). Age and long-term protective immunity in dogs and cats. *Journal of Comparative Pathology* 142 (Suppl 1): S102–S108.

Taylor, L.H. and Woolhouse, M.E.G. (2000). *Zoonoses and the Risk of Disease Emergence. International Conference of Emerging Infectious Diseases*. Atlanta Georgia: Centers for Disease Control and Prevention.

Van Immerseel, F., Pasmans, F., De Buck, J. et al. (2004). Cats as a risk for transmission of antimicrobial drug-resistant *Salmonella*. *Emerging Infectious Diseases* 10: 2169–2174.

WHO (World Health Organization) (2010). WHO Epidemiology. http://www.who.int/topics/epidemiology/en (accessed 6 August 2020).

Wright, J.G., Tengelsen, L.A., Smith, K.E. et al. (2005). Multidrug-resistant *Salmonella* Typhimurium in four animal facilities. *Emerging Infectious Diseases* 11: 1235–1241.

7

Pharmacology

Virginia R. Fajt

Texas A&M University, College Station, TX, USA

7.1 Principles of Drug Decision Making and Therapeutics

The objectives of this chapter are to highlight important principles of applied or clinical pharmacology and therapeutics that impact the drug decision-making process for the veterinarian in the context of infectious disease management in a shelter. This is not meant to be a comprehensive review of therapeutic principles, but rather to highlight characteristics of drugs and drug decision making that are relevant to the treatment of animals in the shelter setting. Drug mechanisms and specific drug formulations will only be discussed if they have an impact on which drug to pick or the drug regimen (dose, route, duration, and frequency).

Making decisions about the therapeutic use of drugs in the shelter setting often involves treating multiple animals at a time. However, decision making in populations of animals may not be much different than that for individual animals. The clinician who treats one animal at a time may be thinking about the individual animal, but the truth is that the rationale for drug decisions comes from evidence in groups of animals. While personalized medicine is the buzzword of the moment, one must start with data from groups. Data from groups define the likelihood of success and allow the comparisons that are the hallmark of evidence: only by comparing across individuals can an accurate assessment be carried out of the difference made by an intervention.

Sometimes veterinarians fail to think analytically when choosing to use drugs and then selecting which drug to use. Good decision making involves less automated, more systematic, or so-called System 2 thinking (Croskerry 2013). The approaches and principles described here are an attempt to encourage systematic thinking about treatment decisions. The general approach to making drug decisions is to search for, and use evidence of, effectiveness (does the intervention result in outcome changes in patients?), consider potential constraints to the potentially effective options (Is it legal? Is it feasible?), make the decision, and then make explicit plans to monitor outcomes in individual patients and across groups to assess outcomes. This is a good time to state that, while the use of clinical impression as the only source of data on which to base treatment decisions is fraught with problems, it is possible that a well-designed evaluation of treatment outcomes within an individual shelter could provide data. If selection, observation, and allocation bias were accounted for,

Infectious Disease Management in Animal Shelters, Second Edition.
Edited by Lila Miller, Stephanie Janeczko, and Kate F. Hurley.

a shelter could generate useful data that are not currently available in the peer-reviewed literature. Please see Chapter 4 on Diagnostic Testing for more information on the use of empirical treatments.

7.2 Searching for and Applying Evidence for Efficacy: Is the Drug Likely to Improve Animal Outcomes?

Whether subconsciously or consciously, veterinarians make decisions about their patients based on some form of evidence about safety, efficacy, and quality, even if that evidence is an opinion from a medical expert whom the veterinarian contacted by phone. There are several ways to find evidence: using free indexes such as PubMed (https://www.ncbi.nlm.nih.gov/pubmed) and paid services such as the Veterinary Information Network (VIN); though not all evidence reported in VIN is peer-reviewed or without significant bias, there is the ability to find peer-reviewed literature on VIN. The Centre for Evidence-based Veterinary Medicine at the University of Nottingham in the United Kingdom (UK) catalogs systematic reviews (http://webapps.nottingham.ac.uk/refbase) and has begun developing knowledge summaries called "best bets" (http://bestbetsforvets.org), which are simple reviews of specific clinical questions. These are great resources offering summaries of the best evidence.

Not all forms of evidence hold the same weight. Evidence should be weighted more heavily if it is unbiased and less heavily if the likelihood of bias is high, bias being anything that might systematically skew results or outcomes. Table 7.1 lists common types of studies of therapeutics in order from lowest to highest potential for bias, and it includes whether a treatment effect can be estimated, which will be described in a later section.

With bias as the key factor in the strength of evidence, clinical impression is the most biased data to use when making a decision, whereas much higher weight is given to randomized controlled data. Clinical impression is an assessment of patient outcome during case management or based on case recall. The reasons for clinical impression being problematic include lack of a comparison group, confounding by indication bias (this means treatments were selected based on different criteria in different groups of animals, such as animals with more or less severe disease, rather than being selected at random), loss to follow up, and biased outcome measurement (the veterinarian doing the treating knows what the treatment was, which can bias their assessment of the outcome) (O'Connor and Fajt 2015). The gold standard of comparisons is the randomized controlled clinical trial, but cohort studies of various kinds can be convincing if of sufficiently high quality.

In addition to the study design, what happened in the study can also impact its value and applicability. For this reason, it is important to specifically assess the quality of the evidence by a careful review for common problems or omissions in reports of an investigation into therapeutics. There are extensive worksheets published by the Centre for Evidence-Based Veterinary Medicine at the University of Nottingham (www.nottingham.ac.uk/cevm/evidence-synthesis/resources.aspx). However, a quick review for the most common issues can be made by answering the questions listed in Table 7.2.

7.2.1 Understanding Statistics

Many veterinarians shy away from trying to grasp the statistical analysis in a published resource because they fear they don't have the skills or knowledge to assess their accuracy or adequacy. Basic understanding of the basis for statistical analysis will help determine whether to trust the source of evidence. While it is beyond the scope of this chapter to review how

Table 7.1 Common study types in veterinary therapeutics ranked in order of potential for bias.

Evidence type	Risk of bias	Treatment effect can be estimated
Systematic review of randomized controlled trials	Low	Yes (sometimes)
Systematic review of other types of studies	Low to variable	Maybe
Large randomized controlled trial	Low	Yes
Small randomized controlled trial	Low	Yes
Cohort study	High	Yes
Case series	High	No
Case reports	High	No
Narrative review	High	No
Expert or other opinions	High	No
Clinical impression or personal experience	High	No
Pharmacokinetic studies	Unknown	No
In vitro studies	Unknown	No

Table 7.2 Questions to uncover common problems or omissions in studies relevant to therapeutics.

Type of evidence or study	Question to ask ("Yes" indicates higher quality; "No" suggests lower quality)
All papers	Were the results discussed critically?
	Were the references complete and up-to-date?
Systematic reviews	Was the literature search exhaustive and reproducible?
Randomized controlled trials (RCTs)	Was the randomization procedure described?
	Was there an adequate number of animals? Was a sample size or power calculation performed?
	Was the control group adequately described and was it appropriate for the study?
	Was the trial blinded?
RCTs, cohort studies, or case series	Were the data complete, and was missing data documented?
	Was essential information about the animals provided (e.g. number, breed, age, sex, housing, inclusion criteria)?
	Were the exposures (such as drugs) and outcomes described in detail?
	Were appropriate statistical assessments used?
Pharmacokinetic studies	Was the regimen comparable to clinical use?
	Is the concentration needed for a therapeutic effect known?
In vitro studies	Were the cells or systems used similar to *in vivo*?
	Were the drugs and concentrations comparable to those achieved *in vivo*?

statistical inferences can be properly made, there are a few principles to keep in mind:

1) All studies in animals represent a sampling of the entire population of animals, and the goal of statistical analysis is to determine if the variables measured in the study differ among groups because of chance or due to the intervention being evaluated.
2) A study being retrospective or prospective does not NECESSARILY mean it is more or less valuable.
3) The fundamental difference among study design types is the degree of bias that is likely as well as the ability to detect such bias. Bias is anything that can systematically skew results or outcomes.

There are very helpful resources online for basic statistics questions, including a site targeting medical students (http://www.students4bestevidence.net/category/appraising-research/statistics-appraising-research) and an excellent tutorial on evidence-based veterinary medicine, "EBVM Learning," (http://www.ebvmlearning.org). An excellent text in an easily digestible format is "Statistics for Veterinary and Animal Science" (Petrie and Watson 2013).

7.2.2 Estimating the Treatment Effect from Published Studies: How Much Difference Did the Drug Make?

In the case of drug interventions, the difference the drug makes can be called the "treatment effect" and is measured by comparing the desired outcome in the treated patients with the outcome in the untreated (or "other" treated) patients. Though it can be challenging to extract this information from published resources, it will provide useful data with which to make treatment decisions, and importantly, it leads to realistic expectations about what treatment success looks like. Here are two examples of estimating treatment effects from published data. The first study compares a drug intervention with a placebo, and the second compares two drugs.

Example 7.1 Robenacoxib for Post-Operative Pain Control in Dogs (Friton et al. 2017)
Dogs undergoing surgical procedures were randomly assigned to receive robenacoxib or a placebo once prior to surgery and for two days post-operatively. One important outcome (the variable used to evaluate efficacy) was the need for rescue therapy to control pain as measured with the Glasgow Composite Measure Pain Scale (CMPS-SF). This was called "treatment success" in the study. Treatment success occurred in 74% of dogs receiving robenacoxib and 58% of dogs receiving a placebo. The treatment effect, therefore, was 74–58 or 16%, meaning that the drug made a difference in 16% of animals. Another outcome evaluated in the study was the pain score at several time points. For example, at three hours post-operatively, the pain score in robenacoxib-treated dogs was an adjusted average of 3.37, whereas the placebo-treated dogs had an average pain score of 4.76. The difference between the two groups, or the actual effect of the drug, was 4.76–3.37, or 1.39 on the pain score scale. It is important to know, or find out when reading the paper, what the scale of the pain score is, so it can be assessed whether the difference in the pain score is clinically significant enough to warrant treatment. (The maximum score on the CMPS-SF is 24.)

Example 7.2 Cefovecin for Abscesses and Wound Infections in Cats (Six et al. 2009)
Cats with naturally occurring abscesses or wound infections were randomly assigned to receive injected cefovecin (8 mg/kg subcutaneously [SC] once) or oral cefadroxil (22 mg/kg (PO) once a day [q24h] for 14 days). Placebos were included with both treatments, so owners were not aware of which drug the animal received; if the cat was assigned to cefovecin, then placebo drops were also administered. The primary outcome was based on clinical signs of purulent discharge, swelling, erythema, nodules, or furuncles, which were scored as nonexistent, mild, moderate, or

severe. Treatment success was defined as all clinical signs being mild or nonexistent 28 days after treatment started. At that time, 97% of the cefovecin-treated cats and 91% of the cefadroxil-treated cats exhibited treatment success. Raw subtraction would suggest that injected cefovecin increases treatment success by 6%. However, the statistical analysis tested "non-inferiority" rather than significant differences between the treatments, making it less clear if the difference could be considered a reasonable estimate of the treatment effect since the paper concluded that cefovecin was "non-inferior" to cefadroxil. Because the difference is relatively small, whether it's real or not, a reasonable approach would be to state that the treatment effect is actually ZERO, which means that the two drugs have essentially the same effect, with neither one being superior to the other.

Therefore, in addition to applying data comparing groups to an individual animal, these treatment estimates can be applied to a group of animals to estimate the likely response rate in the group. From Example 7.1 above, one might predict that using robenacoxib in a group would result in effective pain control over and above spontaneous reduction in pain in approximately 16% of animals.

7.2.3 What if the Drug Formulation and Regimen in the Published Evidence is Not the Same as the One Desired for Use?

In addition to evaluating published evidence for the potential for bias and strength of evidence, the applicability of the information in the study includes making sure that the drug formulation and the drug regimen are the same as the ones intended for use. Both factors can impact how much drug is getting into the animal, and if they are different, there should be different expectations about efficacy. The regimen includes dose, route, duration, and frequency. Lower or higher doses means less or more drug may be delivered to the animal. Longer (or shorter) durations certainly impact how well a drug works. Route of administration can have a significant impact: it should never be assumed that topical is the same as systemic, or that subcutaneous leads to the same amount or rate of drug absorption as intramuscular or intravenous.

7.3 Drug Options Should be Refined Based on Efficacy by Consideration of Constraints on those Options

It is easy to say that drug therapy is about choosing the most effective drug, but that belies the complex nature of medical and surgical decisions. Estimating efficacy or treatment effect is an important step, but drugs that are the most effective are not necessarily the best choice because additional constraints on drug options exist. The most obvious limitations include available formulations and dosages, dose regimens (for example, is the administration of a drug four times a day really feasible?) and cost. Additional constraints include legal and ethical issues, likelihood and severity of potential adverse effects, and public health concerns.

7.3.1 Legal and Ethical Constraints or Restrictions

7.3.1.1 Label and Extra-label Drug Use, Including Compounding

The Animal Medicinal Drug Use Clarification Act of 1994 (AMDUCA) and the regulations promulgated from it in 1997 codified the ability of veterinarians to legally utilize drugs in an extra label (ELDU) fashion, i.e. in a manner not on the manufacturer's label such as in a different species, at a different dose, for a different duration or frequency, or for a different indication (Anonymous 1996). In addition,

ELDU is limited to circumstances when the health of an animal is threatened or suffering, or death may result from failure to treat.

While it seems that many of AMDUCA's provisions apply more often to extra-label use in food-producing animals, there are many requirements for extra-label use that apply to all species. Extra-label use must be in the context of a veterinarian-client-patient relationship (VCPR). Extra-label use by a layperson is not permitted except under the supervision of a licensed veterinarian. (This means that laypersons may not initiate extra-label use.) According to federal regulations, extra-label drugs must be dispensed with a label containing the name and address of the prescribing veterinarian, established name of the drug, directions for use, and any cautionary statements. Additional labeling requirements may also be codified at the state level. Finally, records must be maintained on individual animals that provide condition treated, species of animal, dosage, duration of treatment, and the number of animals treated. These records must be maintained for two years and must be made available to the U.S. Food and Drug Administration (FDA) if requested. The implications of the labeling requirement in a shelter may vary from state to state, depending on the status of the animals in the shelter, given that the drugs are not being dispensed but are instead being administered in the shelter. The author's interpretation is that if the animals are owned by the shelter, a complete label as just described might not be necessary for use within the shelter. However, prudent pharmacy practice dictates the use of relatively complete labels to minimize medication errors and maximize animal health and human safety. Even if animals are owned by the shelter, it would still be judicious to label medications completely. If it is common practice in a shelter to dispense extra-label medications cage-side, a label with the extra-label dosing instructions could be added to the stock medication, and records of individual animal treatments should contain the complete requirements outlined above.

The use of extemporaneous formulations, i.e. compounding, has a long history in veterinary medicine, as drugs that are often approved for limited numbers of species and indications, may be useful in other species and for other indications. In addition, given that there is a large variation in weight among breeds, particularly within the canine species, doses can vary considerably in volume or size. Therefore, veterinarians should be cognizant of state and federal regulations regarding compounding, which are often in flux. The two most common types of compounding, each of which are viewed in quite different ways by regulatory agencies, are: (i) manipulating an approved animal or human drug in a manner not stated on the label, such as reconstituting at a different concentration, or mixing with a flavoring agent; and (ii) making a drug from so-called bulk drug (raw ingredients), such as purchasing raw ivermectin and creating a product.

The first type of compounding has some protection under AMDUCA, provided a valid VCPR exists and there is no approved product in its available dosage form and concentration that could be used in an extra-label manner. This Act does not, however, allow for the second type of compounding, either from unapproved drugs (e.g. drugs approved in other countries but not in the U.S.) or from bulk drugs.

As of this writing, the FDA Center for Veterinary Medicine has published a draft Guidance for Industry #256, which outlines their policy on the acceptability of compounding and was the replacement for a previous Compliance Policy Guide on compounding. Guidance for Industry documents do not hold the force of regulation and are not legally binding, but they provide a sense of how the FDA Center for Veterinary Medicine interprets laws and regulations. This draft guidance focuses on compounding from bulk drug and what violations the FDA will and will not generally take enforcement actions on. A complete enumeration is beyond the scope of this chapter, but important points include that compounded drugs cannot be copies of FDA-approved drugs and that drugs compounded for office stock (i.e., without patient-specific prescriptions) must be on the FDA's "List of Bulk Drug Substances for Compounding Office Stock for Use in Non-Food-Producing Animals or Antidotes for Food-Producing Animals," which can be found at https://www.fda.gov/animal-veterinary/animal-drug-compounding/list-bulk-drug-substances-compounding-office-stock-drugs-use-nonfood-producing-animals-or-antidotes. Compounding pharmacies for veterinary medicine are not immune to regulation and have come under scrutiny legally as well as ethically. The American Veterinary Medical Association (AVMA) has considerable information on how to select a compounding pharmacy on its website (www.avma.org).

For veterinarians who consider compounding under certain circumstances, for example, in shelters where financial constraints may restrict the use of the labeled product, due consideration should be given both to proper compounding (or selection of a good compounding pharmacy) and the liability should an adverse event occur. Products made from bulk drugs are not required to meet the same manufacturing requirements as approved commercial drugs do, and there will always be issues of potency and safety (there is no warranty or guarantee as to how much actual drug is present in the bulk product). For example, compounded itraconazole, (an oral medication that is often recommended for treating fungal infections), was found to result in much lower plasma concentrations than the innovator product that was first authorized for marketing (Mawby et al. 2014). Purchasing one's own bulk drug is fraught with the same problems and must be advised against. The use of a poorly compounded drug to save money may result in an ineffective product that may prolong animal suffering and treatment time and ultimately increase costs. If compounding is being considered, it must be remembered that pharmacists are specifically trained in compounding practices. Their expertise should be consulted to avoid the production of impotent or dangerous products. In addition, there are several published resources with stability data for compounded formulations of many drugs (see Table 7.3). Many of these are available in medical libraries, at veterinary teaching hospitals, or even local human hospitals or pharmacies. Finally, state Veterinary Practice Acts, as well as Pharmacy Practice Acts, should be reviewed for locally acceptable or unacceptable practices when it comes to compounding.

7.3.1.2 How Much Diagnostic Workup is Needed to Justify Therapeutic Intervention?

Other chapters in this textbook address the management of specific infectious diseases, but some general comments can be made here regarding diagnostic and treatment principles. Presumptive diagnoses (those based on physical examination and history) are the norm in many practice settings but are perhaps even more common in resource-poor settings such as some shelters. It may be tempting to consider all other diagnostics as too costly or time-consuming. Though many conditions can be presumptively diagnosed, inaccurate diagnoses may be even more devastating in the shelter than in privately owned animals since larger numbers of animals may be placed at risk. Simple diagnostics such as skin scrapings, cellophane tape impression, cytology, hematocrit/

Table 7.3 Selected references on compounding.

Rita K. Jew, Winson Soo-Hoo, Sarah C. Erush and Elham Amiri, *Extemporaneous Formulations for Pediatric, Geriatric and Special Needs Patients, Third Edition*, American Society of Health-System Pharmacists. Bethesda, MD
Milap C. Nahata and Vinita B. Pai, *Pediatric Drug Formulations*, 6th edition. Harvey Whitney Books Company. Cincinnati, OH
Lawrence A. Trissel and Lisa D. Ashworth, *Trissel's Stability of Compounded Formulations*, 6th edition. American Pharmacists Association Publications. Washington, D.C.

total protein, fecal flotation, and the like can be performed fairly quickly and relatively inexpensively by in-house trained personnel. Gram staining is not hard to implement and can provide useful information for the empirical selection of antimicrobial drugs.

The decision to spend the effort and money on diagnostics requires knowledge of (or assumptions about) the positive and negative predictive value of diagnostic tests. A more expensive test, such as a bacterial culture and antibiotic susceptibility test, may lead to better targeting of an antibiotic, which, in the long run, may save time and money and reduce suffering. This is particularly true for contagious infections or conditions that require prolonged therapy. Bacterial culture may also lead to reduced costs by revealing untreatable infections or an absence of bacteria.

The bottom line is that the professional judgment of the veterinarian is needed to weigh the accuracy of the diagnosis, the consequences if the diagnosis is wrong (or right), and the will of the community supporting the shelter and the shelter management. There are also ethical considerations related to animal welfare and control that cannot be addressed in a simple algorithm, but instead require periodic discussion among veterinary professionals and shelter stakeholders. See Chapter 4 for more information about diagnostic testing.

7.3.1.3 Initiation of Drug Treatment

The initiation of drug administration in the shelter can be problematic, especially in smaller or more rural settings where a full-time veterinarian is not on-site. State-by-state regulations will not be iterated here, but practitioners should familiarize themselves with their state veterinary and pharmacy Practice Acts to determine the latitude allowed and supervision required of personnel administering drugs to patients in a shelter.

Written protocols for managing disease by laypersons are useful in other animal settings, such as for production animals, for common conditions. For example, protocols for managing mastitis or pneumonia are provided so that the veterinarian does not have to examine every animal in order to initiate treatment. This approach can work in shelters, but legal requirements differ from state to state and species to species as to the requirement for a physical examination of individual animals by a licensed veterinarian to establish a VCPR. It may be helpful for the reader to be familiar with the position statements of the Association of Shelter Veterinarians (ASV) regarding the supervision and treatment of shelter animals. The positions can be found at https://www.sheltervet.org/assets/docs/position-statements/Veterinary%20Supervision%20in%20Animal%20Shelters%202018.pdf and https://www.sheltervet.org/assets/docs/position-tatements/medicaltreatmentofanimalsheldinshelters.pdf. Though the ASV statements do not specifically address the VCPR or replace the need to know the law, they help set the tone for responsibly caring for shelter animals.

Controlled substances fall into a different category, as those regulations start at the federal level. However, some states have more stringent regulations than the federal Controlled Substances Act, so the practitioner should also know those laws, which may be in the State Veterinary Practice Act or Pharmacy Act. The Drug Enforcement Administration (DEA) is the ultimate authority, but most states have agencies responsible for state-level management of controlled substance distribution, sales, and prescribing. Many states have enacted laws requiring veterinarians to participate in some manner in state databases for prescriptions of controlled substances. Regardless of whether such a state requirement exists, there are resources that should be consulted about how and where to store, how to label, and how to track controlled substance use in shelters; it would not be a stretch to suggest that controlled substance law is more strictly enforced than almost any other drug laws.

The legal requirements for administering drugs in the shelter, dispensing drugs from the stock for use after an animal leaves the shelter, and writing prescriptions for drugs for an animal leaving the shelter differ by state, so it is important to review State Pharmacy and Veterinary Practice Acts. All State Veterinary Practice Acts can be accessed at www.aavsb.org or www.animallaw.info, in addition to checking each individual state board website. A list of state pharmacy boards is available on the website of the National Association of Boards of Pharmacy (http://nabp.pharmacy). In general, though, it should be assumed that drugs leaving a shelter with an animal should have been ordered by a licensed veterinarian unless it is an over-the-counter (OTC) product that is being used according to the label. (If a drug is OTC for humans, it is by definition extra-label and no longer OTC if being used in an animal—extra-label use requires an order or prescription and a patient-specific drug label.)

There are other resources about writing prescriptions for outside drug dispensing, but veterinarians should be aware of some common miscommunications. Other health professionals are being encouraged to spell out instructions on prescriptions; pharmacists are generally unfamiliar with "SID" for once a day dosing, so veterinarians should instead specify "once per day" (or "q24h") or write "give twice per day" or "administer every 12 hours" rather than BID. There is a movement among veterinary professionals to provide better education to pharmacists about animal drugs, but there are still reports of mistakes being made, so communication is key. It might be important, for example, to state explicitly "no substitutions or generics," or to provide specific instructions and precautions such as "give with food." Veterinarians should also be aware that some pharmacists refuse to fill valid prescriptions because veterinarians lack a National Provider Identifier (NPI). Contacting the state veterinary licensing board or state pharmacy board may help solve this issue.

7.3.2 Other Constraints that Might Limit the Choice of Drug

Other than legal and ethical constraints, several considerations are briefly mentioned here to provide food for thought when narrowing down drug options (or when determining which drugs to stock in the shelter pharmacy). The other side of efficacy is toxicity, so the likelihood and severity of possible adverse drug effects is always on the mind of conscientious veterinarians. Predictions about the likelihood of adverse effects are not generally as easy to calculate from published literature as efficacy, but most drug resources at least provide the most common and catastrophic toxic effects of drugs. The examples provided about estimating treatment effect can be extrapolated to evidence about percent or proportion of animals reported to experience adverse effects.

Cost and logistics are always a consideration; these concerns are often paramount. in the shelter setting, Appropriate management of shelter pharmacies or drug storage areas would include maintaining adequate supplies for dosing, easy-to-follow regimens and treatment sheets or records, and periodic training of personnel. As described above, the cost of an individual regimen might not be the only financial consideration: if the regimen is cheap but less effective or results in lower compliance, the expected savings will be eliminated by the need to re-treat or will result in a reduction in animal welfare.

The third important constraint relates to effects on human health. The handling of some drugs may require safety precautions to protect individuals. In addition, there are public health impacts of some drugs, either a risk to public health (selection for antimicrobial resistance genes by injudicious use of antimicrobial drugs) or an improvement in public health (elimination of zoonotic pathogens). Recent national attention to the opioid epidemic also emphasizes the need for consideration of how controlled substances are managed, stored, and dispensed, and guidance should be sought from local, state, and federal authorities and the AVMA.

7.4 Application of Decision Making to Antibiotics

7.4.1 General Principles of Antimicrobial Drug Therapy

Antimicrobial resistance is a major global public health threat, and all health professionals have a part to play in addressing that threat. Any use of antimicrobial drugs leads to selection for resistant organisms; the only question is which ones, how long do they persist, and how well can they transfer those resistance mechanisms to other organisms? No general rules exist to predict the answer to these questions. Because of this, veterinary professionals have an obligation to be good stewards of antibiotics to preserve their usefulness. According to the AVMA, antimicrobial stewardship "refers to the actions veterinarians take individually and as a profession to preserve the effectiveness and availability of antimicrobial drugs through conscientious oversight and responsible medical decision-making while safeguarding animal, public, and environmental health" (AVMA 2018a). The fundamental consequence of antibiotic use is the selection for antibiotic resistance, so following the principles of antimicrobial stewardship is important to maintain effectiveness and reduce the selection for resistance. An important component of antimicrobial stewardship is maintaining health, using preventive and management strategies, which is core business to animal shelters.

If antibiotics are deemed necessary, stewardship necessitates judicious use with continual evaluation of the outcomes of therapy. In a large shelter, periodic tracking and monitoring of antibiotic use can go a long way in assessing outcomes of antibiotic therapy. Other core principles have been promoted by the AVMA, as well as a task force set up by the AVMA, the Task Force for Antimicrobial Stewardship in Companion Animal Practice. A report from that task force provides some additional guidance (AVMA 2018b).

Antimicrobial resistance can be innate or acquired. Innate resistance is a characteristic of an organism that makes it inherently resistant to a particular antimicrobial. For example, anaerobes are innately resistant to aminoglycosides because there is no transport system in the organism. Acquired resistance can occur through a mutation or transfer of genetic material from one organism to another. In the first case, mutations occur frequently when organisms replicate. These mistakes in replication of genetic material may result in the creation of a protein that is protective for the organism, i.e. resistant to the antimicrobial. The mutation might result in an enzyme that destroys the antimicrobial, or it might change the conformation of the ribosome to which the antimicrobial would normally attach. This change allows this mutated organism to survive when the others are inhibited by the antimicrobial. It then grows and replicates and may potentially continue to cause disease. There are some types of resistance that are "inducible," meaning that they are present in the bacterial cell but not turned on. When exposed to an antimicrobial, however, the mechanism is activated (e.g. an enzyme begins to be produced) that confers resistance. Reports continue to be published of individual resistant organisms among veterinary pathogens, such as methicillin-resistant *Staphylococcus pseudintermedius* (MRSP) (Moodley et al. 2014) and *Escherichia coli* (Thungrat et al. 2015). There are even reports from shelter animals specifically, though not very many (Gingrich et al. 2011); the data from shelter animals suggested that trends mirror those in owned animals. However, trends toward increasing resistance have not been reported for all pathogens. Reports from diagnostic laboratories may be useful to the practitioner in making decisions about antimicrobial use, though a centralized system of data organization has yet to be assembled for all veterinary pathogens in the United States for companion animals.

The most important way to reduce the selection for resistance is to reduce **the need for** and **the use of** antimicrobial drugs. Practically speaking, this means that all antimicrobial drug use should be justified rather than "just in case" (as is sometimes seen in shelters that use antimicrobials for routine spay-neuter surgeries or to indiscriminately treat all upper respiratory infections (URI).). Also, animals should only be treated for as long as necessary and with appropriate regimens to maximize efficacy. For some drugs, there is evidence that the regimen can influence selection for resistance, though this cannot be applied to all antimicrobial drugs. The mutant prevention concentration (MPC) was defined recently as the concentration that inhibits the growth of mutant organisms, i.e. those with stepwise mutations leading to resistance. It is typically measured using a higher number of organisms than used in minimum inhibitory concentration (MIC) testing. In reported experiments so far, the MPC has been higher than the MIC, but the magnitude of the difference varies among drug–bug combinations and even within drug groups. The clinical significance of MPC measurement in veterinary medicine has yet to be determined, but research will likely continue in this area.

The ideal conditions for inhibiting bacterial growth depend on the antimicrobial drug in question. This is often referred to as the pharmacodynamics of the antimicrobial drug (Table 7.4). Empirical laboratory animal studies and retrospective studies in humans have led to the conclusion that drugs in the aminoglycoside class, such as gentamicin and amikacin, are most effective when the peak concentration of drug in the plasma is 8 to 10 times the MIC of the bacterial pathogen. It is also known that drug concentrations do not have to stay above the MIC for long periods of time to be effective. This is **not** true for drugs in the beta-lactam group, which includes all the penicillins (penicillin G, ampicillin, amoxicillin), cephalosporins (cephalexin, ceftiofur, cefpodoxime), and carbapenems (meropenem). For these drugs, plasma drug concentrations must stay above the MIC of the organism for some portion of the dosing interval, usually at least 40–50%. For example, if cephalexin is administered twice a day, then the concentration of drug in the plasma should stay above the MIC of the bacterial pathogen for at least 6 hours, which is half of the dosing interval of 12 hours.

Dogma admonishes that bactericidal versus bacteriostatic drugs may differ in effectiveness, but this has not yet been demonstrated to be true in head-to-head comparisons (Wald-Dickler et al. 2017). More important is the susceptibility of the organism (the concentration needed to effectively inhibit growth) and the location of the infection (protected areas such as the brain and the prostate require the use of drugs demonstrated to penetrate the tissue).

One of the principles touted for prudent antimicrobial use is to treat for the "right duration". Unfortunately, there is very little data to support particular durations of therapy for any given bacterial infection (Lubbers 2017). Data exist to support that one particular regimen was effective in a percentage of patients, but there are very few comparative studies of different durations in animals. On the other hand, an important principle of using antimicrobial drugs is to monitor response in patients and consider stop-by dates when there is no response. There are no generalizable rules of thumb about when to stop therapy since it will vary with the disease, its severity, and concomitant conditions in the patient. It may be helpful to consult other resources for additional information. It is expected that more studies will be conducted to determine the best duration of therapy for antimicrobials since the duration of use has a large impact on total usage.

7.4.2 Specific Steps of Decision Making for Antimicrobial Drugs

Selecting an antimicrobial and a regimen that will be efficacious has become increasingly complicated. The factors below have made the

Table 7.4 Generalized spectra of antimicrobial drugs for use in selecting empirical therapy[a].

Gram-Positive Organisms	
Aerobes	**Obligate anaerobes**
Penicillin G	Penicillins
Aminopenicillins	Aminopenicillins
Penicillinase-resistant penicillins	
Amoxicillin-clavulanate	Amoxicillin-clavulanate
1st generation cephalosporins	1st generation cephalosporins
(2nd generation cephalosporins)	2nd generation cephalosporins
3rd generation cephalosporins (except *Staph. aureus*)	3rd generation cephalosporins
Lincosamides	Lincosamides
Macrolides	Macrolides
Chloramphenicol	Chloramphenicol
Florfenicol	(Florfenicol)
Fluoroquinolones (except for most streptococci)	
Potentiated sulfonamides	
Tetracyclines	(Tetracyclines)
	Metronidazole

Gram-Negative Organisms				
Respiratory and Fastidious Pathogens	**Enterobacteriaceae**	***Pseudomonas***	**Obligate Anaerobes**	**Other gram-negatives (not all drugs listed)**
Aminoglycosides	Aminoglycosides	Aminoglycosides		
(Penicillin G)			Penicillin G	
Aminopenicillins			Aminopenicillins	Aminopenicillins
Carbapenems	Carbapenems	Carbapenems	Carbapenems	
Amoxicillin- clavulanate	(Amoxicillin- clavulanate)		Amoxicillin- clavulanate	

	2nd generation cephalosporins		2nd generation cephalosporins	
3rd generation cephalosporins	3rd generation cephalosporins	3rd generation cephalosporins	3rd generation cephalosporins	
Macrolides			(Macrolides)	Macrolides
Chloramphenicol	Chloramphenicol	Chloramphenicol	Chloramphenicol	
Florfenicol				
Fluoroquinolones	Fluoroquinolones	Fluoroquinolones		Fluoroquinolones
Potentiated sulfas	Potentiated sulfas			Potentiated sulfas
Tetracyclines	(Tetracyclines)		(Tetracyclines)	Tetracyclines
	Polymyxins			
			Metronidazole	
			Lincosamides	

Spirochetes: aminopenicillins, tetracyclines, macrolides

***Mycoplasma*:** tetracyclines, (linconsamides), (macrolides), fluoroquinolones

Penicillin drug group examples

Aminopenicillins: amoxicillin, ampicillin

Penicillinase-resistant penicillins: oxacillin, methicillin, cloxacillin, dicloxacillin

Cephalosporins drug group examples

1st generation: cefazolin, cefadroxil, cephalexin

2nd generation: cefoxitin

3rd generation: cefotaxime, ceftazidime, ceftizoxime, ceftriaxone, ceftiofur, cefpodoxime, cefovecin

[a] Gray areas indicate a relative lack of efficacy of a drug group. Parentheses indicate variable susceptibility.

design of antimicrobial regimens increasingly more complex, requiring more than just an entry in a formulary to adequately describe:

1) Improved knowledge of bacterial species and pathogenesis.
2) More sophisticated diagnostic data available from laboratories performing antimicrobial susceptibility testing.
3) Improved knowledge of the most effective regimens for antimicrobial therapy.
4) Accumulation of pharmacokinetic data.
5) Continuing expansion of the antimicrobial arsenal, at least in terms of new drugs within old classes of compounds.
6) Changes in and spread of genetic material encoding antimicrobial resistance.

The following steps are the idealized clinical approach to making decisions about antimicrobial drugs.

7.4.2.1 Confirm the Presence of a Disease that is Likely to Respond to Antimicrobial Drugs or for which there is Evidence that Antimicrobial Drugs will Influence the Outcome

The first step to successful therapeutic selection is to know (or have solid evidence) that there is a bacterial infection present and that reducing the growth of the bacteria or eliminating the infection will result in the improvement of clinical signs or will prevent other medical sequelae. (Please refer to the section on making diagnoses.)

7.4.2.2 Consider Antimicrobial Drug Options

Based on which bacteria are expected to be present and the expected spectrum of various antimicrobial groups, a drug group or groups might be ruled out or in as possibilities, particularly for empirical therapy. Table 7.4 contains some generalizations about the spectrum of activity of the major groups of antimicrobials, with the major bacterial categories being gram-positive aerobes and anaerobes and gram-negative anaerobes and aerobes. Gram-negative aerobes are further divided into the respiratory fastidious bacteria (mostly Pasteurellaceae), Enterobacteriaceae, *Pseudomonas*, and "others." One way to determine whether a particular drug group is likely to be **ineffective** is to look at the "holes" in each list. For example, metronidazole is not considered effective against aerobes, and lincosamides are generally not considered effective against gram-negative aerobes. (See Table 7.5 for gram-staining characteristics and oxygen requirements of major veterinary bacterial pathogens.) These spectrum categorizations are not absolute. There are organisms within each grouping that may be resistant to the specific drugs within a class, and the changes in resistance patterns worldwide will eventually render some of these generalizations too inaccurate for empirical antimicrobial selection. In addition, some of the drug groups are very general and include drugs with very different spectra. One would not want to look at Table 7.4 and say, for example, that since tetracyclines and beta-lactams are in all four quadrants, the drugs in both groups could be considered equivalent. Individual drugs vary considerably, thus assigning equivalence to doxycycline and amoxicillin-clavulanate would be risky. Specific, potentially successful drug–pathogen combinations can be more accurately determined with antimicrobial susceptibility testing, as discussed in the next step.

7.4.2.3 Determine if there is Information to Support One Drug Option over another

The evidence of the efficacy of antimicrobial drugs can be based on clinical trial data in the appropriate species of animal and indication for treatment in the published literature, or on *in vitro* antimicrobial susceptibility testing, which is, theoretically at least, correlated with *in vivo* efficacy. It is also important to consider whether clinical guidelines have been peer-reviewed and published to support specific options. Guidelines for dogs and cats have been published for URIs (Weese et al. 2019),

Table 7.5 Gram staining and oxygen requirement of major veterinary bacterial pathogens.

	Aerobes	Facultative Anaerobes	Obligate Anaerobes
Gram positive	*Bacillus* *Dermatophilus* *Mycobacterium* *Nocardia* *Rhodococcus*	*Actinomyces* *Trueperella pyogenes* *Corynebacterium* *Enterococcus* *Erysipelothrix Rhusiopathiae* *Listeria monocytogenes* *Staphylococcus* *Streptococcus*	*Clostridium* *Actinobaculum suis*
Gram negative	*Anaplasma* *Bordetella* *Borrelia burgdorferi (microaerophilic)* *Brucella* *Campylobacter (microaerophilic)* *Chlamydia* *Chlamydophila* *Ehrlichia* *Lawsonia intracellularis* *Leptospira* *Moraxella bovis* *Pseudomonas* *Rickettsia*	*E. coli* *Proteus* *Salmonella* *Actinobacillus* *Haemophilus gallinarum* *Haemophilus parasuis* *Histophilus somni* *Klebsiella* *Mannheimia haemolytica* *Nicoletella* *Pasteurella multocida*	*Bacteroides* *Brachyspira* *Dichelobacter* *Fusobacterium*
No gram staining	*Mycoplasma*		

respiratory infections (Lappin et al. 2017), and pyoderma/folliculitis (Hillier et al. 2014).

When systematic reviews, peer-reviewed clinical guidelines, or clinical trial data are not available, *in vitro* susceptibility data can be useful. Information on the concentration of antimicrobial required to inhibit the growth of bacterial organisms has been available in some form for decades. Given the changes in susceptibility patterns of some bacteria, the most current data should be utilized whenever possible to make antimicrobial and dosing decisions. In some clinical settings, this may take the form of submitting a sample to a diagnostic laboratory to determine the inhibitory ability of antimicrobials for the actual isolate from the animal being treated. In other settings, particularly in settings where (i) populations of animals are being treated, and (ii) economic constraints may be significant, culture and susceptibility testing might be performed on a certain percentage of animals, in the case of refractory infections, or not at all. Testing is recommended specifically in shelters during outbreaks of disease caused by pathogens with unpredictable susceptibility patterns, by pathogens causing high mortality, and by pathogens with zoonotic potential (e.g. *Salmonella*). Testing is also recommended when a therapy that has been used successfully in the past is not working as expected.

While cost is often cited as a reason for skipping testing, shelters should consider the cost of drugs and labor associated with therapy that might not be effective; in other words, paying for testing at the onset of disease might save money on ineffective treatments and prevent prolonged shelter stays and longer times to adoption. When susceptibility testing is not performed, for example, in individual cases of bacterial infections, published susceptibility data may be used, or a practitioner may request historical data from the local diagnostic laboratory or veterinary teaching hospital microbiology laboratory. It is the author's opinion that government-run diagnostic laboratories have an obligation to provide data of this nature, especially to agencies with public health functions like shelters, but obtaining this information may be easier said than done.

7.4.2.4 Interpreting Antimicrobial Susceptibility Data from Individual Cases, Populations, or Antibiograms

The purpose of susceptibility testing is to use an *in vitro* method to predict the clinical success of a therapy. The major methods of susceptibility testing include the classic Kirby-Bauer disk diffusion method and the broth dilution method (Walker 2000). While these methods will not be described in detail here, veterinarians are reminded that such testing is not a black box or a magic trick but rather a standardized method of determining how much drug it takes to inhibit the growth of an organism under specific conditions. Diagnostic laboratory personnel do not have any special knowledge of infections that allow them to predict clinical susceptibility but rather rely on published cutoff values, much like making a value judgment on a cholesterol level in a human patient: the level that is called "unhealthy" versus "healthy" is based on the correlation of levels with other unhealthy events. Comprehensive guidance on interpreting antimicrobial susceptibility testing results is now available (CLSI 2019), and veterinarians are encouraged to consider this document as a necessary resource for appropriate clinical application of the results from single case-based isolates, antibiograms, or surveillance isolates. However, some important considerations in the interpretation of antimicrobial susceptibility data are presented here.

The correlation between *in vitro* inhibitory data and *in vivo* clinical response is not usually 100% and is often much less, which should be kept in mind when using susceptibility testing results from clinical cases. *In vitro* testing conditions do not (and cannot) precisely mimic local conditions during a bacterial infection, so this is one major source of difference between *in vitro* and *in vivo* activity. Other reasons for the failure of *in vitro* growth inhibition to predict a clinical response include, but are not limited to:

1) The ability of the drug to penetrate to the site of infection.
2) The inactivation of the drug at the site of the infection (or conditions not conducive to action, such as anaerobic conditions and aminoglycosides).
3) The importance of the organism to the disease process (just because it was cultured does not mean it is the cause of disease or a significant participant).
4) The timing of antimicrobial administration (for some infections, once the pathogenic processes are in place, elimination of the organism will not speed up the healing).

The criteria for correlating a given inhibitory concentration and clinical success are termed "breakpoints." The theory behind the development of breakpoints is to establish a cutoff value of inhibitory concentration such that if a pathogen requires more than that cutoff to inhibit *in vitro* growth, it is highly unlikely that pathogen growth will be inhibited *in vivo* by that antimicrobial, and treatment with it will not result in clinical cures.

Breakpoints have been established and are updated continually by the Clinical and Laboratory Standards Institute (CLSI) Veterinary Antimicrobial Susceptibility Testing

Subcommittee (VAST). The CLSI is a global, nonprofit, standards-developing organization that promotes the development and use of voluntary consensus standards and guidelines within the healthcare community. Two of the publications put together by this subcommittee, and updated on a regular basis, are known as VET 01 and VET 08. These documents outline the standards for performing susceptibility testing, including the breakpoints to use for each drug or representative drug. Breakpoints are ideally determined using a complicated process of evaluating several layers of data, including pharmacokinetics of the antimicrobial in the species of animal, the pharmacodynamics of the antimicrobial, MICs of populations of pathogens isolated from clinical cases, and results from clinical trials of the antimicrobial (Turnidge and Paterson 2007). Access to the most recent table of veterinary breakpoints typically used by diagnostic laboratories to assess susceptibility is free: "Performance Standards for Antimicrobial Disk and Dilution Susceptibility Tests for Bacteria Isolated From Animals" is now available at https://clsi.org/standards/products/free-resources/access-our-free-resources. A review of this document can reveal the sources of breakpoints used by most diagnostic laboratories to categorize bacterial isolates as susceptible or resistant.

It is important to note that these breakpoints are valid for a given animal species, disease, pathogen, drug, and regimen (dose, route, duration, frequency). While the dose is not always noted in the breakpoint table, one should not assume that all doses can be used appropriately for any pathogen. The other important note is that many of the breakpoints have been extrapolated from human medicine. Therefore, while they represent an approximation of a reasonable breakpoint, they were developed using human pharmacokinetic data and human pathogen population data. In other words, when a user gets a report from a laboratory that states a particular pathogen is "susceptible," this is not a guarantee of efficacy but rather an estimate of a prediction.

Users should be aware that not all drugs used clinically are tested separately; some of the drugs tested are class representatives to allow for more drugs to be included in a test panel. Susceptibility to one drug is assumed to represent susceptibility to all drugs within a class:

- Ampicillin: also tests for amoxicillin
- Tetracycline: also tests for doxycycline
- Cephalothin: has been used historically to represent first-generation cephalosporins, but others are now often tested, such as cefazolin
- Trimethoprim-sulfamethoxazole: representative for all trimethoprim-sulfa combinations.

Some organisms do respond differently to different drugs within a class, but they are the exception rather than the rule. For example, a small percentage of isolates will exhibit *in vitro* susceptibility to doxycycline but will be resistant to tetracycline. Whether this correlates to clinical response is unknown, since the breakpoints used for both drugs are based on current human pharmacokinetics.

One of the included datasets underlying a breakpoint is the pharmacokinetics of the antimicrobial drug: where is the drug and for how long? Because a basic tenet of pharmacology is that the dose given is proportional to the concentration of drug in the body, if the concentration of antimicrobial required to inhibit the growth of a pathogen is known, the dose required to achieve that concentration can usually be determined. Pharmacokinetic data are often presented as single values, e.g. the half-life of drug X is four hours. The long version of this statement would likely read as follows:

1) A small number of healthy animals were studied. Applicability to diseased patients is assumed but often not demonstrated.
2) Serum concentrations of the drug were measured at several discrete intervals over time, and the rate of elimination was calculated for each individual animal. If serum

concentration is proportional to tissue concentrations at the site of infection, this parameter is useful; if not, more information may be needed.
3) The average rate of elimination was calculated. As this is an average, it does not capture the variability inherent in all pharmacokinetic data.

The point of this long version is to demonstrate that elimination half-lives or any other pharmacokinetic parameter should not be interpreted as a single data point but rather as estimates of values that generally represent the average animal.

Other pharmacokinetic data whose value is often misunderstood is "tissue concentrations." These data are often gathered to assess the degree to which a drug might penetrate to areas of infection. It is dogma that more lipid-soluble drugs move into cells more easily, but this is not an absolute, as drugs do not enter cells only by diffusion through the cell wall. They can also enter via pores or active or facilitated transport. Other potential barriers to drug entry into parts of the body include physiological barriers such as the blood–brain barrier or the blood-prostate barrier. The veterinarian's interpretation of the importance of knowing tissue concentrations should be tempered by an understanding of how tissue concentrations are determined:

1) Collection of samples from a particular area may be difficult; taking bone samples to measure bone penetration is not straightforward.
2) Antimicrobial drugs may bind to a particular tissue and be detected but may not be available or active in inhibiting the growth of bacteria. For example, tetracyclines bind to bone and may be measured in high concentrations there, but bound tetracyclines are not active.
3) In order to measure the concentration of antimicrobial, the tissue is macerated. A drug that is water-soluble and does not enter cells then becomes underrepresented in terms of concentration in the areas where it actually is (outside cells). A drug that is lipid-soluble and enters cells more readily is overrepresented in cells, but the infection may still be extracellular and might not be inhibited by the antimicrobial concentration present there.

As described in the section above about the ideal conditions for inhibiting bacterial drugs, pharmacodynamics is also a part of selecting breakpoints. Understanding has grown over the years as to which parameters predict success with which chemical class of antimicrobial drug, which suggests that this parameter is at least partly associated with the mechanism of action of the drug and the post-antibiotic effect. These parameters are provided not to suggest that this information can be used in selecting a drug, but the informed user understands the assumptions underlying their diagnostic tools; these data are increasingly being presented in clinical education settings. One example is the now prevalent understanding that most aminoglycoside regimens are for once a day dosing, and the discovery that the peak concentration is more important for efficacy than the time above MIC confirms that. See Table 7.6 for a compilation of the current understanding of how the time-course of drug concentrations impacts antimicrobial drug effectiveness for various groups of antimicrobial drugs.

When evaluating the drugs in a susceptibility report, it is important to know that these test results do not include combinations of antibiotics (with the exception of the fixed combinations of amoxicillin-clavulanate and trimethoprim-sulfamethoxazole), so confirming the efficacy of combinations relies on published research on fractional inhibitory concentrations *in vitro*, clinical trials of combinations, and dogma typically based on extrapolating from human trials. The general rule of thumb should be that unless demonstrated to be additive or synergistic, or when used in the case of polymicrobial infections for which one drug is not expected to

Table 7.6 Pharmacodynamic parameters predicting clinical efficacy by antimicrobial drug group.

Drug Group	Pharmacodynamic Parameter
Beta-lactams (penicillins, cephalosporins, carbapenems)	Time-dependent, or more specifically, plasma concentrations of unbound[a] drug should remain above the MIC of the bacterial pathogen for at least half of the drug dosing interval. This is commonly shortened to Time > MIC
Fluoroquinolones Macrolides Tetracyclines (Possibly Phenicols)	Concentration-dependent, or more specifically, the ratio of the area under the plasma drug-concentration curve for 24 hours to the MIC of the bacterial pathogen should be 30–100. This is commonly shortened to $AUC_{24}/MIC \geq 100$
Aminoglycosides	Concentration-dependent, or more specifically, the ratio of the peak unbound drug concentration to the MIC of the bacterial pathogen should be 8–10. This is commonly shortened to C_{max}: MIC = 8–10

[a] Unbound refers to the fraction of antimicrobial drug that is not bound to plasma proteins since a drug that is protein-bound is not active.Source Turnidge and Paterson (2007).

provide coverage of all suspected bacterial pathogens, combinations of antimicrobial drugs should be avoided. Their use is likely to result in increased expense and increased chances of causing adverse drug events without any additional likelihood of efficacy.

Other caveats for interpreting an antimicrobial susceptibility report include the following:

1) There are no breakpoints for enteric infections, so it is inappropriate to assume susceptibility when "S" is reported for an isolate from enteritis. Breakpoints have not yet been developed that can accurately correlate achievable concentrations of antimicrobial drugs in the intestinal tract with clinical efficacy.
2) There are no breakpoints for topical products used in animals. (There is one validated breakpoint for identifying high-level resistance in human isolates to mupirocin, but it has not been demonstrated to be accurate for animals.) Therefore, no prediction about effectiveness can be made for neomycin, gentamicin, florfenicol in topical or otic products.
3) Particular caution should be taken when believing that an "S" (susceptible) on a report will predict success in a patient if the breakpoint was not established in that species. Several human breakpoints that used to be used for animal pathogens have been shown to be one to two dilutions higher. One concern is the breakpoint for ciprofloxacin, which has not been validated in dogs. The biggest problem with ciprofloxacin is that its absorption is poor and highly variable in dogs. The "S" breakpoint for humans assumes absorption of a level of drug that is not achievable in dogs. Because ciprofloxacin may be cheaper than veterinary fluoroquinolones, especially for large dogs, this is an unfortunate reality, but continuing to use a drug based on what looks like susceptibility *in vitro* is inappropriate.
4) Resistant, "R," is likely to mean resistant, even when human breakpoints are applied. In some cases, veterinarians may have access to antibiograms. Antibiograms are cumulative susceptibility data for a population of animals, such as a hospital, clinic, or diagnostic laboratory. Typical antibiograms report one or more bacteria in a particular species of animal. Similar to studies performed in groups of animals from which one might make predictions about the response in a SINGLE patient, antibiograms

provide group data from which one can attempt to predict the susceptibility of the suspected pathogen in the patient at hand. It is predicting individual responses from population data. An antibiogram will usually report the number of isolates at each MIC tested (or number that were considered susceptible and resistant), and sometimes it will report an MIC_{50} or MIC_{90}, which is a summary statistic attempting to provide median and 90th percentile MICs for the population of bacteria in question.

Important questions to ask when looking at an antibiogram or other types of population summaries of susceptibility data:

1) How many isolates were tested? If fewer than 100 isolates were tested, one would not be confident that the isolate from one's patient is similar to the isolates in the group.
2) What sites of infection are represented? If treating a suspected skin infection and the isolates in the antibiogram are from urine (or worse, their source is not identified), confidence in the similarity between the patient's isolate and the population isolates is lower.
3) What breakpoints were used to categorize susceptibility and resistant isolates? If the breakpoints are not clearly identified or referenced, it would be difficult to trust the designation of "susceptible" or "resistant."

When summarizing the steps of decision making for antimicrobial drugs, it starts with a presumptive or confirmatory diagnosis of bacterial disease for which antimicrobial therapy has been demonstrated to change patient outcomes. Whether empirical therapy is appropriate or whether antimicrobial susceptibility testing leads to better outcomes for specific infections is beyond the scope of this chapter, but an explicit decision should be made that one or the other is more appropriate. If empirical therapy is appropriate, assumptions about which bacteria are present and which antimicrobial drugs are likely to be effective should be based on published clinical trials, drug approval studies, or published antimicrobial susceptibility patterns or local antibiograms. If antimicrobial susceptibility testing of a patient isolate is deemed to be more appropriate, interpretation of results should take into account the integrity and quality of sample collection and submission, as well as whether the breakpoints used to categorize resistance and susceptibility are specific to the patient species, bacterial species, and site of infection, or if they are being extrapolated from other animal species, bacterial species, or infection sites leading to lower confidence in the prediction of clinical susceptibility. Communication with the clinical microbiology laboratory may also help interpret the results.

7.4.3 Completing the Cycle of Antimicrobial Stewardship: Assessing Outcomes and Evaluating Use Practices

Ideally, antimicrobial stewardship includes an evaluation of antimicrobial use practices over time and identification of areas for improvement. The added benefit of considering this type of feedback in the shelter setting is that any use of drugs involves cost, so a review of use practices can also lead to financial stewardship. The AVMA has recently demonstrated a commitment to supporting antimicrobial stewardship efforts, so educational and practice-oriented materials are likely to become available in the future to support the development of antimicrobial stewardship plans. One example is the Veterinary Checklist for Antimicrobial Stewardship now available to AVMA members (see https://www.avma.org/policies/antimicrobial-stewardship-definition-and-core-principles).

7.5 The Shelter Pharmacy

The provision of guidance for establishing a shelter pharmacy that applies to all shelter settings is not appropriate or possible given the broad range of shelter sizes, locations, disease challenges, resources and personnel. However, some general suggestions can be made that are applicable in many settings. Even small shelters that stock and administer drugs can have simple systems or procedures for tracking expiration dates, inventory, and drug use. Shelter management software often includes medication registers or medical records or forms that can be used and reviewed periodically to match drug purchases with drug use in animals. Otherwise, freely available resources for veterinarians for tracking drug inventory are easily found on the Internet from veterinary suppliers and veterinary practice management experts and should be taken advantage of. Inventory should be tracked not only for financial purposes but also to assess disease challenges and prescribing patterns; for example, for antimicrobial stewardship plans and programs, and to identify inappropriate uses or diversion of drugs, particularly opioids and other drugs with a high potential for addiction and substance abuse. Given the current opioid addiction epidemic and increased attention to opioid prescriptions, controlled substance management is of critical importance. There are specific legal requirements for controlled substances related to how to store and who can access drugs, but similar procedures are urged for other drugs as well. In addition to restricting access to drugs to veterinarians, veterinary technicians and authorized and trained individuals only, it is important to ensure that drugs in the shelter pharmacy are never administered or provided to staff for their own personal use.

With the easy availability of next-day shipping and online pharmacies, drug inventories could potentially be relatively small and limited to those likely to be needed on a daily or emergency basis. These basic needs likely include:

1) Oral antibiotics useful for the most common disease challenges in the shelter [e.g. see discussion above about clinical guidelines for simple uncomplicated dermatitis and urinary tract infections (UTIs)].
2) Oral and topical antifungals or antifungal/antiparasitic dips.
3) Topical antibiotic/antifungal combination for wounds and focal dermatitis.
4) Tranquilizers, anxiolytics and anesthetic drugs (depending on shelter protocols).
5) Local anesthetic (for minor procedures).
6) Emergency/ resuscitation drugs: epinephrine, atropine, naloxone (Fletcher et al. 2012), dextrose, doxapram.
7) Nonsteroidal anti-inflammatory drugs for pain management (often better than opioids and not as challenging to manage inventory), e.g. meloxicam and carprofen.
8) Oral prednisolone.
9) Oral and topical anthelmintics.
10) Limited fluids appropriate for intraoperative or resuscitation use.
11) Drugs used for euthanasia.

Drugs used for euthanasia and pre-euthanasia are likely to be kept in stock, but careful attention should be paid to providing protocols for use and maintaining only the necessary amount for relatively short periods of time.

Drugs that are likely not needed or should be very carefully considered include most fluoroquinolones, meropenem, multiple cephalosporins, and a large range of injectable fluids. In some states, euthanasia and pre-euthanasia drugs can be purchased directly by the shelter rather than by a licensed veterinarian, but these drugs must be carefully inventoried, accounted for and stored in accordance with state, federal and DEA regulations.

7.6 Conclusion

It is essential for shelter veterinarians to understand the important principles of applied or clinical pharmacology and therapeutics that impact decisions regarding the use of drugs to maintain and improve the health and welfare of shelter animals. Failure to do so can result in delays in achieving successful clinical outcomes for shelter patients, financial losses due to inappropriate disease treatment, and can create opportunities for increased disease transmission and animal suffering in both the shelter and community's populations. It is impossible to provide a complete review of all the therapeutic principles relevant to treating animals in the shelter in this textbook. Shelter veterinarians are advised to work closely with shelter management to ensure compliance with all federal and local laws regarding acquisition, storage, record-keeping, administration, dispensing, etc. of pharmaceuticals including controlled substances. In addition, they should utilize the resources mentioned in this chapter to help make sound medical decisions, especially when using antimicrobials to treat infectious diseases. Shelters that do not have full-time veterinarians on staff are strongly encouraged to establish a relationship with a practitioner who can provide training and guidelines for proper drug use within the facility.

References

Anonymous (1996). Extralabel drug use in animals; final rule, 21 CFR part 530. *Federal Register* 61 (217): 57731–57746.

AVMA (2018a). Antimicrobial Stewardship Definition and Core Principles. https://www.avma.org/KB/Policies/Pages/Antimicrobial-Stewardship-Definition-and-Core-Principles.aspx (accessed 31 January 2018).

AVMA (2018b). Antimicrobial Stewardship in Companion Animal Practice. https://www.avma.org/KB/Resources/Reports/Pages/Antimicrobial-Stewardship-in-Companion-Animal-Practice.aspx (accessed 31 January 2018).

CLSI (Clinical and Laboratory Standards Institute) (2019). Understanding Susceptibility Test Data as a Component of Antimicrobial Stewardship in Veterinary Settings, 1e CLSI report VET09. Wayne, PA: Clinical and Laboratory Standards Institute.

Croskerry, P. (2013). From mindless to mindful practice--cognitive bias and clinical decision making. *New England Journal of Medicine* 368 (26): 2445–2448.

Fletcher, D.J., Boller, M., Brainard, B.M. et al. (2012). RECOVER evidence and knowledge gap analysis on veterinary CPR. Part 7: clinical guidelines. *Journal of Veterinary Emergency and Critical Care (San Antonio)* 22 (Suppl 1): S102–S131.

Friton, G., Thompson, C., Karadzovska, D. et al. (2017). Efficacy and safety of injectable robenacoxib for the treatment of pain associated with soft tissue surgery in dogs. *Journal of Veterinary Internal Medicine* 31 (3): 832–841.

Gingrich, E.N., Kurt, T., Hyatt, D.R. et al. (2011). Prevalence of methicillin-resistant staphylococci in northern Colorado shelter animals. *Journal of Veterinary Diagnostic Investigation* 23 (5): 947–950.

Hillier, A., Lloyd, D.H., Weese, J.S. et al. (2014). Guidelines for the diagnosis and antimicrobial therapy of canine superficial bacterial folliculitis (antimicrobial guidelines working Group of the International Society for companion animal infectious diseases). *Veterinary Dermatology* 25 (3): 163–175, e142-163.

Lappin, M.R., Blondeau, J., Boothe, D. et al. (2017). Antimicrobial use Guidelines for Treatment of Respiratory Tract Disease in Dogs and Cats: Antimicrobial Guidelines Working Group of the International Society for Companion Animal Infectious Diseases. *Journal of Veterinary Internal Medicine* 31 (2): 279–294.

Lubbers, B.V. (2017). More is better - Reviewing the science behind duration of antimicrobial therapy. 50th American Association of Bovine Practitioners in Omaha, NE, US (14–16 September 2017).

Mawby, D.I., Whittemore, J.C., Genger, S. et al. (2014). Bioequivalence of orally administered generic, compounded, and innovator-formulated itraconazole in healthy dogs. *Journal of Veterinary Internal Medicine* 28 (1): 72–77.

Moodley, A., Damborg, P., and Nielsen, S.S. (2014). Antimicrobial resistance in methicillin susceptible and methicillin resistant Staphylococcus pseudintermedius of canine origin: literature review from 1980 to 2013. *Veterinary Microbiology* 171 (3–4): 337–341.

O'Connor, A. and Fajt, V. (2015). Evaluating treatment options for common bovine diseases using published data and clinical experience. *Veterinary Clinics of North America, Food Animal Practice* 31 (1): 1–15.

Petrie, A. and Watson, P. (2013). Statistics for Veterinary and Animal Science. Chichester, West Sussex, UK: Wiley Blackwell.

Six, R., Cleaver, D.M., Lindeman, C.J. et al. (2009). Effectiveness and safety of cefovecin sodium, an extended-spectrum injectable cephalosporin, in the treatment of cats with abscesses and infected wounds. *Journal of the American Veterinary Medical Association* 234 (1): 81–87.

Thungrat, K., Price, S.B., Carpenter, D.M. et al. (2015). Antimicrobial susceptibility patterns of clinical *Escherichia coli* isolates from dogs and cats in the United States: January 2008 through January 2013. *Veterinary Microbiology* 179 (3–4): 287–295.

Turnidge, J. and Paterson, D.L. (2007). Setting and revising antibacterial susceptibility breakpoints. *Clinical Microbiology Reviews* 20 (3): 391–408, table of contents.

Wald-Dickler, N., Holtom, P., and Spellberg, B. (2017). Busting the myth of "Static vs. Cidal": a systemic literature review. *Clinical Infectious Diseases* 66 (9): 1470–1474.

Walker, R.D. (2000). Antimicrobial susceptibility testing and interpretation of results. In: Antimicrobial Therapy in Veterinary Medicine, 3rde, 12–26. Ames: Iowa State University Press.

Weese, J.S., Blondeau, J., Boothe, D. et al. (2019). International Society for Companion Animal Infectious Diseases (ISCAID) guidelines for the diagnosis and management of bacterial urinary tract infections in dogs and cats. *The Veterinary Journal* 247: 8–25.

8

Sanitation

Cynthia Karsten

UC Davis Koret Shelter Medicine Program, UC Davis School of Veterinary Medicine, Davis, CA, USA

8.1 Introduction

An undesirable consequence for animals seeking safe haven in an animal sheltering facility is to acquire disease while housed there. An effective sanitation plan, as part of the entire wellness plan for all animals in a shelter, is essential to guard against such disasters and must be tailored to each shelter's situation. Shelters often face unique challenges that require particularly stringent disease control considerations. Many animals enter shelters in poor health, malnourished, stressed, and with an unknown history of vaccination or disease exposure. Some animals will already be shedding various harmful pathogens, with or without showing any clinical signs of disease. With the potential for this level of disease present and so many opportunities for transmission, one might think that ubiquitous disease spread is nearly inevitable.

Fortunately, this is not the case. Many factors determine whether infectious disease occurs, including the condition of the host (the exposed animal), the virulence of the pathogen, the amount of the pathogen present, and environmental factors affecting the level of exposure (Hurley and Baldwin 2012). Shelters can support the host's immune response through vaccination, stress reduction, environmental, and behavioral enrichment, a quality diet, fresh water and other measures that support well-being. The amount of pathogen present and the duration of exposure can be controlled through cleaning and using disinfectant products properly. Therefore, in many cases, a researched, well thought out, comprehensive sanitation plan can reduce the dose of exposure to a level the animals' immune system can handle. In the best-case scenario, effective shelter sanitation prevents illness in both animals and humans and creates a pleasant, welcoming environment where people are more likely to come and adopt an animal.

While cleaning and disinfection reduce the number of pathogens on a surface and thus minimize the risk of infection for animals and humans that come into contact with that surface, they do not result in sterility. Additionally, disinfection is non-specific in that it does not inactivate specific pathogens but rather all those that are present and susceptible to the mechanism of action of the method and/or specific product used. Therefore, the goal of sanitation procedures is not to sterilize an environment, but rather to reduce the pathogen load to a level that minimizes the risk of disease transmission between animals and the people who care for them. See Table 8.1 for clarification of commonly used terms.

Infectious Disease Management in Animal Shelters, Second Edition.
Edited by Lila Miller, Stephanie Janeczko, and Kate F. Hurley.

Table 8.1 Definitions of commonly used terms.

Term	Definition
Cleaning	The physical removal of debris and organic matter
Disinfection	The process of reducing the number of pathogens on a surface to minimize the risk of infection for animals and humans who come into contact with that surface, usually with the use of a chemical product
Fomite	An object that can serve as a method to transmit a pathogen from one individual to another, such as hands, clothing, food bowls or toys, etc.
Pathogen	Bacteria, virus, fungus, or other microorganisms that can cause disease
Sanitation	The use of practices involving cleaning and disinfection to promote health and prevent disease
Sterilization	The process of inactivating all microorganisms, such as with surgical instruments in an autoclave

8.2 Components of the Sanitation Process

8.2.1 General Considerations

All sanitation protocols must emphasize the importance of reducing the spread of pathogens and ensuring the safety of all staff while also minimizing stress and harm to the animals during the process. Animal handling should be also be minimized, especially if the animal exhibits fear or aggression or has clinical signs of disease.

A comprehensive evaluation of all the areas and objects in a facility that require sanitation should be undertaken. For each of these, a protocol needs to address the removal of organic matter (cleaning), application of a chemical product to inactivate pathogens (disinfection), if necessary, and drying of the surface afterwards. If animals must be moved from their enclosure during the sanitation process, they should be walked by staff or volunteers or placed in a carrier dedicated to that animal for the duration of their stay, or in a clean enclosure to minimize exposure to pathogens. It is advised not to tether animals or let them run free in the room as this can be dangerous to the animal and staff, and increases the risk of exposure to pathogens.

Animals should not get wet during the sanitation process, nor should they be returned to a wet enclosure. It is unacceptable to spray down kennels or cages with water or chemicals while an animal is inside their housing unit (Newbury et al. 2011). Loud noises, such as slamming cage doors or playing loud music, must also be avoided to help mitigate the stress created by the sanitation process.

All sanitation equipment should be maintained in good working condition and cleaned and disinfected daily. In order to avoid facilitating disease spread, equipment should be kept in the room where it will be used rather than moved around throughout the facility. Staff must also be provided with personal protective equipment (PPE) to be used during all sanitation processes. Additional information on PPE can be found later in this chapter and in chapters 6 and 21.

8.2.2 Cleaning

The first step in the sanitation process includes manual cleaning to remove all visible dirt and debris from all surfaces. In addition to physically removing soiled bedding, newspapers, feces, uneaten food, etc., the surface must be cleaned with a detergent capable of removing hidden dirt and organic debris. Most, if not all, disinfectants must be applied to a clean surface to be effective.

8.2.3 Disinfection

The second step is disinfection. A disinfectant must be capable of substantially reducing the microorganism burden on a surface; this is defined in most test protocols as a reduction in the number of infectious organisms by at least 4 $\log_{10}$ (Addie et al. 2015). Factors to consider when choosing a product include cleaning (detergent) versus disinfecting activity, the spectrum of activity for disinfection, effectiveness in the face of organic matter, speed of action, including surface contact time, and method of preparation, storage, application, disposal and safety.

8.2.3.1 Product Preparation

It is important to follow the manufacturer's instructions for product preparation, as disinfectants must be used at the correct concentration to be effective. The sanitation protocols should include clear instructions on how to correctly dilute, apply, store, and discard all products in use. Measuring equipment should be readily available, as evaluating disinfectants by smell, color, simple visualization or otherwise guessing is *not acceptable.* In addition to written protocols and instructions, staff must be provided with hands-on training on how to prepare, apply, store, and discard the product safely.

Whichever disinfectant and cleaning products are used, they should not be mixed together unless directed by the manufacturer or supported by research. Mixed randomly, disinfectants and detergents can cancel each other's efficacy or even create toxic fumes (e.g. bleach with ammonia or undiluted accelerated hydrogen peroxide). This information, along with all of the health hazards of the material and associated recommended safe work practices on how to handle, use and store the chemical, can be found in the product's Safety Data Sheet (SDS) (formerly known as Material Safety Data Sheet [MSDS]). The Occupational Health and Safety Administration (OSHA) requires that manufacturers supply an SDS to all purchasers of their chemicals and all employers must maintain one for each product used. This information should be referred to when creating all shelter sanitation protocols and made available to all staff who use the product.

Finally, the expiration date, which indicates the time the disinfectant will lose its efficacy after dilution, must be considered. Some disinfectants have a long shelf life (e.g. 90 days for accelerated hydrogen peroxide), while others need to be remixed as often as daily (e.g. bleach stored in an open container) or once a week (e.g. potassium peroxymonosulfate). Storage temperature and method can also affect stability. For instance, bleach stored in a light-proof, sealed container retains its bacterial efficacy for at least a month, while it is more rapidly inactivated when stored in transparent containers (Rutala et al. 1998). The recommended shelf life and storage method should be verified with the manufacturer. Disinfectants should be disposed of properly when the shelf life has passed because not only can they become ineffective; some can become quite noxious.

8.2.3.2 Contact Time

Many, but not all, disinfectants require 10 minutes of wet contact time for effectiveness, especially against the hardiest pathogens (e.g. parvoviruses). Some disinfectants, such as accelerated hydrogen peroxide (Rescue™ Virox Technologies, Oakville, ON), will be substantially effective in as little as one minute under ideal conditions (Omidbakhsh and Sattar 2006), while factors such as low temperature, pH, the hardness of the water and contamination with organic matter will increase the amount of time needed for any disinfectant. Ten minutes contact time at room temperature on a clean surface remains a good general rule, but it may be prudent to leave a disinfectant in contact for up to an hour or more when organic contamination cannot be removed or at very low environmental temperatures, for example, cleaning outdoor runs in the winter. It is important to note which products require rinsing after the appropriate contact time. Failure to rinse certain products before drying can result in caustic residues that can be harmful if in contact with skin or ingested.

It is also important to note that some pathogens, such as parvovirus or *Microsporum canis*

(*M. canis)* can exist in the environment and on objects for months to years under certain conditions (e.g. away from direct sunlight, in organic material or if inadequate disinfection) (Greene and Decaro 2012). Thus, it is not effective or practical to close cages, kennels or full rooms when a known or suspected case of disease involving these pathogens is diagnosed. The disinfection protocol either was effective or it was not: waiting for the pathogen to be inactivated with the passage of time does not increase the protocol's effectiveness. One recommendation is to clean and disinfect three times with a product that has efficacy both in the face of organic material and against un-enveloped viruses (e.g. potassium peroxymonosulfate or accelerated hydrogen peroxide) at the correct dilution for the necessary contact time to help ensure that all surfaces have been sufficiently covered. All three cycles can be completed in one day and animals can be allowed access to the housing unit or area again.

8.2.3.3 Application Systems

The method of application and use of proper equipment are just as important as the choice of disinfectant. In the author's experience, outbreaks of disease or disinfectant toxicity have been traced to lost or broken disinfectant dispensers. The use of mops and buckets in animal shelters should be avoided if possible, as they can actually contribute to the spread of dirt and pathogens. Alternatives to mop use can be found later in the chapter.

For small cleaning jobs, bottles with "squirt tops" rather than spray tops are ideal to decrease the amount of disinfectant aerosolized into the environment, thus helping protect animal and human respiratory health. If a spray bottle is used for spot cleaning, the rag or paper towel should always be sprayed instead of the surface to also help decrease aerosolizing and splashing of the disinfectant. Rescue® and other disinfectant products may also be available as disinfectant wipes for small clean up jobs, however, the active ingredients and contact time must be noted to ensure that the product is effective against the pathogens of concern. For example, Clorox® (The Clorox Company, Oakland, CA) wipes do not contain bleach and the label states that contact time for it to be virucidal is four minutes.

All bottles should be clearly labeled with the identity of the disinfectant, all required safety information, the expiration date of the solution and the date and initials of the person who made up the solution. This is required by OSHA and will permit accountability and retraining should disinfectants be incorrectly formulated.

8.2.3.4 The Importance of Drying

Whatever disinfectant and method of application are used, the final decontamination step that cannot be overlooked is drying the environment. Most pathogens will survive for longer in moist conditions and some that are not otherwise particularly resilient in the environment (e.g. *Giardia* cysts) may persist for hours or days in a damp area. Fatal pathogens can persist in moist and damp environments, even in the presence of disinfectant. For instance, Streptococcus equi subsp. zooepidemicus, associated with a fatal outbreak in dogs (Pesavento et al. 2008), was cultured from pools of water remaining in kennels that had been completely cleaned and disinfected (Personal communication, Kate Hurley, 2018).

Attention to drying is especially important when the surface to be cleaned is uneven and likely to retain pools of water after squeegee use, or in humid climates where effective air drying may not occur. Therefore, drying tools (e.g. squeegees, towels and paper towels) and training on how to use them must be provided to accompany all sanitation protocols. Quiet floor fans can be used on low to expedite drying when needed. Care should be taken to ensure fans are not blowing directly on animals. Minimizing humidity in animal housing areas will also assist in drying.

Again, animals should never get wet during the sanitation process nor returned to enclosures that are still wet.

8.2.4 Other Important Aspects of Sanitation

8.2.4.1 Animal Housing/Facility Design

Consideration of animal housing design and use is an essential component of an effective sanitation plan. Good housing design, along with proper use, facilitates sanitation effectiveness and efficiency. Conversely, poor housing or inappropriate use of good housing can compromise staff's ability to adequately clean and care for animals, which can result in process inefficiencies. This, in turn, can result in the need for more staff, increased cleaning and disinfectant product use, and higher disease rates that all contribute to increased costs and decreased welfare.

Individual animal housing should, at a minimum, meet the basic physical and behavioral needs of the animal, allow for effective and efficient cleaning without the need to remove the animal from the housing unit and limit animal exposure to cleaning procedures. Appropriately sized double-compartment housing (kennels or cages) will generally meet the needs for individually housed dogs and cats adequately for short lengths of stay (up to about two weeks). (See Chapter 2 on Wellness for more details on animal housing). If double-compartment housing is not available or can only be provided to a limited number of animals, new intakes, juveniles and dangerous animals as well as all animals housed in isolation areas should be given the highest priority for use of these enclosures. (See Figure 8.1 for an example of double-compartment housing).

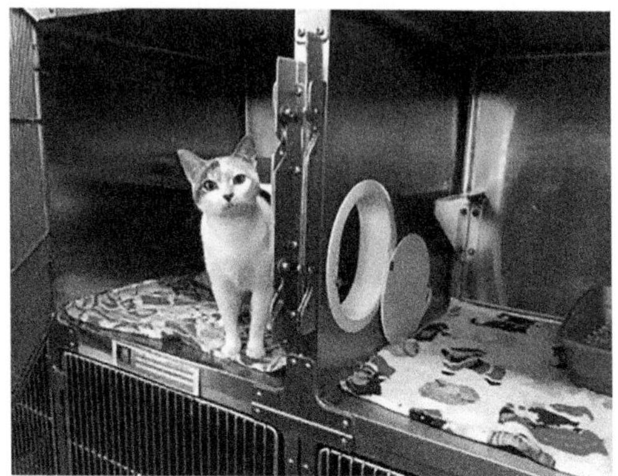

Figure 8.1 Double compartment housing unit.

For sanitation reasons, simple sealed concrete is not recommended in most shelter facilities where animal traffic occurs unless it will be resealed annually. A far better durable, cleanable material for high traffic areas throughout the shelter is polished sealed concrete (colored or not). However, it is not durable enough for use inside dog kennels. Resinous epoxy and urethane coating surfaces over concrete generally meet kennel flooring needs. Other more expensive materials such as non-porous, non-slippery tiles with epoxy grout can be used, however, cost often precludes use in animal shelter facilities. Shelters should consult with contractors who are familiar with the various challenges faced by shelters for the selection of the best materials for use in animal housing areas.

To allow for quick, adequate drying, high water use areas such as dog kennels must have proper drainage. This includes an appropriately sloped floor to a correctly placed drain with adequate flow and properly sized drainpipes to avoid flow back up, and appropriate drain covers to protect animals from injury and the plumbing from clogging. Individual kennel drains or properly designed and covered trench drains prevent cross-contamination from kennel to kennel. Drains should be provided both within the housing unit and in the aisle or walkway.

People and animals should not have to walk through one animal housing area to get to another housing area. To further help disease control, all animal rooms should be designed such that daily cleaning and care can be provided with minimal staff movement into and out of the room. Each animal housing room should be outfitted with its own dedicated cleaning supplies and equipment (identified for use in that room only) and have storage space for it to reduce unnecessary clutter.

8.2.4.2 Population Management

When designing a comprehensive shelter healthcare plan, consideration of the composition, size and management of the population is just as, if not more, important as the sanitation protocols and the design of the shelter building itself. The most thorough sanitation program and best building cannot compensate for the negative consequences suffered when a population is not well managed. Clinical experience and research have shown that the longer an animal remains in the shelter, the more likely they are to develop clinical signs of disease, so shelters must always strive to manage the population so each animal's length of stay (LOS) will be as short as possible to the desired outcome (Dinnage et al. 2009; Edinboro et al. 2004). Strategies such as managed or diverted intake, daily population rounds, identifying and addressing delays in flow-through and removing barriers to adoption can all help with reducing LOS.

When a shelter is crowded, not only is the LOS increased, but the likelihood of direct and indirect contact between animals is also increased, higher pathogen loads are typically present, and animals experience greater stress that negatively impacts their immune system and renders them more susceptible to disease. Additionally, shelter staff are frequently overwhelmed and unable to provide adequate daily care, making it difficult to both monitor and implement good sanitation practices. This can all result in an inability to meet the physical and behavioral needs of the animals which, in turn, can lead to increased health and/or behavioral concerns, diminished quality of life, and longer LOS. Additional information on population management can be found in the Introduction in Chapter 1, Chapter 2 on Wellness and Chapter 3 on Data Surveillance.

8.3 Common Products used in Sanitation Procedures in Animal Shelters

Cleaning and disinfecting agents chosen for usage in a shelter must be effective, safe to use around animals and humans, and practical given each organization's financial resources, ability to provide and monitor staff training and performance, and facility design. Every sanitation protocol must include sufficient information about the products used (e.g. dilution, method of application, storage and disposal, contact time) and be in writing. It is critical that staff are trained on such protocols and that evaluations are made periodically to ensure the whole process is working properly.

8.3.1 Detergents and Degreasers

Detergents and degreasers should be used to maintain clean surfaces that are free of visible dirt and debris. Though some disinfection products have label claims to be effective when organic matter is present, heavily soiled areas should always be pre-cleaned, either with the disinfectant product itself if it has detergent properties or with a separate detergent. Additionally, some disinfection products (e.g. quaternary ammonium compounds) are inactivated by detergents and thus surfaces must be rinsed thoroughly between cleaning and disinfection.

8.3.2 Chemical Disinfectants

Chemical disinfection is the most researched and used form of disinfection in shelters. Factors to consider when choosing a product include demonstrated activity against the pathogens for which the animals are at risk, constraints against efficacy (such as the presence of organic matter or preparation with hard water), method of delivery and time to effect (surface contact time) (Newbury et al. 2011).

There can be disagreement between manufacturer label claims and the efficacy of disinfectants demonstrated through independent testing. This has been illustrated particularly in regard to the commonly used quaternary ammonium class of disinfectants and their efficacy against un-enveloped viruses. In 1980, when researchers at Cornell noted that feline calicivirus spread in their research facility despite using a disinfectant labeled effective against that virus, they conducted a study testing the efficacy of quaternary ammonium products on un-enveloped viruses (e.g. canine parvovirus, feline panleukopenia, feline calicivirus). The study concluded that the product failed to inactivate feline panleukopenia and only partially inactivated calicivirus (Scott 1980). Over the years, quaternary ammonium products were repeatedly reformulated and relabeled as effective against un-enveloped viruses, while subsequent independent studies in 1995, 2002 and 2009 continued to disprove these label claims. (Eleraky et al. 2002; Eterpi et al. 2009; Kennedy et al. 1995). Certain quaternary ammonium disinfectants, especially those reformulated with other ingredients, may eventually be independently proven reliable against the un-enveloped viruses, but data available at the time of publication do not support a recommendation for their use when such pathogens are of concern. Moreover, this history demonstrates the perils of choosing a disinfectant based solely on label claims, and thus scientific research and veterinarians experienced in shelter medicine should also be consulted when choosing a product.

A summary of common disinfectants can be found in Table 8.2.

8.3.2.1 Chlorine Compounds

Sodium hypochlorite, commonly formulated as household bleach (5.25%), is effective at inactivating a wide array of pathogens including un-enveloped viruses and dermatophytes (ringworm), most notably *M. canis*. Historically, the recommendation for disinfection against *M. canis* was sodium hypochlorite at a very strong 1:10 dilution, which is very irritating to both humans and animals and corrosive to cage surfaces. But sodium hypochlorite (bleach 5.5%) at 1:32 and 1:100 dilutions was found to be effective even against a more robust challenge with visible hair and skin debris (Moriello 2015). It is inexpensive and widely available. However, it has numerous limitations, including a lack of any cleaning properties (e.g. detergent), being significantly inactivated by organic matter, and the potential for irritation to animal and human respiratory tracts.

For bleach to be effective, it must be used on a pre-cleaned, surface absent of organic matter, thus requiring a two-step sanitation procedure as well as 10 minutes contact time. Though stable when stored in light-proof containers for 30 days (Rutala et al. 1998), organic matter and exposure to light can substantially compromise the disinfectant properties of bleach solutions. Therefore, bleach solution in an open container should be replaced at least every 24 hours or whenever visibly soiled, whichever comes first. Bleach can be safely mixed together with quaternary ammonium compounds containing detergents; however, it must never be mixed with ammonium or products containing amines (e.g. Dawn dish soap) as this creates a noxious gas. As with any disinfectant, the SDS should be consulted for both bleach and the other product before mixing.

Bleach-related compounds, such as calcium hypochlorite (e.g. Wysiwash®) and sodium dichloroisocyanurate (e.g. Bruclean®), likewise are effective against un-enveloped viruses, do not have any cleaning activity, have limited effect when organic matter is present, and require similar contact times. Wysiwash (Wysiwash, South Daytona, FL) is a patented delivery system for diluted caplets that requires specialized hose-end equipment for use on pre-cleaned surfaces. The dilution occurs inside the caplet container, reducing the potential for mixing error, and it does not require a final rinse.

Poolife Turboshock® (Lonza, Basel, Switzerland), another calcium hypochlorite product, is a powder used for the treatment of swimming pools. It is sometimes used in

Table 8.2 Disinfectant products.

Disinfectant Product	Efficacy	Contact Time	Shelf life once diluted	Forms	Cautions
Sodium hypochlorite (Bleach) Usually used at 1 : 32 (1/2 cup per gallon)	Completely inactivates un-enveloped viruses and dermatophytes when used as directed No detergent activity Inactivated by organic matter	10 minutes	24 hours	Liquid 5.25% household bleach Stronger strengths available commercially	Significantly inactivated by organic matter, exposure to light, or extended storage Surfaces must be pre-cleaned and all organic matter removed prior to disinfection Surfaces must be rinsed after contact Corrosive to metal Respiratory irritant
Calcium hypochlorite (e.g. Wysiwash, https://www.wysiwash.com	Completely inactivates un-enveloped viruses and dermatophytes when used as directed No detergent activity Inactivated by organic matter	2 minutes	N/A	Dry caplet form Requires multiple- step process for cleaning and disinfection Used in a hose-end applicator system specific to this product	Surfaces must be pre-cleaned and all organic matter removed prior to disinfection Rinsing not needed after contact The dry form is hazardous if plastic caplet jacket is removed Disconnect and rinse out the hose-end applicator unit after each use to help maintain the unit
Sodium dichloroisocyanurate (e.g. Bruclean) http://bhcinc.com/our-markets/healthcare/animal-facility-maintenance/	Completely inactivates un-enveloped viruses and dermatophytes when used as directed Some detergent activity if tablet form used Inactivated by organic matter	10 minutes	24 hours	Dry tablet or liquid form Requires multiple step process for cleaning and disinfection Used with a specialized applicator	Surfaces must be pre-cleaned and all organic matter removed prior to disinfection Rinsing not needed after contact The dry form is irritating to mucous membranes if inhaled Less corrosive to metal and less respiratory irritation than bleach Dilute tablet or liquid as needed at time of use

(continued)

Table 8.2 (Continued)

Disinfectant Product	Efficacy	Contact Time	Shelf life once diluted	Forms	Cautions
Quaternary ammonium compounds (Numerous products)	Not proven reliably effective against un-enveloped viruses and dermatophytes Only moderate inactivation by organic matter Some detergent activity Disinfectant activity inactivated by detergents left on the surface	Varies depending on product	Varies depending on product	Most commonly a liquid concentrate that can be diluted	Surfaces must be rinsed of detergents prior to application Surfaces must be rinsed after contact Low tissue toxicity when diluted correctly Potentially toxic to cats causing tongue ulcers if diluted incorrectly
Potassium peroxymonosulfate (e.g. Trifectant) https://tomlyn.com/	Completely inactivates un-enveloped viruses and dermatophytes when used correctly Minimal detergent activity Relatively good activity in the face of organic matter	10 minutes	7 days	Dry powder Not designed for easy application through hose-end applicator systems (can be applied through specialized delivery systems).	Leaves visible residue on some surfaces Damaging to surfaces with routine use if not rinsed
Accelerated hydrogen peroxide (e.g. Rescue ™) https://rescuedisinfectants.com/product-info/	Completely inactivates un-enveloped viruses and dermatophytes when used correctly Good detergent activity Effective in the presence of organic material	1–10 minutes depending on the concentration	90 days	Ready-to-use liquid formula, liquid concentrate, wipes, Various application options - spray bottles, hose-end applicators, centralized systems, pump up foamers	Extremely versatile and safe Rinsing not needed after contact
Alcohol (e.g. Ethanol, Isopropyl alcohol) in hand sanitizers	Not reliably effective against un-enveloped viruses or dermatophytes (spores) Moderately effective against calicivirus at higher concentration (70%) Inactivated by organic matter	1 minute for calicivirus if at least 70%	N/A	Hand sanitizer	Less irritating to tissue than quaternary ammonium or bleach Allow for product to dry completely on hands after use

dilute form as a disinfectant in animal shelters, however, it is not labeled for use in animal care facilities and thus not recommended, as there are other approved products preferable for use around animals.

Bruclean (Brulin Holding Company, Indianapolis, IN) is a premeasured sodium dichloroisocyanurate disinfection tablet or liquid for dilution in water. The Brulin® Company has developed several special applicators for this product that can be used with a degreaser such as Brulin 815MX™ foam. The applicators, available as wall-mounted, portable rolling, or quick-connect foamer/sprayer units, allow for the full three-step process of foam cleaning, a water rinse, and disinfection. This product also does not require a final rinsing step.

8.3.2.2 Quaternary Ammonium Compounds

The quaternary ammonium compounds ("quats") are cationic detergents. Despite their ineffectiveness against un-enveloped viruses and dermatophytes (e.g. *M. canis*), these products do have some strengths. They have some ability to act as a cleaner as well as a disinfectant (depending on concentration and formulation), have some limited activity in the face of organic matter, and are relatively stable once diluted. Dilutions and contact times will vary depending on the product used. Many shelters utilize quaternary ammonium compound products for every day, routine one-step sanitation. If the product is used as both a detergent and disinfectant, it is important to ensure it is prepared and applied in accordance with the manufacturer's directions for each specific use. However, given the long history of disparity between label claims and tested efficacy, it is prudent to use an additional disinfectant when un-enveloped viruses or other resistant pathogens are suspected in an individual case or an outbreak.

8.3.2.3 Potassium Peroxymonosulfate

Potassium peroxymonosulfate (Trifectant®, Vetoquinol, Fort Worth, TX,) is an oxidizing disinfectant with a surfactant that has been proven to be reliably effective against un-enveloped viruses (Eleraky et al. 2002). It is also effective against dermatophytes (2% potassium peroxymonosulfate) (Moriello 2015). The product does have reasonable activity in the presence of organic material, but it is not a very effective stand-alone detergent and does not perform well with hose-end equipment. Potassium peroxymonosulfate comes in a powder form and must be handled carefully using appropriate PPE prior to dilution, as it is a respiratory irritant. The solution is stable for 7 days and requires a 10 minute wet contact time for efficacy against un-enveloped viruses.

8.3.2.4 Accelerated Hydrogen Peroxide

Accelerated hydrogen peroxide (Rescue®, formerly Accel®, Virox Technologies, Oakville, ON), a stabilized buffered oxidizing solution. It is effective against un-enveloped viruses at 1:32 dilution with a 10-minute wet contact time, and at 1:16 dilution with a 5-minute wet contact time (Omidbakhsh and Sattar 2006). It is also effective against dermatophytes (e.g. *M. canis*) at a 1:16 (Rescue™ 4.25% concentrate) dilution (Moriello 2015). It has good detergent activity as well as activity in the presence of organic material. Additionally, accelerated hydrogen peroxide has residual activity; because its residual activity might be negated by rinsing this is not recommended unless the area is extremely soiled. This product comes in ready-to-use liquid form and wipes (1-minute wet contact time), as well as a concentrate that can be diluted to the desired concentration. It is stable for 90 days, a significant advantage especially in areas where frequent remixing is impractical, such as on animal control vehicles. It is also extremely safe.

8.3.3 Disinfectant Toxicity

Like most other chemicals, disinfectants are not without the potential for harm. At a minimum, the use of disinfectants at excessively high concentrations can create respiratory irritation for animals and people, and some chemicals such as quaternary ammonium and phenol disinfectants can actually be fatal when applied incorrectly (Rousseaux et al. 1986; Trapani et al. 1982).

Toxicity resulting from exposure to disinfectants is of particular concern for cats since the idiosyncrasies of the feline metabolism make this species especially sensitive to many substances that are perfectly safe for other species, even when used following the manufacturer's recommendations. This needs to be taken into consideration when choosing the products used directly around animals as well as developing a plan for what steps will be taken if signs of toxicity are observed. Cats are particularly sensitive to phenol-based disinfectants (e.g. Lysol®, Pine-sol®) and these products should be not be used in areas where cats are housed.

Because of their widespread use, quaternary ammonium compounds have been identified as a relatively common cause of disinfectant toxicity in animal facilities. Disinfectant toxicity associated with quaternary ammonium compounds in shelters can cause severe oral and skin ulceration, ocular lesions, high fever, respiratory signs and pneumonia (Figure 8.2). It can present in a single animal or cause dramatic, widespread episodes depending on the source of the problem, e.g. concentrate spilled on one animal's hair coat versus used in a faulty applicator throughout a ward or the entire shelter. Care should be taken to ensure the disinfectant does not drip from one cage into the cage below it. When consistent clinical signs are noted, the disinfection dilution, method of application by staff and equipment should be evaluated carefully to rule out toxicity as a cause. These cases are sometimes reported as suspected virulent calicivirus outbreaks but are much quicker and easier to resolve by revising the sanitation protocols to stop the development of new cases.

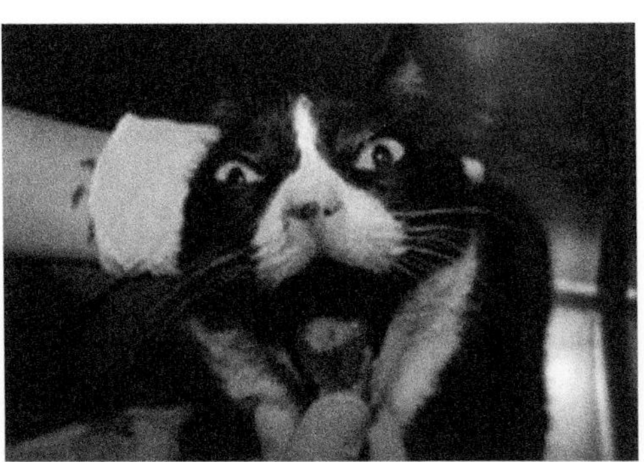

Figure 8.2 A cat with severe oral ulceration from quaternary ammonium toxicity.

If disinfectant toxicity is suspected, the animal should be bathed with warm water and a gentle shampoo, and the environment rinsed and dried to remove all disinfectant residue. Timely veterinary attention and treatment is important and should be provided for any animal with suspected disinfectant toxicity. Treatment will depend on the particular disinfectant and clinical signs observed but may include the administration of broad-spectrum antibiotics and pain control, especially if the animal has oral ulceration. If the animal has ingested disinfectant an animal poison control center or the manufacturer should be consulted for treatment recommendations. Administering emetics may cause more harm than good if the disinfectant is caustic when vomited up, and thus these medications should not be utilized without consultation. Often animals will recover surprisingly quickly from severe clinical signs, and thus treatment should be administered as quickly as possible.

8.3.4 Physical Disinfection

Alternative methods of disinfection such as ultraviolet (UV) light radiation, steam, ozone generators, High Efficiency Particulate Arrestance (HEPA) filters and reliance on freezing during cold weather do not have proven efficacy for all pathogens of concern in shelter facilities. However, while dose and efficacy have not been documented as thoroughly as for chemical disinfectants, UV light and heat, along with mechanical removal, are effective at reducing the dose of many pathogens. These methods may be used as a helpful adjunct, particularly in areas where chemical disinfection is impractical (e.g. lawn areas).

8.4 Order of Cleaning and Disinfection

Even if good application systems and biosecurity precautions (e.g. changing clothes and controlling transmission via fomites such as hands, clothing, and other objects, etc.) are used, some pathogens may still be spread as staff move through the shelter to clean. Ideally, staff should be assigned to care for specific subpopulations within the shelter, but this is not feasible for many organizations. In order to help reduce the risk of disease spread, especially when staff is limited and must clean several areas, areas housing healthy animals should be cleaned and disinfected first (e.g. adoption housing), followed by stray holding areas (e.g. the newly admitted animals), and finally, isolation areas where sick animals are housed. If biosecurity precautions are taken between areas (e.g. gloves, gowns, and dedicated equipment per area), cleaning order becomes less critical though following this order is still recommended whenever possible to further reduce risk. Within each area, biosecurity precautions should be used for enclosures housing juveniles, e.g. gloves changed between handling litters and individuals, etc.

8.5 Where to Focus Sanitation Efforts

Sanitation protocols often focus only on cleaning areas where animals are housed. However, pathogens can be tracked by human and animal traffic throughout the shelter facility. Additionally, pathogens can be spread by people and objects (fomites) such as hands, clothing, carriers, exam tables, instruments and animal transport vehicles. These fomites are a more likely source of disease transmission than direct contact between sick animals or with the cages or kennels themselves. Enclosures must be fully cleaned and disinfected between animals (i.e. every time a new animal occupies the enclosure) so that a housing unit should only contain the pathogens, if any, belonging to the animal(s) housed there at any one time.

Extra care should be taken to fully disinfect surfaces with the following characteristics:

- Frequent contact with many animals, including clothing, hands, countertops, exam-room tables, (e.g. in the medical and intake rooms), equipment and transport vehicles
- Contact with juvenile animals or those not protected by vaccination, including transport vehicles and carriers, intake countertops and clothing of intake staff
- Contact with a sick animal before contact with a healthy one, including clothing or tools that have been worn or used in areas housing sick animals, or during the euthanasia process.

If specific protocols do not exist, it is likely that cleaning some areas will be overlooked or performed improperly, especially in a busy shelter. Even areas that are off-limits to animals can harbor pathogens tracked in by staff and visitors and may need attention beyond general cleaning to avoid fomite transmission, especially during outbreaks of highly transmissible disease.

It must also be acknowledged that some areas, such as those with grass, gravel and dirt surfaces are notoriously difficult, if not impossible, to disinfect completely. Primary enclosures that are in poor condition pose similar challenges. Access to these areas should be evaluated carefully for risk versus benefit to vulnerable populations such as newly admitted and juvenile animals. It is likely an acceptable trade-off for newly admitted adult dogs to go on grassy areas for walks and playgroup when the overall disease level in the population is low and the level of risk is understood and closely monitored. Other biosecurity measures, such as the use of appropriate PPE when providing kennel and behavioral enrichment, should be researched and employed in cases where disease risk is high.

8.6 Sanitation of Animal Housing and Handling Areas

Animals usually spend most of their time within their housing unit while in the shelter. Therefore, sanitation protocols that keep these areas comfortable with a minimal risk for disease exposure and transmission are necessary. Sample protocols for cleaning dog and cat housing units can be found in the appendix.

8.6.1 Cleaning

As explained earlier in the chapter, the first step in the sanitation process includes manually cleaning to remove all visible dirt and debris from all surfaces. In addition to physically removing soiled bedding, newspapers, feces, uneaten food, etc. the surface must be cleaned with a detergent capable of removing hidden dirt and organic debris. Most disinfectants must be applied to a clean surface in order to be effective, as summarized in Table 8.2. Though some products (e.g. quaternary ammonium, accelerated hydrogen peroxide) can be used in a single step to both clean and disinfect, it is recommended to clean and disinfect in a two-step process whenever there is heavy soiling and contamination.

8.6.1.1 Spot Cleaning

Another element of the shelter sanitation plan that needs to be considered is that the actual cleaning process is stressful to animals and more microorganisms may actually be transmitted than removed. In some cases, removing animals from their enclosures for daily cleaning and chemical disinfection is not necessary and may even be detrimental. It has been shown that the stress of rehousing cats for cleaning can cause the recrudescence of the feline herpes virus, resulting in clinical signs of respiratory disease (Gaskell et al. 2007).

For animals that remain in their cage or kennel, spot cleaning is often preferable to thorough daily cleaning and disinfection. Spot cleaning involves leaving the animal in its cage while tidying it and providing fresh food and water daily so that the environment is comfortable for the animal. Bedding, as well as objects with an owner's or the animal's own scent that may bring comfort to an animal, can often be left in place unless visibly soiled. This reduces stress and disruption for the animal and frees up staff time to focus on cleaning and disinfecting thoroughly whenever new animals are introduced to an enclosure.

Spot cleaning works particularly well for cats and kittens because they generally confine their urination and defecation to a litter pan and caregivers do not need to physically enter their cage or condo. Spot cleaning can also be used for dogs in some cases. Full daily cleaning and disinfection of areas and enclosures are recommended for dogs under five months of age and newly admitted dogs with an unknown medical history since these animals may not have adequate protection from pathogens that could be tracked into their kennels on caregivers' clothing, hands or shoes.

For any species, spot cleaning becomes substantially easier and more effective when double-compartment housing that allows animals to move from one side of the enclosure to the other is provided to all animals in the shelter. Figure 8.1 shows an example of double-compartment housing.

Spot cleaning can be utilized in rooms that group house cats and allow them to walk around on the floor. Only vaccinated adult cats should be housed in communal/group rooms, as vaccination should help protect against many of the pathogens that could be tracked in on the shoes of caregivers, volunteers and visitors who enter the room. The room can be cleaned daily to achieve the goals of making the room comfortable for the cat(s) and attractive to visitors. The room should be fully cleaned and disinfected before a new group of cats are housed in the room.

It is important to stress that spot cleaning refers to cleaning only —animals should never be left in the cage if spraying water or applying harsh cleansers or a disinfectant.

8.6.2 Disinfecting

It is important to remember the points made earlier in this chapter concerning product preparation and storage, contact time, application systems, thorough rinsing if indicated, and the importance of drying in order for disinfection to be effective.

In areas that house dogs or other larger species, hose-end foamers, specially designed or built-in room dispensing systems are preferred. Some disinfectants, such as Wysiwash and Bruclean come with specially designed dispensing equipment.

For large facilities, low pressure built-in central systems are available. Disinfectants that come in a liquid concentrate, such as accelerated hydrogen peroxide and quaternary ammonium compounds, are ideal for this use. The use of high-pressure washers should be reserved for when no animals are present in the room or ward; in addition to avoiding stressing or wetting the animals, consideration should be given to the potential for aerosolization of pathogens. For smaller jobs or where the use of a hose is impractical, a hand-held or back-pack style pesticide applicator can be used.

As an alternative to mops, especially where drains are not present, the ANIVAC Pro-Heat System (Ogena Solutions, Stoney Creek, ON) for use with Rescue™ is an option. This is a large, 50-l wet vacuum system with a cleaning wand with changeable brushes for different surfaces that expels a fresh cleaning/disinfecting solution and also removes the soiled solution.

If mops or rags and buckets *must* be used, a disinfectant should be chosen with minimal inactivation by organic matter. Contamination of the disinfectant can be minimized by rinsing the mop or other applicator in a bucket of clean water between each application of a disinfectant. Two-sided buckets are available from janitorial supply houses, or two separate buckets can be used. Separate cleaning supplies should be used for each area to be cleaned and clearly labeled to identify which area they are to be used in.

It is important to apply the disinfection product to all surfaces, including the door and walls of enclosures, leaving it on for the necessary wet contact time and rinsing if necessary before wiping off and drying with a clean rag or paper towel. A separate rag or disposable paper towel should be used for each cage.

8.7 Sanitation of Animal-Related Items

8.7.1 Bowls, Toys and Litter Boxes

Items such as bowls, toys, resting platforms and litter boxes are high-contact surfaces that can readily become contaminated with pathogens. Therefore, these items must be thoroughly cleaned and disinfected between animals, as well as regularly sanitized to provide an enriched, comfortable and healthy environment for the animals.

Whenever disposable products are not used or are not available, high-quality stainless steel is the preferred material for food and water bowls because it is nonporous, durable as well as easily cleaned and disinfected. However, with the availability of new products with good penetration into porous surfaces (e.g. accelerated hydrogen peroxide), other materials such as plastic may be acceptable even though they are less durable over time.

If these items are hand-washed, used litter and uneaten food should be disposed of, items cleaned with a detergent to remove all visible debris and then soaked in a disinfectant at the appropriate dilution for the necessary contact time or longer. Articles should be rinsed unless otherwise indicated by the manufacturer (e.g. accelerated hydrogen peroxide), and allowed to dry completely before re-use. The disinfectant dip should be changed in accordance with the manufacturer's guidelines or whenever visibly dirty. Ideally, bowls and toys should be handled in an area separate from litter boxes, and at a minimum, they should not be handled in the same sink at the same time.

The use of commercial dishwashers or sanitizers are also effective methods to clean/disinfect these items. Visible debris should be rinsed or removed from these items before being put into the machines, and bowls and toys should be washed separately from litter boxes.

All cleaning and disinfecting activities should take place away from areas where human food is handled, consumed or stored.

8.7.2 Laundry

During laundering, microbial decontamination is achieved by a combination of physical removal (due to mechanical action in the wash and rinse cycles) together with inactivation (or killing) of the pathogen, due to thermal or chemical action. Laundry detergents that contain perborate or percarbonate together with a bleach activator release active oxygen in contact with water in a temperature-dependent manner. Though the primary purpose of including activated oxygen bleach (AOB) in the detergent is to enhance stain removal, it also produces some chemical inactivation of pathogens. The surfactant components of laundry detergents can themselves exert some antimicrobial effect as well. It is this complex interaction between physical removal, chemical inactivation and thermal inactivation during laundering that achieves effective sanitization.

All that is usually required for sanitizing most laundry in an animal shelter is the manual removal of visible dirt and debris prior to washing in either a regular or commercial washing machine, using hot water and detergent with AOB or chlorine bleach, and drying in a regular or commercial dryer on a high heat cycle. A half-cup (4 oz or 118 ml) of bleach can be added for an average household washer and is not inactivated by detergent or hot water (Christian et al. 1983; Walter and Schillinger 1975). Large commercial washing machines and dryers are likely better able to meet the needs of most shelters in terms of size and durability. Based on their capacity, a full cup (8 oz or 236 ml) of bleach per load should be used in these machines. Most viruses, bacteria and *Giardia* cysts are inactivated at 60° Celsius(C)/ 140° Fahrenheit (F); parvoviruses are a notable exception. However, it is possible that lower temperatures can be effective if longer wash/agitation cycles (15–30 minutes) and a detergent containing AOB are used (Addie et al. 2015; Honisch et al. 2014). In general, higher temperatures, longer wash cycles, and addition of AOB/bleach all contribute to effectiveness; if one of these factors is not optimal (e.g. only cold water is available; or a particular item cannot be bleached), optimizing the other factors will be helpful.

At this time, the Environmental Protection Agency (EPA) does not allow for the approval of disinfection claims against viruses on soft surfaces such as carpets and bedding. However, some products such as accelerated hydrogen peroxide have a soft-surface sanitation claim of one ounce (29 ml) per gallon (3.8 l) with a three minutes contact time against bacteria. Shelters have reported good results utilizing this product at 4–8 oz (118–236 ml) per load as an alternative for detergent and bleach for laundering.

An additional measure of efficacy is provided by the heat and desiccation caused by drying and for this reason, hanging laundry to dry is not recommended, especially if it would be hung in an area that is not exposed to direct sunlight (e.g. indoors or in cloudy weather). The essential laundry basics are summarized in Table 8.3.

Laundry that has suspected or known exposure to ringworm (e.g. *M. canis*) can be effectively decontaminated by washing twice in cold water (30° C/86° F) on a long wash cycle (longer

Table 8.3 Essential laundry basics.

- Remove solids such as fecal matter and other visible hair, dirt and debris before laundering
- Avoid overloading washers and dryers
- Clean lint traps after every load
- Dry all articles completely in a dryer
- Ensure that clothing and hands do not become contaminated by dirty laundry that can transmit pathogens to freshly laundered articles (fomite contamination)
- Keep the laundry room uncluttered and organized
- Ideally, store clean laundry in a separate room from the washing machines and all of the dirty laundry

than 14 minutes). It is important not to overload the machine to allow for maximal agitation during washing. Always separate exposed laundry from unexposed laundry and routinely clean the environment to prevent fomite contamination. The addition of bleach was not shown to improve decontamination (Moriello 2016).

Though it has not been proven, a similar protocol for laundering articles exposed to un-enveloped viruses will most likely inactivate or remove the viruses along with any organic material. High temperatures of at least 80° C/176° F (Addie et al. 2015) have been shown to be effective at inactivating parvovirus but may be difficult to attain in a non-commercial setting. However, good laundering practices as described above are likely to be effective based on the experience of this author and numerous shelter medicine experts. In some cases, it may be prudent to consider discarding some articles that are heavily soiled with blood or contaminated with highly resistant pathogens such as parvovirus and *M. canis*.

8.7.3 Transport Carriers and Vehicles

The cleaning and disinfection of all carriers and vehicles used to transport animals are of extreme importance to include in the sanitation plan because their surfaces have contact with many animals. A protocol similar to that described for the cleaning and disinfecting of housing units within the shelter after each animal use should be followed for all carriers and transport vehicles. This includes the removal of fecal matter, dirt and other organic debris, application of a product with efficacy against un-enveloped viruses and in the presence of organic matter (e.g. potassium peroxymonosulfate or accelerated hydrogen peroxide) at the proper concentration for the correct contact time, rinsing if indicated, followed by thorough drying. Providing training, the correctly diluted product and the needed application tools in a convenient area for use in the vehicles both on the road and upon return to the shelter will help with compliance.

For disinfection of carriers, large dip buckets or tanks filled with a stable product, such as accelerated hydrogen peroxide, can be used. Carriers should be scrubbed beforehand to ensure removal of any gross organic material and closely inspected to make sure there is no visible hair, body fluids or other debris, allowed to soak in the disinfectant for the appropriate contact time, rinsed if indicated, and then completely dried before the next use. In addition to following the manufacturer's directions for use, the solution should be checked periodically (daily) with test strips to ensure it is still of the desired concentration and changed out when it is not.

8.7.4 Other Equipment

Equipment that is reused by medical staff, such as endotracheal (ET) tubes and breathing circuits, also require a sanitation protocol. Research has shown an effective method of reducing the bacterial load on ET tubes is soaking them in either a chlorhexidine gluconate or accelerated hydrogen peroxide solution for at least five minutes or spraying all tube surfaces with accelerated hydrogen peroxide and letting them sit for at least five minutes and then rinsing (Crawford and Weese

2015). Because chlorhexidine has limited efficacy against un-enveloped viruses, the use of this disinfectant would not be advised if contamination with those pathogens is a concern. Since breathing circuits do not have direct contact with mucosal surfaces of animals, many shelters do not disinfect the systems between patients but rather at the end of each day of use.

Equipment used for handling animals, such as catch poles, muzzles, and leather gloves, should be disinfected regularly, with extra attention and care provided after contact with animals with suspected or known infectious disease.

8.8 Sanitation for the Staff

8.8.1 Hand Sanitation

Cleaning environmental surfaces is only part of the sanitation plan. The benefit of placing an animal on a properly disinfected exam table is negated if the hands that hold the animal are contaminated. Keeping hands clean is also important for the protection of human health. Of all the contact precautions and biosecurity measures used in healthcare settings to help prevent the physical direct or indirect transmission of microorganisms between patients, staff, and the environment, hand hygiene is considered the single most important measure for infection prevention (Mathur 2011). There are three methods for managing hand hygiene: wearing gloves, washing with soap and water, and applying hand sanitizers.

8.8.1.1 Gloves

Gloves are generally the most fool-proof choice for preventing pathogen transfer on hands, provided they are put on, taken off, and changed at the appropriate times. Though gloves can be a nuisance, time-consuming and relatively costly, there are times when it is worth the effort and thus recommended. A change of gloves between every animal is indicated when handling animals that may be infected with particularly environmentally resilient pathogens, when a zoonotic infection is involved (or suspected), or during any outbreak of disease. Hands should always be carefully washed before donning and after removing gloves, especially if handling an animal with a serious or zoonotic illness since hands can become contaminated through small breaks in the gloves or in the process of taking them off. (It should be noted that the Food and Drug Administration [FDA] banned the use of powdered surgeon's gloves, powdered patient examination gloves, and absorbable powder for lubricating a surgeon's gloves in 2017. Though shelter staff would not ordinarily use these types of gloves for sanitation procedures, their use should be avoided for handling animals.)

8.8.1.2 Handwashing

Proper handwashing has the significant advantage over hand sanitizers of mechanically removing even the most resistant pathogens and is therefore required under certain circumstances, such as when hands are contaminated with feces, blood or bodily fluids, are visibly soiled, or after suspected exposure to a durable pathogen such as parvovirus or ringworm (WHO 2009). However, it is important to wash hands correctly but unfortunately, compliance is often lacking.

As with environmental decontamination, the drying step is especially important. Moisture on hands may actually facilitate pathogen survival and transfer (Patrick et al. 1997); paper towels are more efficient for drying and removing bacteria, and they cause less contamination than hand dryers (Huang et al. 2012). Staff, volunteers and visitors should always have ready access to handwashing stations stocked with soap and paper towels. The Centers for Disease Control (CDC) provides very helpful on-line training videos and other resources on handwashing that can be shared and utilized throughout the shelter. These resources can be found at https://www.cdc.

gov/handwashing/index.html. See Table 8.4 for a synopsis of the CDC's guidelines for proper handwashing technique.

8.8.1.3 Hand Sanitizers

The third strategy for dealing with contaminated hands is the use of alcohol-based hand sanitizer gels that kill microorganisms by denaturing proteins and disrupting the cell membrane. It had been widely believed that hand washing was always the next best choice when gloves were impractical. However, current research suggests that hand sanitizers are preferable in some circumstances (Ho et al. 2015; Longtin et al. 2011). Though the spectrum of activity may be limited especially against un-enveloped viruses, a slightly less effective method, used consistently and correctly, will provide better results than the theoretically ideal choice used improperly. In one study that compared the bacterial levels on the hands of veterinary students after performing an examination on a horse, bacterial counts were actually lower on the hands of those who used a hand sanitizer compared to those who washed and dried their hands (Traub-Dargatz et al. 2006). While changing gloves or properly washing hands between animals are the recommended methods to use when handling high-risk animals (such as during the intake process or between litters of juvenile animals), hand sanitizers should be considered as an option for hand sanitation between handling healthy animals. See Table 8.5 for the basics of hand sanitizer use.

It must be noted that no hand sanitizer is effective against the most durable pathogens, such as the parvoviruses or ringworm. When these pathogens are suspected, gloves and handwashing must be used. Additionally, when hands are visibly soiled, hand washing is the necessary method of hand hygiene.

Table 8.4 CDC Guidelines for proper handwashing (CDC 2015).

1) Wet hands with clean running water (warm or cold)—turn off the tap and apply soap[a] from a dispenser (bar soap should be avoided)
2) Lather all surfaces (back of hands, between fingers, under nails) with soap
3) Continue to scrub all surfaces for a minimum of 20 seconds
4) Rinse well under clean running water to remove any contaminants from the hands
5) Thoroughly dry hands using two single-use paper towels for 10 seconds each. Use the towel to turn off the faucet (if not automatic faucet) to avoid direct contact with the handle
6) Total time spent with this method is 30–60 seconds

[a] While antibacterial soap is not recommended in low-risk situations such as homes and general public restrooms, its use is recommended in healthcare settings and thus could extend to veterinary uses as well (Anderson 2015). However, in the shelter setting where antimicrobial resistance is of increased concern and most of the pathogens of serious concern are viral, the routine use of antibacterial soap is not generally recommended.

8.8.2 Personal Protective Equipment (PPE)

OSHA law requires employers to provide their employees with a safe and healthful workplace. As such, PPE that helps to protect the

Table 8.5 The basics of hand sanitizer use.

- Use hand sanitizers that contain 60–80% ethanol or isopropyl alcohol (due to better efficacy against certain un-enveloped viruses such as feline calicivirus). Hand sanitizers should also contain an emollient to protect the skin
- Read the label for other ingredients as some contain phenol (Triclosan) or quaternary ammonium (benzalkonium) compounds, which can be toxic to animals at too high a concentration
- Provide clearly labeled hand sanitizers in all animal areas; position them within 3 ft of animal exam/intake stations and post instructions for proper use
- Apply product to all surfaces of hands for a minimum of a 15-second contact time
- Rub hands until dry
- Total time spent when using these products is 20–30 seconds

staff from exposure to and infection with zoonotic pathogens must be provided. This use of PPE also helps reduce the spread of pathogens between animals. PPE includes such items as disposable gloves, disposable, or reusable gowns, disposable shoe covers, surgical masks and eye protection. Clear instructions and training regarding how, when, and which PPE to use in different situations, such as cleaning, performing intake procedures, and during an outbreak, must be included in all sanitation protocols and must be made readily available to staff. In addition, the PPE must be of good quality and in adequate supply.

8.8.3 Clothing

Disease transmission via clothing is a significant concern in the human healthcare world. For instance, one study found potentially harmful pathogens present on almost half of the doctors' neckties (Nurkin 2004). Clothing-borne disease transmission is a very real concern in veterinary medicine as well. The risk of disease transmission on clothing is enhanced by an animal's propensity to shed hair, which may be contaminated with pathogens from a variety of sources (e.g. dermal, salivary, environmental). Some pathogens may even cluster around hair follicles, facilitating the spread of diseases such as ringworm and virulent systemic feline calicivirus on clothing. This may, in part, explain the ease of fomite spread associated with some strains of calicivirus.

One of the most important and reasonably easy infectious disease control procedures is to have staff change clothing or wear protective garments for "dirty" activities such as cleaning and treatment of sick animals. Though it is not practical to routinely provide a full change of clothing after handling each animal, scrub tops or protective smocks should be freely available and used whenever interacting with a potentially infectious or high-risk animal (e.g. juveniles, ringworm infected animals). Dedicated clothing, just like footwear, should be worn for cleaning and removed if staff perform other activities in the shelter after daily cleaning is complete. Discarded surgery gowns are ideal for this purpose, as the long sleeves provide full coverage for arms that can otherwise escape both hand washing and gloves.

The images in Figures 8.3 (a-d) provide an example of how significant contamination of clothing may be, and how that level of contamination compares to recently washed hands. An instrument designed to measure adenosine triphosphate (ATP) was used to assess the relative cleanliness of an animal shelter caregiver's scrub top (Figure 8.3). Because ATP is the energy source in all living cells, the amount present provides an indirect measurement of the relative quantity of bacteria, yeast, and mold. The measurement was 2362640 reflective light units (RLUs) (Figure 8.3b), compared to a measurement of 66899 RLUs obtained from a hand that was washed and then petted three shelter cats (Figure 8.3c). The hand had 35 times *less* organic matter than the scrub top (Figure 8.3d), which supports the need for all shelter workers to change into a new top after cleaning or performing other "dirty" activities, or to appropriately utilize PPE. It also provides evidence to support the practice of letting potential adopters pet most animals, since they pose a relatively low risk of disease transmission compared to shelter staff, and interacting with the animal could increase the likelihood of adoption.

8.8.4 Footwear

In human healthcare, hands are the primary culprit in infectious disease transmission. In veterinary medicine and animal care, this may also be true but there are additional culprits to consider, such as "foot-borne" disease transmission. For example, animal patients, especially dogs, often sit on the floor of the intake or exam room. Staff often walk in and out of dog kennels for cleaning, potentially contaminating the soles of their shoes and creating a risk of fomite transmission. Cats, on the other hand, are often moved from a carrier to an exam surface or a cage off the ground, consequently

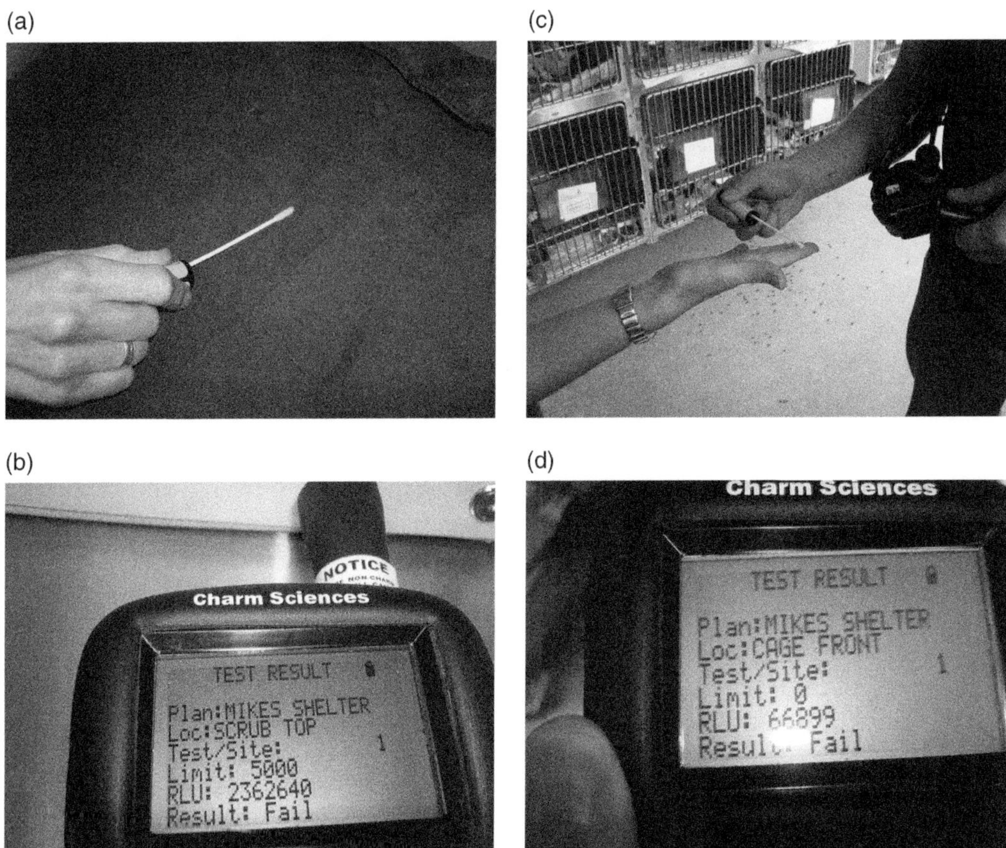

Figure 8.3 (a)Measuring the "cleanliness" of a shelter animal caregiver's scrub top. (b) RLU measurement from the shelter animal caregiver's scrub top. (c) Measuring the "cleanliness" of a simulated potential adopter's hand. (d) RLU measurement from the simulated potential adopter's hand.

leaving them less vulnerable to "foot-borne" disease. However, this is not always the case (e.g. group housing of cats in small rooms) and shelters should critically evaluate the risk of disease transmission via footwear based on their facility design, populations, housing, and standard operating procedures.

If the basic environmental cleaning program is effective, the risk of transmitting disease via footwear is probably relatively low. Because some pathogens may get tracked into a room or kennel when staff enter to clean it, the last step should be the application of a good disinfectant to the floor so that whatever was tracked in will be inactivated. This is most important when dealing with a susceptible population such as new intakes and juveniles. When the infectious disease risk is high, staff should also change footwear after cleaning.

Foot sanitation should be a greater concern under a few special circumstances, such as before entering areas where vulnerable animals (puppies and kittens) are housed (especially if they are on the ground), when entering and exiting isolation areas where animals are being treated for conditions caused by particularly resistant pathogens (e.g. parvovirus or *M. canis*), and during an outbreak of unknown cause.

Footbaths have historically been used in an attempt to provide foot sanitation. However, there are significant, inherent limitations to the use of footbaths and they should not be relied upon as an adequate means of preventing fomite transmission from contaminated footwear. All disinfectants require some amount of contact time for optimal effect, and this will not be achieved with a brief submersion in a footbath. Often disinfectant footbaths are an insufficient depth and are frequently used without prior removal of the gross organic matter contamination present on shoes, making the chemicals used ineffective. One study found that of the products investigated, only potassium peroxymonosulfate was effective in reducing the bacterial count on boots after use, while the more commonly used quaternary ammonium disinfectants did not have that effect (Morley et al. 2005). Even potassium peroxymonosulfate footbaths, correctly used, did not lead to a significant reduction in bacterial contamination of floor surfaces beyond the footbath (Stockton et al. 2006). Furthermore, incorrectly used footbaths have been shown to increase the spread of pathogens (Amass et al. 2008).

Therefore, considering that footbaths can be challenging to use and maintain correctly, and may actually create additional risk, there is little justification to use them in shelter animal housing areas. Instead, the use of dedicated shoes or shoe/boot covers are recommended for use in animal shelters where necessary, particularly in areas housing animals under quarantine or treatment for highly transmissible pathogens such as canine and feline parvovirus and *M. canis*. Rubber over-soles can be kept in a variety of sizes directly outside the areas housing ill or quarantined animals, allowing the staff to easily step in and out of them as they enter and leave the area. Alternatively, disposable shoe covers can be used as a single-use option.

8.9 Developing a Shelter Sanitation Plan

To ensure the development of an effective sanitation plan that also complies with the recommendations in this chapter, a staff member should be designated to be the architect of the plan to oversee its development and implementation. The assigned individual should have a clear responsibility for the process and sufficient knowledge of the shelter facility and disease control to design practical, efficient and effective protocols. They must have adequate time to research and write the plan, train staff and volunteers, and ideally have the capacity to oversee implementation and enforcement of the plan. They must also be willing to make changes to the plan as needed. Ideally, a veterinarian or veterinary technician familiar with shelter medicine should provide advice and input. Certainly, manufacturers of disinfectant and cleaning products can provide input about the proper use of particular products, but it should be remembered that they will probably have some bias toward the products they carry. Additional resources to consult when developing sanitation protocols are included in Table 8.6.

Table 8.6 Shelter Sanitation Resources.

- University of California - Davis Koret Shelter Medicine Program – www.sheltermedicine.com
- University of Wisconsin Shelter Medicine Program – www.uwsheltermedicine.com
- University of Florida Maddie's Shelter Medicine Program – http://sheltermedicine.vetmed.ufl.edu
- Maddie's® Shelter Medicine Program at Cornell – http://www.sheltermedicine.vet.cornell.edu
- The Association of Shelter Veterinarians Guidelines for Standards of Care in Animal Shelters – http://www.sheltervet.org/assets/docs/shelter-standards-oct2011-wforward.pdf
- Shelter Medicine for Veterinarians and Staff 2nd Edition (2013) L. Miller and S. Zawistowski (eds.) https://www.wiley.com/en-us/Shelter+Medicine+for+Veterinarians+and+Staff%2C+2nd+Edition-p-9781118445570
- *Infectious Diseases of the Dog and Cat, 4th Edition (2012)* C.E. Greene (ed.) Published by Saunders Elsevier, St. Louis.
- Veterinary Infection Prevention and Control by Linda Caveney, Barbara Jones, and Kimberly Ellis. (2011) published by John Wiley & Sons, Hoboken, NJ.

8.9.1 Written Protocols

As previously noted, everything that needs to be cleaned/disinfected requires a written protocol that should be made readily available to those who will use it. All staff, and if applicable, volunteers, need to be sufficiently trained on the protocols, and periodic monitoring of all aspects of the sanitation plan is necessary to help ensure continued compliance. It is not uncommon that a shelter has excellent protocols, in theory, only to find that in reality, the practice is quite different, especially when staff turnover is high.

At a minimum, each written sanitation protocol must include:

- How often the area/object is to be cleaned/disinfected (e.g. after each use, daily, weekly, annually, during or after an outbreak)
- What cleaning and disinfection products are to be used, and how they should be prepared, stored and applied, including, in detail, the correct process for dilution, contact time, rinsing if necessary, and disposal following the manufacturer's recommendations and local, state or federal regulations
- Who is responsible for writing the protocol, following the protocol and ensuring the protocol is adhered to
- How and with what frequency the process will be checked to ensure it is being performed correctly.

Staff should be made aware of their individual responsibilities for carrying out sanitation procedures, especially if their schedules or assignments vary periodically. Ideally, they should be trained in all procedures, not just the ones utilized in the areas they may be normally assigned to work in, as staffing shortages may lead to their sudden reassignment to different areas. Supervisors should verify staff have completed training in writing and periodically re-evaluate them. Finally, all members of the management and veterinary teams should be encouraged to praise or reward good disinfection practices when they see it, as well as report any problems.

8.9.2 Achieving and Verifying Success

Occasionally reviewing the efficacy of a shelter sanitation program can be a powerful educational and motivational tool for staff. It can save staff from spending enormous amounts of time on a process that simply does not work, and can help management acknowledge and reward successful efforts or address challenges that may exist.

Education is often the first intervention utilized to improve protocol compliance. But even if the protocols are deemed mandatory and their importance is stressed, providing education alone is generally not enough to change behavior. Change depends on both an individual's ability to perform the behavior and their intention and motivation. Intention includes what one thinks about the practice (attitude toward the action), what one thinks other respected individuals think about the practice (subjective norms), and whether one believes they can effectively perform the required practice (perceived behavior control) (Whitby et al. 2007). Multimodal interventions that address multiple areas of concern and in different ways are likely to be more effective than those that are more narrowly focused (Anderson 2015; Kingston et al. 2016).

The most commonly reported reason for noncompliance with protocols is not having enough time (Ho et al. 2015); thus, maintaining adequate staffing levels to allow individuals sufficient time to complete all assigned tasks with proficiency is paramount to achieving success. A staffing formula has been promulgated by the National Animal Control Association (NACA) to help shelters determine the staffing level necessary to clean and feed the shelter population. As an example, out of the total of 15 minutes recommended per animal for daily husbandry, NACA guidelines (2009) recommend a minimum of nine minutes per animal per day for routine cleaning and six minutes for feeding. Shelters can determine their own formula by observing and timing how long it takes staff members to perform their designated tasks; this is particularly important when facility limitations and constantly changing population numbers require more than the typical amount of labor and time to care for the animals.

Creating awareness about how often staff neglects to perform hand hygiene and its possible impact on disease transmission, and/or providing positive feedback when compliance improves likely provides additional incentive to further improve compliance. When implementing a new protocol, it is important to strike a balance between positive feedback and constructive criticism. Additionally, the use of any kind of penalty system must be done with great caution to avoid creating a negative attitude toward management and the shelter sanitation program itself.

A fun training tool is "Glo-Germ," a powder that fluoresces under UV light and is designed to demonstrate and mimic the spread of pathogens. One way this product can be used is to have staff handle a stuffed or resident shelter cat sprinkled with Glo-Germ, then wash their hands as usual and check for residual "germs." Alternatively, it can be secretly sprinkled in the back of a recently vacated cage and staff can be rewarded if they successfully remove it all in the process of their deep cleaning.

For the sanitation program to be effective, every staff member, including veterinarians, veterinary technicians, shelter directors and managers, kennel staff and volunteers, must receive proper education and training and follow all protocols. Input from staff who must implement the plan should be encouraged when offered to address problem areas, improve the efficacy of the protocols or increase staff compliance and safety. Plan and compliance failures may be due to a variety of reasons, including lack of a realistic plan, failure to update the plan to accommodate new circumstances, crowding that does not permit staff sufficient time to clean, understaffing, damaged, or missing equipment, wrong product selection, poor shelter design, deteriorating physical facility, etc.

Research suggests that involvement and support from upper-level management are necessary for effective implementation of hand hygiene protocols in human healthcare systems (Whitby et al. 2007), and it is reasonable to assume this would also be relevant in animal shelters. The involvement of all individuals, regardless of role, helps to create an overall infection control culture within the shelter.

8.10 Conclusion

The importance of designing and implementing a thorough, well thought out shelter sanitation plan for the health and welfare of the animals cannot be overstated. Not having an effective yet, realistic plan can lead to animal and human illness, increased LOS, decreased welfare for the animals, decreased staff morale, fewer adoptions, and other undesired outcomes (such as an increase in the euthanasia of sick animals). Thankfully, much information is available from experience and research to help shelter veterinarians and managers work together to develop a successful sanitation plan. Managing the population and having appropriate housing and utilizing it properly will work in conjunction with the sanitation plan to keep animals and people in shelters healthy.

References

Addie, D.D., Boucraut-Baralon, C., Egberink, H. et al. (2015). Disinfectant choices in veterinary practices, shelters and households – ABCD guidelines on safe and effective disinfection for feline environments. *Journal of Feline Medicine and Surgery* 17: 594–605.

Amass, S., Vyverberg, B., and Beaudry, D. (2008). Evaluating the efficacy of boot baths in biosecurity protocols. *Journal of Swine Health and Production* 8 (4): 169–173.

Anderson, M.E.C. (2015). Contact precautions and hand hygiene in veterinary clinics. *The Veterinary Clinics of North America. Small Animal Practice* 45 (2): 343–360.

Centers for Disease Control (CDC) (2015). When & How to Wash your Hands. https://www.cdc.gov/handwashing/when-how-handwashing.html (accessed 5 June 2020).

Christian, R.R., Manchester, J.T., and Mellor, M.T. (1983). Bacteriological quality of fabrics washed at lower-than-standard temperatures in a hospital laundry facility. *Applied and Environmental Microbiology* 45 (2): 591–597.

Crawford, S. and Weese, J.S. (2015). Efficacy of endotracheal tube disinfection strategies for elimination of *Streptococcus zooepidemicus* and *Bordetella bronchiseptica*. *Journal of the American Veterinary Medical Association* 247 (9): 1033–1036.

Dinnage, J.D., Scarlett, J.M., and Richards, J.R. (2009). Descriptive epidemiology of feline upper respiratory tract disease in an animal shelter. *Journal of Feline Medicine and Surgery* 11: 816–825.

Edinboro, C.H., Ward, M.P., and Glickman, L.T. (2004). A placebo controlled trial of two intranasal vaccines to prevent tracheobronchitis (kennel cough) in dogs entering a humane shelter. *Preventive Veterinary Medicine* 62: 89–99.

Eleraky, N.Z., Potgieter, L.N.D., and Kennedy, M.A. (2002). Virucidal efficacy of four new disinfectants. *Journal of the American Animal Hospital Association* 38 (3): 231–234.

Eterpi, M., McDonnell, G., and Thomas, V. (2009). Disinfection efficacy against parvoviruses compared with reference viruses. *Journal of Hospital Infection* 73 (1): 64–70.

Gaskell, R., Dawson, S., Radford, A. et al. (2007). Feline herpesvirus. *Veterinary Research* 38: 337–354.

Greene, C.E. and Decaro, N. (2012). Canine viral enteritis. In: Infectious Diseases of the Dog and Cat (ed. C.E. Greene), 67–79. St. Louis: Saunders Elsevier.

Ho, H.J., Poh, B.F., Choudhury, S. et al. (2015). Alcohol hand rubbing and chlorhexidine handwashing are equally effective in removing methicillin-resistant Staphylococcus aureus from health care workers' hands: a randomized controlled trial. *American Journal of Infection Control* 43: 1246–1248.

Honisch, M., Stamminger, R., and Bockmühl, D.P. (2014). Impact of wash cycle time, temperature and detergent formulation on the hygiene effectiveness of domestic laundry. *Journal of Applied Microbiology* 117 (6): 1787–1797.

Huang, C., Ma, W., and Stack, S. (2012). The hygienic efficacy of different hand-drying methods: a review of the evidence. *Mayo Clinic Proceedings* 87 (8): 791–798.

Hurley, K.F. and Baldwin, C.J. (2012). Prevention and management of infection in canine populations. In: Infectious Diseases of the Dog and Cat (ed. C.E. Greene), 1124–1130. St. Louis: Saunders Elsevier.

Kennedy, M.A., Mellon, V.S., Caldwell, G. et al. (1995). Virucidal efficacy of the newer quaternary ammonium compounds. *Journal of the American Animal Hospital Association* 31 (3): 254–258.

Kingston, L., O'Connell, N.H., and Dunne, C.P. (2016). Hand hygiene-related clinical trials reported since 2010: a systematic review. *Journal of Hospital Infection* 92 (4): 9–320.

Longtin, Y., Sax, H., Allegranzi, B. et al. (2011). Videos in clinical medicine: hand hygiene. *New England Journal of Medicine* 362 (13): e24.

Mathur, P. (2011). Hand hygiene: Back to the basics of infection control. *Indian Journal of Medical Research* 134 (5): 611–620.

Moriello, K.A. (2015). Kennel disinfectants for *Microsporum canis* and *Trichophyton* sp. *Journal of Veterinary Internal Medicine* 2015: 853937.

Moriello, K.A. (2016). Decontamination of laundry exposed to *Microsporum canis* hairs and spores. *Journal of Feline Medicine and Surgery* 18 (6): 457–461.

Morley, P.S., Morris, S.N., Hyatt, D.R. et al. (2005). Evaluation of the efficacy of disinfectant footbaths as used in veterinary hospitals. *Journal of the American Veterinary Medical Association* 226 (12): 2053–2058.

National Animal Care and Control Association (NACA) (2009). Determining Kennel Staffing Needs. http://www.nacanet.org/?kennelstaffing (accessed 5 June 2020).

Newbury, S., Miller, L., Patronek, G.J. et al. (2011). Association of Shelter Veterinarians Guidelines for Standards of Care in Animal Shelters. https://www.sheltervet.org/assets/docs/shelter-standards-oct2011-wforward.pdf (accessed 5 June 2020).

Nurkin, S. (2004). Is the Clinicians' Necktie a Potential Fomite for Hospital Acquired Infections? 104th General Meeting of the American Society for Microbiology in New Orleans, LA, US (23–27 May 2004).

Omidbakhsh, N. and Sattar, S.A. (2006). Broad-spectrum microbicidal activity, toxicologic assessment, and materials compatibility of a new generation of accelerated hydrogen peroxide-based environmental surface disinfectant. *American Journal of Infection Control* 34 (5): 251–257.

Patrick, D.R., Findon, G., and Miller, T.E. (1997). Residual moisture determines the level of touch-contact-associated bacterial transfer following handwashing. *Epidemiology and Infection* 119 (3): 319–325.

Pesavento, P.A., Hurley, K.F., Bannasch, M.J. et al. (2008). A clonal outbreak of acute fatal hemorrhagic pneumonia in intensively housed (shelter) dogs caused by Streptococcus equi subsp. zooepidemicus. *Veterinary Pathology* 45 (1): 51–53.

Rousseaux, C.G., Smith, R.A., and Nicholson, S. (1986). Acute Pinesol toxicity in a domestic cat. *Veterinary and Human Toxicology* 28 (4): 316–317.

Rutala, W.A., Cole, E.C., Thomann, C.A. et al. (1998). Stability and bactericidal activity of chlorine solutions. *Infection Control and Hospital Epidemiology* 19 (5): 323–327.

Scott, F.W. (1980). Virucidal disinfectants and feline viruses. *American Journal of Veterinary Research* 41 (3): 410–414.

Stockton, K.A., Morley, P.S., Hyatt, D.R. et al. (2006). Evaluation of the effects of footwear hygiene protocols on nonspecific bacterial contamination of floor surfaces in an equine hospital. *Journal of the American Veterinary Medical Association* 228 (7): 1068–1073.

Trapani, M., Brooks, D.L., and Tillman, P.C. (1982). Quaternary ammonium toxicosis in cats. *Laboratory Animal Science* 32 (5): 520–522.

Traub-Dargatz, J.L., Weese, J.S., Rousseau, J.D. et al. (2006). Pilot study to evaluate 3 hygiene protocols on the reduction of bacterial load on the hands of veterinary staff performing routine equine physical examinations. *Canadian Veterinary Journal* 47 (7): 671–676.

Walter, W.G. and Schillinger, J.E. (1975). Bacterial survival in laundered fabrics. *Applied Microbiology* 29 (3): 368–373.

Whitby, M., Pessoa-Silva, C.L., McLaws, M.L. et al. (2007). Behavioural considerations for hand hygiene practices: the basic building blocks. *Journal of Hospital Infection* 65 (1): 1–8.

WHO (World Health Organization) (2009). *Guidelines on Hand Hygiene in Health Care.* Geneva: World Health Organisation.

9

Canine and Feline Vaccinations and Immunology

Laurie J. Larson[1] *and Ronald D. Schultz*[2]

[1] *CAVIDS Titer Testing Service, University of Wisconsin School of Veterinary Medicine, Madison, WI, USA*
[2] *University of Wisconsin School of Veterinary Medicine, Madison, WI, USA*

9.1 Introduction

Vaccination is an essential component of a comprehensive preventative health management program to minimize disease transmission and maintain and enhance wellness in animal shelters. Effective vaccination programs, in combination with husbandry practices that minimize stress and reduce the risk of exposure to pathogens, help individual animals stay healthy and reduce the severity of clinical disease within the population. This chapter will cover aspects of immunity in relation to individuals, as well as populations of animals within the shelter, and will address special concerns regarding the immunity of juvenile animals. Specific vaccines for dogs and cats will be discussed in the context of vaccination programs designed for optimal effectiveness in the shelter environment. The use of serology for the evaluation of immunity will be described. Finally, diagnostic tests that may be affected by vaccination will be covered.

9.2 Vaccinations and Immunity

9.2.1 Importance of Immunity and Vaccination

Vaccination is critically important for all dogs and cats entering animal shelters to help control the spread of infectious diseases. Many of the significant, potentially deadly viral diseases, such as canine distemper virus (CDV), canine parvovirus (CPV-2), and feline parvovirus (FPV) (the causative agent of feline panleukopenia), are "vaccine-preventable" if animals are effectively immunized prior to exposure to the pathogen (Greene and Schultz 2006). In a shelter setting, where many animals may be susceptible to these diseases and exposure often occurs at the time of intake or very soon after, vaccines form one key part of a foundation for prevention. However, vaccination alone cannot be relied on to protect all animals from illness. Diseases that are not vaccine-preventable, such as canine infectious respiratory disease complex (CIRDC) (kennel cough or canine infectious respiratory disease (CIRD)) and feline upper respiratory tract disease (upper respiratory tract disease (URTD) or feline infectious respiratory disease (FIRD)) can occur even when all animals are vaccinated (Schultz 1998, 1999; Schultz and Conklin 1998). Nevertheless, vaccination provides a helpful adjunct to management even for these diseases by reducing the severity and frequency of clinical signs.

9.2.2 Community Immunity

Currently, in the United States, where probably as many, if not more, dogs and cats are

Infectious Disease Management in Animal Shelters, Second Edition.
Edited by Lila Miller, Stephanie Janeczko, and Kate F. Hurley.

vaccinated than anywhere else in the world, many animals in communities remain unvaccinated and this is reflected in the population of animals entering shelters. Most communities would benefit from programs to vaccinate a much greater percentage of both dogs and cats with core vaccines. Core vaccines are those that are recommended for all cats and dogs with an unknown vaccination history against diseases with significant morbidity and mortality, that are widely distributed, and when, in general, vaccination results in relatively good protection from disease (Stone et al. 2020; Ford et al. 2017). An increase in the percentage of vaccinated animals would have a profound effect on "herd immunity" and provide much better protection for all animals susceptible to these core diseases. It also enhances public health by protecting against rabies. Shelter and low-cost vaccination clinics are one very important way to immunize more animals in the community than might otherwise be vaccinated.

9.2.3 Immune Status of Animals Entering Shelters

Animals entering shelters are either: (i) immunologically naïve and thus susceptible to infection and development of disease if exposed to pathogens; (ii) already immune as a result of natural immunization (e.g. recovery from infection or disease) or previous vaccination; or (iii) already infected. If already infected, they may show clinical signs or possibly incubate disease and/or shed infectious organisms that may infect other susceptible animals. Most animals are immunologically naïve for the vaccine-preventable diseases upon entry into shelters. In serologic surveys of dogs entering shelters nationwide, the authors found that approximately 50 ± 20% of dogs are immunologically naïve (antibody negative) for CDV and approximately 30 ± 15% of dogs are immunologically naïve for CPV-2 (Schultz et al. 2007). A study of dogs in a shelter in Florida showed that 64.5% of 431 dogs sampled were unprotected against CPV-2, CDV or both viruses on intake (Lechner et al. 2010). In more limited surveys of cats entering shelters, the authors found approximately 50% of cats are naïve for FPV, whereas over 75% of the cats entering shelters have antibodies to feline calicivirus (FCV) and feline herpesvirus (FHV-1), many as a result of natural infection and some as a result of previous vaccination (Schultz et al. 2007). It is clear that many of the cats developed FCV/FHV-1 antibody as a result of natural infection because they did not have FPV antibody. If they had been vaccinated, one would expect them to have developed antibody responses against all three viruses that are included in the commonly used trivalent (panleukopenia, herpes, and calicivirus) cat vaccine products.

9.3 Vaccine Characteristics: Efficacy, Onset of Action and Duration of Immunity

9.3.1 Vaccine Efficacy

Vaccines can never be expected to produce more effective or longer-lasting protective immunity than that resulting from natural exposure to infection (whether or not virulent disease develops). In general, when exposure and recovery from a viral infection confer lifelong immunity, (e.g. CDV, CPV-2, and FPV), corresponding vaccine products will have a similar effect on the immune system. For diseases that do not result in long-lived or complete immunity after recovery from infection (e.g. *Bordetella bronchiseptica,* FHV) or cross-protection for varying strains (e.g. FCV), the corresponding vaccines will likely confer similarly limited immunity at best (Schultz 1999).

Vaccines used to prevent CDV, CPV-2, canine adenovirus type 2 (CAV-2) as well as canine infectious hepatitis (CAV-2 vaccine) in the dog, and the FPV vaccine that prevents panleukopenia in the cat are the most effective vaccines. These vaccines can completely prevent infection and clinical disease when properly administered under optimal circumstances, e.g. an adequate time period before exposure and in accordance with the manufacturer's instructions.

In contrast, vaccination cannot entirely prevent feline URTD. This syndrome results from an interaction of environmental factors, stress, and multiple infectious agents, including some bacterial pathogens and mycoplasma that are not included in vaccines. In addition, as noted above, the natural immune response against these pathogens is limited. Finally, cats often arrive at shelters already infected with one or more pathogens associated with URTD, including herpesvirus and calicivirus.

Similarly, vaccines designed to aid in the prevention of CIRD cannot prevent this multifactorial disease. Vaccines, together with good management practices, including attention to husbandry and the environment, should help by reducing the severity or duration of illness in some, but not all, animals.

9.3.2 Onset of Immunity for Modified Live Versus Killed Vaccines

Many animals that enter shelters are susceptible to the viral diseases that the core vaccines protect against. Because the risk of exposure is high, rapid onset of immunity is essential to maintain health for each individual animal and to establish a sufficient level of immunity within the population so outbreaks can be avoided, or their impact minimized. Parenterally administered, modified-live viral (MLV) core vaccines provide rapid immunity against CDV, CPV-2, and FPV with a single dose in the absence of maternally derived antibody (MDA). (See the section later in this chapter on maternal antibody interference with vaccination.) With CDV vaccines, immunity develops within hours after vaccination with MLV and recombinant viral vectored CDV vaccines (Schroeder et al. 1967; Larson and Schultz 2006). Immunity against CPV-2 was verified in 98–99% of dogs without MDA that were challenged experimentally within three days after one dose of MLV vaccine (Schultz 2006). In another earlier study, immunity to FPV was demonstrated when cats were exposed almost immediately after MLV parenteral vaccination. In this case, the exposure dose was lower because the challenge was through the introduction of cats that had just been vaccinated into a contaminated environment rather than through experimental challenge by direct administration. This type of exposure more likely mimics a shelter setting (Brun et al. 1979; Carmichael et al. 1983).

Killed vaccines for CDV, CPV-2, and FPV should not generally be used in the shelter because a significantly longer period of time is required for protective immunity to develop than for the MLV vaccines. Most killed vaccines, including those for CPV-2 and feline panleukopenia, require a minimum of two doses for a protective immune response to develop. An initial dose is administered that primes the immune system, followed in two to four weeks by the second dose, which provides immunity. In general, protection induced by killed vaccines does not develop until at least a week or longer after the second dose is administered. In addition, with most killed vaccines, if the second dose is not given within a maximum of six weeks after the first dose, it is often necessary to begin the series again because the priming effect may be lost and the second dose will not immunize. All subsequent doses of killed vaccines should provide a boost to the immune response. Rabies vaccines, which are killed, are an exception to the requirement for two doses within a six-week interval; most animals over three months of age are protected with a single injection. However, it is recommended by the vaccine manufacturer, and usually required by law, that all animals receive a second dose of rabies vaccine one year after the first vaccination.

9.3.3 Intranasal and Oral Modified Live Vaccines

Intranasal (IN) and oral vaccines, frequently used as an aid in the prevention of "kennel cough" or CIRD in dogs and Feline URTD in cats, are all modified live products that provide local immunity in a shorter period of time than parenteral vaccines. Because herpes and calicivirus IN vaccines are administered at the mucosal surface, maternal antibody interference is not encountered, and these vaccines may be effective at an earlier age in puppies and kittens. This expectation of effectiveness at an early age from IN vaccination does not include immunity for panleukopenia. Parenteral vaccines for panleukopenia are recommended. (Please see specific information on vaccination to immunize against feline panleukopenia in section 9.6.2.1 below.)

CIRD vaccines containing modified live *B. bronchiseptica* and canine parainfluenza (CPi), with or without CAV-2, will stimulate non-specific, innate immunity within hours of administration, due primarily to the adjuvant effect of *B. bronchiseptica*. Bacteria like Bordetella often cause a "shower of cytokines" to be released from cells in the respiratory tract. Among the cytokines released are the type I interferons (IFN) such as alpha and beta IFN. Interferon can restrict the replication of certain viruses, providing rapid, non-specific protection against viruses that contribute to CIRD. Specific humoral and cellular immunity in the respiratory tract will develop in three to seven days to provide local immunity of the upper respiratory tract. That is why mucosal products (administered IN or orally) are recommended for protection against respiratory pathogens, especially in immunologically naïve animals. The authors found that orally administered *B. bronchiseptica* vaccine was as efficacious against bordetellosis as the IN Bordetella vaccine, and was significantly easier to administer (Larson et al. 2013). Animals that have already been naturally immunized as a result of infection with the organisms causing CIRD and URTD (which would likely be common among adult animals entering a shelter) should develop an anamnestic (secondary) response shortly after administration of either a mucosal or a parenteral vaccine. That may explain why it was difficult, if not impossible, for the authors to demonstrate a difference in the protection afforded incoming shelter animals receiving either a parenteral whole-cell killed or antigen extract versus IN CIRD vaccine, or MLV parenteral versus IN URTD vaccines. In those studies, a difference in the development or severity of disease irrespective of the type of vaccine used could not be found (Newbury et al. 2007). Another study found that the use of an IN vaccine for feline URTD containing FHV and FCV was associated with a higher rate of feline URTD in the population (Wagner et al. 2018). Though the association was not found to be causative, the lack of documented evidence for the IN vaccine reducing feline URTD should lead shelters to carefully consider the utility of this vaccine in a given population. If used, URTD rates should be tracked to evaluate whether there is a demonstrable benefit.

9.3.4 Duration of Immunity

Once immunity is established, the duration of immunity (DOI) is not a critical consideration for most shelters as it far exceeds the average length of shelter stay. The canine core (CDV, CPV-2, and CAV-2) and feline core (FPV, FCV, FHV-1) MLV vaccines, properly administered, provide years of protection following effective vaccination (in the absence of maternal antibody interference) (Abdelmagid et al. 2004; Schultz 2006; Scott and Geissinger 1999; Mouzin et al. 2004a.b).

9.4 Vaccination Protocols for Shelters

9.4.1 Core Vaccines for Shelter Cats and Dogs

There are many core and non-core vaccines available for use in cats and dogs (Stone et al. 2020; Ford et al. 2017). They should be administered for privately owned animals in accordance with an evaluation of an animal's risk factors, including age, environment, and lifestyle. A vaccination program for shelter animals differs from that for privately owned pets because the goal is to prevent the spread of diseases most likely to be contracted and/or transmitted within the shelter rather than all the diseases an individual animal may encounter. The program must also consider that animals entering shelters have higher risk factors to contend with, e.g. greater likelihood of exposure to disease, variable states of health, and absence of maternal antibody.

Of all the vaccines available, there are only a few core vaccines that are considered essential to protect individual animals as well as establish "herd" immunity in a shelter population. Vaccination guidelines for cats and dogs were developed specifically for shelters by the American Association of Feline Practitioners (AAFP) and the American Animal Hospital Association (AAHA) respectively and should be considered the standard of care for shelters (Stone et al. 2020; Ford et al. 2017). Every cat should be vaccinated on intake against feline parvovirus (panleukopenia), FCV and FHV type 1 (FHV-1). Every dog should be vaccinated on intake against CDV, CPV-2, CAV-2, CPi and *B. bronchiseptica* (Bb).

The core vaccines required to prevent or reduce the severity of disease caused by viruses will often be found together in the combination products DHPP/DA2PP and Feline Viral Rhinotracheitis, Calicivirus, and Panleukopenia (FVRCP) described below.

- DHPP contains CDV, Hepatitis (CAV-1 and 2), Parvo (CPV-2) and CPi
- FVRCP contains Feline Rhinotracheitis or herpes (FHV-1), Calici (FCV) and Panleukopenia or parvo (FPV)

The following canine *B. bronchiseptica* vaccine products are available:

- a killed monovalent parenteral vaccine
- a modified live (MLV) IN monovalent vaccine
- a bivalent combination vaccine with MLV CPi with or without MLV CAV-2,
- a monovalent oral MLV vaccine.

Each component of the core vaccines for shelter animals is described in greater detail later in this chapter and listed in Table 9.1 at the end of the chapter.

9.4.2 Addition of Non-core Components to Core Vaccines

Because of the type of immune response induced by the core MLV vaccines and the need for a rapid onset of immunity in the face of probable exposure, the use of products that contain any other vaccine components that may cause the immune system to develop a less effective response to the core pathogens should be avoided. Though a discussion of basic immunology is beyond the scope of this chapter, there are certain cell types and components of the immune system that should be stimulated at the time of vaccination in order to provide the most rapid onset and most effective long-term immunity. Combination vaccine (e.g. poly-, bi-, and trivalent) products used to prevent or reduce the severity of disease in shelters should contain only MLV core vaccines. Rabies vaccines are generally monovalent killed products and thus are not mixed with other core vaccines. Core combination vaccines for shelter animals should not routinely contain agents like *Chlamydia felis*, feline *B. bronchiseptica*, *Leptospira* serovars, canine coronavirus, *Lyme* vaccine, etc. Short-term use of a non-core vaccine in the face of diagnostic confirmation of disease may be warranted for documented outbreaks such as feline Bordetella. When it is found beneficial or necessary to use non-core vaccines, they should be given separately (at a different time and site in the animal if possible.) Combination vaccines that contain non-core and core components in conjunction are less than ideal and should only be used when alternative approaches are not available. Vaccines should never be combined in ways not intended by the vaccine manufacturer.

Table 9.1 Core vaccination recommendations for animal shelters.

Basic Core Vaccination Recommendations for Animal Shelters

Species/Age Group	*Recommended Core Vaccines*	*Timing for the first vaccination*	*Re-vaccination*
Adult dogs over 18–20 weeks of age	MLV parenteral DHPP/DA2PP or recombinant CDV combination core vaccine (rCDV+CPV2+ CAV-2+/− CPI)	Prior to or on intake	Two or more weeks after initial vaccination or after adoption (1 dose is immunizing)
Puppies (starting at 4–6 weeks up to 18–20 weeks of age)	MLV parenteral DHPP / DA2PP CDV, CPV-2, CAV-2 with or without CPI	On intake or when they reach 4–6 weeks of age	Every 2–3 weeks until at least 18–20 weeks of age
All dogs and puppies starting as early as 4 weeks	IN or PO CIRD vaccine, *B. bronchiseptica*, CPi with or without CAV-2	On intake	Single-dose adequate for adults and puppies
Adult cats over 18–20 weeks of age	MLV parenteral FVRCP Feline panleukopenia, FHV-1 and FCV	On intake	Two or more weeks after initial vaccination or after adoption
Kittens (starting at 4–6 weeks of age)	MLV parenteral FVRCP Feline panleukopenia, FHV-1 and FCV	On intake or when they reach 4 weeks of age	Every 2–3 weeks until at least 18–20 weeks of age

MLV-modified live vaccine.
IN-intranasal.
PO oral.
SQ- subcutaneous.
CDV-canine distemper.
CPV-2-canine parvovirus.
CAV-1 and 2-canine hepatitis.
CPi-canine parainfluenza.
DHPP-canine distemper, hepatitis (CAV-1 and CAV-2), parvo (CPV-2) and parainfluenza (CPI).
DA2PP-canine distemper, hepatitis (CAV-2), parvo and parainfluenza.
CIRD-canine infectious respiratory disease.
FVRCP-feline viral rhinotracheitis (herpes), calici and panleukopenia.
FHV-1-feline herpesvirus (rhinotracheitis).
FCV-feline calicivirus.

9.4.3 Timing of Vaccination: Vaccination on Intake to the Shelter is Essential

The demonstrably high level of susceptibility in dogs and cats to viral pathogens that are likely to be present in animal shelters highlights and confirms the critical need for the prompt protection provided by vaccines. Vaccination on intake for animals entering animal shelters has been recommended in the aforementioned AAFP and AAHA Vaccination Guidelines; the sections designated specifically for shelters should be considered the standard of care for shelters (Stone et al. 2020; Ford et al. 2017). Timing is extremely important because hours can make a difference in determining whether a vaccine will provide immunity in susceptible (naïve) animals. In all cases, vaccination prior to exposure is the goal.

Vaccination of immune animals provides no benefit, while vaccination of susceptible animals will be one of the most important lifesaving steps that can be taken. Vaccination of already infected animals may not provide protection, but it will not cause the disease to become worse. Since a confirmed vaccination history is often not available for shelter animals, vaccination of all animals helps create a safety net to protect each individual and also promotes good herd immunity (protection of the population). Specific details regarding revaccination for juveniles and adults are given below and in the sections on specific core pathogens.

9.4.4 Special Considerations for Vaccination

9.4.4.1 Vaccination of Puppies and Kittens

Juvenile animals (less than 18–20 weeks of age) cannot be protected by vaccination as reliably as adults can. Modified live parenteral vaccines cannot safely be used on animals less than two to four weeks of age because their immune systems are not fully developed. Maternal antibody interference may prevent effective immunization in animals that are four to approximately 18–20 weeks of age. In general, puppies and kittens in shelters should be vaccinated starting at four to six weeks of age with the core parenteral MLV vaccines, and as early as two weeks of age with IN/oral respiratory vaccines labeled for this use. Juvenile animals should be revaccinated parenterally with core vaccines every 2–3 weeks while in the shelter, until at least 18–20 weeks of age. Additionally, juvenile animals should be protected from exposure to pathogens by physical separation throughout their shelter stay. The rationale behind these recommendations and other details regarding immunization and protection of puppies and kittens are described in greater detail later in this chapter in the section on juvenile animals. Specific strategies or concerns, where applicable, are described in each core vaccine section.

9.4.4.2 Vaccination of Sick or Injured Animals

With few exceptions, every animal four to five weeks of age and older should be vaccinated before or upon arrival to a shelter regardless of their health status at the time of arrival. Vaccines are unlikely to adversely affect sick or injured animals, whereas exposure to a virulent virus is much more likely to cause serious illness in the shelter environment. There is a good chance that much-needed protection will be provided even to animals that are mildly to moderately ill at the time of vaccination. As an extra measure of safety, these animals may be revaccinated after recovery (and no less than two weeks after the previous vaccine). If animals are so ill that vaccination is considered unsafe, they should not remain in the shelter unless appropriate care and treatment can be provided in a physically separate isolation area where they will not be exposed to disease.

9.4.4.3 Vaccination of Pregnant and Nursing Animals

If a pregnant animal arrives at a shelter, the risks and benefits of vaccination must be carefully weighed. Vaccine virus may present a risk to fetuses but, in many cases, the risk of infection and disease from a virulent virus is greater. While there may be a risk to the unborn puppies or kittens from vaccinating the dam if she has not been previously immunized, the risk of disease to an unvaccinated dam entering a shelter environment where there is a high risk of exposure could be very high. By withholding vaccination to protect the fetuses from possible adverse effects of vaccination, the dam and puppies or kittens are often at greater risk of succumbing to disease.

Legal status may be a consideration in deciding whether to vaccinate a pregnant animal. The risks must be weighed against the benefits. When impounding pregnant animals as part of a legal case, every attempt should be made to obtain permission to vaccinate them or confirm valid vaccination records by a licensed veterinarian. Even when animals have an uncertain legal status, an argument could be made that if shelter admission is unavoidable, vaccinating the dam who has an unknown vaccination history is a reasonable course of action to protect against infectious disease.

Checking antibody levels in pregnant animals would be one way of evaluating risk prior to vaccination (see the serologic risk assessment section 9.10 later in this chapter for more details). Pregnant dogs with antibodies will not be infected with the vaccine virus, thus the embryos/fetuses will not be affected. However, in the case of a combination product, one of the antigens (e.g. CAV-2) for which titers cannot be readily evaluated may infect the embryos/fetuses and cause fetal resorption or abortion.

Whenever a combination vaccine product is used, both the benefit and potential risk or adverse consequences associated with each component in the combination, as well as the overall immediate risk from a specific virulent virus in the shelter must always be considered. This is especially true during pregnancy. If pregnant animals are not vaccinated, every effort must be made to physically protect them from exposure to disease by careful isolation or ideally, placing them in foster care or off-site housing. Pregnant animals for whom spay/abortion is planned should always be vaccinated immediately on intake.

Nursing animals should receive core vaccines as usual. Though this will not provide any protection to the offspring, it will not harm the offspring and will confer protection to the dam.

9.4.4.4 Vaccination of Animals Repeatedly Admitted to the Shelter

While vaccination on intake is the recommended standard procedure, routinely revaccinating animals every time they are returned to the shelter without consideration of their vaccination history is neither reasonable nor good veterinary practice. If an animal has a documented history of receiving core vaccines at an age greater than four to five months, vaccination on intake may be waived if the previous vaccination was administered within the expected timeframe that the vaccine is labeled to provide protection (one year or more for commonly administered shelter vaccines, including canine and feline respiratory vaccines).

9.5 Vaccine Handling, Administration, and Adverse Reactions

9.5.1 Care and Handling of Vaccines

In almost all cases, the core vaccines used in shelters should be modified live vaccines (MLV). The only way these vaccines can immunize is when the live vaccine virus/bacteria infects the animal; thus, MLV are referred to as infectious vaccines. In contrast, the killed (KV) vaccines do not infect and are known as non-infectious vaccines.

Because MLV vaccines must remain infectious, careful handling of these vaccines to maintain their infectivity is a critical part of the vaccination program. MLV vaccines should always be refrigerated prior to use at 33–35° F (1–3° C). For long-term storage, they should remain lyophilized (dried cake) and not reconstituted with diluents. MLV should only be reconstituted with the sterile diluent supplied with the vaccine. However, if the diluent contains an unneeded or undesirable component (e.g. Leptospira), an alternate sterile diluent (e.g. water or saline) can be substituted for the diluent supplied with the vaccine. MLV should never be frozen before or after reconstitution with the sterile diluent. Once the vaccine is reconstituted, it should remain at refrigerator temperatures for no more than two hours. If vaccines are kept at ambient (room) temperatures above 70° F (21° C) for more than one hour, they should not be used. In order to be most effective, vaccines should be reconstituted and used immediately; single-dose vials are recommended since multi-dose vials carry a risk of contamination with bacteria that can grow at refrigerator temperatures.

Killed vaccines are more stable than MLV and can be kept in the refrigerator as a liquid for the shelf life of the product. Almost all killed vaccines are sold as liquids, rather than lyophilized as is the case with MLV. However, killed vaccines should also be used within four hours after they have been removed from the refrigerator, especially when ambient temperatures are above 80° F (26° C). Single-dose vaccine vials are preferable because multiple-dose vials can become contaminated.

Killed vaccines should never be mixed with MLV unless they are part of the commercial combination product because preservatives present in some killed vaccines can inactivate the MLV. Different vaccines of any type should never be combined in one syringe. Neither MLV nor KV vaccines should be used beyond the expiration date of the product.

9.5.2 Training for Staff Administering Vaccines

Shelters must be familiar with their state and local laws governing who may administer vaccines. Many states allow veterinary technicians and other trained staff to vaccinate shelter animals against infectious diseases while others may restrict the practice to licensed veterinarians. All staff administering vaccines should receive training in proper vaccine storage, handling, and administration. Staff should be familiar with possible vaccine side effects, and a protocol established and encouraged for reporting if any errors or problems occur in the vaccine handling or administration process (such as giving a vaccine by the incorrect route or to the wrong species). The name of the staff member administering the vaccine should be documented in shelter records or software along with the date and type of vaccination to allow follow-up should any issues arise.

9.5.3 Vaccination Site Guidelines for Cats

If possible, AAFP injection site guidelines should be followed for administering vaccines to cats. These site guidelines help track potential causes of vaccine-associated sarcomas as well as offering some hope of treatment through the possibility of complete tumor removal, to individual animals who may develop these deeply invasive tumors. FVRCP should be given in the right forelimb, rabies in the right hind limb, and feline leukemia virus (FeLV) in the left hind limb. Injection in the scapular region is no longer recommended because removing an invasive tumor from this site can rarely be accomplished. However, if these site guidelines cannot be followed, the vaccines should still be administered subcutaneously.

9.5.4 Adverse Reactions

All vaccines have the potential to cause adverse reactions that range from mild (e.g. stiffness, lethargy, decreased appetite, mild fever) to severe (e.g. tumors, anaphylaxis, autoimmunity, death). The modified live core vaccines recommended for shelter animals are among the least likely to cause adverse reactions, whereas the killed adjuvanted vaccines are among the most reactogenic. Furthermore, considering the high percentage of animals entering shelters that are susceptible to significant disease and death caused by CDV, CPV-2, and FPV, *under no circumstance would the risk of an adverse vaccine reaction ever outweigh or negate the benefit of vaccination with the core vaccines.* Therefore, it bears repeating that every animal entering a shelter should be vaccinated with the core vaccines prior to or at the time of intake. If an animal is considered so severely immunosuppressed that it should not receive a MLV vaccine, then it would be best to avoid shelter entry where it will likely be exposed to more virulent wildtype agents. If shelter entry and housing are unavoidable, then vaccination most likely carries a lower risk than admission with no vaccination.

Though adverse reactions are rare when using only the core vaccine products, veterinarians should provide shelter staff with specific training and written protocols for each species for how to respond should an adverse reaction occur. Adverse reactions should be carefully documented as part of the animal's permanent medical record and adopters should be made aware that the reaction occurred. In addition to adverse reactions, shelter staff should be trained in other risks of incorrectly administered vaccines, such as the risks associated with *B. bronchiseptica* vaccine intended for IN use being administered subcutaneously or the potential for FCV MLV intended for subcutaneous use being taken in orally by the cat (e.g. by licking spilled vaccine from the fur).

9.6 Core Vaccines for Shelter Dogs and Cats

The following sections address each component of the core vaccines individually to describe the expected onset, duration, and efficacy of immunity.

9.6.1 The Canine Shelter Core Vaccines

9.6.1.1 CDV Vaccine

Immunity to CDV has been demonstrated to develop almost immediately after a single vaccination with an MLV or recombinant product if not blocked by MDAs and has been shown to protect from severe clinical signs of CDV, including neurologic disease and death. However, when animals are exposed to CDV within the first few days following vaccination, *it is possible they may only develop partial immunity and become infected, with mild or no clinical signs, and may shed virus into the environment*. These milder infections may also be immunosuppressive, and the infected dogs can show clinical signs consistent with CIRDC, including pneumonia. Though significant benefit and protection from challenge have been demonstrated as early as minutes to hours post-vaccination, ideally, animals should be vaccinated two to three days prior to exposure in order to completely prevent infection and transmission of the virus (Appel 1987; Appel 1999; Larson and Schultz 2006).

When the transmission of CDV is a significant problem in shelters already vaccinating on intake, puppies that cannot be effectively immunized because of MDA will likely develop clinical signs that may progress to neurologic disease or death. Adults who are vaccinated but not effectively immunized (e.g. because exposure occurred concurrently with or very soon after vaccination) may be primarily affected with mild to severe respiratory disease, but they too can progress to severe neurologic disease. Puppies under five months of age must be protected from exposure throughout their stay in shelters by physical separation and careful handling, especially when outbreaks are occurring. (See Chapter 11: Canine Distemper Virus for more information.)

Immunity to CDV can persist for up to the lifetime of the dog, thus dogs need not be revaccinated more often than every three years after the completion of the puppy series at 18–20 weeks of age or older.

The canarypox vectored recombinant (rCDV) and MLV distemper vaccines provide equivalent immunity and will perform similarly (Reed et al. 2003; Hageny et al. 2004), both being highly effective when dogs are vaccinated on intake or prior to infection (Schroeder et al. 1967; Larson and Schultz 2006). All canine distemper vaccines are among the most effective vaccines in any species. Vaccinated dogs that have developed detectable antibodies will resist re-infection and disease even when placed into a shelter with a severe CDV outbreak (Larson et al. 2006).

9.6.1.2 CPV-2 Vaccine

In the absence of MDA, immunity to canine parvovirus that lasts for up to the lifetime of the dog can be demonstrated three or more days after a single MLV vaccination (Carmichael et al.1983). However, even though properly vaccinated, if young dogs are exposed to the virus either before or within the three to five-day period immediately after initial vaccination, they are likely to become infected and develop fulminant clinical disease. Older susceptible dogs are less likely to develop severe disease when compared to dogs less than one year of age. Because environmental persistence of CPV-2 makes exposure likely, it is essential to protect all dogs from fomite transmission or exposure to parvovirus contaminated environments during this early period of time when immunity is developing.

All puppies under 18–20 weeks of age should be considered susceptible regardless of the number of vaccines received, even though it is likely some are effectively protected by vaccination or MDA. There is no early protection induced by the parvoviral vaccine prior to acquired immunity developing. Parvoviral immunity is either complete or non-existent, unlike early partial immunity induced by CDV vaccines. Adult dogs that are immunologically naïve to CPV-2 may become infected and shed the virus without showing signs of disease. However, the virulent virus that is shed can infect young susceptible dogs and cause severe disease and death.

As with CDV, CPV-2 vaccines provide long-lasting immunity, and thus dogs need not be revaccinated more often than every three years after the completion of the puppy series at 18–20 weeks of age or older and revaccination one year later.

Current CPV-2 vaccines from the major manufacturers have been demonstrated by the author's laboratory to induce protective immunity for all current field types of canine parvovirus (CPV 2a, 2b, and 2c) found clinically (Larson and Schultz 1997, 2008). CPV-2c was introduced to the United States in 2005–2006, probably from Europe, as it was detected there in 2001 (Buonavoglia et al. 2001; Martella et al. 2004; Truyen 2006). No vaccine-resistant variants have been found (Larson and Schultz 2008).

9.6.1.3 Canine Adenovirus Type 1 and 2 Vaccine

CAV-1 virus (infectious canine hepatitis) is included in a core vaccine for shelter dogs. Immunity to CAV-1 can be demonstrated as early as seven days after vaccination when the dog is challenged with the CAV-1 virus. It probably takes a similar amount of time (e.g. seven days) for immunity to develop and protect from respiratory disease caused by CAV-2. CAV-2 contributes to CIRD in the dog and alone can cause pneumonia (Greene and Schultz 2006). The DOI against CAV-1 is a lifetime, but the DOI for protection from CAV-2 is approximately three years (Schultz 2006). If CIRD is a significant problem in a shelter, particularly if CAV-2 is found on diagnostic samples, a combination IN CIRD vaccine that includes CAV-2 in addition to the core DHPP parenteral combination viral vaccine may be a helpful adjunct to control the problem.

9.6.1.4 CPi Vaccine

CPi virus is also included in a core vaccine for shelter dogs. The CPi vaccine should be given IN to provide effective immunity from this virus that contributes to CIRD. The DOI is three years for CPI. CPI is often part of the IN CIRD combination vaccines that contain *B. bronchiseptica* with or without CAV-2 (see below). The combination IN vaccines must be given at least annually because of the one year or less DOI for the *B. bronchiseptica* component.

9.6.1.5 *Bordetella bronchiseptica* Vaccine

B. bronchiseptica is considered part of a core vaccine for dogs entering shelters, whereas it is not a core vaccine for cats. IN, oral and parenteral vaccines are available for the dog, but only an IN product is available for the cat. For use in shelters, MLV mucosal (i.e. IN or oral) vaccines are recommended that include either *B. bronchiseptica* alone or in combination with CPi, with or without CAV-2. All currently available IN and oral *Bordetella* products contain modified live bacteria.

The feline monovalent IN *B. bronchiseptica* vaccine should not be given to dogs, just as the canine IN and oral Bordetella vaccines should not be given to cats because these vaccines have only been tested for efficacy and safety in the respective species.

There is a cellular antigen extract of killed *B. bronchiseptica* injectable vaccine available for dogs. This injectable canine product should not be used in cats because it has not been tested for efficacy or safety in the feline species.

Caution must be taken using *B. bronchiseptica* vaccines. The parenteral product should never be administered IN because it will not provide specific immunity to Bordetella. More importantly, IN and oral products containing MLV Bordetella must not be administered parenterally because they can cause a severe local reaction or, rarely, death due to severe acute hepatic failure. If a modified live oral or IN Bordetella vaccine is accidentally given by injection, it should be considered a medical emergency. The injection site will often be painful and swollen due to a local inflammatory reaction. The ASPCA Poison Control Center recommends the following treatment: Injectable gentamicin sulfate, at a standard dose of 2–4 mg/kg every six to eight hours, should be diluted in 10–30 ml of saline (depending on the size of the dog) and injected into the affected area. An oral antibiotic, such as doxycycline, trimethoprim sulfa, or tetracycline, should also be started immediately. Most animals have only injection site swelling and pain, but some animals have been reported to develop injection site abscesses or even hepatic necrosis. Animals should be closely monitored for vomiting, diarrhea, or inappetence. If liver disease develops, hospitalization and intravenous (IV) fluids along with other supportive care may be required. If liver damage does occur, liver enzyme abnormalities can continue for several months.

IN and oral canine respiratory vaccines are living, attenuated products that are administered to mucous membranes where there will be no interference from MDA; therefore, these vaccines can be given at an early age (e.g. four to eight weeks) with no re-vaccination required. Package inserts often recommend re-vaccination of puppies two to four weeks after the initial IN vaccination because it may be difficult to administer the vaccine into the puppy's nose. A second dose may help to protect those who were ineffectively immunized because of vaccine administration issues rather than immunology issues. Most puppies housed in shelters would likely have been naturally exposed to the pathogens the IN products protect against after two to four weeks, so re-vaccination would not be beneficial. IN and oral products can be given to adult dogs once at intake and need not be repeated. In all instances, the entire recommended dose must be administered.

In privately-owned animals, revaccination may be necessary as often as every nine months to a year, as immunity to the *B. bronchiseptica* wanes. In a shelter setting, where natural exposure to Bordetella is very common, immunity will likely persist for at least the average or standard length of stay for most animals. Animals with minimal exposure to newly arriving dogs, such as dogs in quarantine or legal holding, may benefit from annual or every nine months revaccination with the oral/IN vaccines.

The killed parenteral *B. bronchiseptica* product, when used, requires the administration of two doses two to four weeks apart. As with other killed products, the interval between those doses should not exceed six weeks (Appel and Bemis 1978).

Research has shown the IN and oral products are significantly more effective in reducing clinical signs than the parenteral product post-challenge in a research setting (Davis et al. 2007; Larson et al. 2013).

9.6.1.6 Canine Influenza Virus (CIV) Vaccines

As of this writing, two strains of CIV are present in the canine population of the United States. CIV strain H3N8, an equine origin influenza virus, was first seen in dogs in 2003. More recently, CIV H3N2 has caused outbreaks of canine respiratory disease (Newbury et al. 2016). Canine Influenza H3N2 is an avian origin virus that can cause severe disease in dogs. There are currently killed vaccines that can protect both H3N8 and H3N2. There is little or no cross-protection, thus either both vaccines or a bivalent product are recommended for maximum protection. However, neither of these vaccines would be considered core shelter vaccines. If these vaccines are used, two doses given two or more weeks apart are required for protection, thus it takes three weeks or more for protection to be present. This limits the utility of this vaccine in shelters where exposure is likely to occur prior to the completion of the two-vaccine series. Increasing population immunity by encouraging vaccination of pet dogs in communities where canine influenza is present may be a more effective use of the vaccine. (See Chapter 12 for more information.)

9.6.2 The Feline Shelter Core Vaccines

9.6.2.1 Feline Panleukopenia Virus (FPV) Vaccine

Similar to the CPV vaccines, the feline panleukopenia (parvovirus) vaccine provides rapid and long-lasting immunity. Protective benefits of vaccination for susceptible kittens have been demonstrated immediately after vaccination for FPV in one study (Brun et al. 1979). Susceptible kittens vaccinated with a parenteral MLV FPV vaccine and immediately introduced into a contaminated environment developed no clinical signs of disease, while kittens not vaccinated became severely affected. These results most likely represent delayed infection because the authors have demonstrated that kittens challenged experimentally by the IN/oral route must be vaccinated at least three days prior to challenge for protection to occur (Schultz unpublished). These FPV results are similar to vaccination and challenge infection with the closely related CPV-2 in dogs (Larson and Schultz 1997; Schultz 2000). As is the case with CPV, kittens are at risk for FPV infection while in the shelter and should be vaccinated beginning no earlier than four weeks of age, then revaccinated every two weeks (not more often) up to 18–20 weeks of age. The last dose of vaccine must be given at 18–20 weeks of age or older. Cats vaccinated with the last dose after 18–20 weeks of age and revaccinated again one year later need not be revaccinated more often than every three years.

The authors do not recommend either killed or IN administered MLV FPV vaccines in the shelter environment as they are not as effective at immunizing cats as the parenteral (e.g. subcutaneous or intramuscular) MLV vaccines. Though all of these vaccines eventually provide good immunity against FPV, the onset of protection when the killed vaccine is used may not be sufficiently rapid to prevent outbreaks in a shelter setting. It was found that the IN vaccine does not immunize as high a percentage of cats, especially those with MDA (Schultz 2009). There may be inadequate amounts of vaccine virus reaching susceptible cells for virus replication when the vaccine is given IN. MLV vaccines must infect and replicate in the animal to induce immunity.

CPV-2 can cause a panleukopenia-like disease in cats, but MLV parenteral FPV vaccination of cats will prevent infection with both FPV and CPV-2 (Truyen et al. 1996; Olsen et al. 1998).

9.6.2.2 Feline Calicivirus Vaccines

Early immunity develops as soon as seven days after FCV vaccination, reaching full protection after a second dose. The DOI is at least three years; but this immunity is never complete in protecting from infection or disease, especially in high-risk situations like shelters. Immunity is always limited as there are many different strains and/or variants of calicivirus. Unlike protection from FPV, which prevents infection, FCV vaccination does not prevent infection, but hopefully prevents and reduces the severity of disease. Unfortunately, there are an increasing number of FCV strains, against which, vaccination provides limited protection ("vaccine-resistant strains"). The same tendency to mutate that results in the many different clinical manifestations of FCV also means that vaccine-resistant strains are constantly emerging, and at the time of this writing most available FCV vaccines contain strains that have not been updated in years.

Though strategies such as dual-strain vaccines have been shown to induce cross-protective neutralizing antibody and to lessen clinical signs after virulent FCV challenge (Poulet et al. 2005; Huang et al. 2010), it is prudent to assume that even vaccinated cats will be susceptible to infection and potentially severe disease from some strains of calicivirus. Owners with pet cats should take precautions, including isolation, to protect them when they adopt or provide foster care for cats from shelters with signs of feline infectious respiratory disease (FIRD). This is particularly true in any outbreak in which otherwise healthy, vaccinated adult cats have been affected.

9.6.2.3 Feline Herpesvirus Type 1 (FVR) Vaccines

FVR stands for feline viral rhinotracheitis, a formerly common name for herpesvirus infection in cats. Immunity to FHV-1 develops as early as seven days post-vaccination and the DOI is at least three years. Immunity is never complete though, as all vaccinated animals remain susceptible to infection with field virus. When infection occurs, some cats may show clinical signs and virtually all develop latent infections. This is not surprising because, even following natural FHV-1 infection, previously infected cats can become reinfected when exposed to challenge virus. Vaccinates, however, are more likely to be protected from severe disease than unvaccinated animals (Scott and Geissinger 1999; Lappin et al. 2006).

When cats latently infected with FHV-1 become stressed, the latent virulent virus can be reactivated, shed, and transmitted to naive as well as vaccinated animals. Reactivation and shedding of FHV-1 in latently infected cats may cause the recrudescence of disease in stressed animals regardless of vaccination status.

9.6.2.4 Intranasal Combination Products for Cats

IN combination vaccines are available that contain FCV and FHV-1 with or without FPV. These products are used often in pet cats as well as in shelter cats. These vaccines have a theoretical advantage of providing local immunity in a shorter period of time than the MLV parenteral products when given to naïve cats and kittens. They also stimulate immunity to FCV and FHV-1 at an earlier age in kittens with MDA. These IN vaccines have no advantage with regard to FPV. As recommended in the section on FPV, both young and adult cats in shelters should also receive a parenteral MLV FPV, even when the trivalent IN product is used. Though the IN route of administration is theoretically optimal for FCV and FHV-1 vaccine viruses because it provides better local cellular and humoral immunity, use of MLV FCV/FVH-1/FPV parenteral vaccine alone has been shown to be as effective as a combination of both MLV parenteral and IN vaccines for protection against respiratory disease in a shelter setting (Newbury et al. 2007). If used in shelters, respiratory disease levels should be monitored before and after to evaluate effectiveness.

9.6.3 Rabies Vaccines for Dogs and Cats

The rabies vaccine is not necessarily recommended for administration at intake for shelter animals because the disease is unlikely to be contracted in or spread through the facility. However, for public health reasons, rabies vaccination is recommended on intake for cats and dogs staying long term in facilities, and prior to adoption (or release from the shelter) unless local regulations indicate otherwise. Immunity induced by the killed, adjuvanted rabies vaccines can develop as early as two to three weeks after vaccination. Challenge studies have shown immunity to persist for a minimum of three years with most vaccines, and up to four years with one feline vaccine. Though core vaccines should not be administered at intervals of less than two weeks, it is acceptable to administer the rabies vaccine at the time of release from the shelter even if the animal was vaccinated with the core vaccines less than two weeks previously.

Many jurisdictions require that the rabies vaccine be given only by a licensed veterinarian. However, regional regulations vary, so where permitted, vaccines may also be administered by authorized staff under the direct or indirect supervision of a licensed veterinarian.

Only killed rabies vaccines are available for dogs in the United States. A combination of adjuvant and high immunogenicity of rabies glycoprotein G makes this product highly immunogenic. In addition to killed rabies vaccines for cats, a one-year recombinant viral vectored feline rabies vaccine is available. This recombinant rabies product is not labeled for use in dogs, and thus should not be used in this species.

The best products to use in shelters are either one-or three-year rabies vaccines. The cost is likely to be similar for either vaccine. Animals without a history of previous rabies vaccination must legally be revaccinated within the year in most communities regardless of whether a one or three-year product was used initially. Animals must then be revaccinated once every three years, or as often as required by the state or municipality where the animal is living. However, if the dog or cat is not revaccinated after the first dose of rabies vaccine, there may be an increased DOI if a three-year product is used as compared to certain one-year products. Because an increased DOI would benefit the individual animal and the entire community, and many dogs are not re-vaccinated after they leave the shelter, the three-year product is preferred. Regardless of the vaccine strategy used, staff should clearly communicate to adopters the legal need for re-vaccination in one year. The three-year product is as safe or safer than the one-year product.

The three-year product is acceptable for cats, as is the non-adjuvanted one-year recombinant feline rabies vaccine. Just as in dogs, for cats, any initial vaccination, without a documented vaccination history, will require revaccination within one year no matter which product is used.

The age at which the first vaccination must be administered and required re-vaccination intervals is determined by local or state regulations. In most states, vaccination is required after three months of age.

Rabies vaccination documentation is also commonly subject to local regulations. In most cases, the vaccination record must contain the serial and lot numbers of rabies vaccines. Many regions require a veterinarian's signature, and most require a veterinarian to be present or actually administer the vaccine.

Though local regulations and vaccine manufacturer's recommendations vary, all animals should receive at least two doses of rabies vaccine, with the interval between doses being not less than three weeks and not more than one year. This is, in accordance with most local ordinances, that require an animal to be revaccinated either at one year of age or within one year of the initial vaccination. This protocol will allow subsequent revaccination at three or more years to provide excellent protection regardless of whether using a one or three-year product initially. Vaccination for any animal, without an appropriately documented rabies vaccination history, should be considered an initial vaccination. To date, there have been very few animals who were not protected and developed rabies after they had been properly vaccinated twice. However, a higher number of animals who received only one dose of the vaccine have contracted rabies. Also, there are a significant number of dogs that fail to develop adequate antibody titers during the one year after their first vaccine, and only after the second dose is antibody detected. Antibodies are critically important to provide protection from the rabies virus. (See Chapter 22 for more information)

9.7 Optional, Non-core Vaccines for Cats and Dogs in a Shelter

As noted above, administering vaccines in addition to the core vaccines may compromise the immune response to the core pathogens. Therefore, the use of additional vaccines should be carefully considered and justified. The most current AAHA and AAFP Shelter Guidelines should help decide when to use optional, non-core products. Vaccine recommendations for cats and dogs in shelter environments were first included in the 2006 edition of the Canine and Feline Vaccination Guidelines, and these guidelines are updated as needed.

9.7.1 Feline Leukemia Virus (FeLV) Vaccines

One optional vaccine that could be considered for use in shelters is the FeLV vaccine. This is particularly important for kittens in group housing in a shelter for a prolonged period (a scenario that should generally be avoided for many reasons). The risk of FeLV exposure exists even if cats are tested on intake because some early cases may be missed. Several vaccines are available, including an adjuvanted killed virus non-infectious vaccine and a nonadjuvanted canarypox virus-vectored recombinant vaccine, but their efficacy is difficult to assess (Stone et al. 2020). Ideally, the vaccine would only be administered to FeLV negative animals, but it will not harm a FeLV positive cat. If the vaccine is used, kittens should be vaccinated twice: once at eight to nine weeks of age and repeated three to four weeks later. FeLV revaccination must be administered at an interval of three to four weeks (as specified) in order to be effective. The age at the time of the last vaccination is not as crucial a consideration as for other vaccines when attempting to overcome MDA. Instead, with the FeLV vaccine, the second dose or re-vaccination must occur not longer than four weeks following the initial vaccination. Exposure of a kitten to a FeLV viremic cat before or during the vaccination process and up to at least two weeks after the second dose may result in infection, but after that time, protection should be greater than 90% effective when any commercially available vaccine is used. Revaccination at one year of age or one year after the last vaccination is recommended if the cat remains in a high-risk environment, but after that age, revaccination is not necessary. Revaccination intervals depend on the risk of ongoing exposure and product used. A single dose of the FeLV vaccine provides no protection; therefore, unless two doses can be given three to four weeks apart, FeLV vaccines should not be used.

9.7.2 Feline Immunodeficiency Virus (FIV) Vaccines

Feline immunodeficiency virus (FIV) vaccination is not recommended for shelter cats. The immune response to this vaccine is indistinguishable from the antibody response to natural infection with current diagnostic tests. This vaccine requires a minimum of three doses with an interval of two to four weeks between them. When this protocol is followed, cats may have up to 70% protection from some strains (clades) of FIV but have little to no protection from other strains. Considering that most cats, including those in shelters, are at low risk of infection with FIV, the need for multiple doses, a long onset to immunity that is only partial, and interference with diagnostic testing, this vaccine is not recommended for shelter cats.

9.7.3 *Bordetella bronchiseptica* and *C. felis* Vaccines

B. bronchiseptica and *C. felis* vaccines are not recommended for most shelter cats. However, in shelters experiencing severe FIRD, when these pathogens have been specifically identified by laboratory testing as contributing or suspect factors in outbreaks of disease, or these vaccines can be shown to reduce the severity and/or duration of disease when vaccinated and non-vaccinated groups of cats are compared, these vaccines may be helpful. More evidence is needed before these vaccines can be generally recommended.

9.7.4 Other Non-core Vaccines

Feline Infectious Peritonitis (FIP) vaccines are generally not recommended for any cats according to the AAFP Guidelines. As with the Bordetella and *C. felis* products, unless a benefit can be shown through controlled studies for using these vaccines in a shelter environment, their use is not recommended.

The use of canine coronavirus and rattlesnake vaccines is also not recommended for most shelter dogs. Four-way Leptospira and Lyme vaccines are listed in the AAHA Guidelines as optional vaccines for pet dogs at high risk, but not generally recommended for shelter dogs.

9.8 Juvenile Animals

9.8.1 Maternal Antibody Interference with Vaccination

Puppies and kittens in the shelter environment experience unique problems when compared to adult animals with regard to disease prevention through vaccination. This is especially true for CDV, CPV-2 and feline panleukopenia (FPV).

When juvenile animals receive colostrum through nursing in the first hours of life, they acquire varying levels of MDAs. The amount of maternal antibody received is variable and depends on many factors including litter size, frequency of early nursing, and maternal antibody titer. The antibody will have a half-life (50% of it will decay) approximately every two weeks (8–13 days).

Juvenile animals that receive MDA have a "window of vulnerability," also referred to as the "window of susceptibility" that develops with declining levels of these antibodies. A virulent virus is better able to overcome MDA protection than vaccine virus. Levels of MDA may fall low enough to allow infection with a virulent virus while, at the same time, remaining too high to allow effective immunization from vaccination. It is this differential between the onset of susceptibility to virulent virus and the ability of vaccine virus to overcome MDA in order to immunize that creates the "window of susceptibility." The "window" is the period of time or age of the animal when MDA in the puppies' or kittens' serum fails to protect from infection with the wildtype (virulent) virus, while MDA still blocks active protective immunity from developing when the animal receives the vaccine.

With some of the original (pre-1997) CPV-2 vaccines, the "window of susceptibility" persisted as long as 12 weeks in individual animals. It was possible with some of the "old generation" CPV-2 vaccines to show that puppies born to a dam with a very high level of CPV-2 antibody could not be actively immunized until 20–22 weeks of age, while the MDA only provided protection from infection against the virulent virus up to 10–12 weeks of age (Larson and Schultz 1997). That meant that even when the puppy vaccination was started at 4–6 weeks of age and continued every 2–3 weeks until 18–20 weeks of age, those puppies with very high MDA never developed an immune response from the initial vaccination series because the last dose of vaccines had to be given at 20–22 weeks of age. After 1997, the less effective vaccines were either taken off the market or replaced by more effective vaccines (Larson and Schultz 1997).

With the new generation of MLV CPV-2 and FPV vaccines, the "window of susceptibility" for each species rarely exceeds two to four weeks. Because it is rarely known when that two to four week period will occur, this smaller window reduces infection overall but does not diminish the need to physically protect juvenile animals from potential exposure to virulent virus during the entire 18 week (or, rarely, longer) period when the two-week "window" may have opened. While puppies and kittens may still be affected by viral disease during their initial juvenile vaccination series, when the last dose of CPV-2 or FPV vaccine is given at 18–20 weeks in shelter puppies or kittens, few, if any, will have MDA remaining at levels that can block the development of an immune response to current parvovirus vaccines.

Killed vaccines (except rabies vaccines) can also be blocked by MDA. If the first dose is blocked, then the second dose will not immunize and provide protective immunity. It will only prime the immune response and a third dose would be required to immunize. If the second dose is also blocked by MDA, then it will require a fourth dose to provide protection, as the third dose is the priming dose and the fourth is the immunizing one; thus, it can take weeks or more than a month to immunize the animal. This is what the authors found with a commercial killed CPV-2 vaccine that is no longer available (Schultz and Conklin 1998). The same would likely apply to killed FPV vaccines.

9.8.1.1 Variation in Maternal Antibody Levels

As noted previously, a high percentage of animals presenting to shelters have no history of vaccination or maternal exposure to CDV, CPV, or FPV, and thus will have no maternal antibodies to transmit to their offspring. For many puppies and kittens presenting to shelters, therefore, it is likely that passive immunity for CPV, FPV, and CDV has waned or was not present on initial presentation. In that case, the first MLV vaccine that is administered should effectively immunize them, regardless of age. *A single dose of a modified live vaccine, in the absence of MDA or when MDA is low enough to not block vaccination, is sufficient to induce complete immunity against these three pathogens.*

Even for puppies and kittens that did receive MDA, exactly how much is received and when MDA will fall in each individual is variable. Even within a litter of puppies or kittens, individual antibody levels (titers) can be different enough that some animals will become susceptible to infection earlier due to a lower level of MDA than others. MDA can prolong infection within a litter. For example, part of the litter can become infected and die while the other puppies are protected by MDA for another two weeks or more because of their higher level of MDA. These puppies may become infected later and could die if they are not properly immunized prior to infection, as MDA high enough to prevent illness will also have prevented earlier immunization.

While all maternal antibody in a litter will decline at the same rate regardless of the infectious agent it is directed against, the initial titer is highly variable between various viruses. Immune responses to different vaccines (e.g. CDV, CPV-2) in the combination product will generally occur at different ages as the puppy or kitten will rarely have levels of antibody to all viruses that reach low enough levels to allow immunization simultaneously. However, MDA levels to all components of the core vaccines should be at low enough levels in the majority of juveniles by 18–20 weeks of age to permit effective immunization. Because it is never obvious which puppies or kittens have MDA at a level sufficient to interfere with vaccination and which do not, the full series of juvenile vaccinations is recommended for all young animals.

9.8.2 Risk of Vaccine Use in Very Young Animals

While protection from CDV can be safely established using a monovalent rCDV vaccine to actively immunize puppies as early as two weeks of age, modified live canine and feline vaccines should not be administered during the first two weeks after birth. Prior to two weeks of age, the immune system is unlikely to mount an effective immunizing response to many vaccines, and the vaccine virus can cause disease and death at this early age (Schultz et al. 1977).

Both puppies and kittens have limited thermoregulatory control during at least the first seven or more days of life. Thermoregulation may not be fully functional until after two weeks of age in some puppies and kittens. Body temperatures of these neonates rarely, if ever, reach temperatures that are adequate for the immune system to function optimally. This leaves puppies and kittens without a well-functioning, active immune system for at least one week and often up to two weeks or more of age. Thus, MLV vaccines would not be safe to administer, and killed vaccines may not be immunogenic, therefore neither should be given. Vaccination cannot protect against all the potential pathogens that may be covered by passively acquired MDA (Schultz et al. 1977; Schultz and Conklin 1998; Schultz 1998; Greene and Schultz 2006).

9.8.3 Other Issues with Vaccinating Juvenile Animals

The only antibody that blocks active immunity is IgG, which is passed via colostrum from the dam during nursing and absorbed from the intestine into the puppy or kitten's blood during the first three days after birth. Nursing for longer periods will not increase protection, nor will juveniles derive any protection from vaccines administered to nursing mothers (though nursing mothers should still be vaccinated for their own protection). Therefore, young animals can be readily vaccinated before weaning, provided they have no MDA to block vaccination.

Vaccinating puppies when MDA is present will not increase their level of risk by causing MDA to decline more rapidly while responding to vaccine virus. Vaccination should not be delayed in order to conserve MDA.

9.8.4 Biosecurity of Juvenile Animals

Since titer testing is the only reliable way to determine which puppies or kittens received MDA, when the "window of susceptibility" will open, or which puppies and kittens will be effectively immunized by vaccines given prior to four to five months of age, it is crucial to implement management practices that protect juveniles from exposure to the most dangerous infectious agents, i.e. CDV, CPV-2, and FPV. In many cases, the most effective way to protect puppies and kittens from disease is to move them to other low-risk locations such as clean, low-traffic foster homes or well-separated facilities within the shelter (including use of separate equipment, supplies, and protective clothing for staff and volunteers). Foster care is often a more ideal method for biosecurity than isolation within the shelter because it reduces the risk of disease exposure by minimizing the length of stay within the facility. Puppies and kittens can then be raised and vaccinated in a low-stress, disease-free environment while receiving optimal socialization.

9.8.5 Colostrum Replacement for Orphans

As stated earlier, the best form of immunity in the orphaned puppy or kitten is passive immunity (MDA) similar to what they would normally receive in colostrum from their mothers during the first few days after birth. While passive immunity can be problematic because it is likely to interfere with efforts to immunize through vaccination, MDA provides essential protection against bacterial infections that may lead to sepsis as well as protecting against the viral diseases discussed in the sections on the core vaccines. Unfortunately, orphaned neonatal puppies and kittens presented to shelters may have missed the opportunity to nurse and acquire passive immunity. Failure of passive transfer puts kittens and puppies at a very high risk of acquiring a broad range of infectious diseases, especially during the first four weeks after birth, and often minor pathogens will cause disease and death (Levy et al. 2001; Mila et al. 2014). It is likely that the failure of passive transfer of antibody is responsible for much of the neonatal mortality seen in orphaned puppies and kittens.

When kittens or puppies do not get colostrum during the first few days (e.g. puppies or kittens are separated from their mothers, a mother will not allow offspring to suckle, or the mother has no milk or dies at parturition), "artificial colostrum" can be made and administered to correct this failure of passive antibody transfer (Mila et al. 2017). While fostering orphaned kittens to lactating queens or puppies to lactating bitches may have benefits, queens and bitches in mid-lactation or earlier do not have sufficient antibody in their milk to correct this failure of passive transfer. Additionally, replacement colostrum must be provided within 72 hours after birth and before the ingestion of other proteins to be absorbed (Chastant-Maillard et al. 2012).

In order to provide replacement antibodies to colostrum-deprived juveniles, serum from the dam or other adult animals can be collected, preferably from animals housed in the same environment where the puppies or kittens will be housed. Serum should only be obtained from healthy adult animals who have been well immunized and proven to have robust titers against CPV-2 and CDV or FPV through quantitative endpoint titer testing. Adult cats must be FeLV and FIV negative. A donor base of healthy animals known to be free from infectious disease could be established, but this should include clear guidelines and veterinary care and supervision. A pool of potential donors volunteered by their owners can be recruited from home settings and screened in advance. Providing free health screening, vaccination, and titer testing may be an incentive for participation in a donor program. Veterinary health checks should be performed at least yearly on all donor animals.

After blood has been collected and allowed to clot, the serum should be separated and pooled if an insufficient quantity of serum cannot be obtained from a single donor. The serum can be frozen at −20° C (−4° F) for later use. Immune canine serum can also be purchased commercially. For oral administration, one volume of serum (e.g. 10 ml) should be added to an equal volume (e.g.10 ml) of milk replacer (e.g. Esbilac) and the "artificial colostrum" can be fed to the kittens or puppies for the first three days of life. The "artificial colostrum" will provide some protection through passive immunity.

Significant benefits have been demonstrated by administering serum to colostrum deprived kittens parenterally, either by intraperitoneal (IP) or preferably, subcutaneous injection (SQ) (Levy et al. 2001). The SQ route would be the route of choice for most shelter personnel, as IP injection is more difficult and possibly dangerous for those not familiar with the procedure. Administering antibodies by injection, when compared to oral administration, extends the length of time that passive transfer can be accomplished because the transfer is not dependent on gut absorption. In the study by Levy et al. referenced above, the serum was administered either SC or IP to kittens in three doses of 5 ml each—one dose at birth, one at 12 hours and another 24 hours later. However, SQ administration of immune serum could take place at any age because, unlike oral administration, it is not dependent on gut absorption. This parenteral administration resulted in serum antibody concentrations that were equivalent to kittens that nursed continuously with the queen present. Similar procedures could be used for orphaned puppies where 5–10 ml are given, depending on the size of the puppy, every 12–18 hours, with a total of three to five doses to obtain levels of antibody that will provide temporary protection (up to two to four weeks.) Vaccination should proceed as usual when the puppy or kitten reaches the appropriate age (e.g. four to six weeks in shelter environments).

9.9 Use of Hyperimmune Serum for Disease Prevention

Hyperimmune serum has been found to effectively prevent infection in immunologically naïve dogs exposed to CDV, CPV-2, CAV-1, and canine herpesvirus (CHV-1). In naïve cats, hyperimmune serum has prevented infection with FPV. Hyperimmune serum is given before or at the time of exposure and can be administered SQ (serum) or IV (plasma). The use of hyperimmune serum has also been advocated for recently exposed animals before the development of symptoms. While this may be beneficial, the use of serum obtained from vaccinated animals in the environment, rather than commercially prepared hyperimmune serum, is not known to be effective. Due to the cost of immune serum/plasma and the difficulty of obtaining it commercially, the practice of passive immunization is rarely used or recommended today (Greene and Schultz 2006). If exposure has possibly already happened, as is often the case in shelter animals, animals should be vaccinated immediately with an MLV vaccine if this has not already been done. In the case of CDV, CPV-2, and FPV, this will provide immunity in three days or less. Though it will not prevent infection if the exposure occurred prior to vaccination, it will not harm animals that have already been exposed and may prevent illness from future exposures. Passive immunization, either in the natural form of maternal antibody in colostrum or artificially injected or fed antibody, is of greatest importance to protect the newborn puppy or kitten.

9.10 Risk Assessment and Evaluation of Serologic Immunity for Canine Distemper, Canine Parvovirus and Feline Panleukopenia

In recent years, owners and veterinarians have become increasingly cautious about over-vaccinating pet animals. In response, the measurement of antibody titer levels has gained popularity to evaluate protection against certain diseases for which antibody levels correlate well with immunity ((Tizard and Ni 1998; Jensen et al. 2015). In those pets for whom protective levels are documented, revaccination is generally considered unnecessary (Twark and Dodds 2000; Ford et al. 2017). Though not designed or evaluated for risk assessment of recently-exposed animals, the measurement of titer levels also has application in the shelter population.

The following description of a systematic risk assessment process, based on evaluation for serologic immunity, can be used to evaluate individual animal risk after possible exposure to CDV, CPV, or feline panleukopenia. Because antibody levels closely correlate to protection for these three particular diseases, it can be assumed that healthy dogs and cats (no clinical signs of illness) with protective titer levels are very unlikely to become infected or ill, even if exposed. Some animals with no clinical signs and protective titers may actually be subclinically infected but will never develop obvious clinical disease. While these animals may shed virus, they have not posed problems clinically when using this risk evaluation system to resolve outbreaks.

While assigning risk groups never provides an absolute guarantee of whether a particular animal will become infected, defining the level of risk for individual animals and subgroups can substantially help to guide shelter decisions. Serologic risk assessment can be used to minimize euthanasia and other drastic or costly measures taken while still effectively controlling an outbreak. Establishing risk categories for exposed animals also limits the number of animals subject to quarantine, isolation, or special rescue. Because some animals may have strong demonstrable immunity, it is possible to assign these animals to a low-risk group and direct any special precautionary measures only at higher risk animals. Attempting to conserve resources by avoiding diagnostic or titer testing may lead to even greater resource expenditures and euthanasia later. Serologic risk assessment should be used in the context of overall risk assessment and outbreak response. (See Chapters 4 and 6).

9.10.1 Options for Antibody Titer Testing

Antibody testing may be performed by sending serum samples to a commercial diagnostic laboratory or by using an in-house screening test kit. Diagnostic laboratories will most commonly return quantitative (numerical) information while the in-house tests give only qualitative (positive or negative) results. All tests need to be validated initially by a laboratory using challenge testing so that cut-off points for risk categories can be determined through the numerical values. Regardless of whether an in-house test or commercial laboratory is used, the same principles of interpretation apply.

9.10.2 Initial Evaluation for Clinical Signs

Serology for risk assessment can only be interpreted in animals that are *completely free of clinical signs of the illness in question* at the time of testing. Positive titers in animals that have any signs of illness may reflect an active immune response to infection rather than a pre-existing protective titer level. Results must also be interpreted with caution in animals recently recovered from illness. In these animals, positive titers may reflect an immune response to recent infection. While these animals are unlikely to develop severe disease from the condition in the future, they may still be shedding and therefore pose an infectious risk to others. This is particularly a concern for conditions with potentially prolonged post-recovery shedding, such as CDV.

The initial evaluation for illness is critically important. For example, in the face of an outbreak, all dogs showing any clinical signs suggestive of distemper, such as nasal or ocular discharge, respiratory disease, anorexia, or unexplained gastrointestinal disease (GI) must be considered high risk. In the case of parvoviruses, dogs or cats with vomiting, diarrhea, lethargy, or inappetence are considered high risk. An evaluation must include close observation, including the use of daily monitoring sheets and direct observation of fecal quality and output, appetite, and attitude as well as other clinical signs. If clinical signs go unrecognized when a risk assessment is attempted, an infected animal may be improperly identified as having immunity.

9.10.3 Interpretation of Positive Titer Results in Adult Dogs and Cats

Dogs and cats with no clinical signs who test antibody positive on a qualitative kit or are above the protective cut-off for samples sent to a diagnostic laboratory can be assigned to a low-risk category. Because those animals have antibody and no clinical signs, it is most likely that their antibody reflects immunity and not an infection. Dogs and cats in this low-risk category for CPV, FPV, and CDV are unlikely to become infected or develop clinical signs of disease. Because CDV has a long incubation period, there is a small chance that the titer may rise during infection before the onset of clinical signs, thus adding some slight uncertainty to low-risk assessment for antibody-positive dogs. However, in the authors' experience using this system to manage numerous outbreaks of CDV, this theoretically increased risk has not caused a problem clinically.

Animals categorized as low risk based on positive titers may remain in the general population and be adopted with relative safety. It is advisable to make potential adopters aware that there was an outbreak and that the animals were potentially exposed in the shelter while explaining the testing and risk categorization that has been done. *Low risk* does not mean *no risk;* there is always some risk associated with acquiring a new pet from a multi-animal background such as a shelter or pet store. This strategy, to the authors' knowledge, has been used successfully to manage many shelter outbreaks.

9.10.4 Interpretation of Negative Titer Results in Adult Dogs and Cats

In the face of an outbreak, dogs and cats who have no clinical signs and negative titer test results (i.e. no or low antibodies) on qualitative kits or are below the protective cut-off for samples sent to a diagnostic laboratory, must be considered at high risk of becoming infected because they were likely to have been susceptible at the time of exposure. *Not all titer-negative animals will become ill*, especially if they were vaccinated on intake or before. However, these animals are at relatively high risk of becoming ill at any time within the incubation period. They should be removed from the general shelter population immediately. See Chapter 6 on Outbreak Management for more information.

9.10.5 Interpretation of Titer Results in Juvenile Animals

For puppies and kittens under five months of age, it is difficult to differentiate actively produced antibody responses from passive, maternally-derived immunity by testing with a qualitative kit due to its yes/no result based on cut-off values. Quantitative end-point titer testing completed at a diagnostic laboratory is more likely to differentiate an active response from passive immunity if a level of antibody is found that exceeds typical maternal levels seen in juveniles of that age. Titers resulting from active immunity reflect not only the presence of circulating antibodies but also suggest the presence of associated memory cells and ongoing antibody production. On the other hand, titers resulting from passively acquired antibodies represent only those antibodies that were absorbed from colostrum and that degrade over a period of weeks. A passively immune animal who was protected at the time of testing will lose that protection within a short period of time. Memory cells, as part of active immunity, increase immune response in the face of a challenge. Passively acquired antibody titers suggest no such reinforcements and so it is possible that a higher measurable antibody titer may be needed for protection from challenge.

Ideally, a higher bar for titer level should be set for juveniles to suggest low risk. As described above, in-house tests are qualitative and designed to give only a positive or negative result based on a titer level that was shown to be protective for adult dogs with active immunity. Quantitative titer testing for puppies or kittens is a better determinant of risk because a higher cut-off point can be used. However, puppies and kittens (less than 18 weeks of age) with strong positive antibody titers on a qualitative kit most likely have high enough levels of antibodies to protect them from challenge. In most cases, it is probably safe and simplest to assign puppies and kittens with no clinical signs and a qualitatively positive titer result to the low-risk group.

It should be understood, however, that the assignment of juvenile animals to a low-risk group does not reflect the same level of certainty as for an adult because it may be based on MDA titers rather than active immunity. In addition, documented "low risk" status may change rapidly as maternal antibodies wane. Juvenile animals with positive titers have been assigned to an indeterminate risk category in Table 9.2 below for this reason. Puppies and

Table 9.2 Risk factor determination.

High Risk	Indeterminate Risk	Low Risk
No antibody on titer testing, regardless of age	Puppies and kittens <5 months of age, with antibody present	Animals >5 months of age, with antibody
Exposed, with no vaccination history		Known vaccination at >16 weeks of age
Clinical signs present	No clinical signs	No clinical signs

kittens with strongly positive titers should be moved through the shelter system as quickly as possible.

Prolonged waiting time for results and variations between types of testing and cut-off points used by each lab may make outside laboratory testing impractical. While quantitative antibody titer levels are ideal for risk evaluation in puppies and kittens, the use of a qualitative screening kit is often preferable to either waiting for lab results, blindly assigning risk categories or treating all puppies and kittens as equally high risk after exposure.

9.11 Vaccine Effects on Diagnostic Testing

9.11.1 FeLV (Feline Leukemia) and FIV (Feline Immunodeficiency) Vaccine Effects on Diagnostic Testing

FeLV tests detect viral antigen and when positive, demonstrate virus in the blood or other secretions depending on the sample tested. Vaccination with FeLV vaccines will not affect test results (Goldkamp et al. 2008).

In contrast, the commonly used FIV screening test detects antibodies. Since antibodies are produced by vaccination, as well as from infection with virulent virus, it is not possible to consistently differentiate vaccinated animals from infected animals with commonly used point of care tests for FIV. However, FIV PCR testing may be helpful in this regard. See chapter 23 for additional information on retroviral testing and management.

9.11.2 CPV-2 (Canine Parvo) and FPV (Feline Panleukopenia) Vaccine Effects on Diagnostic Testing

The ELISA test for detection of CPV-2 antigen in feces of dogs suspected of having CPV-2 is very helpful in making a diagnosis. This test can also be used for cats when testing for FPV in cats. The two viruses are antigenically similar, and the antibody used to detect the CPV-2 virus will also react with FPV antigens (Larson et al. 2007).

Several studies have examined the likelihood of positive FPV and CPV-2 tests following vaccination and found true positives from vaccination to be extremely rare.

In a study by the authors' laboratory, more than 600 naïve dogs were tested for fecal parvovirus antigen using the IDEXX SNAP test on days three through nine after receiving commercial vaccines. None of those dogs had a positive test. The TiterCHEK™ test (formerly known as Witness™) detected CPV-2 in less than 1% of the samples. Similar results were found with cats. Over 600 naïve cats were tested on days three to nine post-vaccination, with only one positive on the IDEXX test. That cat died after vaccination with FPV and it was believed to be a non-responder to FPV (Larson et al. 2007).

A similar study by others found that, as in the authors' study, of 64 vaccinated, 10-week-old

SPF kittens, only one kitten tested positive (weakly) with the IDEXX SNAP test within two weeks post-vaccination (Patterson et al. 2007). More frequent positive results were found using other test brands in this study.

The authors have conducted several other studies that confirm that true positive reactions due to vaccinations are rare. There was some variation across all the commercially available tests, with the IDEXX tests giving the fewest positive tests after vaccination. This is important information for shelters because many shelters are currently following recommendations to vaccinate all animals on intake. If a positive or weak positive test in an infected animal is mistakenly identified as a false positive test because of recent vaccination, an opportunity may be missed to interrupt the cycle of disease transmission, and needed care and intervention may be delayed because it is believed the animal does not have virulent parvovirus. While it is known that vaccinated animals are, in fact, likely to shed vaccine virus post-vaccination, the level of virus shed is below the range that would be detected as positive on most of the fecal antigen tests. Even when more sensitive methods of viral detection such as hemagglutination (HA) or viral isolation (VI) are used, only a small percentage of animals will have detectable levels of virus in their feces post-vaccination. Therefore, a positive test with antigen detection tests such as HA or ELISA is strongly indicative of virulent viral infection, irrespective of recent vaccination with CPV-2 or FPV.

In contrast, if polymerase chain reaction (PCR) is used to detect CPV-2 or FPV in feces, many fecal samples from vaccinated animals will be positive due to the sensitivity of the assay. Unfortunately, there is no convenient way to determine whether the virus is vaccine or virulent virus. Therefore, negative results on the PCR test for parvovirus are meaningful, but positive results obtained from fecal samples of animals vaccinated during the previous two weeks may result from either vaccination or true infection.

9.11.3 CDV Vaccine Effects on Diagnostic Testing

CDV vaccine virus may be detectable by all common methods of antigen detection including PCR, virus isolation, fluorescent antibody (FA), and immunohistochemistry (IHC) (Appel 1987). Vaccine virus may interfere with diagnostic testing for up to two weeks after vaccination with an MLV vaccine because the MLV virus replicates in a variety of cell types and is present in leukocytes throughout the body. How long vaccine virus may persist in various tissues is individual animal dependent but would not be expected to be detectable beyond two weeks. Interference with testing and false positives would not occur with some tests (virus isolation, FA, IHC) when the canarypox vectored rCDV product is used and is unlikely to occur with PCR testing. The rCDV vaccine does not contain infectious CDV (Noon et al. 1980).

Vaccination could also easily interfere with paired antibody titer testing used as a diagnostic tool for CDV and/or CPV-2 infection. It would be expected that a dog's antibody titer would rise significantly in the three-week period following vaccination with CDV or CPV-2 vaccines if the initial titer was below protective levels.

9.11.4 FHV-1 (Feline Herpesvirus) and FCV (Feline Calicivirus) Vaccine Effects on Diagnostic Testing

FHV-1 and FCV may be shed for two weeks from cats who have recently been vaccinated with an MLV IN vaccine. The first three to seven days are the most common for viral shedding post-vaccination. Shedding would interfere with both VI and PCR, yielding positive test results. Field strain virus cannot be easily differentiated from vaccine virus in most cases; though reverse transcription-PCR (RT-PCR) can distinguish vaccine from field strain FCV, this test is not commercially available (Lappin et al. 2006).

9.11.5 Bordetella/CAV-2/CPi (Canine Parainfluenza) Intranasal Vaccine Effects on Diagnostic Testing

All currently available IN and oral Bordetella vaccines are MLV, thus they can be shed in detectable quantities, generally for not more than two weeks post-vaccination. During this shedding period, vaccine pathogen could give false positives when testing with PCR or culture.

9.11.6 Canine Lyme Vaccine Effects on Diagnostic Testing

Though the Lyme vaccine is not part of the core vaccination program for shelters, it is important to understand its impact on diagnostic testing. There are rapid tests (4Dx®, IDEXX Laboratories, and others) available for use in the shelter to identify dogs that are likely to be infected or that may have previously been infected with *Borrelia burgdorferi*. Positive tests for Borrelia are often an impediment to transfer, transport or adoption because it can be unclear how to interpret the positive result. Some positive dogs do not require any treatment, having already recovered from the disease. However, a positive test may indicate that the animal is infected and should possibly be treated with antibiotics, especially if it is showing clinical signs, such as arthritis. Vaccination against Lyme disease has been shown to not interfere with IDEXX 4Dx which detects a protein (C6) that is only expressed during infection with *B. burgdorferi* (O'Connor et al. 2004). This test also detects heartworm antigen and antibodies to *Ehrlichia canis, E. ewingii, Anaplasma phagocytophilum,* and *A. platys.*

9.11.7 Antibody (Titer) Testing for the Diagnosis of Canine Distemper, Canine Parvovirus and Feline Panleukopenia

Antibody testing for CDV, CPV, and FPV has been discussed in both the context of risk assessment and vaccination of pregnant animals. (Please see the sections on risk assessment (9.10) and vaccination of pregnant animals (9.4.4.2).) In these cases, antibody titers are used as a means of assessing immunity to infection or previous vaccination history. Using antibody titers to help diagnose current CDV, CPV, and FPV infections is, in general, not recommended in shelters since, ideally, shelters will be vaccinating on intake with MLV. It would be expected after receiving an MLV that antibody titers would climb if pre-existing titers were low enough to allow vaccine virus to replicate. Little differentiation could be made between vaccine response and infection when looking at paired titers over time.

9.12 Conclusion

The proper administration of the core vaccines to all dogs and cats upon intake is an essential component of a comprehensive healthcare program to maintain a healthy shelter population. When implemented, along with other good management practices, it protects most animals from the most severe, life-threatening infectious diseases found in shelters, and reduces the severity of clinical signs for others. Most susceptible animals respond very quickly to vaccination with core vaccines (CDV, CPV-2, and FPV), developing immune responses that are protective within hours, in some cases, to just a few days in others. Vaccines are powerful tools but alone cannot be expected to resolve every disease problem in shelters. Additional practices must be put in place to reduce the infectious dose of pathogens and minimize the risk of exposure for susceptible animals. Because so many animals have not been effectively immunized before entering a shelter, every animal, except those who arrive with a valid, documented history of vaccination, should be considered susceptible at admission. Juvenile animals present a unique challenge for shelters and must be presumed to be susceptible until they are over the age of 18 weeks due to unknown levels of maternal antibody that can block vaccination but may or may not prevent disease.

References

Abdelmagid, O.Y., Larson, L.J., Payne, L. et al. (2004). Evaluation of the efficacy and duration of immunity of a canine combination vaccine against virulent parvovirus, infectious canine hepatitis virus, and distemper virus experimental challenges. *Veterinary Therapeutics* 5 (3): 173–186.

Appel, M. (1987). Canine distemper virus. In: *Virus Infections of Carnivores* (ed. M. Appel), 133–159. New York;: Elsevier.

Appel, M.J. (1999). Forty years of canine vaccination. In: *Veterinary Vaccines and Diagnostics - Advances in Veterinary Medicine* (ed. R.D. Schultz), 309–324. San Diego: Academic Press.

Appel, M. and Bemis, D.A. (1978). The canine contagious respiratory disease complex (kennel cough). *Cornell Veterinarian* 68 (7): 70–75.

Brun, A., Chappuis, G., Précausta, P. et al. (1979). Immunization against panleukopenia: early development of immunity. *Compendium of Immunology, Microbiology, and Infectious Disease* 1 (4): 335–339.

Buonavoglia, C., Martella, V., Pratelli, A. et al. (2001). Evidence for evolution of canine parvovirus type 2 in Italy. *Journal of General Virology* 82: 3021–3025.

Carmichael, L.E., Joubert, J.C., Pollock, R.V. et al. (1983). A modified live canine parvovirus vaccine. II. Immune response. *Cornell Veterinarian* 73 (1): 13–29.

Chastant-Maillard, S., Freyburger, L., Marcheteau, E. et al. (2012). Timing of the intestinal barrier closure in puppies. *Reproduction in Domestic Animals* 47 (6): 190–193.

Davis, R., Jayappa, H., Abdelmagid, O.Y. et al. (2007). Comparison of the mucosal immune response in dogs vaccinated with either an intranasal avirulent live culture or a subcutaneous antigen extract vaccine of *Bordetella bronchiseptica*. *Veterinary Therapeutics* 8 (1): 32–40.

Ford, R.B., Larson, L.J., Wellborn, L. et al. (2017). American Animal Hospital Association Canine Vaccination Guidelines. https://www.aaha.org/guidelines/canine_vaccination_guidelines.aspx (accessed 8 September 2019).

Goldkamp, C.E., Levy, J.K., Edinboro, C.H. et al. (2008). Seroprevalences of feline leukemia virus and feline immunodeficiency virus in cats with abscesses or bite wounds and rate of veterinarian compliance with current guidelines for retrovirus testing. *Journal of the American Veterinary Medical Association* 232 (8): 1152–1158.

Greene, C.E. and Schultz, R.D. (2006). Immunoprophylaxis. In: *Infectious Diseases of the Dog and Cat*, 3e (ed. C.E. Greene), 1069–1119. St. Louis: Saunders Elsevier.

Hageny, T.L., Haase, C.J. Larson, L.J. et al. (2004). A comparison between recombinant, naked DNA and modified live canine distemper virus (CDV) vaccines. Poster presented at the 85th Annual Conference of Research Workers in Animal Disease, Chicago (14–16 November 2004).

Huang, C., Hess, J., Gill, M. et al. (2010). A dual-strain feline calicivirus vaccine stimulates broader cross-neutralization antibodies than a single-strain vaccine and lessens clinical signs in vaccinated cats when challenged with a homologous feline calicivirus strain associated with virulent systemic disease. *Journal of Feline Medicine and Surgery* 12 (2): 129–137.

Jensen, W.A., Totten, J.S., Lappin, M.R. et al. (2015). Use of serologic tests to predict resistance to canine distemper virus-induced disease in vaccinated dogs. *Journal of Veterinary Diagnostic Investigation* 27 (5): 576–580.

Lappin, M.R., Sebring, R.W., Porter, M. et al. (2006). Effects of a single dose of an intranasal feline herpesvirus 1, calicivirus, and panleukopenia vaccine on clinical signs and virus shedding after challenge with virulent feline herpesvirus 1. *Journal of Feline Medicine and Surgery* 8 (3): 158–163.

Larson, L.J. and Schultz, R.D. (1997). Comparison of selected canine vaccines for their ability to induce protective immunity against canine parvovirus infection. *American Journal of Veterinary Research* 58: 360–363.

Larson, L.J. and Schultz, R.D. (2006). Effect of vaccination with recombinant canine distemper virus vaccine immediately before exposure under shelter-like conditions. *Veterinary Therapeutics* 7 (2): 113–118.

Larson, L.J. and Schultz, R.D. (2008). Do two current canine parvovirus type 2 and 2b vaccines provide protection against the new type 2c variant? *Veterinary Therapeutics* 9: 94–101.

Larson, L.J., Hageny, T.L., Haase, C.J. et al. (2006). Effect of recombinant canine distemper vaccine on antibody titers in previously vaccinated dogs. *Veterinary Therapeutics* 7 (2): 107–112.

Larson, L.J., Quesada, M., Mukhtar, E. et al. (2007). Evaluation of a CPV-2 fecal parvovirus ELISA (SNAP fecal parvo test®) from IDEXX Laboratories. Poster presented at the 88th Annual Conference of Research Workers in Animal Disease, Chicago (2–4 December 2007).

Larson, L.J., Thiel, B.E., Sharp, P. et al. (2013). A comparative study of protective immunity provided by oral, intranasal and parenteral canine Bordetella bronchiseptica vaccines. *International Journal of Applied Research in Veterinary Medicine* 11 (3): 153–160.

Lechner, E.S., Crawford, C., Levy, J. et al. (2010). Prevalence of protective antibody titers for canine distemper virus and canine parvovirus in dogs entering a Florida animal shelter. *Journal of the American Veterinary Medical Association* 236 (12): 1317–1321.

Levy, J.K., Crawford, P.C., Collante, W.R. et al. (2001). Use of adult cat serum to correct failure of passive transfer in kittens. *Journal of the American Veterinary Medical Association* 219 (10): 1401–1405.

Levy, J.K., Crawford, P.C., Kusuhara, H. et al. (2008). Differentiation of feline immunodeficiency virus vaccination, infection, or vaccination and infection in cats. *Journal of Veterinary Internal Medicine* 22 (2): 330–334.

Martella, V., Cavalli, A., Pratelli, A. et al. (2004). A canine parvovirus mutant is spreading in Italy. *Journal of Clinical Microbiology* 42: 1333–1336.

Mila, H., Feugier, A., Grellet, A. et al. (2014). Inadequate passive immune transfer in puppies: definition, risk factors and prevention in a large multi-breed kennel. *Preventive Veterinary Medicine* 116 (1–2): 209–213.

Mila, H., Grellet, A., Mariani, C. et al. (2017). Natural and artificial hyperimmune solutions: impact on health in puppies. *Reproduction in Domestic Animals* 52 (2): 163–169.

Mouzin, D.E., Lorenzen, M.J., Haworth, J.D. et al. (2004a). Duration of serologic responses to five viral antigens in dogs. *Journal of the American Veterinary Medical Association* 224 (1): 55–60.

Mouzin, D.E., Lorenzen, M.J., Haworth, J.D. et al. (2004b). Duration of serologic response to three viral antigens in cats. *Journal of the American Veterinary Medical Association* 224 (1): 61–66.

Newbury, S.P., Larson, L.J., Schultz, R.D. et al. (2007.) A placebo controlled field trial of an intranasal vaccine for feline calici virus and feline herpes virus to prevent clinical signs of feline infectious respiratory disease complex in an animal shelter. Conference of Research Workers in Animal Diseases, Chicago.

Newbury, S.P., Godhardt-Cooper, J., Poulsen, K.P. et al. (2016). Prolonged intermittent virus shedding during an outbreak of canine influenza A H3N2 virus infection in dogs in three Chicago area shelters: 16 cases (March to May 2015). *Journal of the American Veterinary Medical Association* 248 (9): 1022–1026.

Noon, K.F., Rogul, M., Binn, L.N. et al. (1980). Enzyme-linked immunosorbent assay for evaluation of antibody to canine distemper virus. *American Journal of Veterinary Research* 41 (4): 605–609.

O'Connor, T.P., Esty, K.J., Hanscom, J.L. et al. (2004). Dogs vaccinated with common Lyme disease vaccines do not respond to IR6, the conserved immunodominant region of the VlsE surface protein of Borrelia burgdorferi. *Clinical and Diagnostic Laboratory Immunology* 11 (3): 458–462.

Olsen, L.B., Larson, L.J. and Schultz, R.D. (1998). Canine parvovirus (CPV-2b) infection in cats. Conference of Research Workers in Animal Disease, Chicago.

Patterson, E.V., Reese, M.J., Tucker, S.J. et al. (2007). Effect of vaccination on parvovirus antigen testing in kittens. *Journal of the American Veterinary Medical Association* 230 (3): 359–363.

Poulet, H., Brunet, S., Leroy, V. et al. (2005). Immunisation with a combination of two complementary feline calicivirus strains induces a broad cross-protection against heterologous challenges. *Veterinary Microbiology* 106 (1–2): 17–31.

Reed, T.L., VonMessling, V. Cattaneo, R. et al. (2003). A comparative study of canine distemper vaccines. Poster presented at the 84th Conference of Research Workers in Animal Disease, Chicago (9–11 November 2003).

Stone, A.E., Brummet, G.O., Carozza, E.M. et al. (2020). 2020 AAHA/AAFP Feline Vaccination Guidelines. *Journal of the American Animal Hospital Association* 56: 249–265.

Schroeder, J.P., Bordt, D.W., Mitchell, F.E. et al. (1967). Studies of canine distemper immunization of puppies in a canine distemper-contaminated environment. *Veterinary Medicine/Small Animal Clinician* 62 (8): 782–787.

Schultz, R.D. (1998). Current and future canine and feline vaccination programs. *Veterinary Medicine* 93: 233–254.

Schultz, R.D. (1999). Canine and feline vaccines. In: *Veterinary Vaccines and Diagnostics – Advances in Veterinary Medicine* (ed. R.D. Schultz), 289–358. San Diego: Academic Press.

Schultz, R.D. (2000). Considerations in designing effective and safe vaccination programs for dogs. In: *Recent Advances in Canine Infectious Diseases* (ed. L.E. Carmichael). International Veterinary Information Service http://www.ivis.org. (

Schultz, R.D. (2006). Duration of immunity for canine and feline vaccines: a review. *Veterinary Microbiology* 117 (1): 75–79.

Schultz, R.D. (2009). A commentary on parvovirus vaccination. *Journal of Feline Medicine and Surgery* 11 (2): 163–164.

Schultz, R.D. and Conklin, S. (1998). The immune system and vaccines. *Compendium of Continuing Education for the Practicing Veterinarian* 20: 5–18.

Schultz, R.D., Appel, M.J., and Carmichael, L.E. (1977). Canine vaccines and immunity. In: *Current Veterinary Therapy*, VIe (ed. R.W. Kirk), 1271–1275. Philadelphia: WB Saunders.

Schultz, R.D., Larson, L.J., and Newbury, S. (2007). *Unpublished Data: Surveys of Shelter Dogs and Cats in Multiple States*. University of Wisconsin-Madison.

Scott, F.W. and Geissinger, C.M. (1999). Long-term immunity in cats vaccinated with an inactivated trivalent vaccine. *American Journal of Veterinary Research* 60 (5): 652–658.

Tizard, I. and Ni, Y. (1998). Use of serologic testing to assess immune status of companion animals. *Journal of the American Veterinary Medical Association* 213 (1): 54–60.

Truyen, U. (2006). Evolution of canine parvovirus: a need for new vaccines? *Veterinary Microbiology* 117: 9–13.

Truyen, U., Evermann, J.F., Vieler, E. et al. (1996). Evolution of canine parvovirus involved loss and gain of feline host range. *Virology* 215: 186–189.

Twark, L. and Dodds, W.J. (2000). Clinical use of serum parvovirus and distemper virus antibody titers for determining revaccination strategies in healthy dogs. *Journal of the American Veterinary Medical Association* 217 (7): 1021–1024.

Wagner, D.C., Kass, P.H., and Hurley, K.F. (2018). Cage size, movement in and out of housing during daily care, and other environmental and population health risk factors for feline upper respiratory disease in nine North American animal shelters. *PLoS One* 13 (1): e0190140.

10

Canine Infectious Respiratory Disease (CIRD)

Elizabeth A. Berliner

Maddie's Shelter Medicine Program, Cornell University College of Veterinary Medicine, Ithaca, NY, USA

10.1 Introduction

Canine Infectious Respiratory Disease (CIRD) typically presents as a self-limiting, mild to moderate upper respiratory disease of dogs. Viral and bacterial agents often act synergistically to produce clinical signs. It is a relatively common syndrome in group-housed dogs, including those in animal shelters and kennels. While clinical signs are generally mild and self-limiting for individual dogs, CIRD represents a major animal welfare and management issue for group-housed dogs, including animal shelters with any or all of the following risk factors: crowding; a large proportion of vulnerable dogs; individuals and populations under physiologic stress; insufficient or inconsistent healthcare protocols; poorly managed transport programs; and/or outdated or poorly designed facilities.

CIRD mirrors respiratory syndromes in other animal populations, including bovine "shipping fever" and porcine respiratory disease in that it has a complex, multifactorial etiology with multiple pathogens and environmental stressors acting in the pathogenesis of the disease. Additional risk factors for individual dogs include age and immune status, physiologic stress, co-morbidities, and environmental conditions favoring a high pathogen load; poor conditions contribute strongly to pathogen success. While owned dogs in communities may be exposed to or even harbor CIRD pathogens, they can often resist clinical disease. The same dogs introduced into a stressful shelter environment may become ill, exacerbated by the continuous intake of new dogs from a myriad of sources.

Other terms commonly used to describe this condition include "kennel cough" or "canine infectious tracheobronchitis (ITB)." Agents implicated in this complex have historically included canine parainfluenza virus (CPiV), canine adenovirus type 2 (CAV-2), and canine herpesvirus type 1(CHV), often in conjunction with *Bordetella bronchiseptica*. However, in the last two decades, advances in pathogen detection have resulted in the identification of additional agents in cases of CIRD, including canine respiratory coronavirus (CRCoV), canine influenza (CIV), canine pneumovirus (CPnV), *Streptococcus equi* subspecies *zooepidemicus,* and *Mycoplasma cynos.*

For most individual dogs, clinical signs are mild and pathogen identification is unnecessary. A presumptive diagnosis of an uncomplicated case of CIRD is based on key clinical signs: a hacking, paroxysmal cough, and a mild to moderate nasal discharge with or without mild pyrexia. The majority of CIRD patients are still bright, active, and appetent. Less commonly, dogs demonstrate anorexia and general

Infectious Disease Management in Animal Shelters, Second Edition.
Edited by Lila Miller, Stephanie Janeczko, and Kate F. Hurley.

malaise, though these may also be signs of advancing or more severe systemic illness. For populations affected by CIRD, the implications can be more significant and result in compromised welfare; in outbreaks, diagnostic testing is often warranted.

Two additional significant respiratory agents—canine distemper (CDV) and CIV—are discussed in greater detail in individual chapters because of their unique features and the complexity of their management within the shelter setting. Both can mimic "routine" CIRD, especially early in the course of disease. The index of suspicion for these diseases should be raised based on history, including a high risk of exposure, advancing clinical signs, and the characteristics of animals affected. For example, the index of suspicion for CIV is increased in populations with a high incidence of significant respiratory disease in otherwise fully vaccinated dogs and with a history suggesting possible exposure to the agent. Likewise, though vaccination is protective for CDV, it is still endemic in many areas in the United States, and internationally, and remains a differential in unvaccinated or under-vaccinated adult dogs and all puppies under five months of age from high-risk areas. Longer incubation periods to gastrointestinal (GI) and neurologic components of CDV, as well as the complexity of testing and test interpretation, can delay diagnosis. Specific management of CIV and CDV is critical to prevent spread through an at-risk population and into the community. For a comprehensive discussion of these agents, please see Chapters 11 and 12.

10.2 Etiological Agents, Epidemiology, and Course of Disease

Environmental co-factors are integral contributors to CIRD, appropriately captured in the classic use of "kennel cough" to describe this disease complex. CIRD provides a clear illustration of how host, agent and environmental factors interact to result in disease; successful prevention and control measures for CIRD must address the environment in addition to pathogen and host factors. Many of the pathogens implicated in CIRD can be recovered from clinically healthy dogs (Lavan and Knesl 2015). Without the environmental stressors, most pathogens implicated in routine CIRD pose relatively little risk to immune-competent dogs in homes.

The agents commonly implicated as significant contributors to CIRD, either individually or synergistically, are listed in Table 10.1.

Table 10.1 Canine infectious respiratory disease viral and bacterial agents.

Agent	Abbreviation
Canine parainfluenza virus	CPiV
Canine adenovirus type 2	CAV-2
Canine respiratory coronavirus	CRCoV
Canine herpesvirus	CHV
Canine pneumovirus	CnPnV
Canine influenza	CIV
Canine distemper	CDV
Bordetella bronchiseptica	*B. bronchiseptica*
Mycoplasma cynos	*M. cynos*
Streptococcus equi subsp. *zooepidemicus*	*Strep. zoo*

Debate continues regarding which of these agents are primary versus secondary pathogens; mixed infections are common. Advances in molecular diagnostics unveil agents that may or may not be associated with disease. The rapidly growing availability of polymerase chain reaction (PCR) methods for diagnosis of CIRD has enhanced the sensitivity and speed of testing as well as enabling the detection of multiple infectious agents simultaneously; however, this increased sensitivity greatly complicates the matter of determining their clinical significance.

Co-infections are common in shelter dogs, but multiple studies have also recovered CIRD-agents from dogs demonstrating no signs of respiratory disease. See page 13. A 2015 study looked at the prevalence of canine infectious respiratory pathogens in *asymptomatic, healthy* dogs at the time of intake to shelters in the United States: of 503 dogs tested, 47.7% were PCR positive for at least one CIRD pathogen, and 18.7% had two or more (Lavan and Knesl 2015). This finding lends additional support to the importance of environmental conditions in the development of CIRD in shelter-housed dogs.

10.2.1 Viral Pathogens

While a detailed understanding of the taxonomy or molecular makeup of pathogens is beyond the scope of this text, a basic understanding of virology can be useful in understanding both CIRD pathogenesis and the efficacy of control measures used in shelters. All viruses are obligate intracellular organisms composed of either a DNA or RNA genome protected by a protein coat called a capsid; the nucleic acid genome plus its protein capsid comprises the nucleocapsid. Enveloped viruses are then further surrounded by a lipid bilayer derived from a host cell membrane and studded with virus-coded glycoproteins.

Viruses are classified into families based on shared properties, most notably size and shape, nucleic acid genome, and mode of replication. This classification system also helps to make connections across host species for how viral agents and the immune system may interact to result in (or prevent) disease.

The composition of the nucleic acid genome impacts the stability of a virus over time. RNA viruses show a much higher rate of mutation than DNA viruses due to the innate complexity of RNA replication and the error rate of replication enzymes. Therefore, over time, RNA viruses are more likely to mutate to new variants with potential for new host interactions or vaccine evasion at a rate higher than DNA viruses. Relevant examples of CIRD-associated RNA viruses include coronaviruses, influenzas and parainfluenzas, while DNA viruses include adenoviruses and herpesviruses.

Enveloped viruses are labile and more susceptible to extremes of environmental conditions, including temperature and humidity, and more subject to destruction by standard detergents and disinfectants. Non-enveloped viruses are very stable in the environment and resistant to many products, as well as freezing and cooling cycles. CAV-2 is the only CIRD virus common to shelters that is non enveloped, leaving the rest subject to inactivation with standard detergents and disinfectants used in shelters. Knowledge of the basic science of a virus plays an important role in designing preventive medicine and management protocols in shelter practice.

10.2.1.1 Canine Parainfluenza Virus (CPiV)

CPiV is an enveloped single-stranded RNA virus of the *Paramyxoviridae* family found worldwide and thought to be one of the more common causes of respiratory disease in dogs. Early work demonstrated that CPiV spreads rapidly in group-housed dogs; in military and laboratory dogs, CPiV seroprevalence rose from 3% at intake to 72% after six weeks in group-housing, and CPiV was recovered from 50% of dogs with respiratory signs (Rosenberg et al. 1971; Ellis and Krakowka 2012).

Table 10.2 Prevalence data of CIRD pathogens recovered on PCR ±culture in asymptomatic and CIRD-affected dogs.

References	Agent	Published Prevalence (%)		Comments
		Healthy dogs	CIRD -affected dogs	
Maboni et al. 2019	CAV-2	0	2.5	Prospective study of US veterinary diagnostic lab submissions from deceased dogs at necropsy with no respiratory disease (n = 52) and retrospective study of client-owned CIRD-affected dogs (n = 559); PCR
	CDV	0	2	
	Influenza A	0	11.2	
	CPiV	0	29	
	CRCoV	0.02	4.6	
	B. bronchiseptica	0.02	9	
	M. cynos	0	24.5	
	M. canis	2.9	23.6	
	Strep. zoo	0	0	
Lavan and Knesl 2015	CAV-2	12.5	N/A	Prospective study of asymptomatic dogs sampled on intake to 7 US shelters (n = 503); PCR
	CDV	7.4		
	CHV-1	0.8		
	CIV	0.4		
	CPiV	3.2		
	CRCoV	1.8		
	B. bronchiseptica	19.5		
	M. cynos	29.2		
	Strep. zoo	1.8		
Schulz et al. 2014	CAV-2	1.1%	0	Prospective study of healthy dogs (n = 61) and CIRD-affected dogs (n = 90) in Southern Germany; PCR
	CDV	0	0	
	CHV-1	0	0	
	CIV	0	0	
	CPiV	7	23	
	CRCoV	0	9.8	
	B. bronchiseptica	45.6	78.7	
Acke et al. 2015	*Strep. zoo*	2	N/A	Prospective study of healthy dogs (n = 197) in New Zealand; culture
Chalker 2005	*M. cynos*	0.9	0	Prospective study of healthy (n = 109) and CIRD-affected dogs (n = 43); tonsillar swabs; culture with PCR typing

The incidence of CPiV has been thought to have declined over time with the initiation of aggressive vaccination programs (Ellis and Krakowka 2012; Ford 2012). However, CPiV is still regularly identified in diagnostic laboratory samples, with prevalence rates reported as high as 29% and a significant association with mild and moderate/severe clinical signs in at least one study; most commonly it occurred in co-infections with *M. cynos* and *B. bronchiseptica* (Maboni et al. 2019). CPiV continues to be implicated in respiratory disease outbreaks in dogs and remains a concern for group-housed populations, including those in veterinary clinics (Weese and Stull 2013). Though related to the simian virus 5 that infects humans, there are no reports of CPiV causing disease in humans (Randall et al. 1987).

CPiV is considered a primary pathogen in CIRD. Characteristically, CPiV causes acute onset cough of short duration but high transmissibility. Infection is primarily confined to the upper respiratory tract, where it causes cytolytic replication and destruction of respiratory epithelium. Laryngeal inflammation results in a characteristic honking cough which, in turn, contributes to viral shedding in aerosolized respiratory secretions. A serous nasal discharge, pharyngitis, and tonsillitis may also be present.

Shedding persists for 8–10 days following infection, and sub-clinically infected and recovering animals can be a source of ongoing infections in a kennel environment if a "clean break" is not established (Ellis and Krakowka 2012). See Chapters 6 and 11 for more information about establishing a clean break. Natural infection produces circulating antibody at detectable levels, but this does not reliably confer protection; IgA at the level of the respiratory mucosa affords more reliable immunologic protection (Ford 2012). In the absence of other complicating pathogens or underlying medical conditions, clinical resolution occurs within 14 days.

A 2014 study found dogs diagnosed with CIRD were significantly more likely to test positive on reverse-transcriptase polymerase chain reaction (RT-PCR) for CPiV than healthy dogs (37.7% compared to 7.8%); healthy dogs had not been vaccinated within four weeks of the study, but 60% of the CIRD-affected dogs had been previously vaccinated at some point in their lifetime (Schulz et al. 2014). Another study of healthy dogs entering shelters recovered CPiV from RT-PCR of nasal and oropharyngeal swabs in 3.2% of dogs. These molecular studies suggest CPiV has a subclinical or carrier state (Lavan and Knesl 2015).

10.2.1.2 Canine Adenovirus Type 2 (CAV-2)

CAVs are non-enveloped DNA viruses of the *Adenoviridae* family. Both canine infectious hepatitis virus type 1 (CAV-1) and CAV-2 cause respiratory signs; however, of the two, CAV-2 is the predominant virus recovered from dogs with CIRD (Ford 2012). CAV-2 was first reported in 1962 as the cause of an outbreak in a group of university-housed laboratory dogs (Ditchfield et al. 1962). CAV-2 replicates in the epithelium of the nasal and pharyngeal cavities and the goblet cells of the trachea, causing acute onset laryngotracheitis. Similar to CPiV, CAV-2 causes damage to the upper airway resulting in a characteristic honking cough. Viral replication peaks within a week and then declines rapidly. Though CAV-1 resembles adenoviruses causing respiratory infections in humans, it is not thought to be zoonotic.

Clinical signs with CAV-2 are generally mild and self-limiting unless complicated by other pathogens. Experimentally, however, CAV-2 has been shown to induce lower respiratory tract lesions in the lung and distal airways, resulting in bronchitis and interstitial pneumonia even though clinical signs of these lesions were not seen (Fairchild et al. 1969). Additionally, severe disease and mortality occurred in young puppies infected with CAV-2, though hemolytic *Escherichia coli* was also present in three of the five deaths (Almes et al. 2010). A 2015 study of healthy dogs entering US shelters recovered CAV-2 in 12.5% of dogs (Lavan and Knesl 2015).

10.2.1.3 Canine Respiratory Coronavirus (CRCoV)

CRCoV is an enveloped RNA virus from the family *Coronaviridae* and first detected in 2003. It is important to note CRCoV is a *Betacoronavirus* distinct from the GI canine coronavirus (CCoV), an *Alphacoronavirus*; other *Alphacoronaviruses* include feline coronavirus (FCoV) and porcine transmissible gastroenteritis (TGE). CRCoV is genetically similar to both bovine (BCoV) and human respiratory coronaviruses (HCoV); the human variant is often implicated in the "common cold." Natural exposure to CRCoV appears to be widespread: a 2006 study reported that testing of serum samples from 1000 dogs in North America revealed 54.7% to be seropositive for antibodies to CRCoV (Priestnall et al. 2006). Additionally, it appears to be highly infectious, with almost 100% of dogs testing positive for antibodies three weeks after intake to a shelter with endemic CIRD, compared to 30% on the day of entry (Erles et al. 2003).

CRCoV has been called the "lawnmower virus" due to its characteristic denuding of the respiratory cilia, resulting in classic CIRD clinical signs. CRCoV has been recovered from trachea and lung samples from both affected and unaffected dogs, though it is most often recovered from the trachea of dogs with a mild cough (Erles et al. 2003). Experimental challenge studies administering CRCoV to dogs produced clinical signs consistent with an upper respiratory infection (URI), including nasal discharge, coughing and sneezing (Erles and Brownlie 2005; Mitchell et al. 2013a). In two prevalence studies of healthy and CIRD-affected dogs, CRCoV was recovered at a significantly greater frequency from dogs with clinical signs of CIRD (Schulz et al. 2014; Maboni et al. 2019). However, a study of healthy dogs entering US shelters recovered CRCoV from 1.8% of dogs (Lavan and Knesl 2015).

Currently, CRCoV is not thought to be a primary pathogen in CIRD, but to play a role in co-infections. Concurrent infection of CRCoV with *B. bronchiseptica* has been most commonly reported in the literature (Erles and Brownlie 2008; Schulz et al. 2014). At the time of this publication, there is no vaccine against CRCoV, and the product for the enteric canine coronavirus provides no cross-protection against the respiratory pathogen. There is no evidence CRCoV is zoonotic.

10.2.1.4 Canine Herpesvirus (CHV)

CHV is a varicellovirus of the subfamily *Alphaherpesviridae*; it is an enveloped DNA virus with worldwide distribution. CHV causes a systemic fatal infection in neonatal puppies. In mature dogs, CHV affects respiratory epithelium; experimentally infected dogs demonstrate conjunctivitis, rhinitis, and pharyngitis (Ford 2012; Ledbetter et al. 2012). In a 2009 case–control study, CHV was identified using PCR on conjunctival swabs more frequently in dogs with conjunctivitis (5/30) than those without the disease (0/30) (Ledbetter et al. 2012). CHV has been sequenced in lung and tracheal samples from shelter-housed dogs with respiratory disease, though more frequently in severely affected dogs with lower respiratory tract signs than in those with classic, mild CIRD (Erles and Brownlie 2005). Serologic studies of both shelter-housed and owned dogs report a relatively high prevalence of antibodies in both the United States and Europe, suggesting natural exposure is frequent and results in immune response (Erles and Brownlie 2005).

As with other herpesviruses, dogs with CHV remain latently affected and can recrudesce under stress; however, even though CHV has been recovered from coughing dogs, it is not thought to be a primary pathogen in typical cases of CIRD.

10.2.1.5 Canine Pneumovirus (CnPnV)

CnPnV is in the family *Paramyxoviridae*, subfamily *Pneumoviridae*, and genus *Pneumovirus* (Renshaw et al. 2010). It is an enveloped RNA virus closely related to murine pneumovirus (MPV), as well as human syncytial virus (hRSV) and bovine syncytial virus (bRSV). In humans, RSV is associated with significant morbidity and mortality, particularly in infants and immune-compromised adults. BRSV is more commonly known as "shipping fever" and acts in the bovine respiratory disease complex, which presents significant economic and welfare challenges for herds in cattle and dairy industries (Brodersen 2010). The parallels to shelter-housed dogs, especially with increased dog transport in the United States, are noteworthy.

CnPnV is currently considered an emerging disease and the extent of its pathogenicity is not well understood. It was first described in a 2010 study of respiratory disease in two US animal shelters when researchers were alerted to the presence of uncharacteristic cytopathic changes on PCR amplification of nasal and pharyngeal swabbed specimens from dogs with clinical signs of CIRD (Renshaw et al. 2010). A subsequent retrospective study in the United Kingdom, of tissue and serum samples, found seroprevalence rates to be 50.2% in owned and kenneled dogs (n = 314/625). In paired serum samples from kenneled dogs, seroprevalence rose from 26% at admission, to 93.5% three weeks later (n = 215), indicating expedient transmission to naïve dogs (Mitchell et al. 2013b). CnPnV seroconversion was significantly associated with the development of respiratory disease when compared to dogs that were already seropositive at admission. This suggests a vaccine for CnPnV would be efficacious as it has been for pneumovirus in other species, but a vaccine does not exist at this time. However, the significance of the pathogen in the development of respiratory disease in these dogs is still not clear because co-infections were common on examination of archived respiratory tissues. Most commonly, CRCoV and CPiV were also detected in tissues of CnPnV affected dogs (Mitchell et al. 2013b).

10.2.1.6 Canine Distemper (CDV)

CDV is a relatively large single-stranded, enveloped RNA virus of the family *Paramyxoviridae* and genus *Morbillivirus*. During natural exposures, it is transmitted by aerosolized droplets to the respiratory epithelium. Infection can be inapparent, mild, severe or fatal. Respiratory signs including conjunctivitis occur within days to weeks following exposure, followed by GI signs, and then neurologic abnormalities. CDV has a relatively long shedding period—up to 16 weeks—compared to other CIRD agents.

CDV is a disease for which vaccination is protective. Widescale use of vaccination has made it rare in many regions: the vast majority of owned dogs presenting to veterinary hospitals have protective antibody titers (as high as 97.6%) (Twark and Dodds 2000). However, unvaccinated and young dogs are highly susceptible to disease and in a study of 431 dogs entering a Florida shelter, only 64.5% had protective antibody levels for CDV (Lechner et al. 2010). Furthermore, vaccination can confound diagnosis and, in the face of many causes of respiratory and GI disease, suspicion for CDV can be delayed until neurologic signs appear, especially in regions where it is not common.

Due to all of these factors, management of CDV in a shelter involves a very different approach than other causes of CIRD: this may include protective antibody titer testing as part of a risk assessment, as well as significantly longer quarantine and isolation periods in exposed and affected dogs, respectively. Though it is often believed CDV only presents in its most severe form and is easily distinguished from CIRD, it should be considered on the differential list. Please see Chapter 11 for a comprehensive discussion of CDV in animal shelters.

10.2.1.7 Canine Influenza (CIV)

CIVs are single-stranded, enveloped RNA viruses of the *Orthomyxoviridae* family which are classified as type A, B, or C. Influenza viruses affect a vast variety of mammals and birds, with A having the broadest host range and the highest rate of mutability. Subtypes of A are specified by two surface glycoproteins—hemagglutinins (HA 1–18) and neuraminidases (NA 1–11) —and these are incorporated into nomenclature for different influenza strains. Frequent point mutations in the viral genome allow for genetic drift, contributing to influenza's impressive ability to jump species and evade vaccination strategies. CIV is not zoonotic.

Historically, dogs have been sporadically diagnosed with influenzas from other species (humans, pigs, birds) but there was no evidence of sustained transmission between dogs. In 2004, an H3N8 influenza virus closely related to an equine strain was isolated from an outbreak in racing Greyhounds (Crawford et al. 2005). This host-adapted CIV-H3N8 was subsequently implicated in multiple shelter outbreaks, confirming true canine influenza with a dog-to-dog transmission.

In 2007, a host-adapted H3N2 avian influenza strain was similarly implicated in an outbreak in dogs in South Korea (Song et al. 2008). In 2010, an outbreak in shelter cats in South Korea was also attributed to CIV-H3N2 (Song et al. 2011). In 2015, CIV-H3N2 was diagnosed in an outbreak of dogs in the Midwest region of the United States (Voorhees et al. 2017).

Clinically, CIV resembles many of the other causes of CIRD, particularly early in the course of the disease. Shedding precedes signs by up to two days, and in the case of CIV-H3N2, shedding can occur for up to 28 days. The vast majority of dogs are naïve to CIV and therefore susceptible to disease. Though a killed vaccine (KV) product exists for CIV, due to delayed onset of immunity and lack of cross-protection between strains its use is not widespread in shelters at this time. Therefore, risk factors for and management of CIV outbreaks in shelters are different than for other causes of CIRD. See Chapter 12 for a comprehensive discussion of CIV in animal shelters,

10.2.2 Bacterial Pathogens

10.2.2.1 *Bordetella bronchiseptica* (*B. bronchiseptica*)

B. bronchiseptica is a gram-negative aerobic bacterium acting as both a primary and secondary pathogen in CIRD. *B. bronchiseptica* is one of nine species of *Bordetella* —three of which cause respiratory tract disease in varying species. *B. bronchiseptica* is infectious for many other mammals, most notably cats. Cats may also act as carriers of the agent, particularly in shelters and other settings with high rates of dog exposure (Binns et al. 1999). Additionally, *B. bronchiseptica* can be found in ferrets, guinea pigs, and rabbits. Though very rare, *B. bronchiseptica* has also been shown to cause infection and disease in humans, particularly in immune-compromised individuals or those with underlying respiratory illness. Depending on the species, infection with *B. bronchiseptica* infection may lead to a subclinical carrier state or result in severe lower airway disease; please see Chapter 24 for additional information on this pathogen in species other than dogs and cats.

As a single agent, *B. bronchiseptica* primarily produces rhinitis, nasal discharge, and a paroxysmal cough. However, co-infections are common and may result in more severe, systemic signs as well as progression to lower respiratory tract disease. Once it has colonized the respiratory epithelium, chronic shedding can occur; dogs may continue to shed the bacteria for several weeks to months following recovery from clinical disease.

Research into the virulence patterns of *Bordetella spp.* have elucidated how the bacterium acts on a spectrum from commensal to highly virulent pathogen; virulence is often multiplied by the presence of a viral pathogen. In the presence of co-infections or favorable host factors, *B. bronchiseptica* causes disease by binding to receptors on ciliated epithelia, attaching to and colonizing these cells, eluding destruction by the immune system, and causing tissue injury. Additionally, they induce ciliostasis, dismantling the mucociliary apparatus which would otherwise aid in the clearance of the bacteria and mucus (Anderton et al. 2004). Finally, *B. bronchiseptica* releases exotoxins and endotoxins, which lead to further direct cell injury (Ford 2012).

B. bronchiseptica can be isolated from the upper respiratory tract of normal dogs at a relatively high rate. One study recovered *B. bronchiseptica* in 19.5% of samples from healthy dogs entering US animal shelters (Lavan and Knesl 2015). Another study recovered high rates of *B. bronchiseptica* from both CIRD-affected and healthy dogs (78.7 and 45.6%, respectively) (Schulz et al. 2014). Given the high prevalence of *B. bronchiseptica* recovered from healthy dogs, it is sometimes difficult to interpret its impact as a pathogen, though its interference with ciliostasis likely makes it a significant co-factor as well as a primary pathogen.

10.2.2.2 *Mycoplasma* Spp.

Mycoplasma is a genus of bacteria lacking a cell wall. Because they are fastidious organisms requiring complex growth media in order to be cultured, mycoplasmas likely have been under-recognized historically. Newer molecular diagnostics employing PCR testing have contributed to greater recognition of the organism's presence in dogs but have not elucidated its role.

M. cynos is transmitted via droplets from nasal and ocular secretions, as well as saliva (Chalker 2005; Priestnall et al. 2014). They colonize both upper and lower respiratory epithelium, but this colonization does not always result in clinical signs. *M. cynos* has demonstrated sialidase activity, a virulence factor that enables adherence to epithelial cell surfaces and results in direct cytotoxic effects on host cells (May and Brown 2009). Natural and experimentally induced infections produce purulent bronchitis and can lead to interstitial pneumonia (Rosendal and Vinther 1977). Antibody titers to *M. cynos* in dogs occur within three weeks of exposure, corresponding to a decrease in clinical signs and an ability to recover the organism from affected dogs (Chalker 2005; Rycroft et al. 2007).

Several species of *Mycoplasma* have been recovered from the respiratory tracts of both healthy and CIRD-affected dogs, including *M. cynos and M. canis. M. cynos* is frequently identified in CIRD outbreaks, often in combination with other agents. A study of samples submitted to a veterinary diagnostic laboratory found *M. cynos* to be one of the most prevalent pathogens, identified in nearly 25% of all samples. *M. cynos* was more frequently identified in symptomatic dogs and there was a significant association between its presence and moderate or severe clinical signs. The same study also found a significant association between the severity of clinical signs and the presence of *M. canis*, which had not previously been found to be significantly associated with respiratory disease. Both species were reported in this study to be common co-infections with other agents, particularly with CPiV (Maboni et al. 2019).

There is also a high prevalence of *M. cynos* recovered from clinically healthy dogs: one study recovered *M. cynos* from 29.2% of asymptomatic dogs entering US shelters (Lavan and Knesl 2015). The clinical significance of this pathogen in a case or an outbreak of CIRD can be difficult to interpret and needs to be considered in light of other diagnostic findings.

10.2.2.3 *Streptococcus equi Subsp. zooepidemicus (Strep. zoo)*

S. equi subsp zooepidemicus is a beta-hemolytic Lancefield group C bacterium that is a commensal organism of horses associated with upper respiratory disease and lower genital tract infections. In addition to dogs, *Strep. zoo* has been reported in cows, pigs, monkeys, seals, llamas, and humans, as well as implicated in outbreaks of respiratory disease in cats (Blum et al. 2010; Priestnall et al. 2014). *Strep. zoo* is distinct from group G bacteria such as *Streptococcus canis* more commonly considered commensal in dogs and implicated in chronic upper respiratory infections in cats

(Pesavento and Murphy 2014). It is also distinct from *Strep. equi.* ssp. *equi* which causes strangles in horses (Greene and Prescott 2012).

Current thinking is that *Strep. zoo* can act as a primary pathogen in dogs. Both mild and chronic upper respiratory infections in dogs have been infrequently attributed to *Strep. zoo.* In densely-housed kenneled dogs, however, *Strep. zoo* has been implicated in outbreaks of acute, hemorrhagic, fibrinosuppurative pneumonia followed by sudden death (Kim et al. 2007; Pesavento et al. 2008; Byun et al. 2009). Early signs may be non-specific, including mild respiratory signs. However, the disease progresses rapidly to include depression, anorexia and fever, and then epistaxis, hematemesis, dyspnea, and death over the course of 24–48 hours. Exotoxins such as those identified in "toxic shock" streptococcal-associated syndromes in humans are thought to be responsible for its rapid destruction of pulmonary vasculature and subsequent fibrin leakage, edema and hemorrhage (Priestnall et al. 2014).

Though a laboratory challenge study failed to produce clinical disease in healthy dogs inoculated with *Strep. zoo* as a solo agent, there have been outbreaks of *Strep. zoo* in shelters in which no additional agents were identified (Pesavento et al. 2008; Larson et al. 2011). Treatment for *Strep. zoo* alone has successfully controlled transmission in shelter outbreaks (Kim et al. 2007).

This observed variation in virulence of the pathogen may be due to the clonal nature of *Strep. zoo.* At least one outbreak has been due to transmission of a single, highly virulent clone between dogs in the presence of environmental conditions favoring pathogen proliferation and transmission (e.g. densely-housed dogs, wet environment) (Pesavento et al. 2008). Co-morbidities are likely to contribute to its virulence in certain settings, and co-infections with other viral and bacterial agents have been reported (Priestnall et al. 2010).

Strep. zoo has also been recovered from clinically healthy dogs, though the prevalence was less than 2% in multiple studies (Acke et al. 2015; Lavan and Knesl 2015). The presence of *Strep. zoo* in healthy dogs supports there may be an aclinical carrier state that does not result in disease (Chalker et al. 2003; Acke et al. 2015; Lavan and Knesl 2015).

The reservoir host for *Strep. zoo* is the horse, with presumed transmission from horses to all other affected species, including humans and dogs. There is one report of transmission of *Strep. zoo* from a dog to a human handler, confirmed by molecular sequencing (Abbott et al. 2010). Based on this case, protective equipment including clothing, gloves, safety glasses, and masks are advised when handling *Strep. zoo* suspects.

10.2.2.4 Additional Bacterial Agents

Other bacterial pathogens commonly isolated from the respiratory tracts of dogs with signs of CIRD include *Pasturella* spp., *Pseudomonas* spp., *Staphylococcus* spp., *Streptococcus* spp., and coliforms. These are all interpreted to be opportunistic infections by commensal organisms, though in densely housed, compromised populations they may act as primary pathogens (Priestnall et al. 2014; Lappin et al. 2017; Sykes 2017).

10.3 Prevalence

CIRD is generally associated with low mortality, as the disease is primarily limited to the upper respiratory tract and self-limiting. However, in a shelter environment morbidity can be high, especially if preventive measures are not in place: these include timely vaccination, population monitoring, capacity for care management, and biosecurity. All breeds of dogs are susceptible to CIRD, though young animals and immune-compromised animals are more at risk. Dogs with additional risk factors include unvaccinated and under-vaccinated dogs and dogs that come into contact with many other dogs (i.e. in shelters, dog parks, daycare centers, boarding kennels, and veterinary hospitals). Shelter-specific risk factors for the development of respiratory disease include crowding, inefficient population management, prolonged length of stay (LOS), inadequate isolation of affected animals, poor air quality, inadequate housing, and lack of preventive care, both medical and behavioral (Holt et al. 2010). Environmental and population management factors play a significant role in the incidence of CIRD in populations.

While shelters are encouraged to track the frequency of common medical conditions as a means of assessing welfare and to measure the effectiveness of preventive medicine protocols, this is not commonly reported and no collective data exists on the occurrence of CIRD in US shelters. Shelters are encouraged to use their shelter software programs to monitor population-level statistics for CIRD in their shelter over time and as a means to measure the efficacy of control measures and alterations to practices and facilities (Scarlett et al. 2017).

10.4 Diagnosis

Clinical diagnosis of CIRD is based on clinical signs, a history of recent exposure, and response to therapy. In the animal shelter, where populations are transient and histories are often unavailable, a presumptive diagnosis of CIRD is most commonly based on clinical signs: a "honking" or paroxysmal cough, recurrent sneezing, and either serous, mucoid or mucopurulent nasal discharge with or without ocular discharge and conjunctivitis. The terminal retch and production of phlegm associated with coughing in dogs can be confused with vomiting, particularly if respiratory secretions are found in the dog's enclosure and the cough is not observed. Mild pyrexia may be present, sometimes accompanied by inappetence thought to be related to decreased olfaction as well as overall malaise (Ellis and Krakowka 2012). Classically, observation of a cough or elicitation of cough on tracheal palpation has been used to diagnose a case of CIRD. Mild cases of CIRD generally lack systemic signs such as marked pyrexia, anorexia, depression, or lethargy and are self-limiting over the course of approximately 10–14 days.

Routine hematology and biochemistry profiles are not diagnostic for CIRD, though they can help determine the underlying health status of an individual dog. The presence of a stress leukogram characterized by mild neutrophilia, lymphopenia and eosinopenia may be present in some cases of CIRD. However, a more severe inflammatory leukogram with accompanying fever is more indicative of lower respiratory disease with bacterial pneumonia (Ford 2012). Additional diagnostics for individual dogs with more severe signs can include thoracic radiographs, as well as sedated sterile endotracheal or bronchoalveolar lavage tracheal washes followed by cytology and culture. In some regions, fungal and parasitic organisms are additional causes of pneumonia.

Knowing the etiologic agent(s) present in an individual CIRD case may not affect the treatment course for that individual. However, testing may be useful if the animal is experiencing an unusual course of the disease or prolonged recovery, or as part of a risk assessment to expedite placement (e.g. adoption, foster care). For populations, diagnostic testing aids in confronting unusual infections either more severe or more widespread than respiratory disease typically seen in the facility, when multiple species (including humans) are affected, or when a novel agent is suspected. The severity of clinical signs observed in an individual animal does not necessarily correlate with the potential severity of the pathogen.

The most appropriate and timely testing modality for identifying pathogens in CIRD cases is PCR of nasal, conjunctival, and/or oropharyngeal swabs. For respiratory disease, PCR testing is best done within one to two days of the onset of clinical signs; blood samples for serology should be drawn at the same time whenever possible in the event paired samples are desired at a later date.

PCR may be followed by culture, virus isolation, or additional sequencing to distinguish more information about an agent. *B. bronchiseptica* is experiencing an increase in multi-drug-resistant (MDR) strains, and so culture and sensitivity can help target anti-microbial therapy (Sykes 2017). Culture is also a helpful sequela when *Strep. zoo* has been identified. Virus isolation is useful to confirm the presence of live virus, and additional sequencing can provide further information regarding variant and virulence. If a patient has shown CIRD signs for more than five to seven days, PCR becomes less useful and serology is likely indicated, as some inciting agents such as CIV-H3N8 may no longer be present.

Instructions for the collection and submission of PCR samples vary per laboratory, so veterinarians are advised to check with their diagnostic facility before sample collection. Standard instructions are to use 6-inch plastic-handled polyester-tipped sterile swabs and empty sterile red top tubes. Some labs request dry swabs only, while others prefer 0.5–1 ml of sterile saline or viral media added to tubes; when in doubt, it is useful to provide both dry and moistened swabs. For oropharyngeal swabs, good restraint is required and clean gloves should be worn and changed between patients. The head should be tipped back and the mouth opened widely, while the investigator cleanly and vigorously swabs the deep, oropharyngeal area. The swab should be placed in the sterile red top tube, and the handle broken off. The tube should be capped sterilely. For nasal swabs, a similar process is followed except that the swab is passed deeply into the nasal passages and spun to remove epithelial cells; this is less tolerated by many patients as it causes irritation and sometimes bleeding. For CDV, conjunctival swabs of the inside of the eyelid are also requested. Swabs should be held under refrigeration or shipped on ice packs overnight. Many diagnostic labs have smaller-sized swabs and other specialized diagnostic supplies helpful in collecting effective samples in smaller dogs.

Interpretation of molecular test results can be challenging. PCR is a highly sensitive testing modality. A positive result is based on the amplification of minute amounts of nucleic acids from a pathogen and indicates the presence of the organism but does not necessarily confirm it to be the cause of clinical signs; quantitative PCR, when available, can help make the distinction by estimating pathogen load. Additionally, as previously mentioned, many organisms implicated in CIRD have been recovered from healthy dogs, most notably *M. cynos* and *B. bronchiseptica*; it can be difficult to judge when a positive result for these agents is clinically significant.

Positive PCR results must also be interpreted in light of vaccination history, particularly if modified-live vaccines were administered within four weeks prior to testing. Many respiratory pathogens are included in standard intake vaccination protocols and IN respiratory vaccinations (*B. bronchiseptica* + CPiV ±CAV-2) will result in positive PCR results for these pathogens; parenteral products are likely less to do so, at least from pharyngeal and oral swabs (Ruch-Gallie et al. 2016). Quantitative PCR (qPCR), when available, can be useful in distinguishing between wild-type and vaccine virus, though the distinction is not clear in every case. Inaccurate positive results can result from contamination of the sample either at the point of collection or the point of testing. Positive PCR results should be interpreted as a part of the larger picture of clinical history, clinical signs, disease progression, and risk factors for the population.

Negative results on PCR indicate that the pathogen was not detected; however, these results can be falsely negative due to sampling or handling errors, variant strains, an undetectable level of organism on the swab, or sample degradation (particularly relevant for RNA viruses). For bacterial agents, recent administration of antibiotics may also impact results.

An outbreak of CIRD without clear etiology warrants representative PCR testing in a population. Shelter veterinarians are frequently asked how many dogs should be tested when confronted with a CIRD outbreak. In a traditional approach to production animal disease diagnosis, sample-size calculations to detect disease in populations depend on herd size, the minimum expected prevalence of a disease (if it is present), and the level of confidence for detecting that disease. Both affected and unaffected animals are tested and large sample sizes are needed to diagnose agents with low prevalence. Applying this approach in a shelter is more of an academic exercise as it would require relatively expensive testing of high numbers of both healthy and sick dogs and would not necessarily be as helpful in a transient multi-source population. Therefore, CIRD investigations commonly target diagnostic testing on small representative groups of affected dogs followed by careful interpretation of results that takes into consideration clinical history, the biological behavior of agents, risk factors (i.e. prevalence and signalment), and test accuracy (i.e. sensitivity and specificity).

In the case of an outbreak or a high level of endemic disease, shelters are advised to test, at a minimum, 10–30% of the population, or at least 5–10 dogs (Hurley 2012). Larger sample sizes are likely to be more informative on a population level. It is best to test acutely ill dogs since some agents (such as CIV-H3N8) have short shedding periods.

Diagnostic interpretation of CIRD PCR testing may be helped by known prevalence data for agents recovered using PCR testing methods. See Table 10.2. For example, results revealing a high prevalence of a rare pathogen in the test population, such as 25% with *Strep. zoo* or CRCoV or CPiV, suggest a more meaningful association between agents and the disease in question. On the other hand, recovery of *B. bronchiseptica* or *M. cynos* from 20 to 30% of the test population may be unremarkable given the high prevalence of these agents in studies of healthy dogs. Recovering more than one agent can be informative since many of the agents are symbiotic in their pathogenesis.

For emerging pathogens such as CIV, any single positive test in a previously naïve population is likely significant (though false positives occur rarely so single positive tests without clinical support should be questioned). It is also important to note that it is only through submission of samples that previously unrecognized agents have been discovered, and shelters play an important sentinel role in identifying emerging companion animal diseases.

In the event of CIRD-related deaths, a necropsy should be performed and oropharyngeal swabs and fresh respiratory tissues submitted for histopathology, virus isolation, and bacterial culture and sensitivity. Care should be taken to collect samples for culture early in the necropsy procedures using sterile technique to avoid contaminating the samples.

Many diagnostic laboratories as well as academic and large non-profit shelter medicine programs offer consultation on diagnostic testing and interpretation; shelter veterinarians are encouraged to reach out for assistance with diagnostic testing procedures and interpretation as recommendations can change as modalities evolve.

10.5 Prevention and Control

Pathogens traditionally associated with CIRD are most commonly spread in aerosolized droplets from coughing and sneezing and through contact with fomites such as hands, clothing, and cleaning tools. Control methods for CIRD include solid husbandry and biosecurity principles along with timely vaccination. Given the majority of shelters do not have "true isolation" as represented by a separate building or even separate entrance for CIRD patients, vaccination at intake provides one important line of defense for incoming animals in the face of a population with potential disease. However, given that vaccination for most CIRD agents only reduces signs and severity, rather than protecting against disease, its efficacy is limited in the shelter environment.

Environmental design, housing, and husbandry are key factors in how animals fare in shelters in the face of disease; recent research around stress and housing in kenneled dogs indicates they benefit from more humane design and enrichment than traditional long runs of single-compartment kennels can offer. Population management in animal shelters must balance the challenges of admitting transient populations of dogs with widely varying vaccination histories, secondary medical conditions, and ongoing physiologic stressors with environmental and behavioral health and welfare. The modern shelter is generally best served by minimizing the use of quarantine procedures and other traditional management models that prolong the LOS of healthy animals in the animal shelter. Instead, active population management strategies to minimize the time dogs spend in shelters, coupled with enriched and supportive environments and active surveillance, are the most effective means to reduce CIRD in shelters.

10.5.1 Housing

Double-compartment housing units with guillotine doors provide many benefits for kenneled dogs: efficient cleaning without exposing dogs to water or chemicals; minimal handling and intermingling of dogs during cleaning and daily care; and increased safety for staff, especially if dogs are aggressive. This design is critical for dogs with infectious disease and has additional behavioral benefits for all dogs.

Dogs in double-sided kennels have demonstrated they will preferentially use both sides of the enclosure and segregate their elimination functions from resting and eating areas when both compartments are available to them. In a study of kenneled beagles in four different laboratories, dogs were found to frequently use indoor resting areas and elevated beds, as well as to demonstrate preferential use of outside runs for defecation (Döring et al. 2016). A shelter-based study of dogs housed in indoor double-compartment runs also demonstrated they will preferentially urinate and defecate in the compartment not used for bed, food, and water (Wagner et al. 2014). Double-compartment housing is advised in shelters as a best practice for medical and behavioral welfare, especially in areas with prolonged lengths of stay such as isolation wards for CIRD-affected dogs.

Housing design can also aid in preventing CIRD outbreaks. Shelter intakes generally involve a steady stream of unrelated animals. When possible, facilities designed with smaller housing wards of six to eight double-compartment enclosures allow for cohort-grouping of dogs that aids in disease and risk management, deep cleaning between cohorts, and flexible usage dependent on current needs. Smaller wards also greatly reduce noise levels from barking and provide increased opportunities for in-kennel enrichment and training opportunities; these conditions result in better cage presentation and overall behavioral health (Coppola et al. 2006; Luescher and Medlock 2009). Shelters that group-house dogs are advised to avoid arbitrarily mixing dogs from a myriad of sources or with varying risk factors for CIRD (e.g. age, vaccination status, co-morbidities, etc.). Segregation by risk factors, including potential disease exposure or community of origin, is considered a better practice.

Enclosure construction and materials are also important for controlling disease transmission and pathogen load in the environment. Solid barriers are advised between dogs for both medical and behavioral reasons. Enclosure surfaces and materials should be in good repair and easily cleaned, disinfected and dried. Concrete surfaces should be sealed, not painted. Floors should slope toward drains for cleaning and drying purposes. Shelters are discouraged from using high-pressure hoses or power sprayers for cleaning kennels, as they aerosolize pathogens and contribute to high humidity.

10.5.2 Air Quality

CIRD pathogens are primarily spread through aerosolized droplets. Therefore, ventilation, humidity, temperature, and air handling are important considerations in controlling CIRD transmission in an animal shelter. Heating, ventilation, and air conditioning (HVAC) systems should de-couple temperature control measures from ventilation. Humidity also varies significantly by region and season, for which HVAC systems should compensate. Separately zoned HVAC systems are ideal for preventing cross-circulation between isolation and healthy housing areas; theoretically, systems that share air between areas could allow for the circulation of pathogens from sick animals to healthy populations. However, the implications of shared HVAC are likely not as important as other mechanisms that allow for maintenance of the pathogens in the environment—namely crowding, poor quality enclosures, excessive moisture, poor sanitation and other environmental factors.

Ideally, animal housing spaces are advised to have 10–12 air changes per hour with 100% outdoor air for optimal air quality and prevention of disease (Schlaffer and Bonacci 2013). This demand is significantly higher and more costly than in human housing areas. Maintaining adequate air quality also encompasses minimizing moisture and the accumulation of waste materials and gases, along with the provision of fresh air. While zoning restrictions and aspects of the architectural design may at times impact the use of outdoor spaces for shelters, increased access to the outdoors and fresh air is thought to be of benefit to most dogs in temperate seasons. This can be accomplished through the use of indoor/outdoor runs as well as time in outdoor play yards and on walks. As much as possible, outdoor spaces should be segregated similarly to indoor spaces: ideally separate play yards and traffic patterns will exist for healthy dogs, CIRD-affected dogs, new intakes, and puppies. See Chapter 2 for more information.

10.5.3 Population Management and Capacity for Care

Shelters in the United States have evolved in the last few decades to minimize euthanasia as a means of population control, leading to longer-term stays. Managing population density is essential to any shelter preventive medicine program. Crowding is a profound risk factor for CIRD. Daily animal inventory is a product of intake numbers and length of stay (LOS) for each dog. As LOS increases in a shelter, the risk of CIRD increases (Edinboro et al. 2004; Holt et al. 2010).

Capacity for care management for shelters is a proactive system of preventing crowding in shelters: this is accomplished by managing intake, planning efficient pathways to humane outcomes, and providing preventive care (Karsten et al. 2017). Managed intake includes scheduling dogs as space allows and providing alternatives to relinquishment. Shelters are encouraged to utilize services to prevent relinquishment to shelters as often as they can: spay/neuter, behavior training, pet food pantries, or referrals to other services can keep pets in homes; these services benefit not only individual pets, but the population of pets in the shelter. A lower daily inventory of dogs contributes to shorter LOS overall, as well as decreased pathogen loads and lower rates of disease.

LOS can also be greatly reduced by effective pathway planning for dogs through the facility, starting at intake. Shelters should incorporate methods with demonstrated success in minimizing LOS: examples include daily rounds, fast-tracking of healthy adoptable dogs, open viewing and selection of dogs while on holds, and addressing bottlenecks in the system that increase hold times (e.g. surgery or behavior assessments) by providing staff time and resources to perform necessary services efficiently.

10.5.4 Behavioral Enrichment

Balancing biosecurity with behavioral enrichment, including interactions with people and conspecifics, is important for shelter animal welfare. Research indicates dogs entering shelters have a spike in cortisol levels at intake which decreases to original, at-home levels over three to five days (on average). Correlation between cortisol levels and behavioral indicators of stress has not been found to be reliably consistent so interpreting welfare from cortisol levels or other physiologic parameters is complex (Protopopova 2016). However, inferring welfare status from behavioral indicators is an essential part of animal welfare science and crucial to ensuring the Five Freedoms. See Chapter 2 for more information about the Five Freedoms. In humans and mice, chronic stress has been demonstrated to impair immune function and increase susceptibility to infection (Frank and Griffin 1989; Glaser and Kiecolt-Glaser 2005).

It is widely believed that dogs in shelters benefit from environmental and behavioral enrichment, and this contributes to their overall state of well-being and good health, as well as adoptability. Activities can include enrichment activities within enclosures, training opportunities, exercise, food puzzles, toys, positive interactions with conspecifics, and sensory stimulation through olfactory and visual cues. Performing behavioral preference assessments and then using preferred items in dog introductions to adopters has been shown to increase adoption success (Protopopova et al. 2016). Similarly, displaying more desirable in-kennel behaviors on the adoption floor has been demonstrated to decrease LOS for shelter dogs (Protopopova et al. 2014). Enrichment activities and preference provisions should be employed for all dogs, including those affected by CIRD; managing this means identifying staff and methods for providing enrichment without compromising biosecurity or exposing healthy dogs to disease.

One shelter-based study aimed to investigate associations between behavioral indicators of stress and the development of CIRD. The study struggled with numerous confounding factors, including a high rate of disease across the population, a very low rate of vaccination for CIRD (13% of dogs), overall poor husbandry, poor sanitation, and random co-mingling of dogs. Only 19% of dogs completed the study, with 83% of the study dogs euthanized. Not surprisingly, time in shelter was a risk factor for CIRD and behavioral indicators of stress were common; however, due to numerous confounding variables, associations between behavioral markers of stress and CIRD were unable to be elucidated. After the study, steps were taken to improve welfare in that shelter, including improved compliance with recommendations for intake vaccinations, medical care, and improved sanitation. (Protopopova et al. 2019).

Interaction with conspecifics is also desirable for many shelter dogs. Playgroups are one way to enrich dogs' lives in shelters, especially those with longer stays and high energy levels. Though research is lacking at this point on their efficacy, anecdotally, many shelters report great success in improving outcomes and welfare of shelter dogs with well-executed playgroups. Resources for utilizing playgroups include on-site training opportunities, conferences, and on-line materials (Sadler n.d.; Center for Shelter Dogs n.d.). Specific to CIRD, playgroups have the added advantage of getting dogs outside and exposing them to fresh air for scheduled periods of time. Playgroups have also been used for cohorts of dogs mildly affected with CIRD; this will be discussed as well in the treatment section. See Chapter 2 for additional information.

10.5.5 Surveillance

Many dogs carry pathogens potentially associated with CIRD, but shedding is increased in conjunction with clinical signs. Monitoring and prompt isolation of clinically affected dogs is key to lowering environmental load and transmission from affected to unaffected dogs. In a shelter population, daily monitoring and frequent visual inspection of animals are crucial for controlling disease. Daily population rounds capture and communicate important developments in the status of individual animals and can be an important aspect of early recognition. Staff trained to recognize early signs of disease alert medical staff to the need to assess and isolate animals displaying signs of respiratory disease. Standing protocols written by a veterinarian with direct knowledge of the shelter and the population should specify isolation, testing, and treatment procedures in order to avoid delays in addressing suspect cases. The frequency of CIRD cases in the shelter should be tracked, a process made easier by shelter software systems that allow for the capture of the disease by individual animal conditions and then for the generation of population-level reports (Scarlett et al. 2017). Recognizing a high or increasing cumulative incidence of disease may be the first step prompting the analysis of CIRD-related risk factors and the need to improve practices.

10.5.6 Quarantine Recommendations

Shelter medicine practitioners strive to minimize the LOS for each animal entering the animal shelter. For CIRD this is a key consideration, as studies have shown LOS in the shelter to be the single greatest risk factor for infection and clinical disease (Edinboro et al. 2004; Holt et al. 2010). Therefore, healthy animals without known exposure to, or clinical signs of, infectious disease are not placed routinely under quarantine in shelters.

However, there are some cases when quarantine of certain animals or distinct populations is advised in the shelter. The most obvious of these include animals with a history of recent exposure to CIRD or susceptible dogs relocated from facilities or areas identified as high risk for more serious pathogens such as CIV or CDV. Incubation periods for the most common CIRD pathogens are 3–10 days; a minimum 14-day quarantine is indicated for cases at high risk for CDV (some strains can take up to six weeks to result in clinical signs but quarantine of that length is seldom possible or advised in the shelter. See Chapter 11 for more information on CDV). In shelters at high risk for overcrowding and compromised care due to poor housing and other environmental factors, "open selection" protocols that allow dogs in quarantine to still be seen by the public for adoption while mitigating the risk of disease transmission can be life-saving.

10.5.7 Isolation Recommendations

Any dogs demonstrating clinical signs of CIRD should immediately be moved to a separate isolation area or facility, ideally with its own HVAC and high-quality double-sided enclosures (for more information on isolation housing design, see sections 10.5.1 on housing and 10.6.3 on environmental enrichment during treatment). Shelter staff should be trained to recognize even mild clinical signs and empowered to move suspected cases to isolation without delay. A timely examination by a trained medical staff member or veterinarian to confirm a diagnosis and assess the need for treatment is critical to maintaining both individual and population health and welfare. In the absence of a veterinarian on-site, a standing protocol written by a veterinarian detailing clinical signs of disease and a standard treatment protocol may be employed in most shelters unless the law specifically prohibits such action (Newbury et al. 2010; AVMA 2019).

Because shedding periods of pathogens associated with CIRD vary from weeks to months, some caution should be exercised introducing recently recovered dogs into susceptible populations. Most viral components—including CPiV and CAV-2 and CIV H3N8—have relatively short shedding periods of less than two weeks; CDV and CIV H3N2 are notable exceptions. Bacterial agents such as *B. bronchiseptica* and *Mycoplasma* continue to be recovered from dogs for weeks to months following infection and are actually recovered at a fairly high rate from healthy dogs (Lavan and Knesl 2015). Because *Strep. zoo* outbreaks have been infrequent, shedding periods are not entirely understood, though treatment appears to clear the infection in treated dogs (Greene and Prescott 2012).

Though some organisms can be recovered from recovered dogs for prolonged periods, this does not imply that dogs should be isolated for extended periods of time (CDV and CIV-H3N2 are exceptions to this rule; see Chapters 11 and 12). Decisions regarding releasing recovered dogs from isolation should be based on the resolution of clinical signs and, when testing has been performed, what is known about shedding periods and severity of particular agents in combination with a risk assessment regarding where dogs will be housed upon release. For example, given that transmission of the most common CIRD agents is primarily through aerosolized droplets, recovered dogs no longer coughing are much less likely to be infectious to other dogs as long as direct contact and fomite transmission are managed. Likewise, for agents such as CIV-H3N8 coughing may persist beyond the seven-day shedding period.

In typical cases of CIRD, dogs that have shown clinical improvement can be released after 7–10 days of isolation/treatment, and potentially earlier if they have had resolution of clinical disease or have managed-risk housing options.

Shelters are encouraged to strategize methods for minimizing LOS in isolation while also minimizing the risk of exposing healthy dogs. An example of this may include "open selection" adoption policies that allow adopters to view and apply for dogs in isolation housing. In these cases, shelters may even elect to release dogs from isolation to adoption (or foster care) while under treatment, with care instructions and full-disclosure about the disease. Another approach is to create designated pathways and wards for recovered dogs within adoption housing to minimize interactions between recovered dogs and healthy and incoming dogs. These creative examples aren't appropriate for every shelter, but for mild cases of CIRD and challenged or crowded shelter environments, adoption or foster care may offer significant improvements in environmental conditions and husbandry and result in faster resolution of signs. This should always be done with full-disclosure and recommendations to prevent the spread of disease in household pets or the community (see section 10.7 on implications for foster care and adoption).

10.5.8 Vaccination

An understanding of the immunologic mechanisms of the respiratory system is important to understanding the efficacy of particular products and the challenges of protecting shelter-housed dogs against CIRD. The viral and bacterial pathogens associated with CIRD primarily infect dogs through the mucosa of the respiratory epithelium. Protection is provided by two branches of the immune system: innate immunity which is composed of physical barriers such as epithelial tight junctions and the mucociliary apparatus, and adaptive immunity which is the antigen-specific branch of the immune system enacted by B and T lymphocytes. Innate immune responses are non-specific and require no prior exposure to a pathogen. In contrast, adaptive immunity involves a systemic response to a specific antigen, employing immunoglobulins (IgA, IgG, IgM) at various levels of the respiratory system (Tizard 2012).

For mucosal infections, intact respiratory barriers and serum IgA concentrations in nasal secretions are more critical than serum IgG or IgM antibody responses; the innate immunity provides the critical first line of defense (Mitchell and Brownlie 2015). Vaccination protocols that activate both the innate and adaptive pathways are likely more capable of preventing the onset and progression of disease, especially in the acute challenge posed upon entry into an animal shelter. Additionally, environmental controls that protect the health of the respiratory epithelium through air quality and reduction of irritants play a role in the resistance posed by the innate immune response to infection.

Vaccination is available for many of the agents implicated in CIRD: CDV, CPiV, CAV-2, CIV (H3N8 and H3N2) and *B. bronchiseptica*. See Table 10.3. Standard core vaccinations in the United States commonly referred to as "canine distemper" vaccinations (DHPP or DA_2PP) include respiratory agents CDV, CAV-2, and CPiV (as well as canine parvovirus, CPV). Intranasal (IN) "kennel cough" vaccinations may only include *B. bronchiseptica,* but a bivalent product (*B. bronchiseptica* and CPiV) and trivalent product (*B. bronchiseptica*, CPiV and CAV-2) are available. Additionally, a parenteral as well as an oral vaccine product exists for *B. bronchiseptica* as a solo agent. Of all the respiratory pathogens described here, CDV vaccination is the only one to induce a sterilizing immunity; vaccinations for all other CIRD agents do not prevent colonization, shedding of organisms, and clinical signs of disease in vaccinated dogs. However, vaccination against CIRD agents reduces infection rates, duration of shedding, and severity of signs.

For most respiratory pathogens, vaccines delivered to the mucosal surfaces have been demonstrated to have greater efficacy and faster onset of immunity than parenteral products, which is particularly relevant for dogs at imminent and acute risk of exposure in group settings like shelters, boarding kennels, and dogs shows. The exception to this rule is CAV-2, for which the parenteral vaccination results in prolonged immunity. Vaccines for CAV-2 and CPiV include the combination modified live parenteral product containing CDV and CPV considered core. In the case of CAV-2, the adenovirus component is included primarily to protect against the more severe effects of canine infectious hepatitis (CAV-1); however, the vaccine also protects against the respiratory pathogen CAV-2.

For CPiV, the level of protection induced by parenteral administration in the core vaccine is not as strong as IN administration; therefore, in shelters, IN vaccination products containing CPiV are recommended in addition to the parenteral CPiV vaccine (Ellis and Krakowka 2012; Ford et al. 2017).

Furthermore, at least two studies indicate IN vaccination for *B. bronchiseptica* is superior to parenteral administration. In one challenge study, dogs vaccinated with IN *B. bronchiseptica* had significantly lower cough scores and shed significantly fewer challenge organisms than dogs administered parenteral vaccination or controls (Davis et al. 2007). In a 2013 study comparing the efficacy of IN, oral, and parenteral vaccinations for *B. bronchiseptica*, the IN and oral groups scored significantly lower in the experience of clinical signs after challenge with the pathogen than those receiving the parenteral product or a placebo (Larson et al. 2013).

The combination of mucosal and parenteral vaccination, otherwise known as the "heterologous prime/boost" approach to immunization, is an area of emerging research in human medicine and is thought to provide better clinical response than either route alone (Ellis and Krakowka 2012; Ellis 2015). This is supported by both experimental and field trials demonstrating a significant reduction in clinical signs of CIRD in response to the use of the *combination* of both IN and parenteral products for CPiV (Ellis and Krakowka 2012). Likewise, in a 2001 study of *B. bronchiseptica* vaccination, administration of both parenteral and IN *B. bronchiseptica* vaccines to specific pathogen-free puppies was more effective at reducing clinical signs of infection than either vaccination alone (Ellis et al. 2001).

In shelters, IN vaccines containing *B. bronchiseptica* and CPiV (with or without CAV-2) are generally preferred, in addition to parenteral delivery of CPiV and CAV-2 in the core DHPP or DA_2PP vaccine. This is consistent with recommendations of the World Small Animal Veterinary Association (WSAVA) and the American Animal Hospital Association (AAHA) regarding vaccination of shelter-housed dogs, though both guidelines consider the parenteral CPiV optional (Day et al. 2016; Ford et al. 2017).

Table 10.3 Vaccination recommendations for CIRD in shelter-housed dogs.

Vaccine information	Route of Administration	Shelter Protocol	Comments
Recommended			
CAV-2 (MLV) CPiV (MLV) CDV (MLV, rCDV) plus CPV (MLV)	Subcutaneous	• On or prior to admission • As early as 4 weeks of age, and repeated every 2–3 weeks until 18–20 weeks of age	• Reconstituted vaccines should be discarded after one hour • Usually administered as DHPP or DA_2PP
B. bronchiseptica (avirulent live) plus CPiV (MLV)	Intranasal	• On or prior to admission • As early as 3 weeks of age. • Single dose per label • Two doses, 2–4 weeks apart are recommended by some guidelines. • Repeat annually	• Provides fast onset to immunity; 48–72 h for *B. bronchiseptica* • Maternally derived antibodies do not interfere with mucosal immunity • DO NOT administer orally or parenterally (see text)
B. bronchiseptica plus CPiV and CAV-2	Intranasal	• Same as Bb plus CPiV	• Same as Bb plus CPiV above • Parenteral adenovirus vaccine preferred for CAV-1 protection and is protective for CAV-2, so the CAV-2 component may not be necessary
Alternative products			
B. bronchiseptica (avirulent live)	Intranasal Oral	• Same as Bb plus CPiV	• Use of intranasal product + CPiV is preferred to the parenteral or oral product • Duration of immunity for oral is not known
B. bronchiseptica (cellular antigen abstract)	Subcutaneous	• Two initial doses, 2–4 weeks apart	• Recommended only when intranasal or oral is not possible • May be used in combination with intranasal product in high-risk populations
CIV-H3N8 (killed) CIV-H3N2 (killed)	Subcutaneous	• Two initial doses, 2–4 weeks apart • As early as 6 weeks of age	• Use in shelters based on risk assessment of population • Not cross-protective • See Chapter 12 for a broad discussion

Sources: Ford et al. (2017); Day et al. (2016).

At least two challenge studies have demonstrated that the duration of immunity after a single IN dose of vaccine is 12–13 months for *B. bronchiseptica* and CPiV (Jacobs et al. 2005; Lehr et al. 2008). Duration of immunity for parenteral CAV-2 has been demonstrated to be at least four years (Abdelmagid et al. 2004).

Vaccines are not currently available for CHV, CRCoV, CnPnV, *Strep. zoo.* and *Mycoplasma* spp. The vaccine for canine GI coronavirus does not offer cross-protection for CRCoV.

10.5.8.1 Vaccine Safety and Efficacy

Shelters should have standard protocols written by a veterinarian for monitoring, recognition, and treatment of vaccine reactions. Shelter staff administering vaccinations should be well-trained in the handling and administration of vaccine products, as well as in monitoring for signs of adverse events.

Vaccine safety has been of increasing concern in human and veterinary medicine. In private practice, triennial vaccination protocols for dogs and cats have become common in response to research demonstrating a prolonged duration of immunity for many agents. However, in animal shelters, vaccination for common infectious disease agents, including CIRD pathogens, is recommended for all animals at intake due to often unknown or unreliable vaccine histories and increased risk of exposure in the shelter setting. The most common adverse events to vaccination occur within three days, with hypersensitivity reactions being most common. Higher rates of reaction occur with multiple antigen products and KV that rely on adjuvants.

It is important to recognize that overall rates of vaccine reactions are very low, and vaccine technology continues to improve. In a retrospective study of 1,226,159 dogs vaccinated at 360 veterinary hospitals, type 1 adverse events (coded as a nonspecific vaccine reaction, allergic reaction, urticaria, or anaphylaxis) occurred in only 0.38% (38.1/10000) of dogs in the three days following vaccination. Risk factors for reactions included increased age, neutered status, decreased body weight, and the administration of multiple vaccines at one time. Parenteral *B. bronchiseptica* vaccines had the lowest rate of adverse effects of all vaccine products, but IN vaccines were not administered in the hospitals in this study (Moore et al. 2005).

IN vaccination for CIRD agents has been associated with mild clinical signs lasting up to three days, including cough and/or serous nasal discharge. This has been reported to be more common in puppies, though a 2016 study did not find this to be true (Ruch-Gallie et al. 2016). Another shelter-based study found no difference in vaccine-associated clinical signs between dogs receiving IN vaccination (Bb + CPiV ±CAV-2) and those receiving a placebo (Edinboro et al. 2004).

Perhaps the most significant risk associated with vaccination for CIRD in shelters is the inadvertent administration of an IN *B. bronchiseptica* vaccine subcutaneously. Complications range from local cellulitis and abscessation at the injection site to rare but life-threatening hepatocellular necrosis. In the event such a mistake occurs, the supervising veterinarian should be notified immediately, and at minimum, systemic antibiotics effective against *B. bronchiseptica* (e.g. doxycycline at 5 mg/kg BID or 10 mg/kg SID) should be administered for no fewer than five days (Ford et al. 2017). Additional treatment protocols suggest infusing appropriate injectable antibiotics (e.g. gentamicin) diluted with sterile fluids subcutaneously in the area of the vaccination, but there is no evidence this is more effective than systemic antibiotics alone. The dog should be monitored closely for a week following the inadvertent injection for clinical signs of injection-site necrosis or liver damage requiring additional supportive care.

It is important to remember no currently licensed vaccine can claim 100% efficacy. In addition to the inherent limitations of the respiratory vaccines described above, several factors can contribute to vaccine failure, including inappropriate handling and administration of products, or failure of individuals to respond to vaccination due to immunosuppression, immunodeficiency, or the presence of maternally derived antibodies (Day 2006).

Dogs vaccinated against *B. bronchiseptica* will shed attenuated bacteria for two weeks following vaccination, potentially immunizing the dogs around them. However, there is no evidence to support administering IN or parenteral vaccines to currently vaccinated dogs already showing clinical signs of disease in an outbreak of CIRD. Likewise, there is no evidence to support the therapeutic vaccination of dogs with chronic or lingering signs of CIRD (Ford 2012). See Chapter 9 for more information on vaccinations and immunology.

10.5.9 Sanitation and Disinfection

The most significant methods to prevent high incidence of CIRD in shelters include effective pathway planning and population management, creation of humane housing facilities to include enriched isolation wards, and prompt identification and relocation of suspect cases to isolation housing. Additionally, enacting standard protocols to halt transmission by establishing a "clean break" between CIRD cases and incoming animals is critical. Cleaning and disinfection remain important elements in controlling fomite transmission and decreasing overall pathogen load in the shelter, but without attention to population management and environmental factors such as air quality, traffic patterns, and ongoing exposure of new dogs to affected and recovered dogs, shelters are unlikely to be successful in controlling ongoing transmission of CIRD.

Many of the pathogens involved in CIRD are transmitted via aerosolized droplets which dogs propel up to 6 m in the act of coughing and sneezing, leading to widespread contamination in open dog kennels and common spaces (Stull et al. 2016). Further contamination is accomplished via direct contact or fomite transmission on hands, clothing, and equipment. However, all CIRD pathogens are inactivated by many disinfectants used in animal shelters, including sodium hypochlorite (bleach™), accelerated hydrogen peroxide (Rescue®), and potassium peroxymonosulfate (Trifectant®). Hand sanitizers containing at least 60% alcohol are also effective against the primary viral and bacterial pathogens in CIRD, with the exception of CAV-2 (Sykes and Weese 2014). Quaternary ammonium compounds are likely less to be effective in the face of CIRD pathogens because they have a limited antimicrobial spectrum against gram-negative bacteria (*B. bronchiseptica),* are not effective against non-enveloped viruses (CAV-2), and are inactivated by hard water, organic debris, and detergent.

Key principles for infection control include prompt removal of gross debris, cleaning with detergent and water, rinsing and drying surfaces, and application of disinfectant with adherence to product specifications (i.e. surface selection, dilution, and contact time). Cleaning must include the removal of organic debris for disinfectants to be effective. Newer one-step products, including some accelerated hydrogen peroxides, may be labeled for cleaning and disinfection in one step, but this assumes the presence of only very minimal debris. Both *Strep. zoo* and *B. bronchiseptica* have been recovered from inoculated endotracheal tubes following cleaning and disinfection with common protocols, including spraying and soaking with accelerated hydrogen peroxide or triclosan detergent (Crawford and Weese 2015).

Cleaning and disinfection are not without risk when it comes to the management of CIRD. Exposure to chemicals used for disinfection can irritate respiratory tissues, leaving animals more vulnerable to infection. Excessive moisture associated with cleaning can facilitate the survival and transfer of pathogens. For example, *Strep. zoo* has been cultured from standing water in a shelter after cleaning (Pesavento et al. 2008). *Bordetella* spp. also thrive in standing water (Kirilenko 1965).

To minimize the risk of amplifying the proliferation and transmission of CIRD agents through cleaning procedures, shelters should employ equipment that limits aerosolization (such as hose-end foamers rather than pressure sprayers). Products should be used at recommended metered dilutions, as over-concentrated chemicals are irritating to respiratory tissues and often caustic to surfaces and equipment. Organic debris should be removed prior to disinfection and all areas should be promptly and thoroughly dried after cleaning. For the protection of both human and animal health, cleaning staff are advised to utilize attire and equipment specific to different areas of the shelter: for example, staff cleaning dog kennels should wear coveralls or other protective garments and rubber boots that are not then worn throughout other areas of the shelter or into the community. Double-compartment enclosures should be used to house sick animals in order to minimize the handling of animals during cleaning procedures. See Chapter 8 for more detailed information on sanitation.

Unlike agents such as canine parvovirus, CDV, and CIV, most pathogens associated with CIRD have a carrier state and can be found in healthy dogs. Creating an environment that is entirely free of CIRD agents is not possible.

10.6 Treatment

For veterinarians working with cases of individual dogs with CIRD, a discussion of medical treatment is primarily concerned with the administration of appropriate pharmaceuticals at an effective dose and duration. However, the shelter veterinarian must reach well beyond prescribing medications to include comprehensive treatment recommendations encompassing housing and husbandry, behavioral enrichment, stress management, and environmental controls. Successful treatment of CIRD patients in the shelter environment depends on a team approach and can include enlisting adopters and volunteers, especially in outbreaks, to ensure adequate welfare during treatment.

10.6.1 Antimicrobials

For the individual dog in a private home, treatment of mild clinical signs of CIRD with antimicrobials may not be warranted, especially in the first 10 days; this is consistent with treatment recommendations for acute respiratory infections in children that dictate antibiotics only if signs are worsening after 5–7 days, or not improved within 10 days (Wong et al. 2006). Given many CIRD infections are viral in origin and self-limiting, the administration of antibiotics in otherwise healthy animals in homes is of questionable benefit and may contradict principles of judicious use of antibiotics in veterinary practice (Lappin et al. 2017).

On the other hand, given a subset of patients are likely at risk of developing opportunistic bacterial infections, sometimes with severe results, the initiation of antibiotic therapy at the time of clinical diagnosis is not unreasonable when there are complicating factors or when a primary bacterial pathogen is suspected. This is especially true in animals with underlying medical conditions or other stressors; in the animal shelter, environmental conditions place marked physiological and immunological stress on dogs, and antibiotics may be used more frequently for CIRD cases in the shelter than in the general population. Even under the best of circumstances, shelter-housed dogs are often immune-compromised, with limited vaccination prophylaxis, less than ideal housing conditions, higher levels of exposure to multiple agents, and a myriad of stressors. Given these factors, early empirical use of antimicrobials in clinically affected shelter dogs is often warranted to minimize risk both to the individual and the population. Issues in population management and environmental conditions should be addressed to decrease the incidence of disease in shelters: attention to air quality, humane enclosures, behavioral health, and biosecurity; management of population density; and minimizing the length of stay will reduce the need for routine antimicrobial use in most uncomplicated CIRD cases.

It is not unusual for shelter veterinarians to be pressured by management to place ALL dogs on antibiotics prophylactically to control CIRD, but it must be remembered any use of antimicrobial drugs leads to selection for resistant organisms. According to the American Veterinary Medical Association (AVMA), antimicrobial stewardship "refers to the actions veterinarians take individually and as a profession to preserve the effectiveness and availability of antimicrobial drugs through conscientious oversight and responsible medical decision-making while safeguarding animal, public, and environmental health" (AVMA 2016). If antibiotics are deemed necessary by the veterinarian, stewardship necessitates judicious use with continual evaluation of the outcomes of therapy; see Table 10.4. The use of antibiotics prophylactically in exposed dogs is strongly discouraged in the management of CIRD in shelters, with the exception of dogs exposed to *Strep. zoo*.

If a decision is made to start antimicrobial therapy, several drugs are appropriate first-line selections for uncomplicated CIRD, including doxycycline, amoxicillin-clavulanate, and amoxicillin (Ford 2012; Sykes 2013; Lappin et al. 2017). Of these, doxycycline is much preferred in shelters for its efficacy against *B. bronchiseptica* and *Mycoplasma spp.* and its ability to be administered once daily (Sykes 2013; Lappin et al. 2017). Either hyclate or monohydrate forms are effective. Minocycline has also been used in times of doxycycline shortage and is effective. Most commonly, a 7–10-day course of doxycycline is initiated as a first-line anti-microbial option (Lappin et al. 2017). If clinical signs resolve, dogs may be discharged from isolation and treatment discontinued after seven days.

All *Mycoplasma* spp. and some *B. bronchiseptica* isolates have demonstrated resistance to amoxicillin-clavulanate (Lappin et al. 2017). Therefore, while amoxicillin-clavulanate is included as a first-line antibiotic for CIRD, it is actually better reserved for cases non-responsive to doxycycline and/or when opportunistic commensal pathogens have been identified as the source of infection.

Second-line drugs for the treatment of CIRD, which include fluoroquinolones and azithromycin, are usually reserved for non-responsive cases and/or pneumonia and are best used based on culture and sensitivity testing of endotracheal or bronchoalveolar lavage samples (Weese 2006; Sykes 2013; Lappin et al. 2017). Generally, more advanced cases are treated to the resolution of clinical signs, though some cases of bacterial bronchitis or pneumonia may require extending treatment for up to one week after the resolution of clinical signs (Lappin et al. 2017). Unlike in cats, CIRD has not been associated with chronic respiratory disease in dogs.

When *Strep. zoo* is suspected or confirmed, two critical exceptions apply. First, *Strep. zoo* strains have demonstrated resistance to doxycycline, but have demonstrated susceptibility to penicillin, ampicillin, and amoxicillin; these should be considered first-line antibiotics for suspected cases of *Strep. zoo*. Second, unlike other respiratory pathogens, the recommendation in the face of a *Strep.* zoo outbreak is to prophylactically treat all exposed dogs with antibiotics. Disease progression is rapid and deadly, and waiting for the presence of signs in exposed dogs is likely to increase morbidity and mortality in a shelter population. Injectable penicillin procaine G is inexpensive and efficacious but requires daily dosing; longer-acting deposition forms of cefovecin sodium are more expensive but have demonstrated efficacy in controlling outbreaks and minimizing additional patient losses. It is suggested to follow molecular confirmation of *Strep. zoo* with culture and sensitivity to verify the efficacy of the selected antibiotic in an outbreak scenario.

CIRD treatment protocols should include that once antibiotics are initiated a patient must be monitored daily for a response to treatment. A failure to demonstrate improvement after a

Table 10.4 Anti-microbial treatment options for CIRD in animal shelters.

Drug	Dose	Comments
First-line antibiotics		**Uncomplicated CIRD**
Doxycycline	10 mg/kg PO q24hr (recommended) or 5 mg/kg PO q12hr	Effective against CIRD associated *B bronchiseptica* or *Mycoplasma* spp. Much preferred over other options in shelters.
Minocycline	5 mg/kg PO q12hr	Similar to doxycycline
Amoxicillin-clavulanate	11 mg/kg PO q12hr	Effective against CIRD caused by secondary commensals, including *Pasturella, Staphylococcus,* and *Streptococcus* spp. Ineffective against beta-lactamase bacteria, including most *B. bronchiseptica* isolates. Ineffective against *Mycoplasma* spp.
Second-line antibiotics		For use in non-responsive or cases progressing to pneumonia. Preferably based on culture and sensitivity of endotracheal wash or bronchoalveolar lavage samples. Culturing nasal swabs not recommended.
Azithromycin	5–10 mg/kg PO q 24 hr. for 3–7 days (dosing varies greatly between sources)	Primary bacterial pneumonia including *Mycoplasma* spp. Also treats *Neospora* pneumonia in puppies.
Enrofloxacin	5–20 mg/kg PO, IM, IV q24hr	Effective against most isolates of *B. bronchiseptica* and *Mycoplasma* spp.
Marbofloxacin	2.7–5.5 mg/kg PO q 24 hr	Effective for *B. bronchiseptica* and *Mycoplasma* spp. and many secondary Gram-positive and Gram-negative organisms.

PO – orally.
q – every.
hr – hour.
IV – intravenously.
IM – intramuscularly.
Sources: Sykes (2013); Plumb (2015); Lappin et al. (2017).

few days is indicative that the selected antibiotic treatment may not be appropriate and should warrant additional veterinary assessment, including diagnostic testing and/or a change or addition to antibiotic administration.

In some cases, primary CIRD pathogens, respiratory compromise, and environmental co-factors, such as poor air quality, can allow for overgrowth of commensal organisms and require a combination protocol (e.g. administration of both doxycycline and amoxicillin-clavulanate). Additionally, if CIRD cases are worsening in the face of standard antibiotic treatment (e.g. developing signs of pneumonia or other advanced sequelae), it may be necessary to reach for additional broad-spectrum or second-line antibiotics without advanced testing in a shelter environment.

The length of time to recovery may be impacted by the quality of the housing, air quality, and the density of dogs housed in isolation areas. Treatment plans should aim to minimize the length of time to recovery. This will potentially reduce individual and population disease severity. LOS in isolation is minimized by choosing effective drugs dosed at appropriate levels and frequency, monitoring daily progress, and adapting treatment accordingly. Shelter veterinarians are encouraged to practice judicious use of antibiotics while also ensuring patient health and welfare by providing comprehensive treatment plans for patients. Additional supportive measures ensuring behavioral and medical supportive care are discussed later in this section. Also, see Chapter 7.

10.6.2 Antitussives

Antitussives are sometimes used in private practice to decrease cough and secondary inflammation from coughing in uncomplicated cases of CIRD. These are of limited efficacy and not without complications, especially in the animal shelter. Each administration of medication can be another event causing stress, fomite transmission, or inappetence in already compromised shelter patients. Additionally, suppression of cough, commonly thought to be a protective mechanism to aid in the clearance of secretions, may increase opportunities for opportunistic colonization of lower airways by CIRD pathogens. Therefore, the use of antitussives in CIRD should be reserved for cases in which coughing is severe or debilitating, when the benefits outweigh the risks, and only in combination with antimicrobial therapy.

Other than butorphanol, all antitussives used in dogs fall under extra-label usage. Over-the-counter human cough suppressants and expectorants such as dextromethorphan/ guaifenesin (2 mg/kg q 8 hr) have been used to offer clinical relief for CIRD-induced cough in the dog with mixed results. Narcotic cough suppressants include hydrocodone bitartrate/homatropine MBr (0.2–0.5 mg/kg PO q 6–12 hr) and butorphanol (0.5 mg/kg PO q 6–12 hr); in the United States, these drugs are usually subject to controlled substance handling laws, which have made them more difficult to attain and can be a particular challenge in a shelter environment. Maropitant (0.5 mg -1 mg/kg q 24 hr) has been reported to be effective in cough suppression in cats, dogs and humans through its inhibition of the tachykinin NK1 receptor and Substance P (this is extra-label usage) (Chapman et al. 2004; Otsuka et al. 2011; Grobman and Reinero 2016).

10.6.3 Supportive Care and Environmental Enrichment

Supportive treatment for CIRD includes maintenance of adequate caloric and fluid needs; prevention of secondary or opportunistic bacterial infections; and reduction of physiologic and emotional stressors, including in both macro- and micro-environments. The macro-environment is that of the room and the facility around the dog's primary enclosure and includes elements such as adequate ventilation and environmental temperature controls, sanitation, provision of an overall low-stress environment, and utilizing enrichment to minimize barking and excitement. The micro-environment includes the dog's primary enclosure, and care should be taken to ensure temperature and ventilation, sanitation, and immediate provisions such as bedding are adequate within each enclosure.

Isolation housing for CIRD patients should be separated from other animals, humane, and enriched. Dogs with CIRD are likely to be isolated a minimum of seven days, and sometimes significantly longer as in the case of CIV-H3N2. Isolation facilities should include double-sided housing for dogs to allow for more natural feeding, resting and elimination behaviors and to minimize handling during routine procedures, such as cleaning and feeding, that can act to increase fomite transmission by staff (Wagner et al. 2014). Isolation enclosures should be enriched and as large as reasonably possible and, in some cases, may even exceed the quality of housing offered in public areas of the shelter or areas where LOS is significantly shorter.

Shelters are strongly encouraged to develop isolation protocols that enable humane handling and behavioral enrichment without compromising biosecurity. This may involve the recruitment and training of specific staff and volunteers in aspects of the donning and removal of personal protective equipment (PPE) including over garments such as coveralls and exam gloves, low stress-handling techniques for husbandry and medical procedures, and isolation-friendly behavioral enrichment activities. The use of a neck collar for walking dogs is discouraged during this time to reduce physical pressure on the upper airway; harnesses are preferred. Dogs should be provided access to separate areas for elimination from eating and resting areas, as well as exercise outside of their enclosures during this time.

The creation of an exercise yard and isolation traffic pattern to get CIRD-affected dogs outside for enrichment is recommended. Likewise, in organizations employing playgroups as part of their behavioral enrichment program, behavior and medical teams may collaborate to appropriately select mildly affected CIRD dogs for pairing during their convalescence. Given that most dogs with CIRD are minimally impacted in terms of their overall activity levels, maintaining mental stimulation and quality of life is essential for the individual dog, even as one works to prevent the spread of the disease through the facility. Trained volunteers specific to this function may be useful in executing enrichment procedures for dogs in isolation wards.

10.7 Implications for Foster Care and Adoption

Getting animals out of the shelter is sometimes the best way to provide appropriate supportive care. When considering the placement of clinically ill CIRD patients outside of the shelter, it is critical to remember several things. First, vaccines for most CIRD pathogens (outside of CDV) do not induce sterilizing immunity, and so vaccinated animals in the community can still contract many CIRD pathogens, though usually with less intensity and milder clinical signs. Second, some pet species for whom vaccines are not available are susceptible to select CIRD pathogens: notable examples of animals susceptible to *B. bronchiseptica* include cats, ferrets, rabbits, and other small mammals. Immune-compromised owners may also be susceptible to *B. bronchiseptica*: risk factors include long-term steroid therapy, organ transplantation, peritoneal dialysis, human immunodeficiency virus (HIV), splenectomy, chemotherapy due to malignancy, and pre-existing respiratory disease (Ford 2012). Third, in the absence of diagnostic testing, shelters cannot be sure they are not introducing rare or emerging agents into naïve populations or environments.

If risks can be mitigated for particular homes through screening and risk assessment (potentially to include diagnostic testing in high-risk dogs), some shelters may find that care through foster care or adoption of CIRD-affected dogs is a reasonable alternative to prolonged stays in isolation facilities. This is particularly true for mild or recovering cases of CIRD and/or when shelter isolation facilities are full, inadequate, or inhumane.

Steps in this process must involve a risk assessment of both the affected dog as well as the home to minimize public health risks. Dog factors include a risk assessment for more problematic agents such as CIV or CDV (this can be accomplished through history, clinical signs, and/or testing), the severity of current clinical signs, the progression of the disease, and the overall state of welfare. Home care factors include housing type as it relates to the risk of exposing community dogs (e.g. apartment vs. house; urban vs. rural), presence and type of other pets in the home, and the caretaker's self-assessment and comfort level in providing treatment and managing clinical signs. Though unlikely in many homes, if separation can be provided from other pets for the duration of treatment, this would be preferable. However, in the high likelihood that pets will interact, a risk assessment can help to elucidate the actual risk.

Shelter medical staff should verify up-to-date vaccinations for respiratory pathogens and overall health status of any pets in the home—or ask that the foster/ adoptive owner does so with their own veterinarian —prior to placing CIRD affected dogs in the home. Caretakers should be advised dogs should not come into contact with community dogs for the duration of clinical signs, and dogs should be returned to the shelter for rechecks and/or access follow-up care as deemed necessary by the course of treatment and the shelter's policies. Instructions for minimizing the pathogen load through standard cleaning practices should include the use of household disinfectants in housing areas, regular washing of food and water bowls, and laundering of bedding and toys. If a foster home is likely to be used again for additional shelter animals, more complete instructions for animal containment to spaces that can be disinfected such as laundry rooms, kitchens, or bathrooms may be warranted.

Caretakers should be advised to regularly wash their hands and change garments (or use over-garments) before interacting with other susceptible animals during the duration of treatment. They should also be provided with information about the limited risks to immune-compromised humans, so they can assess whether placement is an appropriate choice for their home given inhabitants and interactions with others.

For severe cases of CIRD, or early in the course of the disease when its progression is uncertain, care in isolation facilities is often the best choice. However, as cases are recovering, private homes can be a reasonable option if the aforementioned complicating factors are addressed.

10.8 Implications for Relocation Programs

Transport of animals between shelters raises the risk that disease may be transmitted between animals and potentially into new populations. Responsible relocation programs prioritize the health of populations at both source and destination shelters and take measures to reduce the spread of disease. Such efforts require strong preventive healthcare programs: these should include administration of core vaccines at or before intake to the source shelter; following strong biosecurity measures before, during, and following transport; limiting the intermixing of animals from multiple locations; setting limits for the length and duration of transport; and monitoring and following-up on reported issues, including instances of disease, following transport (AAWA 2019; AVMA-ASV 2020).

Dogs that are healthy prior to transport may break with CIRD acutely after travel; thus, the common use of "shipping fever" to describe this disease process in other species. In most cases, identification, isolation, management, and treatment of these dogs can follow standard protocols as outlined earlier in the chapter. However, since CIRD signs can be caused by a myriad of pathogens, including some that may be new to the receiving shelter, relocation of infected dogs can introduce new agents to the shelter and potentially the community. Of particular concern is transporting dogs with CIV, including H3N8 and H3N2, into areas where dogs are naïve.

Shelters receiving animals from other organizations should have veterinary services available to perform an inspection of animals on arrival. Furthermore, receiving shelters should have adequate isolation facilities and protocols prepared for dogs showing clinical signs of respiratory disease at or shortly after their arrival. Standard operating protocols (SOPs) outlining CIRD management strategies in their facility, and, particularly for transport animals, should include diagnostic testing when the source community may have a higher incidence of pathogens not common in the receiving community. An outbreak of CIRD, during or following the transport of dogs, can be a good indication of the need for proactive diagnostic testing to enable the recognition of risks to not only the involved dogs but other animals at the receiving shelter and in the community. An example of this would be the introduction of CIV-H3N2, with its prolonged 28-day shedding period, to a shelter and a community where it has not been diagnosed previously.

Relocation of dogs with clinical signs of CIRD can be highly problematic and may not be legally permissible, particularly if dogs cross over state lines. Laws of interstate transfer for most states in the United States require a valid Certificate of Veterinary Inspection (CVI) or health certificate. This requires an examination and signed statement from a veterinarian that the animal in question was inspected for transport and the dog "appeared to be free of any infectious disease or physical abnormality which would endanger the animal(s) or other animals or endanger public health." Additional regulations are determined by the specific requirements of the state in which the receiving shelter is located. A database of requirements by state can be found at the USDA APHIS website (https://www.aphis.usda.gov/aphis/pet-travel/interstate-pet-travel). Some states, such as Massachusetts and Connecticut, have created very specific procedures and documentation requirements for shelter and rescue relocation programs with clear implications for dogs affected with CIRD. When in doubt, organizations are advised to communicate with their state veterinarian before transporting dogs across state lines.

The veterinary profession discourages the movement of sick animals between organizations but acknowledges it may be appropriate under certain circumstances. Guidelines from professional organizations advise that animals who pose a significant risk of transmitting infectious diseases should not be transported. They also acknowledge that transporting ill animals may be justified when transport allows access to life-saving resources at the destination. Applicable state laws and regulations must be followed. Receiving shelters should have veterinary services available on arrival for any animals requiring care and provide for isolation of sick animals who break with infectious disease (AAWA 2019; AVMA-ASV 2020).

Consistent, transparent communication between destination and source shelters is crucial to prevent or promptly address any concerns that may arise; ideally, receiving shelters will be aware of the source shelter's preventive medicine protocols, the general prevalence of disease, and any particular concerns, and vice versa. Collectively, these steps can help ensure successful, life-saving programs that minimize CIRD outbreaks for shelters and communities.

10.9 Euthanasia Guidelines

An uncomplicated case of CIRD rarely warrants euthanasia from a medical perspective. If the working definition of CIRD is a mild to moderate, self-limiting upper respiratory infection with potential for secondary complications, most CIRD cases can be managed humanely in an animal shelter or foster home.

Dogs with CIRD with additional complications, including pneumonia or sepsis, may deteriorate to a point when euthanasia is the most humane course of action. Dogs displaying more severe clinical signs—including severe weakness, inappetence, pyrexia, and dyspnea—should be evaluated by a veterinarian immediately and emergency care provided. Severe cases may require advanced treatment—including intravenous antibiotics, supplemental oxygen, and fluid therapy—and if this cannot be provided euthanasia needs to be considered a humane outcome. Cases resulting in death or euthanasia warrant necropsy and additional diagnostic testing to determine if a more severe infectious disease is present. CDV, CIV, and *Strep. zoo* can have deadly consequences for populations, and recognition and appropriate management of these pathogens are critical to containing disease and suffering in the shelter.

Outbreaks of CIRD rarely warrant euthanasia of affected populations of shelter dogs; the depopulation of healthy animals is not considered an appropriate response to a CIRD outbreak (ASV 2020). Shelters experiencing an outbreak or high level of endemic disease are strongly advised to work with a veterinarian with shelter-specific training to perform a risk assessment and employ short- and long-term management solutions.

Successful management relies on establishing a clean break between affected populations and new intakes, as well as performing a wide-scale assessment of housing and husbandry measures to institute preventative measures discussed earlier in this chapter. A comprehensive approach includes a review of intake procedures, vaccination, husbandry, surveillance, treatment, housing, quarantine, isolation and environmental control protocols and procedures. Population monitoring and thorough documentation are critical at all times.

10.10 Conclusion

CIRD is typically a disease of high morbidity and low mortality. Though select pathogens such as *Strep. zoo*, CDV and CIV have the potential for greater virulence, the majority of CIRD presentations are mild and self-limiting. Prevention CIRD in shelters is the goal; vaccination is only one important element of a broad comprehensive approach. Rapid implementation of mitigation measures then follows when disease occurs.

Population management to minimize the LOS of each animal and avoid crowding is likely the single most important aspect of controlling respiratory disease in shelters. As population density increases, pathogen load and stress increase and control measures become severely challenged. Other important activities include environmental control measures, effective use of isolation facilities, daily population rounds, disease surveillance, staff training, and stress reduction and behavioral enrichment. Additional information can be found in this textbook in the introduction and chapters on wellness, vaccinations, diagnostic testing, data surveillance, sanitation and outbreak management.

Though CIRD can be common in animal shelters, a high level of endemic disease or any occurrence of epidemic disease should be cause for veterinary investigation. State-funded diagnostic labs are typically tasked with herd health investigations for food production and wildlife populations; small animal populations do not have the same level of support for infectious disease research and management. However, with the increasing availability of advanced training and board certification in shelter medicine practice—as well as the existence of comprehensive shelter medicine programs at veterinary colleges and some large national animal welfare organizations—shelters are encouraged to solicit consultation and diagnostic assistance. The prevention of disease is the prevention of suffering, and proactive approaches through management and design are preferable to reactive crisis interventions. Nonetheless, assistance is available for both types of scenarios, and the reduction of CIRD in shelters is an attainable goal.

References

AAHA (2017). Canine Vaccination Recommendations – Shelter-Housed Dogs. https://www.aaha.org/aaha-guidelines/vaccination-canine-configuration/vaccination-recommendations--shelter-housed-dogs (accessed 17 April 2020).

Abbott, Y., Acke, E., Khan, S. et al. (2010). Zoonotic transmission of Streptococcus equi subsp. zooepidemicus from a dog to a handler. *Journal of Medical Microbiology* 59 (1): 120–123.

Abdelmagid, O.Y., Larson, L., Payne, L. et al. (2004). Evaluation of the efficacy and duration of a canine combination vaccine against virulent parvovirus, infectious canine hepatitis virus, and distemper virus experimental challenges. *Veterinary Therapeutics* 5: 173–186.

Acke, E., Midwinter, A.C., Lawrence, K. et al. (2015). Prevalence of Streptococcus dysgalactiae subsp. equisimilis and S. equi subsp. zooepidemicus in a sample of healthy dogs, cats and horses. *New Zealand Veterinary Journal* 169 (February): 1–19.

Almes, K.M., Janardhan, K.S., Anderson, J. et al. (2010). Fatal canine adenoviral pneumonia in two litters of bulldogs. *Journal of Veterinary Diagnostic Investigation* 22 (5): 780–784.

American Veterinary Medical Association (2016). Antimicrobial Stewardship in Companion Animal Practice. https://www.avma.org/KB/Resources/Reports/Pages/Antimicrobial-Stewardship-in-Companion-Animal-Practice.aspx (accessed 17 April 2020).

American Veterinary Medical Association (2019). Model Veterinary Practice Act. https://www.avma.org/sites/default/files/2019-11/Model-Veterinary-Practice-Act.pdf (accessed 20 April 2020).

American Veterinary Medical Association (2020). Non-emergency Relocation of Dogs and Cats for Adoption Best Practices. https://www.avma.org/sites/default/files/2020-03/AWF-TransportAdoptionBestPractices.pdf (accessed 3 April 2020).

Anderton, T.L., Maskell, D.J., and Preston, A. (2004). Ciliostasis is a key early event during colonization of canine tracheal tissue by Bordetella bronchiseptica. *Microbiology* 150 (9): 2843–2855.

Association for the Advancement of Animal Welfare (2019). Companion Animal Transport Programs Best Practices. https://cdn.ymaws.com/theaawa.org/resource/resmgr/files/2019/BP_Updated_March2019.pdf (accessed 16 February 2020).

Association of Shelter Veterinarians (2020). Position statement: Depopulation. https://www.sheltervet.org/assets/docs/position-statements/Depopulation%20PS%203.20.pdf (accessed 17 April 2020).

Binns, S.H., Dawson, S., Speakman, A.J. et al. (1999). Prevalence and risk factors for feline Bordetella bronchiseptica infection. *Veterinary Record* 144: 575–580.

Blum, S., Elad, D., Zukin, N. et al. (2010). Outbreak of Streptococcus equi subsp. zooepidemicus infections in cats. *Veterinary Microbiology* 144: 236–239.

Brodersen, B.W. (2010). Bovine respiratory syncytial virus. *The Veterinary Clinics of North America. Food Animal Practice* 26 (2): 323–333.

Byun, J.W., Yoon, S.-S., Woo, G.-H. et al. (2009). An outbreak of fatal hemorrhagic pneumonia caused by *Streptococcus equi* subsp. *zooepidemicus* in shelter dogs. *Journal of Veterinary Science* 10 (3): 269–271.

Center for Shelter Dogs (n.d.). Doggie social hour: how to run a playgroup in your shelter. http://centerforshelterdogs.tufts.edu/wp-content/uploads/2016/03/Website-CSD_Playgroup_Manual-11.11-1.pdf (accessed 17 April 2020).

Chalker, V.J. (2005). Canine mycoplasmas. *Research in Veterinary Science* 79 (1): 1–8.

Chalker, V.J., Brooks, H.W., and Brownlie, J. (2003). The association of *Streptococcus equi* subsp. *zooepidemicus* with canine infectious respiratory disease. *Veterinary Microbiology* 95 (1–2): 149–156.

Chapman, R.W., House, A., Liu, F. et al. (2004). Antitussive activity of the tachykinin NK1 receptor antagonist, CP-99994, in dogs. *European Journal of Pharmacology* 485 (1–3): 329–332.

Coppola, C.L., Enns, R.M., and Grandin, T. (2006). Noise in the animal shelter environment: building design and the effects of daily noise exposure. *Journal of Applied Animal Welfare Science* 9 (1): 1–7.

Crawford, S. and Weese, J.S. (2015). Efficacy of endotracheal tube disinfection strategies for elimination of *Streptococcus zooepidemicus* and *Bordetella bronchiseptica*. *Journal of the American Veterinary Medical Association* 247 (9): 1033–1036.

Crawford, P.C., Dubovi, E.J., Castleman, W.L. et al. (2005). Transmission of equine influenza virus to dogs. *Science* 310 (5747): 482–485.

Davis, R., Jayappa, H., Abdelmagid, O.Y. et al. (2007). Comparison of the mucosal immune response in dogs vaccinated with either an intranasal avirulent live culture or a subcutaneous antigen extract vaccine of Bordetella bronchiseptica. *Veterinary Therapeutics* 8 (1): 32–40.

Day, M.J. (2006). Vaccine side effects: fact and fiction. *Veterinary Microbiology* 117 (1): 51–58.

Day, M.J., Horzinek, M.C., Schultz, R.D. et al. (2016). WSAVA (world small animal veterinary association) guidelines for the vaccination of dogs and cats. *Journal of Small Animal Practice* 57 (January): E1–E33.

Ditchfield, J., Macpherson, L.W., and Zbitnew, A. (1962). Association of a canine adenovirus (Toronto A 26/61) with an outbreak of laryngotracheitis (and kennel cough). *Canadian Veterinary Journal* 3 (8): 238–247.

Döring, D., Haberland, B.E., Bauer, A. et al. (2016). Behavioral observations in dogs in 4 research facilities: do they use their enrichment? *Journal of Veterinary Behavior: Clinical Applications and Research* 13: 55–62.

Edinboro, C.H., Ward, M.P., and Glickman, L.T. (2004). A placebo-controlled trial of two intranasal vaccines to prevent tracheobronchitis (kennel cough) in dogs entering a humane shelter. *Preventive Veterinary Medicine* 62 (2): 89–99.

Ellis, J.A. (2015). How well do vaccines for Bordetella bronchiseptica work in dogs? A critical review of the literature 1977–2014. *The Veterinary Journal* 204 (1): 5–16.

Ellis, J.A. and Krakowka, G.S. (2012). A review of canine parainfluenza virus infection in dogs. *Journal of the American Veterinary Medical Association* 240 (3): 273–284.

Ellis, J.A., Haines, D.W., West, K.H. et al. (2001). Effect of vaccination on experimental infection with Bordetella bronchiseptica in dogs. *Journal of the American Veterinary Medical Association* 218 (3): 367–375.

Erles, K. and Brownlie, J. (2005). Investigation into the causes of canine infectious respiratory disease: antibody responses to canine respiratory coronavirus and canine herpesvirus in two kenneled dog populations. *Archives of Virology* 150 (8): 1493–1504.

Erles, K. and Brownlie, J. (2008). Canine respiratory coronavirus: an emerging pathogen in the canine infectious respiratory disease complex. *The Veterinary Clinics of North America. Small Animal Practice* 38 (4): 815–825.

Erles, K., Toomey, C., Brooks, H.W. et al. (2003). Detection of a group 2 coronavirus in dogs with canine infectious respiratory disease. *Virology* 310 (2): 216–223.

Fairchild, G.A., Medway, W., and Cohen, D. (1969). A study of the pathogenicity of a canine adenovirus (Toronto A26/61) for dogs. *American Journal of Veterinary Research* 30: 1187–1193.

Ford, R.B. (2012). Canine infectious respiratory disease. In: Infectious Diseases of the Dog and Cat, 4e (ed. C.E. Greene), 55–65. St. Louis: Elsevier.

Ford, R.B., Larson, L.J., McClure, K.D. et al. (2017). 2017 AAHA canine vaccination guidelines. *Journal of the American Animal Hospital Association* 53 (5): 243–251.

Frank, J. and Griffin, T. (1989). Stress and immunity: a unifying concept. *Veterinary Immunology and Immunopathology* 20: 263–312.

Glaser, R. and Kiecolt-Glaser, J.K. (2005). Stress-induced immune dysfunction: implications for health. *Nature Reviews. Immunology* 5: 243–251.

Greene, C. and Prescott, J. (2012). Gram-positive bacterial infections. In: Infectious Diseases of the Dog and Cat, 4e (ed. C. Greene), 325–340. St. Louis: Elsevier.

Grobman, M. and Reinero, C. (2016). Investigation of neurokinin-1 receptor antagonism as a novel treatment for chronic bronchitis in dogs. *Journal of Veterinary Internal Medicine* 30 (3): 847–852.

Holt, D.E., Mover, M.R., and Brown, D.C. (2010). Serologic prevalence of antibodies against canine influenza virus (H3N8) in dogs in a metropolitan animal shelter. *Journal of the*

American Veterinary Medical Association 237 (1): 71–73.

Hurley, K.F. (2012). Prevention and management of infection in canine populations. In: Infectious Diseases of the Dog and Cat, 4e (ed. C. Greene), 1124–1130. St. Louis: Elsevier.

Jacobs, A.A.C., Theelen, R.P.H., Jaspers, R. et al. (2005). Protection of dogs for 13 months against *Bordetella bronchiseptica* and canine parainfluenza virus with a modified live vaccine. *Veterinary Record* 157: 19–23.

Karsten, C.L., Wagner, D.C., Kass, P.H. et al. (2017). An observational study of the relationship between capacity for care as an animal shelter management model and cat health, adoption and death in three animal shelters. *The Veterinary Journal* 227: 15–22.

Kim, M.K., Jee, H., Shin, S.W. et al. (2007). Outbreak and control of haemorrhagic pneumonia due to *Streptococcus equi* subspecies *zooepidemicus* in dogs. *Veterinary Record* 161: 528–530.

Kirilenko, N.I. (1965). Survival of *Bordetella pertussis* in the air and on some objects. *Zhurnal Mikrobiologii, Epidemiologii, i Immunobiologii* 42: 39–42.

Lappin, M.R., Blondeau, J., Boothe, D. et al. (2017). Antimicrobial use guidelines for treatment of respiratory disease in dogs and cats: antimicrobial guidelines working group of the international society for companion animal infectious diseases. *Journal of Veterinary Internal Medicine* 31: 279–294.

Larson, L.J., Henningson, J., Sharp, P. et al. (2011). Efficacy of the canine influenza virus H3N8 vaccine to decrease severity of clinical disease after co-challenge with canine influenza virus and *Streptococcus equi* subsp. *zooepidemicus*. *Clinical and Vaccine Immunology* 18 (4): 559–564.

Larson, L.J., Thiel, B.E., Sharp, P. et al. (2013). A comparative study of protective immunity provided by oral, intranasal and parenteral canine *Bordetella bronchiseptica* vaccines. *International Journal of Applied Research in Veterinary Medicine* 11: 153–160.

Lavan, R. and Knesl, O. (2015). Prevalence of canine infectious respiratory pathogens in asymptomatic dogs presented at US animal shelters. *Journal of Small Animal Practice* 56 (9): 572–576.

Lechner, E., Crawford, P.C., Levy, J.K. et al. (2010). Prevalence of protective antibody titers for canine distemper virus and canine parvovirus in dogs entering a Florida animal shelter. *Journal of the American Veterinary Medical Association* 236 (12): 1317–1320.

Ledbetter, E.C., da Silva, E., Kim, S.G. et al. (2012). Frequency of spontaneous canine herpesvirus-1 reactivation and ocular viral shedding in latently infected dogs and canine herpesvirus-1 reactivation and ocular viral shedding induced by topical administration of cyclosporine and systemic administration of corticosteroids. *American Journal of Veterinary Research* 73 (7): 1079–1084.

Lehr, C., Jayappa, H., Erskine, J. et al. (2008). Demonstration of 1-year duration of immunity for attenuated *Bordetella bronchiseptica* vaccines in dogs. *Veterinary Therapeutics* 9: 257–262.

Luescher, A.U. and Medlock, R.T. (2009). The effects of training and environmental alterations on adoption success of shelter dogs. *Applied Animal Behaviour Science* 17: 63–88.

Maboni, G., Seguel, M., Lorton, A. et al. (2019). Canine infectious respiratory disease: new insights into the etiology and epidemiology of associated pathogens. *Public Library of Science One (PloS one)* 14 (4): e0215817.

May, M. and Brown, D.R. (2009). Secreted sialidase activity of canine mycoplasmas. *Veterinary Microbiology* 137 (3–4): 380–383.

Mitchell, J.A. and Brownlie, J. (2015). The challenges in developing effective canine infectious respiratory disease vaccines. *Journal of Pharmacy and Pharmacology* 67 (3): 372–381.

Mitchell, J.A., Brooks, H.W., Szladovits, B. et al. (2013a). Tropism and pathological findings associated with canine respiratory coronavirus (CRCoV). *Veterinary Microbiology* 162 (2–4): 582–594.

Mitchell, J.A., Cardwell, J.M., Renshaw, R.W. et al. (2013b). Detection of canine pneumovirus in dogs with canine infectious respiratory disease. *Journal of Clinical Microbiology* 51 (12): 4112–4119.

Moore, G.E., Guptill, L.F., Ward, M.P. et al. (2005). Adverse events diagnosed within three days of vaccine administration in dogs. *Journal of the American Veterinary Medical Association* 227 (7): 1102–1108.

Newbury, S., Blinn, M.K. Bushby, P.A. et al. (2010). Association of Shelter Vets Guidelines for Standards of Care in Animal Shelters. http://www.sheltervet.org/assets/docs/shelter-standards-oct2011-wforward.pdf (accessed 4 April 2020).

Otsuka, K., Niimi, A., Matsumoto, H. et al. (2011). Plasma substance P levels in patients with persistent cough. *Respiration* 82: 431–438.

Pesavento, P.A. and Murphy, B.G. (2014). Common and emerging infectious diseases in the animal shelter. *Veterinary Pathology* 51 (2): 478–491.

Pesavento, P.A., Hurley, K.F., Bannasch, M.J. et al. (2008). A clonal outbreak of acute fatal hemorrhagic pneumonia in intensively housed (shelter) dogs caused by *Streptococcus equi* subsp. *zooepidemicus*. *Veterinary Pathology* 45: 51–53.

Plumb, D. (2015). Plumb's Veterinary Drug Handbook, 8e. Ames: Wiley-Blackwell.

Priestnall, S.L., Brownlie, J., Dubovi, E.J. et al. (2006). Serological prevalence of canine respiratory coronavirus. *Veterinary Microbiology* 115 (1–3): 43–53.

Priestnall, S.L., Erles, K., Brooks, H.W. et al. (2010). Characterization of pneumonia due to *Streptococcus equi* subsp. *Zooepidemicus* in dogs. *Clinical and Vaccine Immunology* 17 (11): 1790–1796.

Priestnall, S.L., Mitchell, J.A., Walker, C.A. et al. (2014). New and emerging pathogens in canine infectious respiratory disease. *Veterinary Pathology* 51 (2): 492–504.

Protopopova, A. (2016). Effects of sheltering on physiology, immune function, behavior, and the welfare of dogs. *Physiology and Behavior* 159: 95–103.

Protopopova, A., Mehrkam, L.R., Boggess, M.M. et al. (2014). In-kennel behavior predicts length of stay in shelter dogs. *Public Library of Science One (PLoS One)* 9 (12): e114319.

Protopopova, A., Brandifino, M., Wynne, C.D.L. et al. (2016). Preference assessments and structured potential adopter-dog interactions increase adoptions. *Applied Animal Behaviour Science* 176: 87–95.

Protopopova, A., Hall, N.J., Brown, K.M. et al. (2019). Behavioral predictors of subsequent respiratory illness signs in dogs admitted to an animal shelter. *Public Library of Science One (PLoS One)* 14 (10): e0224252.

Randall, R.E., Young, D.F., Goswami, K.K. et al. (1987). Isolation and characterization of monoclonal antibodies to simian virus 5 and their use in revealing antigenic differences between human, canine and simian isolates. *Journal of General Virology* 68 (Pt. 11): 2769–2780.

Renshaw, R.W., Zylich, N.C., Laverack, M.A. et al. (2010). Pneumovirus in dogs with acute respiratory disease. *Emerging Infectious Diseases* 16 (6): 993–995.

Rosenberg, F., Lief, F.S., Todd, J.D. et al. (1971). Studies of canine respiratory viruses. I. Experimental infection of dogs with an SV5-like canine parainfluenza agent. *American Journal of Epidemiology* 94 (2): 147–165.

Rosendal, S. and Vinther, O. (1977). Experimental mycoplasmal pneumonia in dogs: electron microscopy of infected tissue. *Acta Pathologica Microbiologica Scandinavica Section B Microbiology* 85: 462–465.

Ruch-Gallie, R., Moroff, S., and Lappin, M.R. (2016). Adenovirus 2, *Bordetella bronchiseptica*, and parainfluenza molecular diagnostic assay results in puppies after vaccination with modified live vaccines. *Journal of Veterinary Internal Medicine* 30 (1): 164–166.

Rycroft, A.N., Tsounakou, E., and Chalker, V. (2007). Serological evidence of *Mycoplasma cynos* infection in canine infectious respiratory disease. *Veterinary Microbiology* 120 (3–4): 358–362.

Sadler, A. (2020). Dogs Playing for Life! https://dogsplayingforlife.com (accessed 17 April 2020).

Scarlett, J.M., Greenberg, M.J., and Hoshizaki, T. (2017). Medical data: from the individual to the population. In: Every Nose Counts: Using Metrics in Animal Shelters, 110–135. CreateSpace Independent Publishing Platform.

Schlaffer, L. and Bonacci, P. (2013). Shelter design. In: Shelter Medicine for Veterinarians and Staff (eds. L. Miller and S. Zawistowski), 21–35. Ames: Wiley/Blackwell.

Schulz, B.S., Kurz, S., Weber, K. et al. (2014). Detection of respiratory viruses and Bordetella bronchiseptica in dogs with acute respiratory tract infections. *Veterinary Journal* 201: 365–369.

Song, D., Kang, B., Lee, C. et al. (2008). Transmission of avian influenza virus (H3N2) to dogs. *Emerging Infectious Diseases* 14 (5): 741–746.

Song, D.S., An, D.J., Moon, H.J. et al. (2011). Interspecies transmission of the canine influenza H3N2 virus to domestic cats in South Korea, 2010. *Journal of General Virology* 92 (10): 2350–2355.

Stull, J.W., Kasten, J.I., Evason, M.D. et al. (2016). Risk reduction and management strategies to prevent transmission of infectious disease among dogs at dog shows, sporting events, and other canine group settings. *Journal of the American Veterinary Medical Association* 249 (6): 612–627.

Sykes, J.E. (2013). Antimicrobial therapy in cats and dogs. In: Antimicrobial Therapy in Veterinary Medicine, 5e (eds. S. Giguere et al.), 473–494. Ames: Wiley-Blackwell.

Sykes, J.E. (2017). Update on canine infectious respiratory tract disease. OVMA Midwest Veterinary Conference, Columbus.

Sykes, J.E. and Weese, J.S. (2014). Chapter 11 – infection control programs for dogs and cats. In: Canine and Feline Infectious Disease, 1e (ed. J.E. Sykes), 105–118. St. Louis: Elsevier.

Tizard, I.R. (2012). Veterinary Immunology: An Introduction, 9e. St. Louis: Elsevier/Saunders.

Twark, L. and Dodds, W. (2000). Clinical use of serum parvovirus and distemper virus antibody titers for determining revaccination strategies in healthy dogs. *Journal of the American Veterinary Medical Association* 217 (7): 1021–1024.

Voorhees, I.E.H., Glaser, A.L., Toohey-Kurth, K.L. et al. (2017). Spread of canine influenza A(H3N2) virus, United States. *Emerging Infectious Diseases* 23 (12): 1950–1957.

Wagner, D., Newbury, S., Kass, P. et al. (2014). Elimination behavior of shelter dogs housed in double compartment kennels. *Public Library of Science One (PloS one)* 9 (5): e962545. http://journals.plos.org/plosone/article/file?id=10.1371/journal.pone.0096254andtype=printable (Accessed April 26, 2020).

Weese, J.S. (2006). Investigation of antimicrobial use and the impact of antimicrobial use guidelines in a small animal veterinary teaching hospital: 1995–2004. *Journal of the American Veterinary Medical Association* 228 (4): 553–558.

Weese, J.S. and Stull, J. (2013). Respiratory disease outbreak in a veterinary hospital associated with canine parainfluenza virus infection. *The Canadian Veterinary Journal* 54 (1): 79–82. https://www.ncbi.nlm.nih.gov/pmc/articles/PMC3524821/pdf/cvj_01_79.pdf (Accessed April 26, 2020).

Wong, D.M., Blumberg, D.A., and Lowe, L.G. (2006). Guidelines for the use of antibiotics in acute upper respiratory tract infections. *American Family Physician* 24 (6): 956–966. https://www.aafp.org/afp/2006/0915/p956.pdf (Accessed April 26, 2020).

11

Canine Distemper Virus

Sandra Newbury

Shelter Medicine Program, Department of Medical Sciences, University of Wisconsin-Madison School of Veterinary Medicine, Madison, WI, USA

11.1 Introduction

Canine distemper virus (CDV) causes a highly contagious infection in dogs that was once considered the most common and deadly infectious disease in dogs. Though largely preventable through immunization, CDV remains a significant cause of morbidity and mortality in shelters because many dogs and puppies are susceptible at the time of shelter intake and disease is often unrecognized when introduced. While the disease is less common in owned pets, communities with low rates of vaccination may similarly see disease more frequently. Shelters in communities where the disease is more common are more likely to be affected. Infection can be inapparent, mild, severe, or fatal in some cases. CDV may cause obvious, acute outbreaks with high morbidity and mortality or, perhaps most confusing, CDV in shelters can smolder at low levels, going unrecognized for long periods of time. In recent years, great strides have been made in preventing illness and managing outbreaks without resorting to depopulation. If shelters are experiencing problems with CDV related illnesses, life-saving solutions can often be found.

11.2 Agent and Epidemiology

CDV is an enveloped ribonucleic acid (RNA) virus in the genus Morbillivirus in the family *Paramyxoviridae*. The other viruses in the same genus include the closely related measles virus of primates, rinderpest of ruminants and pigs, and the peste des petits ruminants virus found in certain small ruminants. Animals susceptible to CDV that are most likely to be present in shelters or have contact with shelter animals are dogs, ferrets, coyotes, skunks, and raccoons. Many other species are also susceptible to infection; however, zoonotic transmission (to humans) of CDV has not been demonstrated. While dogs are the primary host for CDV, and dog-to-dog transmission is the most likely source of infection, it is likely that the raccoon population acts as a substantial reservoir and is responsible for much of the exposure and maintenance of CDV in some communities. A significant source of infection in at least one major CDV outbreak in shelter dogs was found to be infected raccoons. The exposure apparently occurred when both species were placed in the same animal control vehicles (Hurley 2005).

Infectious Disease Management in Animal Shelters, Second Edition.
Edited by Lila Miller, Stephanie Janeczko, and Kate F. Hurley.

Confusion about cats sometimes occurs because feline panleukopenia virus infection is sometimes referred to as "feline distemper." Panleukopenia or "Feline distemper" is actually caused by feline parvovirus (FPV) which is the ancestral virus of canine parvovirus type 2. CDV does not infect domestic cats nor cause disease in that species, however, it does cause disease in large felids (e.g. lions, tigers) (Ikeda et al. 2001; Spencer 1995).

11.2.1 Biotypes of CDV

There are a variety of biotypes of CDV. The biotypes have different incubation periods as well as different disease patterns in the animal. The classic, acute biotype of CDV that was originally isolated and characterized is often referred to as the "Snyder Hill" strain of virus because it was isolated and characterized at the Veterinary Virus Research Institute (now the James A. Baker Institute for Animal Health) at Cornell University, which is located on Snyder Hill Rd. in Ithaca, New York. Today, the acute virus biotype Snyder Hill has been replaced by a subacute virus biotype referred to as R252. A very similar, if not identical, virus, A75 has also been isolated. These two isolates are of the same or similar biotypes and probably are the more common biotype in the field since the 1980s.

Importantly, though there are multiple biotypes, there is only one serotype (antigenic type) of CDV, and thus the modified-live virus vaccines made in the late 1950s and early 1960s remain highly effective in limiting infection and preventing disease. Similarly, current diagnostic testing appears to effectively detect CDV in infected dogs. Outbreaks and disease are seen because of gaps in vaccination rather than because new biotypes are breaking through effective immunization. In communities where vaccination is common, the disease caused by CDV is rarely seen because vaccinated dogs are immune to infection and/or disease. Even in outbreak settings, dogs with adequate antibodies do not develop clinical signs or shed the virus. If this cross-protection were not effective, many more dogs would be infected. CDV-induced disease remains common, or at least sporadic, in regions where vaccination is less common, and in environments such as shelters where infected dogs or wildlife may enter unrecognized and cause exposure to unvaccinated or recently vaccinated dogs. This has happened even in shelters in communities where CDV is rarely seen in private practice and, in each case, lapses in vaccination correlate well with the development of the disease. CDV should be considered at least on the list of differentials anytime unusually severe or frequent respiratory disease is seen in a shelter.

11.3 Transmission

CDV may be shed in virtually all body secretions and excretions depending on the stage of infection. A lower cycle threshold (Ct) or higher viral load on quantitative reverse transcription-polymerase chain reaction (RT-PCR) suggests the dog may be more likely to contribute to transmission. (See the section (11.7) on diagnostics in this chapter for more information.)

CDV is a labile (unstable) virus. While fomite or environmental transmission of CDV is possible, the virus is easily killed by most disinfectants and does not remain infectious outside the body for more than a few hours to a few days, depending on ambient temperature and other conditions.

Transmission probably occurs most commonly through direct contact between sick dogs and susceptible dogs, making recognition and isolation of animals with infectious respiratory disease especially important in shelter settings where dogs will be housed together or come into contact with each other. Aerosol transmission between susceptible and actively infected dogs also occurs via inhalation of airborne virus (Appel 1987). Mildly affected and recovering animals may play an important role in maintaining transmission cycles in shelters.

Fomite and environmental contamination are of less importance for disease transmission than for a hardier virus such as canine parvovirus but, since the virus only needs to survive for minutes on contaminated fomites, this route of transmission may become significant in a shelter environment through staff handling or if equipment, kennels or holding pens are not thoroughly disinfected between dogs. Fomite transmission becomes even more likely when the disease is not recognized or identified and infectious dogs are housed or otherwise comingled in the same area as healthy dogs.

11.4 Pathogenesis

Virus replication initially occurs in lymphoid tissues when CDV first enters the body (Appel 1987; von Messling et al. 2004). In all likelihood, phagocytic cells transport the virus from the respiratory tract to local lymph nodes or other respiratory lymphatic tissues, where CDV actively replicates in an immunologically naïve dog. Once the virus begins to replicate in the macrophage/monocyte and the T and B lymphocytes, it is rapidly transported to peripheral lymphoid tissues throughout the body, including lymph nodes, spleen, bone marrow, Kupffer cells of the liver, etc. (Appel 1987).

During this early phase of the infection, the animal becomes immunosuppressed with severe T and *B lymphocytopenia*, interference with macrophage function, as well as other immune function impairment (Krakowka et al. 1975; Schobesberger et al. 2005). Immunosuppression can last for weeks, depending on the biotype of CDV infecting the dog. This immunosuppression probably contributes to many of the signs of disease seen in shelters as infected dogs become vulnerable to secondary infections.

11.5 Risk Factors for Infection

Evaluations of titers from dogs entering shelters throughout the United States have shown wide variation from region to region, but approximately 50 ± 20% of dogs were antibody negative for CDV at the time of intake, suggesting that those dogs have never been vaccinated or naturally infected, are susceptible to infection, and have a high probability of becoming infected if exposed prior to or near immunization (Lechner et al. 2010). Age offers no specific benefit or protection from the development of the disease; susceptible dogs in any age group may develop severe clinical signs of CDV. This contrasts with canine parvovirus, where adult dogs tend to have at least some age-related defense against the development of severe clinical signs. More obvious clinical signs as well as higher morbidity and mortality may be seen in puppies because young dogs are more likely to be immunologically naive and, because of maternal antibodies, are more difficult to effectively immunize. Because of the possibility of maternal antibody interference with vaccination, puppies under 18–20 weeks of age must be considered potentially susceptible, regardless of their vaccination history. (See Chapter 9 on Canine and Feline Vaccinations and Immunology for more information about maternal antibody interference.)

11.6 Incubation Period, Clinical Signs and Disease Course

There is significant variation in the course of the disease, clinical signs, and severity of illness dogs experience with CDV infections. The time until onset of clinical signs, the duration of infection and disease, and the severity of disease are virus strain and host (dog) dependent, as is the case for many viral infections/diseases (Appel 1987; Summers et al. 1984). The infectious dose or viral load the dog is exposed to likely also plays a role. The incubation period, depending on the strain of the virus and the dog, may range from less than one week up to six weeks post-infection. Longer incubation periods can be a reality but are much less common. In the author's experience, in the field, clinical signs most often develop more quickly and only rarely develop as late as six weeks.

Importantly, the morbidity and severity of the disease seen in shelters can be dramatically lowered through the vaccination of dogs immediately on or prior to intake. Vaccination for CDV provides early partial protection from the development of severe clinical illness and neurologic disease (Schroeder et al. 1967; Larson and Schultz 2006). Many dogs exposed to CDV after vaccination on shelter intake will develop only mild to moderate signs of illness while still posing a significant risk of transmission. In this situation, CDV often goes unrecognized until a dog who was not vaccinated or a puppy who was not effectively immunized develops more fulminant disease.

Clinical signs of CDV have frequently been described as bi-phasic. The earliest sign of infection with CDV would normally be an initial febrile response within a few days to a week after infection. This often goes unrecognized, especially in shelter settings. The initial febrile response often coincides with the onset of a period of immunosuppression that can occur as early as three days post-infection and persist for weeks to a month or more.

The earliest recognized clinical signs of CDV infection are usually non-specific signs of malaise and respiratory disease, including coughing and a mucopurulent nasal discharge. Ocular involvement is fairly common, usually characterized by a mucopurulent ocular discharge or squinting. These signs occur early in the first to third week after infection and can be difficult to differentiate from more benign disease but should be recognized as potentially suggestive of CDV. See Figures 11.1 and 11.2.

These early signs may be followed or accompanied by vomiting and diarrhea. Gastrointestinal (GI) signs may be associated with tenesmus and bloody feces. Intussusception is a risk. Dramatic body wasting can occur with or without anorexia and should be considered a key clinical sign. Dehydration and systemic

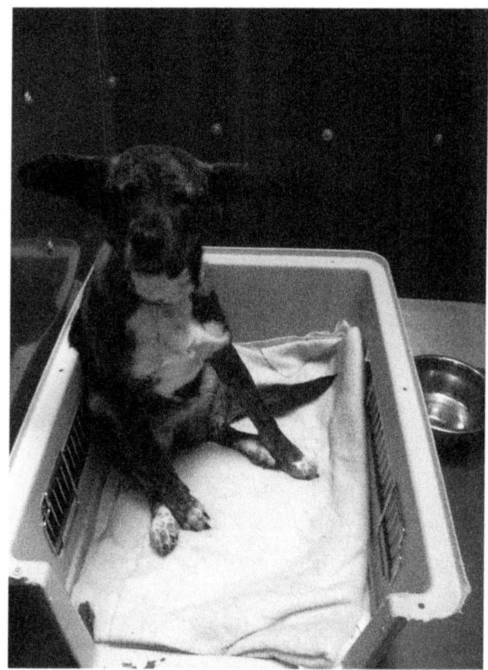

Figure 11.1 A young dog exhibiting squinting that can be a characteristic sign of distemper.

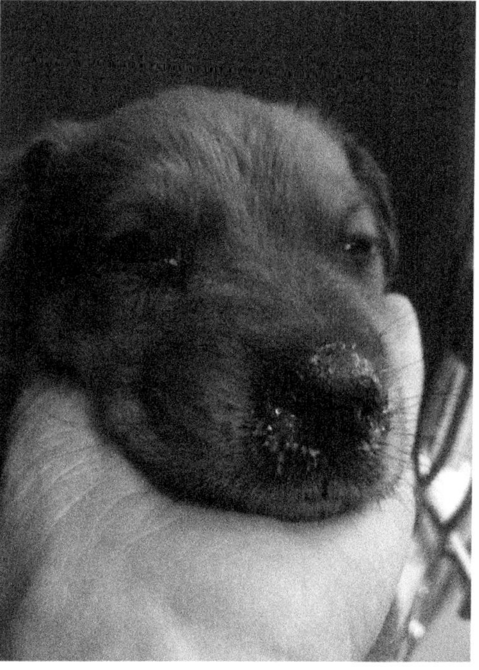

Figure 11.2 A puppy with canine distemper exhibiting marked mucopurulent nasal discharge and squinting.

collapse are a significant risk without timely and proper medical support and intervention. As a result of viral infection of the pulmonary tissues, and opportunistic bacterial infection, lower respiratory tract disease (e.g. pneumonia) may also be seen during this later phase.

Skin disease (pustules) or a rare, measles-like rash may be seen in a small percentage of infected dogs. Digital and nasal hyperkeratosis have also been well described and are most often associated with varying levels of neurologic disease. Distemper was once known as "hardpad disease" a reference to the digital hyperkeratosis that is less commonly seen today.

A careful ocular exam is indicated in all cases of suspected distemper because ocular signs are relatively common. The most common ocular signs are crusting, mucopurulent ocular discharge and conjunctivitis as described above. Dogs may also be seen squinting or blinking their lids. (See Figures 11.1 and 11.2.) Keratoconjunctivitis sicca ("dry eye") may result in ulcer formation and perforation of the cornea, as first described by Dr. Henri Carré in what may have been one of the earliest descriptions of distemper in 1905. Though rarely seen by the author, other ocular signs of CDV may result from viral effects on the optic nerve and the retina. Lesions that develop on the retina, secondary to degeneration and necrosis, appear as gray-pink densities. Post-infection, these lesions can be identified as hyper-reflective areas suggestive of previous infection with CDV. Optic neuritis, sudden blindness and retinal detachment can also occur but are rarely reported.

Clinical signs of neurologic disease may develop concurrently with other systemic signs, in the absence of other signs or, very rarely, develop one to three weeks or even longer after the resolution of other systemic signs of illness. Neurologic signs may range from only very subtle twitching to severe seizure activity. Most commonly, dogs who develop neurologic signs will do so near the time of infection. This neurologic disease results from the viral invasion of neurologic tissue.

Neurologic signs are characterized by salivation and chewing movements (petit mal, chewing gum seizures) and seizures that may become more frequent and severe (grand mal). Though the development of central nervous system (CNS) signs is a poor prognostic indicator, some dogs may recover. Prognosis worsens with increased severity of neurologic signs. Some dogs who recover will clear their clinical signs, while others may have neurologic signs that persist but do not progress (e.g. persistent myoclonus.)

11.6.1 Secondary Infections Associated with Immunosuppression

As described above, CDV can cause a period of immunosuppression with or without concurrent typical signs of canine distemper. In shelters, this immunosuppression most often leads to clinical signs of canine infectious respiratory disease (CIRD). This disease complex is caused by a variety of bacteria (*Bordetella, Streptococci, Pasteurella*), Mycoplasma, and viruses (Canine Adenovirus-2, Canine Parainfluenza Virus (CPiV) and others) and is described in Chapter 10. When present in dogs co-infected by canine distemper, CIRD may cause severe clinical signs including pneumonia and death. In shelters, respiratory disease from secondary pathogens may appear more quickly than actual pulmonary infection with CDV. Immunosuppression may also contribute to other opportunistic infections.

Subclinical infections are possible. Fortunately, these subclinical infections have not generally been of great concern in transmission or outbreak management. More importantly, clinical signs of mild CDV infections may be missed or may mimic many of the clinical signs associated with more mild forms of infectious respiratory disease. These mildly affected dogs shed virus which, if unrecognized, can be associated with a substantial risk of transmission.

11.6.2 Recovery

CDV remains a potentially fatal disease and can lead to profound illness and mortality in some dogs. Outbreaks can cause devastating problems for shelters; resolution can require thousands of dollars in resources for treatment and diagnostic testing. But the situation for individual dogs and shelters facing problems with CDV has improved dramatically in recent years. While neurologic disease still carries a poor prognosis, this clinical manifestation is uncommon, especially when even partial vaccine protection is present. In the numerous outbreaks managed by the author and others involving hundreds of dogs, the vast majority of animals had uncomplicated recoveries when treated effectively with prompt supportive care. Mortality from outbreaks tends to be lowest in shelters that vaccinate on intake. Once recovered from clinical signs, dogs will normally be immunocompetent and can be vaccinated and spayed/neutered without additional precautions for the individual dog. It is important to reiterate that vaccination for CPV should not be delayed because of CDV infection.

11.6.2.1 Viral Shedding, Carrier State and Confirming Recovery

Viral shedding begins by one-week post-infection, sometimes before the development of clinical signs, and usually resolves within a short period of time following the resolution of clinical signs. In some cases, however, viral shedding may persist for as long as 16 weeks.

Though there is no carrier state per se for CDV, recovered animals may remain infectious even after the resolution of clinical signs. Shedding is most common in respiratory secretions but is possible from all tissues and bodily excretions. Defining recovery and developing confidence that dogs are no longer an infectious risk is essential to disease control and outbreak resolution and can be achieved through diagnostic testing.

For defining recovery, polymerase chain reaction (PCR) testing is probably best performed starting soon after the resolution of clinical signs. A positive PCR suggests the animal may remain contagious to others, while a negative PCR suggests the dog is less likely to be infectious. Viral load normally drops significantly as clinical signs resolve. (See the diagnostic section 11.7 for more details.)

In the author's experience, a small fraction of dogs may remain RT-PCR positive at low quantitative levels for extended periods of time (months) after recovery. It remains unclear at the time of publication if the genetic material being detected in these dogs represents viable virus or a transmission concern. In the author's preliminary investigations, virus isolation from swab samples collected from these "long shedders" yielded no viable virus. (Research is currently underway.) There is no one right answer for how to manage the rare dogs who remain RT-PCR positive. General recommendations involve keeping the dogs away from susceptible dogs and housing in foster or adoption homes with immunized dogs.

11.7 Diagnosis of Canine Distemper

Diagnostic testing can be utilized to confirm infection and determine if recovered dogs are still infectious. Diagnostics can also be used to make risk assessments that identify dogs who are likely to be protected from infection.

In the early stages of the disease, it is often difficult to recognize distemper, as the signs may resemble CIRD (or Kennel Cough) or other diseases depending on the system affected. As described above, clinical signs of CDV encompass a wide range of disease symptoms that frequently overlap with other conditions commonly seen in shelters. Oculo-nasal discharge, upper and lower respiratory tract disease, and gastrointestinal (GI) disease such as inappetence, vomiting, and diarrhea are the most common early signs of disease. While neurologic disease is the most distinctive late phase clinical sign, it is, thankfully, seen less commonly.

Neurologic disease suggestive of CDV in any individual animal in a shelter setting warrants further investigation. Neurologic disease suggestive of CDV in animals within the population or after adoption, or markedly increased severity or frequency of CIRD is cause for diagnostic evaluation of both the individual and the population. In addition, diagnostic evaluation for any dogs with signs or history suggestive of CDV at intake will help to identify infection and diminish the risk of transmission.

11.7.1 Diagnostic Tests

Isolation of the wildtype (virulent) virus has always been difficult because the virulent virus does not readily replicate in tissue culture cells, either primary cells or cell lines. Appel found that primary cultures of alveolar macrophages could be used to isolate wildtype virus, but the cells did not grow well, fresh lung tissue was required, and the cells could not be passed (Appel and Jones 1967; Appel et al. 1992).

Because of the difficulty of growing CDV in tissue culture, fluorescent antibody (FA) tests were adapted for detection of CDV in tissue sections and in various other sources where cells could easily be obtained (e.g. conjunctival swab, rectal mucosa swab, leukocytes, etc.) These assays are used on cells from conjunctival, rectal, buccal, mucosal, and vaginal swabs, tracheal washes, cerebral spinal fluid (CSF), and buffy coats, as well as tissue biopsy imprints or sections (Damian et al. 2005; Saito et al. 2006). FA tests were used for years before the development of other more reliable and sensitive diagnostic methods.

The most commonly used diagnostic test is now reverse transcriptase-polymerase chain reaction (RT-PCR). RT-PCR may be used on samples taken either from living dogs or on postmortem tissue.

Postmortem testing may involve multiple tissue samples tested by RT-PCR, FA, or immunohistochemistry (IHC). Also, histologic tissue changes and the presence of viral inclusion bodies in cells are diagnostic for CDV (Appel 1987).

11.7.1.1 Reverse Transcriptase-Polymerase Chain Reaction (RT- PCR) Assay

RT-PCR assay is commonly used to detect viral nucleic acid in samples from suspect animals. Since CDV is shed in all body secretions/excretions during the acute systemic disease, a variety of samples can be tested and would be expected to be positive in infected dogs depending upon the phase of infection. Nasal, deep pharyngeal, and conjunctival swabs are most commonly collected. Conjunctival swabs tend to yield the least amount of virus and are the most objectionable to the dogs so are often omitted by the author when designing a sampling plan.

The sampling technique is especially important since the sensitivity is so high. False positives are possible from sampling contamination. Careful control of cross-contamination from one dog or swab to the next is essential and requires training, a glove change between each sample collected, and diligence to ensure all sampling instructions are followed.

It is also possible that samples tested from recently vaccinated animals may be positive because the modified live vaccine (MLV) CDV replicates in most of the same cell types as the virulent virus. Though vaccine virus replication is transient and non-pathogenic and the virus is not shed at sufficient levels to infect in-contact naïve animals, the sensitivity of RT-PCR may detect the vaccine virus in certain samples. It is not known with certainty how long after vaccination the individual animal would remain positive, what exact quantitative level would be seen, or how commonly positive results occur after vaccination. It is likely the animal would be positive as soon as three to four days after vaccination and viral nucleic acid could be detectable, at least in certain samples (those with leukocytes), for up to two weeks. The only vaccine that should not be detected would be the canarypox vectored recombinant CDV vaccine found in the Recombitek® vaccine.

Quantitative RT-PCR can help to differentiate mild infections, highly infectious animals, and vaccine positives. Positives may be reported out as either a Ct or a viral load that is estimated from the Ct. When a Ct is reported, a higher number means less genetic material was present and more cycles were run before the virus was detected. Estimates of viral load turn the Ct around into an estimated quantity of viral particles so the higher values indicate more virus was present. Some laboratories will provide a quantitative cut point above which they believe the virus more likely results from infection rather than from vaccination. Because recent vaccination is so common in many shelters, it should be verified that this information is available before selecting a laboratory to submit samples. In general, it is expected that vaccination would only result in positives with relatively low viral load or high Ct, within only about two weeks after vaccination, and only in dogs who were not previously immunized. It is important to recognize that mild, early, or late infections may also have a low viral load or high Ct that is not related to vaccination. Interpretation is needed to evaluate the results in conjunction with clinical signs, dates of vaccination, and possible exposure for the dog.

While RT-PCR is an extremely sensitive test, viral shedding may be intermittent, especially in the late or recovery phase of the illness. A single negative test result from a single sample may not completely rule out distemper. Because of this, repeat testing may be prudent in some cases, especially when suspicion is high or when attempting to define recovery. However, in outbreak settings, the resource investment required to obtain two negative tests to assign risk groups or define recovery must be carefully weighed with the additional care days needed and additional financial burden.

11.7.1.2 Serology

Serologic testing as a tool for diagnosis is not particularly valuable in a shelter setting. Serologic tests that measure IgM (early in infection) versus IgG (later in infection) have been used but are not reliable in the field or in a shelter where dogs are vaccinated at entry (Blixenkrone-Møller et al. 1991). Paired serology must be completed over a period of weeks. It is expected that rising titers will be seen in recently vaccinated dogs. More informative tests are available for diagnosis (e.g. IHC, FA, and PCR).

In contrast to its relatively limited value in diagnosing disease in individual dogs in a shelter setting, serologic testing is of great value in determining the immunologic status of dogs *entering shelters or that are present at the time of a CDV outbreak* and is described in the section on outbreak management in this chapter.

11.7.1.3 Postmortem Testing

Postmortem testing can be the most reliable means to definitively diagnose distemper in an individual animal and a population because multiple tissue samples can be examined. Also, histologic changes and the presence of viral inclusion bodies are diagnostic.

11.7.1.4 Immunohistochemistry and Fluorescent Antibody Tests

Immunohistochemistry (IHC), and to a lesser extent today, immunofluorescence can be used primarily on tissue sections after postmortem examination for detection of CDV in situ but RT-PCR is now more commonly performed as part of necropsies. Because these assays are designed to detect intact virus, with viral protein associated with the envelope antigens, these techniques have a reduced sensitivity and a shorter period of detection time compared to RT-PCR, which detects viral RNA. They are unlikely to detect CDV from the MLV for more than a few days, with a peak time of three to seven days after vaccination. This is in contrast to the presence of nucleic acids that are produced at higher levels and detected at higher sensitivity with PCR. Because CDV is widespread in tissue in infected dogs, IHC or FA of tissue sections are sensitive methods for postmortem diagnosis.

IHC can be performed on cells from antemortem samples, including conjunctival scrapes, urine sediment or buffy coat. These are not believed to be affected by recent vaccination so specificity is high, but due to variable shedding in these tissues, sensitivity is low and negative results do not rule out infection.

11.7.2 Initial Diagnostic Strategy

Recognizing disease and differentiating CDV infection from other potential pathogens is essential to provide appropriate treatment and effectively control disease in a shelter setting, as well as to identify concerns for rescue groups or adopters. Diagnostic testing also plays a key role in defining when an outbreak investigation or response is necessary, assigning risk groups, and determining when dogs are no longer a risk.

Diagnostics for an individual animal or population problem, such as a new arrival with suspicious signs, a shelter with endemic levels of disease or an outbreak of CDV, should be a priority whenever suggestive signs are present in an individual or within a population. Organizations having problems with the CIRD complex should always be wary of the possibility that CDV may be playing a role. Some additional criteria for heightened suspicion that CDV is present in a shelter population include:

- shelter and community history of problems with CDV
- vaccination practices that do not ensure ALL dogs are vaccinated immediately on intake
- development of neurologic disease in any dogs either in the shelter or after release
- markedly increased frequency or severity of CIRD
- management practices that favor transmission by allowing potentially infected dogs to remain in the general population or to have contact with healthy susceptible animals, especially very soon after intake and vaccination.

Evaluating samples from multiple dogs by PCR testing is a great beginning point for diagnostic inquiry if these risk factors are present. Ideally, a mix of dogs in varying stages of clinical illness would be sampled, including acutely affected dogs and some that have been sick a little longer (at least about 10 dogs or a good proportion of the population that has clinical signs).

Positive results on PCR should be carefully evaluated with consideration for both the quantitative value, the presence of illness in the population as a whole, and the individual animal's history including vaccination date, intake date, and severity of clinical signs. Additional diagnostics may be necessary as part of that evaluation process. If animals have died or are euthanized, necropsy testing of suspicious cases should be undertaken to permit definitive diagnosis and rule out cofactors.

11.8 Treatment

Treatment recommendations for CDV focus largely on supportive care. Detailed information about the treatment of canine distemper can be found in other veterinary textbooks; only the basics will be covered in this chapter. As mentioned earlier, systemic disease may lead to severe dehydration and emaciation, respiratory disease may progress to pneumonia, and immunosuppression facilitates invasion by secondary pathogens. Supportive care primarily revolves around intensive nursing care, fluid replacement and systemic vascular support, nutrition, and treatment or prevention of secondary bacterial infection. Supportive care and treatment for secondary infections are essential as the viral infection runs its course. Dogs who have not developed neurologic disease have the best prognosis for recovery. The prognosis becomes more guarded to grave for dogs who develop severe neurologic signs depending on severity. Mild neurologic signs, such as myoclonus, may be more manageable, but neurologic disease is often progressive during the course of illness and is often irreversible. In every case where treatment is being considered, both risk of contagion to other animals, prognosis, and welfare of the individual animal should be considered carefully.

The judicious use of broad-spectrum bactericidal antibiotics is recommended when treating respiratory disease associated with CDV. Viral pneumonia is often accompanied by secondary bacterial infections, or a primary bacterial pneumonia may be present due to CDV immunosuppression. Bacteria associated with primary or secondary pneumonia include *Bordetella bronchiseptica*, Streptococcal species, *Pasteurella multocida*, *Escherichia coli*, Staphylococcal species and Mycoplasma. Secondary infections may be susceptible to different antibiotics than those most commonly used in shelters to treat suspected primary Bordetella or mycoplasma infections.

When GI signs are present, broad-spectrum parenteral antibiotic therapy is essential. Fluid replacement therapy in the form of polyionic fluids such as Lactated Ringers solution corrects dehydration and helps prevent systemic collapse. B vitamins are also recommended. Anti-emetics should be given when vomiting is present. For dogs who are unable or unwilling to eat, other forms of nutritional support should be considered since treatment may be prolonged and body wasting is common.

Treatment for the neurologic disease is commonly less successful than supportive care for respiratory and systemic signs and is beyond the scope of this chapter.

11.9 Prevention, Management, and Response to Disease in the Shelter

11.9.1 Vaccination

Vaccination of all dogs and puppies at the time of, or prior to, intake is probably the most important method to prevent CDV from causing disease in shelters. Modified live virus vaccines for CDV are among the most effective vaccines available, inducing strong, protective immunity rapidly after administration. Even so, vaccination must be combined with planning and management strategies that focus on prevention.

Implementing programs designed to increase vaccination rates for dogs in the community, especially those who may not receive regular veterinary care, would be quite helpful in increasing overall population immunity. Please refer to Chapter 9 on Canine and Feline Vaccinations and Immunology for more information on this topic.

11.9.1.1 Vaccine Types

There are two types of vaccines available as of this writing: (i) modified live viral (MLV) CDV vaccine; and (ii) recombinant (r)CDV vaccine. The CDV vaccine from Boehringer Ingelheim has a canarypox vectored recombinant CDV component, whereas all the other products are conventional MLV. A small study suggested that the canarypox rCDV has the potential advantage of providing more rapid protection in the face of maternal antibody (Pardo et al. 2007). However, most puppies entering shelters do not have maternally derived antibody (MDA), likely because being an unsterilized bitch, having a litter of puppies that ends up in a shelter, and being unvaccinated, are risk factors arising from similar circumstances (Lechner et al. 2010). The MLV are generally lower cost than recombinant vaccines and have the theoretical advantage of being able to competitively occupy viral binding sites, generating protection even before humoral immunity is induced. Therefore, MLV are generally preferred in shelters for puppies as well as adults.

11.9.1.2 Vaccine Efficacy and Safety

MLV CDV and rCDV vaccinations provide significant protection even when dogs are challenged with exposure almost immediately following vaccination. One study (Schroeder et al. 1967) showed significant benefit from MLV CDV vaccination of susceptible puppies compared to those who were unvaccinated even when puppies were placed immediately into a CDV contaminated environment. Recombitek™, the rCDV vaccine product by Boehringer Ingelheim, provided protection against IV challenge one week after vaccination, and protected dogs placed in a distemper contaminated environment within hours of administration (Larson and Schultz 2006).

It is important to recognize that the very early benefits from vaccination described in the studies above are not likely to confer the same sterile immunity that can be expected a little later from vaccination for CDV. Full immunity does develop quite quickly but may not be reached for three to five days. Instead, the very early post-vaccine immunity provides protection from the development of severe neurologic disease and death. Dogs challenged by exposure within 72 hours of vaccination may become infected, shed virus, and be a risk to other susceptible dogs in the population even if they do not develop fulminant disease.

When vaccinations are administered on intake; preventative management practices are put in place to minimize co-mingling, exposure and stress; and sick animals are promptly isolated, the short lag between vaccination and onset of sterile immunity does not often lead to clinical problems. However, in environments where susceptible and potentially infectious dogs are housed or allowed to co-mingle together or share common space, the disease may still occur in dogs who are vaccinated at intake and exposed shortly afterward. This can create some confusion and be associated with ongoing, endemic disease that may mimic unusually frequent or severe CIRD.

11.9.1.3 Vaccine Handling

Because CDV is relatively labile, it is critical that the vaccine is reconstituted only shortly before use, taking care not to leave the vaccine at room temperature. If the room or ambient temperature is elevated, it is especially important that vaccines are reconstituted just prior to administration. The vaccine can be administered subcutaneously or intramuscularly. If any portion of the vaccine fails to be administered subcutaneously (e.g. part of it is injected onto the skin or hair coat), a second full dose should be given immediately.

11.9.1.4 Vaccine Timing and Revaccination

Every animal over four to five weeks of age should be vaccinated prior to or upon arrival to a shelter, regardless of their health status at the time of arrival. Vaccines are unlikely to cause harm, whereas virulent virus is likely to be present. For animals who are sick, it is possible, though not likely, the animal will be unable to mount an immunizing response. It is unlikely the vaccine will adversely affect the animal, while there is a good chance much needed protection will be provided.

Provided maternal antibody interference is not present, the majority of dogs over 16–20 weeks of age will be protected by a single vaccination. However, because of the severity of the illness, the low risk associated with the vaccine, and the small chance of vaccine failure due to factors such as incorrect handling or errors in administration, an initial series of two vaccines two to three weeks apart is generally recommended (Welborn et al. 2011). Dogs who remain in the shelter for long periods of time need not be re-vaccinated more often than every three years as per the American Animal Hospital Association (AAHA) vaccination guidelines.

11.9.1.5 Vaccination of Puppies

As with other diseases, interference from MDA can hinder effective immunization of puppies under 20 weeks of age. While many puppies will not have sufficient MDA to interfere and will be effectively immunized by the initial vaccine, it can never be certain which puppies may not be effectively immunized. Therefore, regular vaccination for puppies with combination vaccine products should begin at four to six weeks of age and be repeated every two weeks if puppies are in a high-risk environment such as a shelter or high population volume foster home, until 20 weeks of age. After adoption or transfer to a low-risk environment, the interval of revaccination can be extended to three weeks, but even after adoption, puppies should receive a final vaccine at or after

20 weeks of age. The rationale for giving the final vaccine for shelter puppies at a later age than has commonly been recommended for purposely-bred puppies is two-fold: the possibility that the dam recovered from field strain infection leading to higher than average levels of maternal antibodies, and the difficulty of accurately aging puppies when the exact birth date is unknown (as is often the case in shelters).

Again, it should be emphasized that vaccination alone will never be a sufficient intervention when disease and exposure risk is high. Vaccination programs must work in concert with management plans that decrease infectious dose and risk of exposure, especially for puppies who may remain susceptible even after vaccination. The best management plan for susceptible juvenile animals is almost always housing outside of the shelter in an alternate, low-risk environment.

11.9.1.6 Special Considerations for Pregnant Dogs in a Shelter

If a pregnant animal arrives at a shelter, the risks and benefits of vaccination must be carefully weighed. The safest CDV vaccine to use in pregnant dogs is the canarypox rCDV vaccine, as the MLV in immunologically naïve (CDV antibody negative) dogs has the potential to infect the fetuses, very rarely causing death and absorption or abortion. While there may be a small risk to the unborn puppies from vaccinating the dam, if she has not been previously immunized, the risk to the dam entering a shelter environment unvaccinated and susceptible, followed by likely to almost certain exposure, could be very high. As a result of an effort to protect the fetuses from the possible adverse effects of vaccination, the dam and the puppies could all be lost to the disease.

Regardless of the vaccine type used (recombinant or MLV), pregnant dogs that have antibodies will not be infected with the vaccine virus, thus the embryos/fetuses will not be affected. Because canine parvovirus is likely also a risk, a monovalent product for CPV should also be strongly considered if the ferret rCDV product is used.

11.9.1.7 CDV Vaccination of Other Species

For species other than dogs (e.g. raccoons, ferrets), the PureVax® Ferret rCDV vaccine (1.0 ml dose) should be used rather than a MLV vaccine because of the adverse reactions the MLV vaccine may cause in these species. MLV CDV vaccines should only be used in the species for which they were licensed.

11.9.2 Environmental Control

Because CDV is an RNA virus that is enveloped, the virus is rapidly inactivated outside the body by a variety of disinfectants, many of which are commonly used in shelters. (See Chapter 8 on Sanitation for more information.) CDV is also rapidly destroyed by heat. At temperatures of 56° C (130° F), it has a half-life of four to five minutes, at 45° C (113° F), 10 minutes, at body temperature and room temperature, 37° C (99° F) and 21° C (68° F) respectively, about one to three hours, and 9–11 days at 4° C (42° F). Therefore, unlike canine parvovirus-2, which is very stable in the environment and resistant to many disinfectants and heat, CDV is very labile and can be readily destroyed in the environment.

Notwithstanding this, even the short-term persistence of the virus in the environment can contribute to transmission. Efforts at decontamination in the face of an outbreak or persistent endemic disease concerns should focus on identifying points of common contact, especially surfaces likely to be in contact with sick and newly admitted, susceptible animals. This should include consideration of animal control vehicle compartments, intake pens that are also used for housing sick animals prior to transfer or euthanasia, and staff clothing if biosecurity precautions are not followed between handling sick and healthy individuals or populations.

11.9.3 Isolation and Separation

As mentioned above when describing transmission, infected dogs serve as the primary reservoir for the virus. When infected dogs are intermixed with susceptible dogs, transmission is very likely to occur. This makes isolation or separation of all dogs with clinical signs of disease an essential component of distemper prevention and control. This is especially true for respiratory disease because of the strong potential for aerosol transmission and the frequent overlap of signs of canine respiratory disease complex and early or milder to moderate canine distemper. However, as a general practice, dogs with any clinical signs of potentially infectious disease (e.g. GI, neurologic) should also be isolated from the general population.

Isolation for CDV ideally is achieved by the use of a separate building or ward, including separate airflow. Proper protective garments should be provided as well as separate equipment for use in the isolation area exclusively. Staff must be trained in isolation procedures and either designated to work in that area only, sequenced so that healthy animals are never handled or cared for after sick animals, or full biosecurity must be utilized, including a change of coveralls, gloves, and footwear between affected and susceptible populations.

In some cases, a separate ward is difficult to establish. In that case, creating separation where sick animals are promptly identified and moved, housed in a designated area separated by at least two empty kennels from the susceptible population, and never cared for ahead of healthy animals are strategies that have been effectively implemented to bring an end to disease transmission. Even simple measures to create separation between healthy animals and those with clinical signs can have a dramatic effect on improving animal health. Housing and/or treating sick animals in the general population will ensure exposure of the entire population, and if CDV is present, it will lead to severe disease in at least some susceptible animals.

Isolating or separating sick dogs removes the greatest source of exposure in the shelter. Subclinically affected dogs may still shed virus and go unrecognized as infectious, but this tends to be less clinically relevant. The reduction in infectious dose in the environment that results from isolating the dogs who are most obviously a potential risk has a substantial effect on clinical disease reduction.

Separation of sub-populations of apparently healthy dogs and puppies works hand in hand with isolation to protect susceptible animals as they enter the shelter. In many cases, transmission can be interrupted by establishing defined housing areas and order of care for specific susceptible groups.

Special handling practices to reduce transmission should be targeted toward the most susceptible animals. In general, separation is most important for puppies, since MDA may cause interference with vaccination that leaves many of them susceptible even post-vaccination. Healthy puppies should be housed in double-sided kennels that can easily be cleaned while the puppies remain protected within the enclosure, with designated equipment for use exclusively in that area and handling by staff wearing clean protective garments. Identifying clinical signs and isolating or separating sick animals promptly helps protect incoming animals during the first several days after admission when they have been vaccinated but have not had sufficient time to develop full immunity.

11.9.3.1 Planned Co-mingling and All-In All-Out Housing

Group housing dogs randomly at intake because there is insufficient housing in the shelter is an enormous risk factor for the transmission of many infectious diseases and creates poor welfare. Shelters with this practice should evaluate their intake and flow-through practices as well as housing capacity to implement change. If a shelter does plan to group house recently admitted dogs, screening carefully for signs of illness and planning co-mingling of apparently healthy dogs can reduce the risk of transmission presented in group housing by defining cohorts or subgroups within the general population; this reduces both the viral load and the number of animals to which each animal is exposed. To implement planned co-mingling, a system must be put in place defining which incoming healthy animals will be co-housed and interact with each other in playgroups or other activities. The simplest method is to identify behaviorally and physically compatible dogs who are entering the shelter at the same time (e.g. the same day). Only those dogs who are part of the planned cohort would interact with each other.

Though in general, co-mingling is not recommended, when undertaken, all-in all-out housing is an essential component of planned co-mingling. All-in all-out housing dictates that when co-mingling is necessary, all dogs will be removed from the housing unit or housing area before new susceptible dogs are brought in. Ideally, animals are moved through the shelter in cohorts. New animals should not be added once the group has been established. When all-in all-out practices are not used, it is possible that one subclinically infected animal could remain in an area long enough to expose another susceptible animal and so on, creating a cycle that allows persistence of the virus in the population. All-in all-out housing interrupts that cycle by creating small groups in which all dogs are less likely to have been infected. Each time one group leaves, the risk of exposure for the new group begins with just those dogs who have entered together, with no risk carried over from the previous group. All-in all-out housing is an important component of halting a cycle of transmission.

11.10 CDV Outbreak Management

If an outbreak of distemper does occur in a shelter, it is possible to control the outbreak and bring the shelter back to a healthy state by using life-saving evaluation and response tactics. Once an outbreak occurs, it becomes even more essential that all dogs are vaccinated prior to or at entry. Response measures, beyond vaccination, must also be taken when the disease has been identified in the general population. This consists primarily of assigning risk categories, creating a sanitary environment for incoming dogs (clean break) and isolating or removing exposed potentially infectious animals.

Please see Chapter 6 on Outbreak Management for more information.

11.10.1 Outbreak Risk Factors

Population health management practices play an important role in the prevention of CDV transmission in the shelter setting. Common risk factors in shelters experiencing outbreaks or ongoing problems with CDV in their populations include sporadic or delayed vaccination; failure to examine or vaccinate animals on intake; crowding beyond the capacity for care; kennels that are used inappropriately or in ways other than intended when designed (e.g. guillotine doors closed in double-sided housing units); group housing that is not all-in all-out; lack of separation between sick and healthy animals; poor or infrequent use of disease detection methods and lax response to respiratory disease that is believed to be "kennel cough." Animals transferred from other shelters may also increase the risk of CDV if the source shelters are in CDV endemic communities or have any collection of these risk factors.

11.10.2 Risk Assessment

Through a combination of careful observation of clinical signs and antibody testing, risk categories can be assigned to dogs. Risk categories help management to move dogs who are not likely to be affected by the disease through the shelter quickly, leaving a much smaller, more easily managed group for outbreak response or treatment.

While assigning risk groups never provides an absolute guarantee of whether a particular animal will become infected or not, defining the level of risk for individual animals and subgroups can at least guide informed decisions. Risk assessment can be used to clear animals for rescue or adoption and help guide efforts to create effective isolation and separation. Establishing risk categories for exposed animals limits the number of dogs subject to quarantine, isolation, or special rescue. Because some animals may have strong immunity to distemper demonstrable via serologic assessment, it may not be necessary to treat all who have been exposed as potentially infectious or "at-risk."

Serologic risk evaluation is a valuable tool, especially as an alternative to quarantine for CDV because its long incubation period, in many cases, makes quarantine of all exposed dogs difficult to impossible for many shelters to implement. Antibody testing correlates well with immunity for CDV, and both commercial and in-house tests (Vaccicheck™ and Synbiotics TiterCheck™) are available for this purpose. Those dogs that are free of clinical signs and have sufficient antibodies can be considered protected and are very unlikely to become infected or develop the disease. One caveat is that when disease detection and monitoring have not been consistently or effectively performed, it may be necessary to pair serologic testing with RT-PCR testing even in dogs with no clinical signs to be sure clinical signs weren't missed and the dogs are not in the recovery phase of illness and still shedding virus. In the author's experience, it is not uncommon in complex outbreaks to find apparently healthy dogs whose immune status and PCR testing together suggest they were recently infected and continue to shed some level of the virus as the outbreak intervention gets underway. It is important to identify and isolate these dogs when establishing a clean break to stop the cycle of transmission.

Using serologic testing sparingly on dogs recovering from clinical signs who tested positive on PCR can also save resources in an outbreak setting. It is almost certain that dogs who were infected will develop protective antibody titers, so serologic testing in these dogs should be a low priority for resource investment.

In-house serologic tests have great value because they can be run fairly quickly and simply and provide immediate answers about immunologic status. Samples for serology can also be sent to diagnostic labs, but turnaround time for results is important in an outbreak response setting. When attempting to identify low risk, clinically healthy animals for adoption or transport, it is more financially frugal to test for antibody first and pair positive antibody results with a PCR that suggests the dog is not currently shedding virus. If the dog is antibody negative or insufficient antibody is present to suggest protection, then a PCR should be repeated at the time the next antibody test was collected to suggest that the titer was rising because of vaccination and not as the result of infection.

Many questions arise about serology testing in puppies. Puppies under five months of age may have MDA present. This passive immunity is detectable on most serologic tests but can't be well differentiated from active immunity. Passive immunity does not have the backup system of antibody-producing memory cells that active immunity provides, which suggests it may be somewhat less protective. Also, maternally derived antibodies are constantly degrading, so antibody levels from passive immunity are likely to drop with time, making the puppies more at risk of infection. Adding to this complication is the potential for MDA interference with immunization from vaccination. With all of this being true, clinically, puppies with sufficient antibody titers appear to be protected from infection just as adult dogs are. The difference in terms of management is that while the immune status of adult dogs who are antibody positive will not change, it is probable that the immune status of puppies changes over time. While adult dogs who are known to be protected can remain in an environment where the virus is present, *it is essential that puppies identified as low-risk through antibody testing be removed from the risk of continued exposure as quickly as possible.*

When titer testing cannot be used to assign risk groups, dogs can be assigned to risk groups based on vaccination dates and the likelihood of exposure. However, this method will mean that many will be considered high risk unless a known start date can be identified for possible exposure or excellent management practices were in place to prevent transmission. If complete veterinary vaccination records are available, dogs who had been vaccinated when older than 20 weeks and prior to admission or possible exposure should be considered low-risk but revaccination is likely still the safest course of action. Verbal assertions by owners relinquishing dogs that they are "current on their vaccinations" are inadequate to ensure protection.

11.10.3 Quarantine Requirements for High-Risk/Exposed Dogs

If high-risk dogs must remain in the shelter, they should be separated from other dogs, especially those who have been recently admitted, recently vaccinated and all puppies under 20 weeks of age. In the past, it has been recommended that these dogs should be held for a quarantine period of at least four to six weeks to ensure that they are not incubating the disease. In many cases, this long holding time is impossible for the shelter; it also creates welfare concerns or runs the risk of actually contributing to more disease in the shelter due to crowding. Quarantine areas should have safety procedures equivalent to those described for isolation areas above in the section on isolation and separation. As an alternative, the development of positive serology paired with a negative RT-PCR can provide good evidence that a dog has developed immunity usually much sooner than the full incubation period.

11.10.4 Creating a "Clean Break": Protection of Incoming Dogs During an Outbreak

When responding to an outbreak, all dogs, without exception, must be vaccinated prior to or within minutes of entry. All incoming dogs should be placed into clean, disinfected kennels. Housing for incoming dogs should be located at least 25 ft away from moderate to high-risk dogs (based on titers, exposure history or clinical signs) and from other dogs coming in with clinical signs of disease; ideally, this should be a separate building or at least a separate ward. If necessary, this can be a separate set of runs with clear visual barriers delineating at-risk versus clean areas. As described above for isolation, separate staff and supplies should be used for new incoming dogs versus exposed/at-risk dogs. Dogs designated as low-risk based on titer testing can be housed with new incoming dogs, if necessary, based on space considerations.

When separate housing for exposed versus new incoming dogs is not possible, a "snaking clean break" has been used successfully to resolve an outbreak. While not ideal, this method can reduce risk and overall mortality. A snaking clean break is created by establishing a separation of exposed versus incoming dogs of at least 25–40 ft (7.7–12.2 m). This can be achieved, if necessary, by leaving several empty kennels between exposed and incoming dog housing areas. Clear visual markers designate each area, such as signage, rope, or chain barriers, and full-width curtains hung across aisleways. Designated equipment and biosecurity precautions must be used for each area just as would be the case if truly separate buildings or wards were available. However, as the population of exposed/at-risk dogs dwindles (e.g. through transfer or clearance of quarantine) and the population of newly admitted dogs grows through ongoing intake, the location of the clean break can be changed to accommodate this dynamic flow.

Initially, most of the dogs in the shelter may be considered exposed/at-risk and just a few kennels will be designated for new intakes, while late in the resolution of an outbreak the reverse will be true. Of course, thorough cleaning of kennels that are transitioning from housing exposed to newly admitted dogs is critical in this circumstance.

11.10.5 Summary of Outbreak Control

Outbreaks within the shelter can be brought under control with careful attention to the measures described above. Clinical cases may continue to occur, but they should be limited to dogs infected before entering the shelter. If timely preventive management practices are put into place as part of the outbreak response, disease transmission from these cases can be controlled and future outbreaks avoided.

11.11 Considerations for Adoption

Decision making and safety surrounding adoptions or transfers of dogs during or after an outbreak can be greatly aided by the use of diagnostic testing. Diagnostic testing can help assess if dogs continue to shed virus or are safe to interact with other dogs. A combination of RT-PCR testing for antigen and antibody testing can help to clear dogs for adoption or transfer. A negative RT-PCR test in combination with a positive antibody test suggests the dog is very unlikely to pose an infectious risk.

As noted earlier, some recovered dogs may continue to test positive on RT-PCR for prolonged periods. It is unknown at this time if dogs testing positive on RT-PCR for very prolonged periods actually continue to be an infectious risk, but until clarity is gained, it is important to proceed with caution. This rare prolonged timeframe for positive results is possible even for dogs where clinical signs have not been noted. In shelters that were not vaccinating at intake, viral shedding within the group tends to last longer.

Adopters or shelters receiving recovered or exposed/at-risk dogs **who have not been cleared using diagnostics** should be made aware that the dog may have been exposed or infected with CDV and advised to keep the dog away from areas frequented by puppies, due to disease progression or development of infection. These concerns arising from failure to utilize diagnostic testing to help define risk can create significant welfare concerns for all concerned, (i.e. the shelter, adopter and the dog), and is also likely a false economy compared with the cost of testing. In the author's experience, clearing dogs through diagnostic testing to allow for adoption and transfer without additional precautions has been a safe and powerful life-saving tool. After managing hundreds of dogs with this systematic process, we have not had any reports of a cleared dog going on to cause infectious problems or develop new clinical signs related to CDV.

11.12 Conclusion

Canine distemper remains an important and challenging disease, especially in animal shelters, throughout the United States and world. Fortunately, this potentially devastating disease is vaccine-preventable and if effective vaccination programs are used in shelters and, more importantly, if more dogs in the community were properly vaccinated, CDV could be substantially reduced as an important cause of disease. Until that time, meticulous examination and vaccination of animals on intake, careful monitoring, separation and isolation of symptomatic animals, and prompt diagnosis and response when the disease is suspected can greatly minimize the damage inflicted by this once-relentless disease.

References

Appel, M. (1987). Canine distemper virus. In: *Virus Infections of Carnivores* (ed. M. Appel), 133–159. New York;: Elsevier.

Appel, M. and Jones, O.R. (1967). Use of alveolar macrophages for cultivation of canine distemper virus. *Proceedings of Society for Experimental Biology Medicine* 126: 571–574.

Appel, M.J., Pearce-Kelling, S., and Summers, B.A. (1992). Dog lymphocyte cultures facilitate the isolation and growth of virulent canine distemper virus. *Journal of Veterinary Diagnostic Investigation* 4 (3): 258–263.

Blixenkrone-Møller, M., Pedersen, I.R., Appel, M.J. et al. (1991). Detection of IgM antibodies against canine distemper virus in dog and mink sera employing enzyme-linked immunosorbent assay (ELISA). *Journal of Veterinary Diagnostic Investigation* 3 (1): 3–9.

Damian, M., Morales, E., Salas, G. et al. (2005). Immunohistochemical detection of antigens of distemper, adenovirus and parainfluenza viruses in domestic dogs with pneumonia. *Journal of Comparative Pathology* 133 (4): 289–293.

Hurley, K.F. (2005). Canine distemper in the shelter: lessons learned from a Chicago outbreak. *Animal Sheltering* (September), pp. 39–43.

Ikeda, Y., Nakamura, K., Miyazawa, T. et al. (2001). Seroprevalence of canine distemper virus in cats. *Clinical and Diagnostic Laboratory Immunology* 8 (3): 641–644.

Krakowka, S., Olsen, R.G., Confer, A. et al. (1975). Serologic response to canine distemper viral antigens in gnotobiotic dogs. *Journal of Infectious Disease* 132: 384–392.

Larson, L.J. and Schultz, R.D. (2006). Effect of vaccination with recombinant canine distemper virus vaccine immediately before exposure under shelter-like conditions. *Veterinary Therapeutics* 7 (2): 113–118.

Lechner, E.S., Crawford, P.C., Levy, J.K. et al. (2010). Prevalence of protective antibody titers for canine distemper virus and canine parvovirus in dogs entering a Florida animal shelter. *Journal of the American Veterinary Medical Association* 236 (12): 1317–1321.

Pardo, M.C., Tanner, P., Bauman, J. et al. (2007). Immunization of puppies in the presence of maternally derived antibodies against canine distemper virus. *Journal of Comparative Pathology* 137 (Suppl 1): S72–S75.

Saito, T.B., Alfieri, A.A., Wosiacki, S.R. et al. (2006). Detection of canine distemper virus by reverse transcriptase-polymerase chain reaction in the urine of dogs with clinical signs of distemper encephalitis. *Research in Veterinary Science* 80 (1): 116–119.

Schobesberger, M., Summerfield, A., Doherr, M.G. et al. (2005). Canine distemper virus-induced depletion of uninfected lymphocytes is associated with apoptosis. *Veterinary Immunology and Immunopathology* 104 (1–2): 33–44.

Schroeder, J.P., Bordt, D.W., Mitchell, F.E. et al. (1967). Studies of canine distemper immunization of puppies in a canine distemper contaminated environment. *Veterinary Medicine/ Small Animal Clinician* 62 (8): 782–787.

Spencer, L.M. (1995). CDV infection in large, exotic cats not expected to affect domestic cats. *Journal of American Veterinary Medical Association* 206 (5): 579–580.

Summers, B.A., Greisen, H.A., and Appel, M.J. (1984). Canine distemper encephalomyelitis: variation with virus strain. *Journal of Comparative Pathology* 94 (1): 65–75.

Von Messling, V., Milosevic, D., and Cattaneo, R. (2004). Tropism illuminated: lymphocyte-based pathways blazed by lethal morbillivirus through the host immune system. *Proceedings of National Academy of Science USA* 101 (39): 14216–14221.

Welborn, L.V., DeVries, J.G., Ford, R. et al. (2011). 2011 AAHA canine vaccination guidelines. *Journal of the American Animal Hospital Association* 47 (5): 1–42.

12

Canine Influenza

Stephanie Janeczko

Shelter Medicine Services, American Society for the Prevention of Cruelty to Animals (ASPCA), New York, NY, USA

12.1 Introduction

Canine influenza virus (CIV) is an important pathogen that causes acute respiratory infection and must be considered in the diagnostic workup for canine infectious respiratory disease (CIRD). CIV typically causes mild to moderate upper respiratory signs, but more serious or even fatal disease may occur in a small proportion of cases. Since the identification of H3N8 CIV in 2004 and the introduction of H3N2 CIV to the United States in 2015, the virus has been an important health issue for shelter veterinarians to understand and address. While the prevalence of CIV in the general dog population remains low, high-density housing is clearly an important risk factor, and the introduction of an infected dog to a shelter is likely to have a significant impact on the entire population. A large outbreak can have serious long-term implications for animal shelters and can ultimately impact an entire community.

Active efforts are necessary to break the infection cycle in shelter environments. While many of the strategies employed to prevent and manage CIRD in shelters are applicable to CIV, others are unique to this pathogen. Prompt isolation of clinically ill animals and timely diagnostic testing, along with quarantine of exposed dogs, are critical tools in the management of this virus. (See Chapter 10 for more information on Canine Infectious Respiratory Disease).

The purpose of this chapter is to provide veterinarians with current information on diagnosis, therapy, and basic strategies for managing CIV in shelter environments.

12.2 Epidemiology of Canine Influenza Virus

12.2.1 Etiologic Agent

Influenza A viruses are negative-sense, single-strand ribonucleic (RNA) viruses (family *Orthomyxoviridae)* that can cause acute respiratory disease in humans, horses, pigs, and domestic poultry (Webster et al. 1992). Influenza A viruses are subtyped based on the hemagglutinin (H) and neuraminidase (N) proteins on the virion surface (Webster et al. 1992). To date, 18 hemagglutinin and 11 neuraminidase subtypes have been identified, each of which is antigenically distinct (Kosik and Yewdell 2019). As examples, human seasonal influenza is typically caused by subtype H3N2 or H1N1 viruses, while equine influenza is caused by subtype H3N8 virus. Canine influenza is a highly contagious

Infectious Disease Management in Animal Shelters, Second Edition.
Edited by Lila Miller, Stephanie Janeczko, and Kate F. Hurley.

respiratory infection of dogs caused by a novel influenza A subtype H3N8 or H3N2 virus.

12.2.1.1 H3N8 Subtype

The H3N8 subtype of CIV was first isolated from the lungs of racing greyhounds that died from pneumonia during outbreaks of acute respiratory disease at tracks in Florida in March 2003 and January 2004 (Crawford et al. 2005). A retrospective seroprevalence study found evidence of an H3N8 canine influenza-like virus circulating in racing greyhounds as early as 1999 (Anderson et al. 2012). Subsequently, CIV has been associated with respiratory disease outbreaks involving thousands of racing greyhounds and non-greyhound dogs across the United States and in Florida, Colorado, New York, and other northeastern states in particular (Crawford et al. 2005, 2006; Yoon et al. 2005; Payungporn et al. 2008; Parrish and Voorhees 2019).

Phylogenetic analyses of H3N8 CIVs indicate that they are closely related to equine lineage H3N8 viruses isolated from horses in the United States since 2000 (Crawford et al. 2005; Payungporn et al. 2008). The close genetic relationship suggests the interspecies transmission of influenza viruses from horses to dogs at some point in the recent past, followed by viral adaptation to the dog with sufficient replication in the respiratory tract to cause clinical disease and sustained dog-to-dog transmission (Crawford et al. 2005; Payungporn et al. 2008). Retrospective analysis of a respiratory disease outbreak in 2002 in foxhounds in the United Kingdom also documented infection of the dogs with equine influenza H3N8 virus, but there is has been little evidence of ongoing influenza infections in dogs in the United Kingdom (Daly et al. 2008).

Despite the potential for widespread community transmission, after 15 years of circulation within the US dog population, H3N8 CIV now has a patchy distribution with a low level of transmission. There is evidence that in a small number of endemic hot spots in large animal shelters, CIV has a high reproductive potential within these facilities, which act as a persistent source of viral transmission to the larger dog population in which sustained spread does not seem to occur in an ongoing or efficient manner (Dalziel et al. 2014; Parrish and Voorhees 2019). Lack of evolution to increase transmissibility within the dog population coupled with improved control measures in shelters, including the availability of vaccination against CIV, may explain the limited circulation of H3N8 in recent years (Voorhees et al. 2017).

12.2.1.2 H3N2 Subtype

The H3N2 subtype of CIV is of avian origin and was first detected in South Korea in 2007 in both individually owned dogs as well as in dogs housed in an animal shelter (Song et al. 2008). Subsequent investigations confirmed that the virus had been circulating in South Korea and China since at least 2005–2006 (Li et al. 2010; Lee et al. 2012) and may have existed as early as 1999 (Zhu et al. 2015). The virus remains in circulation in Asia, including Thailand (Bunpapong et al. 2014).

This subtype was first reported in the United States in February–March 2015, with rapid spread through high-density housing environments (i.e. animal shelters and boarding facilities) and veterinary clinics of the Chicago area. The virus was detected in neighboring states by early April, outside the Midwest by May, and in several eastern and southeastern states within a year of its introduction despite the implementation of control measures. Whole-genome sequencing confirmed the virus to be most similar to the H3N2 CIV circulating in South Korea, and phylogenetic analysis showed that the outbreaks were the result of a single virus introduced in the Chicago area that was then broadly dispersed (Voorhees et al. 2017). Additional smaller, limited outbreaks have been reported since 2015, each stemming from separate and single introductions of the virus in the United States from China and South Korea. Many of these subsequent outbreaks were associated with dog shows. In at least one incident, the virus was introduced to Canada via the United States by dogs originally imported from South Korea (Weese 2018). The exact point of introduction to the United States remains unknown but it has been hypothesized to be the result of the importation of infected dogs rescued from meat farms or animal markets in Asia.

Despite multiple introductions, H3N2 CIV in the United States has been characterized by sporadic outbreaks and then fade-out of the virus. As result, it has been suggested that the virus is poorly transmissible within the general dog population and that introduction to, and spread within and from higher density populations (i.e. animal shelters and boarding kennels) is necessary for ongoing, sustained transmission (Voorhees et al. 2018).

12.2.2 Susceptible Species

Because CIV is still a relatively novel pathogen, virtually all dogs are susceptible to infection due to the lack of preexisting immunity, unless they have been previously exposed to and recovered from the specific subtype in question. Vaccines are available to protect dogs against both H3N2 and H3N8, but they do not induce sterilizing immunity, so even previously vaccinated dogs may still be susceptible to infection, if not obvious clinical disease.

There has been no evidence of zoonotic transmission of H3N8 CIV from dogs to people (Krueger et al. 2014). Despite the initial jump from horses to dogs, there has been no evidence of H3N8 CIV transfer back to horses or transmission to other species, and no evidence that this subtype has been involved in reassortments with other influenza viruses (Dalziel et al. 2014).

Interspecies transmission of H3N2 CIV remains a greater possibility, however, as this subtype appears to have a much broader host range than H3N8 CIV. In one study, ferrets and guinea pigs were found to seroconvert, shed virus, and develop lung lesions in the absence of clinical disease (Lyoo et al. 2015), while in another study, cats and ferrets were shown to develop clinical signs, viral shedding and serologic responses when inoculated with H3N2 CIV experimentally or through direct contact with infected conspecifics (Kim et al. 2013). Airborne interspecies transmission of H3N2 CIV from dogs to cats was demonstrated in one experimental study (Kim et al. 2013), and there are at least two reports of infection and clinical disease in cats following natural exposure to H3N2 CIV-infected dogs in animal shelters (Song et al. 2011; Jeyoung et al. 2013).

There are no documented cases of zoonotic transmission of H3N2 CIV from dogs to people, and it is believed that further adaptation is likely necessary for this virus to pose a threat to humans. However, dogs are a potential mixing vessel for mammalian and avian influenza viruses, and naturally occurring reassortants of H3N2 CIV and both the swine and pandemic H1N1 subtype have been reported (Song et al. 2012; Na et al. 2015; Chen et al. 2018). These occurrences highlight the potential for dogs to act in an intermediate role in the transmission of zoonotic and/or pandemic influenza viruses and thus the need for ongoing surveillance (Zhu et al. 2015; Sun et al. 2017).

12.2.3 Prevalence

Since its initial identification in 2004, H3N8 CIV has infected thousands of dogs in the United States. Its distribution, however, remains patchy with a prevalence in the general dog population that is almost certainly less than 3–5% based on the limited studies conducted to date (Barrell et al. 2010; Anderson et al. 2013; Wiley et al. 2013; Jang et al. 2017). Certain areas have had enzootic disease, most notably Florida, Colorado, and New York, but even this has changed in recent years with H3N8 CIV infections occurring at a relatively low rate at the time of this writing. Similarly, the overall prevalence of H3N2 CIV in the general dog population in the United States appears to be quite low (Voorhees et al. 2018;

Gutman et al. 2019; Parrish and Voorhees 2019), with occasional sporadic introductions of the virus followed by limited outbreaks that have not been sustained or become more widely dispersed. It is likely that some low level of transmission may still occur within the canine population, and it is important to note that serologic evidence supports a much higher prevalence of infection in countries from which the importation of H3N2 CIV to the United States is believed to have occurred (Lee et al. 2009).

Activities that put dogs in close contact with other dogs, including attending dog shows or doggie daycare programs, or spending time in a boarding facility are risk factors for CIV infection. Shelter facilities are also at higher risk for CIV; following the introduction of the virus to a facility by a community dog, endemic disease resulting from continued spread to newly introduced naïve dogs is likely to occur in the absence of concerted measures to interrupt the transmission cycle (Pecoraro et al. 2014). It has been proposed that a small number of animal shelters with endemic H3N8 CIV serve as the reservoir for this subtype; sustained transmission in small facilities and within the general population would not be possible otherwise (Dalziel et al. 2014).

12.2.4 Morbidity, Mortality, and Prognosis

Like most influenza A viruses, canine influenza is a disease with high morbidity but low mortality. Nearly all exposed dogs become infected, and most have clinical disease while some have a subclinical infection. Most dogs with the clinical disease develop mild upper respiratory tract signs and recover within 10–14 days, with resolution of the clinical signs in nearly all dogs by 30 days. More severe disease manifestations are typically the result of co-infection with one or more other viral or bacterial pathogens in the CIRD complex, or due to other co-morbidities affecting individual patients.

12.2.5 Transmission

Influenza viruses are rapidly transmitted between animals by a combination of aerosols, droplets, and direct contact with respiratory secretions or contaminated fomites (Tellier 2006). Coughing and sneezing generate substantial amounts of virus in droplets and aerosols, forming suspensions that remain airborne for prolonged periods and travel long distances before settling down on surfaces (Tellier 2006). As demonstrated for influenza in other species, aerosols are important contributors to the spread of CIV in shelters and may account for the explosive onset of disease in many dogs over a short period of time. Distances traveled by CIV-containing aerosols are unknown, but aerosol transmission of human influenza viruses has been documented at distances over 50 ft. Direct dog-to-dog transmission and fomite-associated transmission are two other important means of CIV transmission. CIV spread within shelters has anecdotally been attributed, in part, to human handling of infected dogs followed by contact with other dogs without decontamination of hands and clothing. Sustained transmission of CIV appears far more likely to occur in a shelter setting where high infection pressures result from the density of animal housing and the continual introduction of naïve animals. As stated earlier, it has been posited that endemic disease within a relatively few large animal shelters act as a reservoir for H3N8 CIV, as the reproductive number (R_0) in the general dog population is close to 1.0. Thus, it is the heterogeneity in dog-to-dog contact rather than transmission efficiency that limits the spread of this subtype (Dalziel et al. 2014). The H3N2 subtype has similarly been shown in multiple US outbreaks to have an $R_0 = 1.0–1.5$, suggesting that ongoing infection within high-density populations and/or reintroduction from other populations is necessary for continued circulation in the dog population in this country (Voorhees et al. 2018).

12.2.6 Incubation and Shedding Periods

The incubation period is approximately two to five days from exposure to onset of clinical signs. This relatively short incubation period is typical for influenza in other species and is shorter than for some other causes of acute respiratory diseases such as canine distemper virus and *Bordetella bronchiseptica*.

Studies in naturally and experimentally infected dogs have shown that H3N8 CIV may be shed for up to seven days in most dogs, and to 10 days in some dogs (Crawford et al. 2005; Rosas et al. 2008; Larson et al. 2011). Peak viral shedding from the upper respiratory tract occurs two to four days post-infection; since this overlaps with the incubation period, infected dogs may be most contagious before or at the onset of clinical signs.

Influenza A viruses do not establish persistent infections, and no carrier state has been described. Though some dogs have a subclinical infection, there is no true carrier state. Once virus replication and shedding cease, the dog is no longer contagious to other dogs. Shedding usually ends by 7–10 days post-infection for the H3N8 subtype, but intermittent shedding has been reported to extend beyond 21 days in some dogs infected with the H3N2 subtype (Hong et al. 2013; Newbury et al. 2016). Thus, when managing CIV in a shelter environment, it is critical to recognize and address the fact that outwardly healthy dogs may serve as a source of infection for other dogs before the onset of clinical signs or due to subclinical infection, and that dogs clinically recovered from H3N2 infection may continue to shed virus for an extended period of time.

12.3 Clinical Signs

Distinguishing canine influenza from other causes of acute respiratory disease can be very difficult and is not possible solely based on the clinical presentation. Laboratory testing is necessary to confirm a clinical suspicion of CIV infection, and to determine which subtype is present. In a population of dogs with CIV, there may be a sudden increase in the prevalence of acute respiratory disease, the severity of illness, or a prolonged to complete lack of response to antibiotic therapy for *B. bronchiseptica*. When introduced into a naïve population, CIV typically causes an explosive onset and spread of "kennel cough" in most dogs in the shelter within a short period of time, usually less than two weeks. Once CIV has become established in a population, the classic rapid spread of disease is less apparent. Dogs of all ages are susceptible to infection with CIV and prior vaccination against canine distemper virus, adenovirus type 2, parainfluenza virus, and *B. bronchiseptica* does not diminish introduction and spread of CIV within the shelter population.

Approximately 80–90% of infected dogs develop clinical disease. A small percentage (10–20%) of dogs are subclinically infected and appear healthy yet are shedding virus. Therefore, all exposed dogs in the facility should be considered an infectious risk, whether or not they are showing signs of respiratory illness. Mild upper respiratory symptoms are most commonly seen. Coughing is the predominant clinical sign and can persist for several weeks, even with antibiotic and antitussive therapy. Fever is common, and dogs may have mild anorexia and a mucopurulent to purulent nasal discharge due to secondary bacterial infections. Approximately 1–20% of dogs may progress to more severe illness resulting from lower respiratory tract involvement, characterized by high fever, lethargy, inappetence, tachypnea or dyspnea, productive cough, and prolonged recovery. The fatality rate related to pneumonia is reported to be 5–8%, but with rapid diagnosis and aggressive therapy, it may be much lower. Peracute fatal hemorrhagic pneumonia has only been reported in the literature in greyhounds, though there have been some anecdotal reports of this clinical presentation where CIV has been confirmed and no other pathogens were identified.

Canine influenza cannot be distinguished from respiratory disease caused by other infectious agents based on clinical signs alone. Also, coinfections with other respiratory pathogens may occur, all producing similar clinical signs. Ultimately, diagnostic testing must be performed to differentiate the cause(s) of "kennel cough" or CIRD in individual animals or larger populations. The reader is directed to Chapter 10 for further information on CIRD.

12.4 Diagnosis

There are multiple laboratory methods available for the detection of influenza infection, including virus isolation, virus antigen detection by immunoassays, virus nucleic acid detection by polymerase chain reaction (PCR), and serology for virus-specific antibody. Each method has strengths and weaknesses that are important for shelter practitioners to understand. The timing of sample collection relative to viral shedding relates directly to test performance. To institute optimal control measures, it may be necessary to combine several diagnostic approaches to identify the etiological agent accurately and rapidly.

12.4.1 Swabs for Immunoassays, PCR, and Virus Isolation

During the first few days following infection, clinical signs are generally inapparent to mild, but viral shedding in nasal secretions is high. It is during acute influenza infection that achieving a diagnosis is often most critical for case management and outbreak control. Diagnostic methods aimed at detection of the virus (i.e. antigen detection methods, PCR-based assays, and virus isolation) are the preferred tests for early cases. Nasal and/or caudal pharyngeal swabs can be used for these tests. Swabs should be collected from exposed subclinical dogs or those with early clinical signs (one to three days) to coincide with peak virus shedding. To maximize the detection of CIV, swabs should be collected from multiple dogs in the population. If testing is being done through a commercial reference laboratory, it is recommended to contact the laboratory in advance for collection, handling and shipping preferences.

Patient-side immunoassay kits for human influenza A infection can be used for diagnosis of CIV. These kits detect the highly conserved nucleoprotein of influenza A viruses, but the sensitivity is unknown. Some shelters have these kits on-site for in-house use. The tests do not require special equipment, are easily performed, and provide rapid results. Positive results are most likely correct, but negative results may be "falsely negative" due to the critical timing of swab collection with peak virus shedding. Nasal and/or caudal pharyngeal swabs are also used for the detection of CIV nucleic acid by PCR tests (Spindel et al. 2007; Payungporn et al. 2008).

PCR testing is inexpensive and fast and is now offered by most reference and university diagnostic laboratories as stand-alone tests or as part of a respiratory PCR panel. The laboratories should be contacted in advance for collection, handling, and shipping preferences, and practitioners are advised to confirm the exact pathogens (including which CIV subtype(s)) are being tested for as part of that specific laboratory's panel. An outbreak of unknown infectious respiratory disease warrants laboratory investigation. A representative sampling of dogs within the population for PCR testing of multiple CIRD pathogens is generally the most efficient and cost-effective means of obtaining a diagnosis and implementing a targeted management plan, particularly when multiple pathogens are present.

PCR tests are highly sensitive and specific and are more likely than virus antigen immunoassays to yield positive results when low amounts of virus are present. However, the assay's high sensitivity can produce false-positive results due to DNA contamination during sample collection as well as during sample processing in the laboratory. Shelter personnel should wear clean examination gloves for each dog and only touch the swab tip to the area sampled to avoid contamination by nucleic acid on hands and in the environment. False-negative results may occur due to inappropriate sample collection and handling or inappropriate timing of sample collection (i.e. several days or longer after the onset of clinical signs). Other diagnostic samples such as transtracheal washes, bronchoalveolar lavage fluid, and tissues can be submitted for CIV PCR and should be considered particularly when clinical signs of lower respiratory disease are present.

Virus isolation from clinical samples is critical for epidemiologic investigation, but it may have limited use for routine diagnostic purposes as it is a slow and specialized test. Laboratories that offer virus isolation should be contacted in advance for collection, handling, and shipping preferences.

In general, the best results for virus isolation are often achieved by collecting nasal and/or pharyngeal swabs using polyester-tipped swabs. Cotton swabs should be avoided, as influenza viruses can adhere to the cotton fibers, thus decreasing the likelihood of virus isolation. The swabs should be placed in sterile dry tubes or tubes containing viral transport medium (depending on laboratory preference) and kept on ice packs for shipping to a laboratory. Depending on the amount of viable virus present in the sample and sample handling, virus isolation can take three to five days for the initial growth of CIV.

12.4.2 Serology

Serology is a reliable diagnostic test for confirmation of CIV infection and ideally should be performed in conjunction with other tests to confirm canine influenza infection and rule other CIRD pathogens in or out of consideration. CIV-specific antibodies can be detected in a hemagglutination inhibition assay as early as seven days post-infection, but reliable detection occurs after 10 days of clinical signs (Anderson et al. 2006). Therefore, a negative antibody titer for serum samples collected before day 10 does not rule out infection. Because the presence of antibodies indicates exposure, but not necessarily active infection, comparing an acute titer and a convalescent titer (two weeks apart) to confirm a four-fold rise in antibody titer (seroconversion) is necessary to prove recent active infection. However, because most dog populations remain naïve to CIV, a single positive titer in a dog that had consistent clinical signs and was not previously vaccinated against CIV may be sufficient for an initial or presumptive diagnosis. The relationship of timing of sample collection and performance of various diagnostic methods for H3N8 CIV is shown by results from one Florida shelter in 2007 (see Table 12.1).

12.4.3 Ancillary Diagnostic Work-Up

Once a diagnosis of canine influenza is confirmed, further workup may be very different in a single dog compared to a population of many dogs. Facilities with large numbers of symptomatic animals may not have the resources to perform a complete work-up on multiple dogs. Alternatively, veterinary decisions may be made that best utilize resources and allow for maximal numbers of dogs to be treated.

A complete blood cell count (CBC) with differential, serum biochemistry profile, urinalysis, and thoracic radiographs can yield important information. The CBC may be normal or show mild leukopenia suggestive of viral infection. If pneumonia is developing, leukocytosis consisting of neutrophilia with or without a left shift may be detected. Thoracic radiograph findings range from mild broncho-interstitial infiltrates to the consolidation of all lung lobes.

CIV replicates in the epithelial layer lining the nasal passages, trachea, bronchi, and bronchioles, resulting in sloughing of the damaged epithelium and exposure of underlying tissues to potential bacterial infection. Bacterial cultures performed on nasal swabs from dogs

Table 12.1 Diagnostic test results for a canine influenza outbreak in an animal shelter[a].

Dog ID	Clinical Signs	Duration	Influenza A Nucleoprotein	Influenza A Matrix Gene PCR	Virus Isolation	Acute Antibody Titer	Convalescent Antibody Titer
1	None – exposed	1 day	negative	negative	not done	4	64
2	Sneeze/cough	1 day	positive	positive	positive	4	256
3	Cough	1 day	negative	negative	not done	4	512
4	None – exposed	1 day	negative	positive	positive	4	128
5	None – exposed	1 day	negative	negative	not done	4	256
6	None – exposed	1 day	negative	negative	not done	4	128
7	Nasal discharge	1 day	negative	negative	not done	4	512
8	Cough	1 day	negative	negative	not done	4	512
9	Cough/nasal discharge	1 day	positive	positive	positive	4	1024
10	Cough/nasal discharge	1 day	negative	positive	positive	4	512
11	Cough/nasal discharge	1 day	negative	positive	positive	4	1024
12	Cough/nasal discharge	1 day	negative	negative	not done	4	1024
13	Cough/nasal discharge	1 day	negative	negative	not done	4	512
14	Cough	3 days	negative	positive	positive	4	1024
15	Cough	3 days	positive	positive	positive	4	1024
16	Cough/nasal discharge	3 days	positive	positive	positive	4	1024
17	Cough	4 days	negative	positive	positive	4	1024
18	Cough	4 days	negative	suspect	positive	4	1024

[a] Nasal swabs were collected between days one and four of clinical signs for the detection of influenza A nucleoprotein (Directigen Flu A®) and nucleic acid (matrix gene PCR). Virus isolation was performed on PCR-positive samples. Paired acute and convalescent serum samples were collected for CIV antibody titers using the hemagglutination inhibition test. Antibody titers <32 are negative.

with a purulent nasal discharge and on transtracheal and endotracheal washes of dogs with pneumonia have revealed secondary infections with a variety of commensal gram positive and gram negative bacteria, including *Staphylococcus* spp., hemolytic and nonhemolytic *Streptococcus* spp., *Pasteurella multocida, Klebsiella pneumoniae, Escherichia coli*, and *Mycoplasma* spp.

The value of a necropsy should not be overlooked in the diagnostic work-up for respiratory infections, including canine influenza. If dogs are euthanized or die during respiratory disease outbreaks, a prompt necropsy with the submission of tissues to diagnostic laboratories for histopathology, bacterial and viral cultures, and PCR can provide very valuable information. At a minimum, sections of trachea, lung, liver, spleen, kidney, and urinary bladder should be fixed in 10% buffered formalin for histopathology. For cultures and PCR, sections of fresh trachea and lung should be placed in a sterile container, refrigerated, and shipped to a diagnostic laboratory as soon as possible.

12.5 Treatment

Not all dogs with canine influenza require therapeutic intervention. Therapy relies mainly on supportive care while the viral infection runs its course. There is little evidence to support the use of antitussives for reducing the frequency and duration of coughing. In addition, antitussives are contraindicated in dogs with productive cough. Antibiotics are indicated for dogs with secondary bacterial infections (or co-infection with a primary bacterial pathogen, such as *B. bronchiseptica* or *Streptococcus equi* subsp. *zooepidemicus*) evidenced by mucopurulent discharge along with fever, lethargy, or inappetence. Ideally, bacterial culture and antibiotic sensitivity tests should be performed on each dog to determine the most effective antibacterial therapeutic plan. The use of a reference for proper procedure and accurate interpretation of susceptibility results is recommended (CLSI 2008).

Bacterial cultures for each dog may not be practical or financially feasible in a population of many affected dogs, so many shelters opt for empirical treatment. If there is no clinical evidence of pneumonia (i.e. crackles or wheezes on thoracic auscultation), a 7–10-day course of doxycycline has been recommended as a first-line antimicrobial option. Most dogs with a bacterial component to their CIRD will respond quickly to treatment. Thus, if a bacterial infection is still suspected after the first seven days and the initial treatment was ineffective, a more extensive diagnostic workup is indicated before initiating treatment with other antibiotics such as azithromycin or a fluoroquinolone (Lappin et al. 2017). For pneumonia, empiric treatment with a combination of antibiotics that provide coverage against gram-positive, gram-negative, aerobic, and anaerobic bacteria have been effective in many cases; however, patterns of response may vary. Dogs with pneumonia usually require intravenous (IV) fluids in addition to antibiotics. Oxygen supplementation and nebulization with coupage have been very beneficial. Despite aggressive therapy, severe pneumonia may lead to death or become a criterion for euthanasia.

There is no specific antiviral treatment for canine influenza at this time. Though treatment with oseltamivir (Tamiflu®, Roche Pharmaceuticals) has been suggested, the doses, frequency of dosing, and efficacy and safety of this human drug have not been determined for use in dogs with canine influenza. For best effect in humans, the drug needs to be started within 48 hours of infection; canine influenza is rarely diagnosed this early. Most importantly, Tamiflu® represents a primary line of defense against human seasonal influenza and pandemic influenza, so veterinary use of this drug should be reserved for the protection of human health. Limited data exists on other antiviral treatments; nitazoxanide and tizoxanide were shown to inhibit viral replication of H3N8 *in vitro* (Ashton et al. 2010) but no data has been published on their efficacy *in vivo*. Supportive care remains the mainstay of treatment for clinically ill dogs.

12.6 Prevention and Management

Many of the strategies employed to prevent and manage CIRD, which are discussed in Chapter 10 on CIRD, are broadly applicable to CIV. Unique considerations for CIV are discussed below.

12.6.1 Risk Assessment

As with any infectious disease outbreak, the management of CIV requires breaking the cycle of transmission between exposed, infected, and naïve (new intake) dogs. The short incubation and virus-shedding periods make this a more manageable proposition with H3N8 CIV compared with canine distemper and *B. bronchiseptica*, which have prolonged incubation and shedding periods; the longer quarantine period necessary for H3N2 CIV poses additional challenges. Because of the high transmissibility of CIV, all dogs in the shelter at the time a case is suspected or diagnosed should generally be considered exposed/at risk.

Whenever possible, owned dogs with respiratory illnesses should be isolated at home for two weeks prior to intake. For dogs with clinical evidence of respiratory disease that must be admitted, appropriate isolation and diagnostic testing procedures are important for the early detection and containment of CIV as well as other pathogens. Additional precautions, including a mandatory 14-day quarantine and aggressive testing protocol, are indicated for any dogs originating from South Korea and China (particularly those rescued from the meat trade) due to the relatively high prevalence of H3N2 circulating in those countries.

12.6.2 Quarantine and Isolation

Exposed dogs pose a risk of infection for 7–12 days for H3N8 CIV and a risk of infection to other dogs, cats, ferrets, and guinea pigs for more than 21 days for H3N2 CIV, considering both the incubation and shedding periods of each subtype. Though it may be difficult to implement a quarantine in shelters, to be safe, exposed dogs should be quarantined for a minimum of 14 days. Ensuring that fomite, aerosol, and direct-contact transmission do not occur between the exposed and unexposed populations of dogs is crucial in breaking the transmission cycle. Exposure of just one naïve dog can defeat the quarantine. It is also critical that shelters carefully monitor the quarantined population for any signs of illness (especially coughing) in individual dogs. If clinical signs are identified, dogs must be promptly moved to an isolation area and the quarantine clock restarted. Where resources allow, dogs in quarantine may be PCR tested four to seven days after exposure; negative dogs can be released from quarantine.

For shelters that can discontinue intake and the adoption of dogs for several weeks, quarantine of the entire population is ideal. The movement of dogs in and out of the facility should remain suspended until the virus is eliminated from the population. When discontinuation of intake is not an option, efforts should be made to limit canine intake to the facility to the greatest extent possible. This may include diversion of dogs to other facilities and/or a waiting list for owner relinquished canines. For those dogs that must enter the shelter, a clean area should be created for the intake of unexposed dogs. Whenever possible, this should be a physically enclosed room with separate ventilation. When a separate area like this is not available or cannot be created, exposed dogs can be housed together in one ward located as far as possible from wards used for new intakes. Alternatively, though a challenging task, the exposed population can be transferred to an off-site location. Foster care in a household with no other dogs is another option for holding exposed dogs for the quarantine period, especially adoptable dogs that have completed their stray holding period.

The quarantined population should be managed with strict biosecurity procedures to minimize CIV transmission, including the use of personal protective equipment (PPE) (gown or jumpsuit, gloves, boots, and hair covers) by staff. Ideally, personnel caring for dogs in the facility would be separated into distinct groups: one caring for sick dogs in isolation, one caring for exposed dogs in quarantine, and one caring for unexposed/newly admitted dogs. If this is not possible, then personnel should manage the unexposed population first, wearing PPE for the exposed and sick populations, and taking care to safely remove PPE and wash hands in between areas and prior to entering common use spaces. Care should be taken to prevent any inadvertent exposure of cats to dogs exposed to or infected with H3N2 CIV. There should be no visitors to the quarantined area unless they are reclaiming their dogs. In this circumstance, if possible, the owner and dog should try to leave by an exit that does not risk contamination of the facility.

Shelters in communities where CIV is endemic may have continual reintroduction of CIV into their population. In this situation, quarantines, diversion of new admissions, and shutdown of adoptions may become impractical or financially unreasonable. Shelters may have no choice but to continue intake and the release of dogs since CIV is a treatable disease with a good prognosis for recovery. However, this may contribute to the spread of infection to other facilities or households and perpetuate the endemicity of the virus in the community. Clients should be educated about CIV, advised to quarantine outwardly healthy dogs leaving the facility for 7–14 days, and informed about follow-up medical care. Similarly, clients should be advised to isolate dogs that are ill or recovered dogs for either a seven day or 21–28-day period for H3N8 and H3N2, respectively. This information should be provided in a written document. While shelters may opt to release dogs only after their quarantine, thus ensuring that the shelter is not serving as a continual source of community infection, it is important to balance the impact such practices would have on overall shelter density and capacity for care. Longer lengths of stay (LOS) have been shown to be a risk factor for seroconversion to H3N8; reducing exposure by minimizing the amount of time dogs spend in the shelter may be a more effective and practical strategy for some organizations (Holt et al. 2010). It must be acknowledged that many of these choices may be very difficult, if not impossible, for some shelters to implement. Please see the Introduction in Chapter 1 and Chapter 6 on Outbreak Management for more information on population management and biosecurity measures.

12.6.2.1 Post-infection Immunity

CIV-specific antibodies have been shown to persist in naturally infected dogs for at least five to six years (Anderson et al. 2007; Daly et al. 2008). Theoretically, dogs that recover from infection should be immune to reinfection with the same viral strain. However, the correlation of post-infection antibody titers with protection against reinfection and duration of protective immunity has not been established for natural infection with CIV. Furthermore, influenza viruses possess remarkable ability to mutate, so antibodies induced by infection with one strain may not be protective against infection by future strains that have mutated or against infection with new strains that are introduced from other parts of the world.

12.6.2.2 Euthanasia Criteria

CIV is a disease from which most dogs recover either on their own or with appropriate supportive treatment. However, some shelters have elected euthanasia of the entire or majority of the population in an effort to eliminate CIV from the facility. Many shelters have also euthanized individual dogs affected by CIV, particularly those with pneumonia. Treatment costs for large numbers of dogs, lack of space and staff to maintain quarantine, and lack of resources for isolation or intensive care of dogs with pneumonia have contributed to these decisions. Euthanasia guidelines for individual dogs and shelter populations with CIRD are presented in Chapter 10.

12.6.2.3 Community Education

Shelters that experience outbreaks of CIV should consider open and rapid communication with other local sheltering facilities, veterinarians, adoption/rescue groups, boarding kennels, adopters, the media and the public to provide increased awareness of virus activity in the community. Proactive communication provides a beneficial "advisory" so that other potentially affected parties can step up surveillance and biosecurity measures; this enhances the shelter's reputation as a valuable and considerate member of the animal welfare community.

12.6.3 Environmental Contamination and Disinfection

Influenza A viruses are enveloped viruses that do not persist in the environment for an extended period of time. These viruses can survive for 24–48 hours on nonporous surfaces (e.g. stainless steel, concrete, plastic), for 8–12 hours on porous surfaces (cloth, paper), and for minutes on hands (Bean et al. 1982). For CIV, routine cleaning and disinfecting are sufficient to inactivate infectious virus. Kennel surfaces should be cleaned first with a detergent to remove dirt and organic debris, followed by application of virucidal disinfectants such as an accelerated hydrogen peroxide product (Rescue™), sodium hypochlorite (household bleach), quaternary ammonium compounds, or potassium peroxymonosulfate (Trifectant®) at an appropriate concentration and contact time effective against enveloped viruses. The kennel surface should be dried before returning the dog. All potential fomites (e.g. bowls, bedding, toys, etc.) should also be cleaned and disinfected. The reader is referred to Chapter 8 for additional information on sanitation.

12.6.4 Vaccination

Vaccines against H3N2 and H3N8 subtypes are available as monovalent or bivalent products. As with most respiratory pathogens and similar to human influenza vaccines, vaccination against H3N2 and/or H3N8 provides only partial protection as it does not produce sterilizing immunity and does not prevent infection. At the time of publication, all commercially available vaccines were killed products, with limited information published about potential live-attenuated bivalent CIV vaccines (Rodriguez et al. 2017). For all available vaccines, two injections must be administered two to three weeks apart, with an additional one to two weeks after the second dose necessary for the development of a complete immune response to the vaccine. The vaccines will lessen the severity and duration of clinical signs and, perhaps most importantly in a shelter setting, reduce viral shedding. CIV is not a vaccine-preventable disease.

Widespread vaccination within the general dog population can help increase herd immunity and reduce community-based transmission, but vaccination upon entry to an animal shelter is less likely to have a significant impact on disease transmission within the facility. Vaccination against CIV is considered to be non-core for both pet and shelter-housed dogs, with its use typically reserved for those facilities that (i) encounter suspected or confirmed CIV infections, and (ii) house dogs long enough that administration of both doses in the initial vaccine series will typically be possible (Ford et al. 2017). When possible, the administration of both doses before entry to a sheltering facility is preferred to allow for the development of an immune response. When this is not possible, some shelters have developed systems to help ensure dogs receive both vaccine doses by administering the first dose 14 days prior to intake and giving the second dose upon entry to the facility, or by administering the first dose upon intake and partnering with veterinarians, adopters, and other shelters and rescue groups in the community to ensure the dog receives the second dose at the appropriate time. However, it is important to realize that even in such cases, vaccination will be of limited use in reducing transmission within the facility unless newly arrived animals can be protected from exposure for at least one to three weeks after intake. An additional consideration is that the costs to administer the vaccination to all arriving dogs against CIV are significant; shelters should carefully weigh this use of resources to determine if the benefits are sufficient to warrant its use. If a decision is made to proceed, it is recommended that any dog deemed at risk for exposure to CIV be vaccinated against both H3N2 and H3N8, recognizing that infection with H3N2 CIV is of greater concern for most shelter populations given the current prevalence and distribution of infections and the extended shedding period that occurs with this subtype.

To minimize coinfections with other respiratory pathogens and the possibility of more severe disease, all dogs, regardless of age or health status, should be vaccinated before or at intake against canine distemper, adenovirus-2, parainfluenza virus, and *B. bronchiseptica*.

12.7 Conclusion

CIV is an important cause of acute respiratory infection in dogs. High-density housing is an important risk factor and the introduction of just one infected dog to a shelter can have significant implications for the larger population. Though most infected dogs develop only mild to moderate upper respiratory signs, more serious or even fatal disease may occur in a small proportion of cases.

Continued vigilance for potential CIV infection is warranted, and early recognition of infected dogs will minimize the impact on individual animal health and welfare as well as that of the larger shelter and community populations. When CIV is present, active efforts are necessary to break the infection cycle including timely diagnostic testing and aggressive quarantine and isolation protocols for exposed and infected dogs. CIV is not a vaccine-preventable disease, but vaccination may be a helpful tool in some shelter populations. Ongoing surveillance for mutations, further introductions of circulating CIV subtypes, or the emergence of new influenza viruses capable of infecting dogs will be necessary to minimize the impact on animal and human health.

References

Anderson, T.C., Katz, J.M., Gibbs, E.P.J. et al. (2006). Development of a hemagglutination inhibition assay for diagnosis of canine influenza virus infection. *110th Annual Meeting USAHA and 49th Annual Conference of the American Association of Veterinary Laboratory Diagnosticians*, Minneapolis, MS, US (12–18 October 2006).

Anderson, T.C., Grimes, L. et al. (2007). Serological evidence for canine influenza virus circulation in racing greyhounds from 1999 to 2003. *Journal of Veterinary Internal Medicine* 21: 577.

Anderson, T.C., Bromfield, C.R., Crawford, P.C. et al. (2012). Serological evidence of H3N8 canine influenza-like virus circulation in USA dogs prior to 2004. *The Veterinary Journal* 191 (3): 312–316.

Anderson, T.C., Crawford, P.C., Dubovi, E.J. et al. (2013). Prevalence of and exposure factors for seropositivity to H3N8 canine influenza virus in dogs with influenza-like illness in the United States. *Journal of the American Veterinary Medical Association* 242 (2): 209–216.

Ashton, L.V., Callan, R.L., Rao, S. et al. (2010). in vitro susceptibility of canine influenza A (H3N8) virus to nitazoxanide and tizoxanide. *Veterinary Medicine International* 2010 https://doi.org/10.4061/2010/891010.

Barrell, E.A., Pecoraro, H.L., Torres-Henderson, C. et al. (2010). Seroprevalence and risk factors for canine H3N8 influenza virus exposure in household dogs in Colorado. *Journal of Veterinary Internal Medicine* 24 (6): 1524–1527.

Bean, B., Moore, B.M., Sterner, B. et al. (1982). Survival of influenza viruses on environmental surfaces. *Journal of Infectious Diseases* 146: 47–51.

Bunpapong, N., Nonthabenjawan, N., Chaiwong, S. et al. (2014). A. Genetic characterization of canine influenza A virus (H3N2) in Thailand. *Virus Genes* 48 (1): 56–63.

Chen, Y., Trovão, N.S., Wang, G. et al. (2018). Emergence and evolution of novel reassortant influenza A viruses in canines in southern China. *mBio* 9 (3): e00909–e00918.

Clinical and Laboratory Standards Institue (2008). *Performance Standards for*

Antimicrobial Disk and Dilution Susceptibility Tests for Bacteria Isolated from Animals. Approved Standard – Third Edition. CLSI document M31-A3. Wayne, PA: Clinical and Laboratory Standards Institute.

Crawford, P.C., Dubovi, E.J., Castleman, W.L. et al. (2005). Transmission of equine influenza virus to dogs. *Science* 310: 482–485.

Crawford, P.C., Gibbs, E.P.J. Anderson, T.C. et al. (2006). Emergence of influenza virus in pet dogs. *International Conference on Emerging Infectious Diseases*, Atlanta, GA, US (19–22 March 2006).

Daly, J.M., Blunden, A.S., Macrae, S. et al. (2008). Transmission of equine influenza virus to English foxhounds. *Emerging Infectious Diseases* 14: 461–464.

Dalziel, B.D., Huang, K., Geoghegan, J.L. et al. (2014). Contact heterogeneity, rather than transmission efficiency, limits the emergence and spread of canine influenza virus. *PLoS Pathogens* 10 (10): e1004455.

Ford, R.B., Larson, L.J., McClure, K.D. et al. (2017). 2017 AAHA canine vaccination guidelines. *Journal of the American Animal Hospital Association* 53 (5): 243–251.

Gutman, S.N., Guptill, L.F., Moore, G.E. et al. (2019). Serologic investigation of exposure to influenza A virus H3N2 infection in dogs and cats in the United States. *Journal of Veterinary Diagnostic Investigation* 31 (2): 250–254.

Holt, D.E., Mover, M.R., and Brown, D.C. (2010). Serologic prevalence of antibodies against canine influenza virus (H3N8) in dogs in a metropolitan animal shelter. *Journal of the American Veterinary Medical Association* 237 (1): 71–73.

Hong, M., Kang, B., Na, W. et al. (2013). Prolonged shedding of the canine influenza H3N2 virus in nasal swabs of experimentally immunocompromised dogs. *Clinical and Experimental Vaccine Research* 2 (1): 66–68.

Jang, H., Jackson, Y.K., Daniels, J.B. et al. (2017). Seroprevalence of three influenza A viruses (H1N1, H3N2, and H3N8) in pet dogs presented to a veterinary hospital in Ohio. *Journal of Veterinary Science* 18 (S1): 291–298.

Jeoung, H., Lim, S., Shin, B. et al. (2013). A novel canine influenza H3N2 virus isolated from cats in an animal shelter. *Veterinary Microbiology* 165 (3–4): 281–286.

Kim, H., Song, D., Moon, H. et al. (2013). Inter-and intraspecies transmission of canine influenza virus (H3N2) in dogs, cats, and ferrets. *Influenza and Other Respiratory Viruses* 7 (3): 265–270.

Kosik, I. and Yewdell, J.W. (2019). Influenza hemagglutinin and neuraminidase: Yin–Yang proteins coevolving to thwart immunity. *Viruses* 11 (4): 346.

Krueger, W.S., Heil, G.L., Yoon, K.J. et al. (2014). No evidence for zoonotic transmission of H3N8 canine influenza virus among US adults occupationally exposed to dogs. *Influenza and Other Respiratory Viruses* 8 (1): 99–106.

Lappin, M.R., Blondeau, J., Boothe, D. et al. (2017). Antimicrobial use guidelines for treatment of respiratory tract disease in dogs and cats: antimicrobial guidelines working group of the International Society for Companion Animal Infectious Diseases. *Journal of Veterinary Internal Medicine* 31 (2): 279–294.

Larson, L.J., Henningson, J., Sharp, P. et al. (2011). Efficacy of the canine influenza virus H3N8 vaccine to decrease severity of clinical disease after cochallenge with canine influenza virus and Streptococcus equi subsp. zooepidemicus. *Clinical and Vaccine Immunology* 18 (4): 559–564.

Lee, C., Song, D., Kang, B. et al. (2009). A serological survey of avian origin canine H3N2 influenza virus in dogs in Korea. *Veterinary Microbiology* 137 (3–4): 359–362.

Lee, Y.N., Lee, D.H., Lee, H.J. et al. (2012). Serologic evidence of H3N2 canine influenza virus infection before 2007. *Veterinary Record* 171: 477–479.

Li, S., Shi, Z., Jiao, P. et al. (2010). Avian-origin H3N2 canine influenza a viruses in southern China. *Infection, Genetics and Evolution* 10 (8): 1286–1288.

Lyoo, K.S., Kim, J.K., Kang, B. et al. (2015). Comparative analysis of virulence of a novel, avian-origin H3N2 canine influenza virus in various host species. *Virus Research* 195: 135–140.

Na, W., Lyoo, K.S., Song, E.J. et al. (2015). Viral dominance of reassortants between canine influenza H3N2 and pandemic (2009) H1N1 viruses from a naturally co-infected dog. *Virology Journal* 12 (1): 134–138.

Newbury, S., Godhardt-Cooper, J., Poulsen, K.P. et al. (2016). Prolonged intermittent virus shedding during an outbreak of canine influenza A H3N2 virus infection in dogs in three Chicago area shelters: 16 cases (March to May 2015). *Journal of the American Veterinary Medical Association* 248 (9): 1022–1026.

Parrish, C.R. and Voorhees, I.E. (2019). H3N8 and H3N2 canine influenza viruses: understanding these new viruses in dogs. *Veterinary Clinics: Small Animal Practice* 49 (4): 643–649.

Payungporn, S., Crawford, P.C., Kouo, T.S. et al. (2008). Influenza A virus (H3N8) in dogs with respiratory disease, Florida. *Emerging Infectious Diseases* 14 (6): 902–908.

Pecoraro, H.L., Bennett, S., Huyvaert, K.P. et al. (2014). Epidemiology and ecology of H3N8 canine influenza viruses in US shelter dogs. *Journal of Veterinary Internal Medicine* 28 (2): 311–318.

Rodriquez, L., Nogales, A., Reilly, E.C. et al. (2017). A live-attenuated influenza vaccine for H3N2 canine influenza virus. *Virology* 504: 96–106.

Rosas, C., Van de Walle, G.R., Metzger, S.M. et al. (2008). Evaluation of a vectored equine herpesvirus type 1 (EHV-1) vaccine expressing H3 haemagglutinin in the protection of dogs against canine influenza. *Vaccine* 26 (19): 2335–2343.

Song, D., Kang, B., Lee, C. et al. (2008). Transmission of avian influenza virus (H3N2) to dogs. *Emerging Infectious Diseases* 14 (5): 741.

Song, D.S., An, D.J., Moon, H.J. et al. (2011). Interspecies transmission of the canine influenza H3N2 virus to domestic cats in South Korea. *Journal of General Virology* 92 (10): 2350–2355.

Song, D., Moon, H.J., An, D.J. et al. (2012). A novel reassortant canine H3N1 influenza virus between pandemic H1N1 and canine H3N2 influenza viruses in Korea. *Journal of General Virology* 93: 551–554.

Spindel, M.F., Lunn, K.F. et al. (2007). Detection and quantification of canine influenza virus by one-step real-time reverse transcription PCR. *Journal of Veterinary Internal Medicine* 21: 576.

Sun, H., Blackmon, S., Yang, G. et al. (2017). Zoonotic risk, pathogenesis, and transmission of avian-origin H3N2 canine influenza virus. *Journal of Virology* 91 (21): e00637–e00617.

Tellier, R. (2006). Review of aerosol transmission of influenza A virus. *Emerging Infectious Diseases* 12: 1657–1662.

Voorhees, I.E., Glaser, A.L., Toohey-Kurth, K. et al. (2017). Spread of canine influenza A (H3N2) virus, United States. *Emerging Infectious Diseases* 23 (12): 1950.

Voorhees, I.E., Dalziel, B.D., Glaser, A. et al. (2018). Multiple incursions and recurrent epidemic fade-out of H3N2 canine influenza A virus in the United States. *Journal of Virology* 92 (16): e00323–e00318.

Webster, R.G., Bean, W.J., Gorman, O.T. et al. (1992). Evolution and ecology of influenza A viruses. *Microbiology Review* 56: 152–179.

Weese, S. (2018). Canine Influenza: Ontario. Worms and Germs Blog. https://www.wormsandgermsblog.com/2018/01/articles/animals/dogs/canine-influenza-ontario (accessed 1 July 2020).

Wiley, C.A., Ottoson, M.C., Garcia, M.M. et al. (2013). The seroprevalence of canine influenza virus H3N8 in dogs participating in a Flyball tournament in Pennsylvania in 2010: a follow-up study. *Journal of Veterinary Internal Medicine* 27 (2): 367–370.

Yoon, K.-Y., Cooper, V.L., Schwartz, K.J. et al. (2005). Influenza virus infection in racing greyhounds. *Emerging Infectious Diseases* 11: 1974–1975.

Zhu, H., Hughes, J., and Murcia, P.R. (2015). Origins and evolutionary dynamics of H3N2 canine influenza virus. *Journal of Virology* 89 (10): 5406–5418.

13

Feline Infectious Respiratory Disease

Annette Litster

Zoetis Petcare, Chicago, IL, USA

13.1 Introduction

Feline infectious respiratory disease (upper respiratory tract disease or URTD) is a very common cause of illness in US shelters, threatening the health and adoptability of individual cats and the entire feline population (Litster et al. 2012). The labor and material costs of caring for sick cats for prolonged periods also reduce the lifesaving capacity of the shelter and it can be difficult to find permanent adoptive homes for cats with ongoing clinical signs (Litster et al. 2011). While the etiology of the problem is infectious, its solution is more complex than just isolation or treatment of clinically affected cats, effective sanitation and appropriate vaccination protocols. Furthermore, the development of disease in shelter cats often occurs without actual pathogen transmission (e.g. recrudescence of herpesvirus infections) and thus a holistic approach is necessary to minimize disease. Active population management and attention to individual cat well-being are required to reduce stress and minimize the transmission of infectious agents to susceptible cats. Carefully planned management of the feline population can dramatically reduce disease prevalence, increase life-saving success and enhance the reputation of the shelter. Published shelter-based studies from the United States and the United Kingdom have reported quite different risks for the development of clinical URTD in cats after shelter admission, possibly attesting to different management styles, housing types and intake rates that impact disease frequency and expression.

The major causative pathogens in feline infectious respiratory disease are feline herpesvirus (FHV-1), feline calicivirus (FCV), *Mycoplasma* spp., *Chlamydia felis* and *Bordetella bronchiseptica* (Bannasch and Foley 2005). There is evidence for an association between each of these infectious agents and clinical disease, though each agent can also be present in subclinically infected cats (McManus et al. 2014). Though theoretically possible, it appears that asymptomatic carrier animals pose a minimal risk for transmission, in most cases, as evidenced by many shelters that do not isolate healthy appearing cats from one another, yet do not experience high levels of upper respiratory disease. Bacterial strain or viral biotype, route of exposure, host age and immune/vaccination status, and the presence of concurrent disease are important factors in determining the outcome of infection. Typical clinical signs include conjunctivitis, ocular or nasal discharge, gingivitis, and oral and/or corneal ulcers. These signs are often more severe if more than one agent is present.

Infectious Disease Management in Animal Shelters, Second Edition.
Edited by Lila Miller, Stephanie Janeczko, and Kate F. Hurley.

Additionally, secondary bacterial infection with *Pasteurella* spp., *Escherichia coli*, *Staphylococcus* spp., *Streptococcus* spp., or *Micrococcus* spp. has been reported (Litster et al. 2012), usually secondary to primary viral infection.

The overlap in clinical signs between infectious agents can pose challenges for the diagnosis of specific pathogens on clinical grounds alone, but similar strategies for the control of disease transmission and shelter population management apply across infectious agents. Major priorities include allowing adequate space to meet the individual physical and behavioral needs of each cat; protecting incoming cats by prompt vaccination and minimizing exposure to shedding cats; effective environmental decontamination, including fomite control; and treatment and isolation of sick cats (McManus et al. 2014; Wagner et al. 2018b). Diligent attention to these principles can dramatically reduce the prevalence of URTD and facilitate the welfare and adoptability of shelter-housed cats.

13.2 Causative Agents, Pathogenesis and Clinical Signs

Most URTD pathogens are associated with a similar array of clinical signs, including serous to mucopurulent ocular and/or nasal discharge, photophobia, sneezing, fever, inappetence or anorexia and submandibular lymphadenopathy (Gaskell et al. 2012). See Figures 13.1a and b. While clinical signs of URTD are generally mild, severe disease can occur, especially in at-risk groups such as kittens, elderly cats, and purebreds (Dinnage et al. 2009), or when infection spreads to the lower respiratory tract. More severe clinical signs may also be associated with a higher dose of exposure, as in a crowded shelter environment with high disease levels. Clinical signs of severe disease include anorexia, dehydration, fever, and dyspnea (Radford et al. 2009; Thiry et al. 2009).

(a)

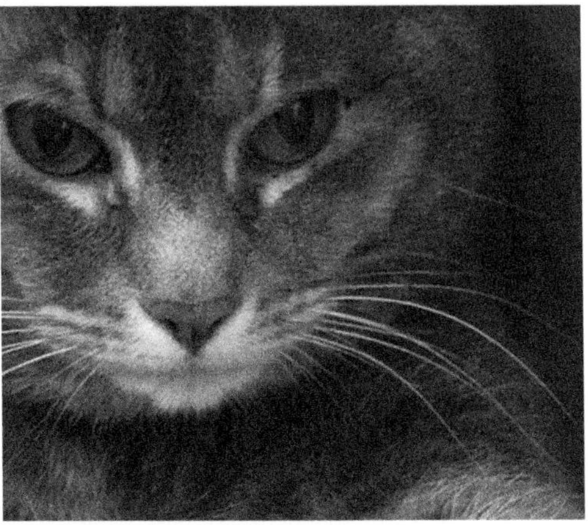

(b)

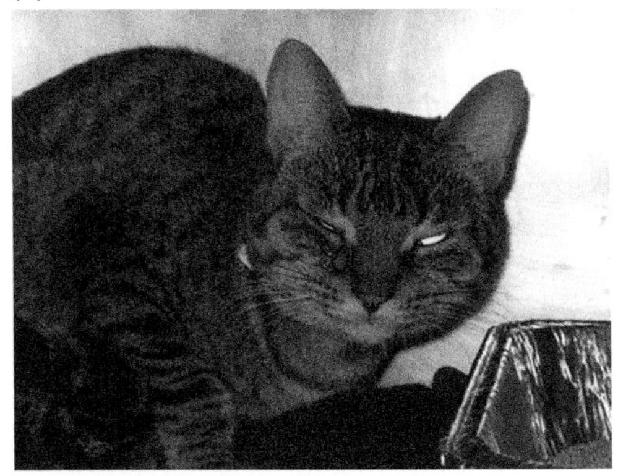

Figure 13.1 (a) and (b) Ocular discharge and photophobia are common non-specific clinical signs of infection with feline infectious respiratory pathogens.

Incoming cats commonly carry URTD pathogens into the shelter environment, either subclinically or clinically and often as co-infections. Subclinical infections create challenges for the identification of infected cats. One Canadian study reported that 28% of incoming cats were polymerase chain reaction (PCR) positive for at least one URTD infectious agent (Gourkow et al. 2013), while a California study reported a rate of 61.6% (Bannasch and Foley 2005). In the Canadian study, *Mycoplasma felis* infections predominated (21%), while in the US study, FHV-1 (3–38%) and FCV (13–36%) were the most common agents. A Chicago-based study of cats with clinical URTD entering a large adoption-guarantee shelter reported mostly FHV-1 (94%) and *M. felis* (83%) infections, while *B. bronchiseptica* and FCV recovery rates were 44% and 11%, respectively. Co-infections with multiple respiratory pathogens were common (Litster et al. 2015a).

13.2.1 Feline Herpesvirus (FHV-1)

FHV-1 is a double-stranded, enveloped DNA virus that is a common cause of respiratory and ocular disease in animal shelters. The disease is also known as feline rhinotracheitis. The virus is relatively genetically stable; differences in severity can reflect variation in virulence between field isolates of the same strain of FHV-1, dose and individual immune response (Gould 2011). After initial infection, in at least 80% of cats, the virus becomes latent in relatively low-temperature areas of the upper respiratory tract (URT), such as the nasal mucosa, turbinates and nasopharynx, and in neural tissue such as the trigeminal ganglia. This persistent viral carrier state explains the estimated seroprevalence of 50–97% in feline populations worldwide. The virus is shed by infected cats in oral, nasal, and ocular secretions and transmitted by direct contact, through sneeze droplets over short distances, or by fomites. True aerosol transmission, however, is considered unlikely. The virus is relatively easy to inactivate using many common disinfectants. Viral shedding in acutely infected cats peaks at seven days post-infection (Reubel et al. 1992) and lasts for two to three weeks; FHV-1 is shed intermittently in carrier cats after viral reactivation (Gaskell and Povey 1982).

Stress can be associated with FHV-1 reactivation, usually within three weeks of the stressful event, with clinical signs of respiratory infection appearing approximately 4–11 days after the stress (Contreras et al. 2017). Stress can not only induce reactivation of FHV-1 but also inhibit the production of mucosal antibodies, such as IgA, predisposing to clinical URTD; therefore, proactive management of emotional stress could be an important tool in shelter management of URTD (Gourkow et al. 2014). Stressful events, such as pregnancy and nursing; relocation from one housing environment to another (including shelter admission if not carefully managed); and grouping with unfamiliar cats in shared housing can all act as triggers for viral reactivation (Gaskell and Povey 1982). Techniques designed to reduce stress, such as providing adequate housing size, hiding spaces, minimally invasive daily cage cleaning, and minimizing stressful handling, are vital (Bannasch and Foley 2005). Beyond reducing stressful interactions, gentle handling to actively promote the well-being of cats may be beneficial in reducing herpes recrudescence.

Clinical signs of infection are fairly uniform and include depression, sneezing, conjunctivitis and chemosis, corneal or conjunctival ulceration, nasal and ocular discharge and, less commonly, dermatologic lesions (Persico et al. 2011). Ocular signs can include conjunctivitis and signs of erosion and ulceration of mucosal surfaces, such as superficial and deep corneal ulcers and dendritic ulcers. Severe systemic signs, such as depression, fever, anorexia, and pneumonia, can sometimes lead to fatalities in kittens. One recent study of 59 FHV-1 infected client-owned cats presented to a veterinary medical teaching hospital reported the following common clinical findings: conjunctivitis (n = 51/59; 86%), keratitis (n = 51/59; 86%), blepharitis (n = 19/59; 32%), nasal discharge or sneezing (n = 10/59; 17%), and dermatitis (n = 4/59; 7%) (Thomasy et al. 2016). In the longer term, chronic rhinosinusitis can occur due to osteolysis and permanent destruction of the nasal turbinates and bone, followed by secondary bacterial infection leading to chronic sneezing with mucopurulent discharge, especially in short-nosed breeds (Thiry et al. 2009). There is some evidence that viral shedding can occur in the absence of clinical signs (Gould 2011), though this has not been definitively documented in shelter-housed cats.

13.2.2 Feline Calicivirus (FCV)

FCV is a single-stranded non-enveloped RNA virus that can mutate rapidly, resulting in a diversity of biotypes. Though all FCV isolates are currently grouped into a single serotype, these isolates differ antigenically, creating challenges for the development of broadly protective vaccines (Radford et al. 2006) and resulting in a variety of clinical presentations. Most commonly, FCV infection can cause acute upper respiratory signs such as conjunctivitis and/or rhinitis and tongue/oral ulceration. Less commonly, clinical outcomes can also include bronchointerstitial pneumonia (Radford et al. 2009); vesicular lesions on the nasal philtrum or footpads (Pesavento et al. 2008); and/or chronic gingivitis/stomatitis, which is thought to be immune-mediated, or faucitis (Belgard et al. 2010). Numerous studies have documented the impact of experimental FCV infection, with variable consistency in reproducing disease, suggesting that co-factors are involved (Pesavento et al. 2008). Self-limiting lameness and fever have been reported in some young cats after infection with or vaccination against FCV (Dawson et al. 1994; Radford et al. 2009); this "febrile limping syndrome" has not been associated with any of the other URTD pathogens (Gaskell et al. 2012).

Outbreaks of a highly contagious, virulent systemic disease characterized by fever, subcutaneous (SC) edema of the head and paws, severe oral ulceration, epithelial necrosis, and multi-organ failure (virulent systemic feline calicivirus, virus VSFCV) have been reported. Mortality rates from the virulent systemic form of the disease are high (33–50%; up to 67%), adult cats are more likely to have more severe clinical disease than kittens, and the prognosis is guarded. Crowded, high-stress environments select for VSFCV. Fomite transmission is extremely important and contaminated cat hair is a common source of the virus. Routine FCV vaccines are not protective, and each outbreak is likely to be due to a different biotype (Pedersen et al. 2000; Hurley et al. 2004; Radford et al. 2009; Litster 2015). Additionally, because it is a non-enveloped virus, FCV is not susceptible to many routinely used disinfectants, such as quaternary ammonium products.

In most cases of FCV infection, clinical signs resolve in days to weeks. Ongoing oral inflammation has been associated with FCV infection, however, and the development of a chronic viral carrier state with viral shedding is relatively common (Radford et al. 2009), which facilitates the development of clinical disease and viral transmission on reactivation.

13.2.3 Influenza Viruses

Influenza A viruses are endemic in humans, and serologic surveys have suggested that cats can be infected with, and develop antibody responses against, human seasonal and highly pathogenic avian influenza viruses. Most feline infections appear to be self-limiting and cats are not considered an important reservoir of influenza A infection (Hatta et al. 2018). While cats are susceptible to infection with various avian (including H3N7 and H5N1), swine (H1N1), and canine (H3N2) influenza viruses, clinical infection is rarely documented (Song et al. 2011; Cornell Feline Health Center 2016). However, in December 2016, an outbreak of low pathogenic avian influenza A (H7N2) virus infection occurred among hundreds of cats in a New York City shelter. Clinical signs were generally mild, such as lethargy, nasal congestion and nasal discharge, though some affected cats developed more severe signs of lower respiratory disease (Shelter Medicine, School of Veterinary Medicine, University of Wisconsin-Madison 2017). H7N2 is transmissible by cats to humans and a veterinarian who handled infected cats was also diagnosed with the infection, though the risk of zoonotic transmission is thought to be low (NYC Health 2016; Hatta et al. 2018).

13.2.4 *Mycoplasma* Spp.

Mycoplasma spp. are among the smallest free-living bacterial species; they are unable to survive outside a host and usually establish persistent infections that can cause chronic disease (Browning et al. 2011). They are commonly isolated from conjunctival and nasal swabs in healthy cats as well as shelter cats with clinical signs of URTD (Litster et al. 2012). Though infection can be carried subclinically for years (Waites et al. 2008; Browning et al. 2011), *Mycoplasma* can be part of the normal flora of the feline upper respiratory tract, conjunctiva, and genital tract (Tan and Miles 1974; Haesebrouck et al. 1991). *Mycoplasma* spp. also have the potential to be a primary or secondary pathogen of shelter cats. Because *Mycoplasma* can be present in healthy cats or as a secondary/opportunist pathogen in cats with clinical URTD, caution should be taken when interpreting upper respiratory PCR panels from shelter cats; a positive *Mycoplasma* result does not confirm that the primary infection responsible for clinical signs is *Mycoplasma*.

LeBoedec (2017) reported significant associations between *Mycoplasma* spp. isolated from oropharyngeal swabs and clinical URTD in non-shelter cats, but not for cats housed in a shelter environment. While there was an improvement of clinical signs in association with treatment and a reduction of *Mycoplasma* carriage in the feline study by Hartmann et al. (2008), the potential roles of secondary bacterial infections and/or co-pathogens were not investigated. In the shelter study by Bannasch and Foley (2005), *Mycoplasma* was more frequently identified in cats with clinical URTD, but the study was unable to document a primary relationship between clinical signs and *Mycoplasma* infection.

13.2.5 *Bordetella bronchiseptica*

B. bronchiseptica is a Gram-negative coccobacillus that is a primary respiratory pathogen of dogs, cats, guinea pigs and rabbits. Though uncommon, it has been shown to also cause infection and disease in humans. However, it should be noted that transmission to humans is more likely to occur from dogs, who are more likely to aerosolize it than cats.

B. bronchiseptica has been detected in both healthy cats and those with signs of URTD. Clinical signs in cats are usually minor and can include fever, coughing, lymphadenopathy, sneezing and ocular discharge. However, severe pneumonia with dyspnea and cyanosis can occasionally occur, especially in high-density environments or in cats with co-morbidities (Egberink et al. 2009). While some authors have reported significant coughing in feline bordetellosis, infection is less frequently associated with coughing than in dogs (Foley et al. 2002). Once established in the epithelium of the respiratory tract, the organism destroys the cilia, thereby removing an important primary immune defense and predisposing to co-infections (Egberink et al. 2009). The presence of clinically affected dogs is a risk factor for infection in cats and molecular studies have confirmed cross-species transmission (Dawson et al. 2000; Foley et al. 2002); see Figure 13.2. One study reported that *B. bronchiseptica* was isolated frequently from shelter-housed dogs and cats during outbreaks of canine and/or feline URTD. It was suggested that if infected cats served to maintain or further amplify *B. bronchiseptica* in the shelter environment, this could pose a risk for much more serious URTD in dogs (Foley et al. 2002).

13.2.6 *Chlamydia felis*

C. felis is an obligate intracellular Gram-negative rod-shaped coccoid bacterium that is very short-lived outside the host, therefore requiring direct cat-to-cat contact for transmission of infection (Gruffydd-Jones et al. 2009). The primary site of infection is the conjunctiva, and ocular fluids are the most common source of infection. Kittens are more likely to be infected than adults, though they can be

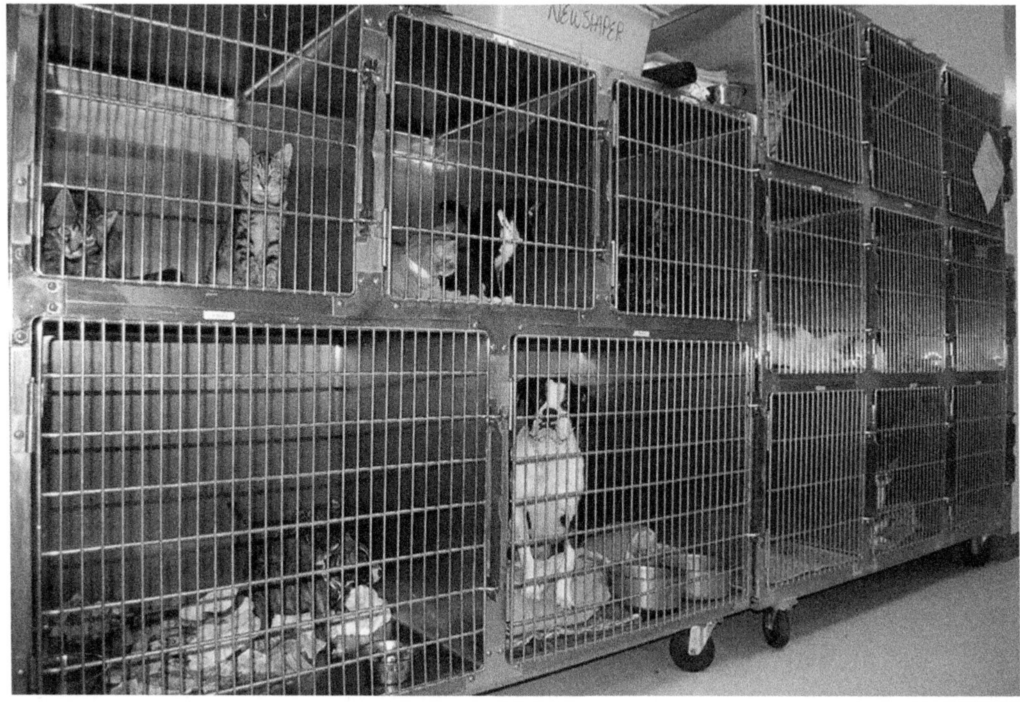

Figure 13.2 Housing cats near dogs should be avoided as it is stressful for cats and poses a risk factor for transmitting *B. bronchiseptica* infection.

protected by maternal antibodies for the first one to two months of life. Conjunctivitis is the most common clinical sign, initially unilateral and with serous discharge, progressing to bilateral mucoid or mucopurulent discharge. Transient fever, inappetence and weight loss can also occur in the early stages of infection. Since *C. felis* has very poor environmental persistence, individual housing and routine hygiene measures should be sufficient to prevent infection in shelters (Gruffydd-Jones et al. 2009). One recent study of four different shelter management models reported that clinically affected cats in foster-care programs and trap-neuter-return programs were more likely to carry *C. felis* infection than healthy cats (McManus et al. 2014). While conjunctival shedding usually ceases after about two months, some cats develop persistent infections and can shed for many months (Gruffydd-Jones et al. 2009). Since prolonged treatment (four weeks) is required to clear the infection, PCR testing should be used to confirm infection before treatment is commenced. *C. felis* infection is responsive to a limited number of antimicrobial agents; tetracyclines such as doxycycline are the treatment of choice (Gruffydd-Jones et al. 2009). Cats are no longer contagious once clinical signs resolve and can be made available for adoption.

13.2.7 Other Bacterial Agents

Bacterial infections with *Pasteurella* spp., *E. coli*, *Staphylococcus* spp., *Streptococcus* spp., or *Micrococcus* spp. often occur secondary to primary viral infections in cats with clinical signs of upper respiratory infection (Schultz et al. 2006; Hartmann et al. 2010; Litster et al. 2012). There is also anecdotal evidence that, at least in some settings, some of these bacterial species have appeared to act as primary pathogens (S. Janeczko, Personal communication, 2018).

13.2.7.1 *Streptococcus canis*

Of particular note in shelter housed cats is *Streptococcus canis*, which is a Gram-positive bacterial species in the group G beta-hemolytic species of *Streptococcus*. While typically considered a commensal and extracellular pathogen in cats, *S. canis* has caused outbreaks of rapidly progressive necrotizing sinusitis, meningitis and skin ulceration, or necrotizing fasciitis and toxic shock syndrome, with fatality rates of up to 30%. In some cases, shelters were crowded, or affected cats had chronic upper respiratory infections before succumbing to *S. canis* infection. In other cases, infection may have been linked to oral and tissue trauma associated with handling and housing methods (use of a rabies pole and housing on slatted floors). However, other specific management factors predisposing to highly pathogenic strains of *S. canis* remain unidentified (Pesavento et al. 2007).

13.2.7.2 *Streptococcus equi* subspecies *zooepidemicus*

Another streptococcal species, *Streptococcus equi* subspecies *zooepidemicus*, has been isolated in cats with or without clinical signs of respiratory disease. Its role as a primary pathogen or opportunist co-infection in feline URTD is poorly understood, but it has been reported in association with purulent nasal discharge, dyspnea, coughing, pneumonia, rhinitis, meningoencephalitis; infection can be fatal. *S. zooepidemicus* is likely to be an under-recognized cause of severe feline URTD since commercially available PCR panels for feline respiratory pathogens do not routinely include it and the clinical presentation is similar to other common pathogens (Polak et al. 2014). Therefore, if *S. zooepidemicus* infection is suspected, a special request should be made for the laboratory to include specific PCR testing for the organism. Bacterial culture can also be requested on oropharyngeal and/or nasal swabs; selective culture media for Gram-positive bacteria is ideal. If fatalities occur, necropsies should be performed, and lung specimens submitted for histopathology. Since zoonotic infection from a dog to a handler has been reported, it is important to wear personal protective equipment and observe hand hygiene when handling infected animals and their bodily fluids (Priestnall and Erles 2011).

13.3 Transmission

The main mode of transmission for all the major feline respiratory pathogens is by direct contact with infected cats that are actively shedding. However, in a shelter where direct contact between cats can generally be controlled, transmission by fomites on contaminated surfaces, objects, clothing or hands is likely more important (Edwards et al. 2008). Additionally, sneezed (aerosolized) respiratory droplets from infected cats spread up to 1–1.3 m (3–4 ft) (McManus et al. 2014). FHV-1 is relatively fragile in the environment, surviving up to 18 hours in a damp environment; survival is reduced in dry conditions. FCV is relatively long-lived outside the host, surviving at least 28 days at room temperature (Gaskell et al. 2012).

Feline URTD is not thought to be airborne; therefore, separate ventilation per cage or room is not necessary (Wardley and Povey 1977; Gaskell and Povey 1982). However, air quality in the environment, and particularly within the housing unit, is important to support respiratory health. For large, grate or wire-front cages, natural air circulation may be sufficient, while active ventilation may be required in a more enclosed housing environment. Required air change rates vary depending on population density and pollutants (such as litter dust and cleaning chemicals) in the air. If banks of cages face one another, they should be separated by at least 1.3 m (4 ft) to prevent sneeze droplet spread of URTD pathogens (Scarlett 2009).

Though droplet transmission can theoretically play a role, fomite transmission is by far the most common means of URTD spread in shelters (other than the recrudescence of latent

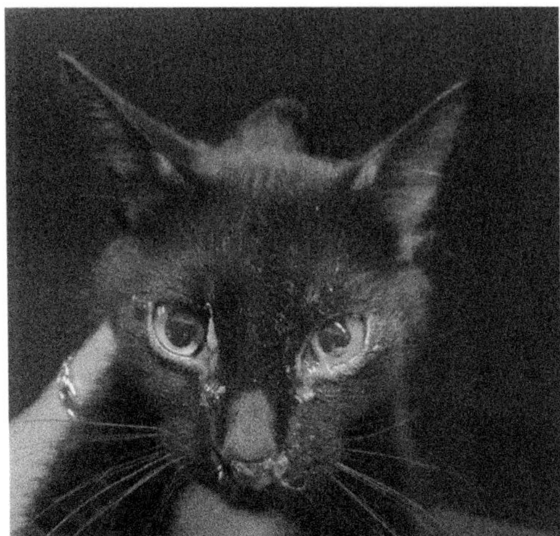

Figure 13.3 Prompt antimicrobial treatment is required if signs of bacterial infection, such as mucopurulent ocular and/or nasal discharge, are present.

FHV-1 infections due to stress). In addition to playing a role in stress and feline well-being, housing type and arrangement will strongly affect fomite disease transmission opportunities. Double-compartment housing facilitates cleaning without extensive handling of the cat, reducing transmission opportunities as well as lowering the stress associated with environmental change. See Figure 13.3. If single-compartment housing is sufficiently large, a carrier within the housing unit can serve a similar function, allowing the cat to be safely confined while the environment is tidied and cleaned. Housing that encloses the cat behind a solid front may seem beneficial to reduce fomite transmission but might not be a good strategy to reduce feline URTD. The bulk of fomite transmission likely occurs via shelter worker hands and clothing, along with shared equipment (especially that used while cleaning) and surfaces, particularly from heavy foot traffic by newly admitted and/or sick animals. Adopters and shelter visitors, by contrast, arrive in a relatively uncontaminated state and likely transmit relatively little between healthy cats on the adoption floor. (See Chapter 8 for more information on sanitation.) Meanwhile, a solid front may prevent the cats from displaying the type of approach and greeting behavior preferred by many adopters, as well as compromising air quality within the housing unit (Wagner et al. 2018a; Weiss et al. 2012).

13.4 Clinical Epidemiology

The shelter environment can predispose cats to the development of clinical URTD because of high population turnover, crowding, stress, and relatively high numbers of cats with comorbidities, poor nutrition, and no previous vaccinations against relevant pathogens (Bannasch and Foley 2005). While shelters are not necessarily the source of infection, the shelter environment can amplify pathogen shedding and enhance transmission rates between infected and non-infected cats (Pedersen et al. 2004). Since the incubation period for feline respiratory pathogens is approximately one to six days, cats that develop clinical signs in the first three to four days after intake are more likely to have been infected prior to shelter admission, whereas those that develop signs of URTD after five days or more have probably been infected as a result of shelter exposure (Dinnage et al. 2009).

Interestingly, the reported proportions of cats with clinical URTD in shelters vary widely. In a large urban shelter in the northeastern United States, Dinnage et al. (2009) reported that the cumulative probability of developing signs of infectious respiratory disease by day seven after admission was approximately 26–32% for litters, individual kittens and adult cats. By contrast, in a longitudinal, year-long study in five UK feline shelters, the risk of clinical URTD actually decreased with time since shelter admission (Edwards et al. 2008). In the UK study, shelter-related factors were more important determinants of risk than cat-related factors. In a comparison of nine North American animal shelters, the risk of URTD varied nearly 50-fold between shelters. This variation was associated with environmental risk factors at the shelter level rather than variation in pathogen frequency in cats at the time of admission (Wagner et al. 2018b).

13.5 The Effect of Environment and Shelter Type on Pathogen Prevalence

The type of population being cared for, the housing environment, level of population density, length of stay (LOS) and other management practices can make important differences in the patterns of feline URTD pathogens that are likely to dominate. Because of its close association with stress, FHV-1 may be relatively common where poor housing, high turnover, or other stressful conditions predispose to recrudescence and spread; this information should be used to help inform preventative care programs or initial empiric therapeutic choices for cats with clinical signs of URTD before more specific diagnostic information is available.

The prevalence of feline URTD pathogens has been compared in four different types of shelters: short-term shelters, long-term sanctuaries, home-based foster-care programs, and trap-neuter-return programs for community cats. FHV-1 and *B. bronchiseptica* dominated in short-term shelters, while FCV and *M. felis* were more prevalent than other pathogens in long-term sanctuaries. Clinically affected cats in foster care were more likely to carry FHV-1, *M. felis* or *C. felis* than healthy cats in the same housing model, while in trap-neuter-return schemes, cats with upper respiratory signs were more likely to carry FCV or *C. felis* than healthy cats (McManus et al. 2014). Another study of infectious diseases in large-scale cat hoarding investigations reported that FCV, *M. felis* and *S. zooepidemicus* were the most commonly detected respiratory pathogens among those cats with clinical respiratory disease (Polak et al. 2014). However, it is important to remember that there are not strong correlations between the detection of feline URTD pathogens and the presence of clinical signs, suggesting that population management needs to be multifaceted and that simply isolating unwell cats is unlikely to be successful (McManus et al. 2014; Polak et al. 2014).

While the scientific literature provides some general suggestions on the prevalence of URTD pathogens in different settings, it is likely that variation within these categories and over time within a given shelter is also significant. Therefore, these general findings can be used to provide context for interpretation of shelter-specific testing but should not take the place of further diagnostics on an individual shelter level in the event of unusually frequent or severe disease.

13.6 Risk Factors for Clinical Respiratory Disease

Reported individual-level risk factors for clinical URTD in shelter cats include being a kitten, older (>11 years old), purebred, neutered, being housed close to dogs and testing PCR-positive for an infectious agent (Bannasch and Foley 2005; Dinnage et al. 2009; Gourkow et al. 2013). Study results have varied on whether stray or abandoned cats are at greater risk (Bannasch and Foley 2005; Edwards et al. 2008; Dinnage et al. 2009).

LOS has been implicated as the single greatest risk factor for individual cats in multiple studies, regardless of other risk factors (Edinboro et al. 1999; Bannasch and Foley 2005; Edwards et al. 2008; Dinnage et al. 2009). The probability of developing clinical URTD gradually rises over the first two weeks after admission, coinciding with increased URTD pathogen shedding rates, but can stabilize after approximately three weeks (Bannasch and Foley 2005; Dinnage et al. 2009; Gourkow et al. 2013).

Population-level risk factors for clinical respiratory disease have also been described, including the level of hygiene (sanitation), number of cats present, household or shelter type, housing type and the number of moves within the shelter (Binns et al. 2000; Helps et al. 2005; Wagner et al. 2018a). As noted above, substantial variation in URTD levels has been reported among shelters, ranging from an incidence of over 30% to under 2% (Edwards et al. 2008; Dinnage et al. 2009). The variation in levels between and within shelters indicates that a dramatic reduction of URTD is an achievable goal and will depend on a combination of mitigating individual and shelter risk factors.

13.7 Diagnostics

While clinical signs of primary or secondary bacterial infection in feline URTD are often similar, consisting of mucopurulent conjunctivitis, rhinitis and sneezing, some differentiating signs are more likely to be associated with specific infectious agents. It must be noted, however, that none is pathognomonic for an individual bacterial pathogen. One shelter-based study of cats with URTD reported that coughing was rarely observed (Litster et al. 2012), but another review paper advised that if acute or chronic coughing occurs, *B. bronchiseptica* infection should be considered (Egberink et al. 2009). Another shelter-based study reported that there was more severe ocular discharge, conjunctivitis and nasal discharge in cats infected with *Mycoplasma* spp. than in those that tested PCR-negative for *Mycoplasma*. In those shelter populations, cats with the most severe ocular and nasal discharge with conjunctivitis were infected with *C. felis*, while those infected with both FHV-1 and FCV presented with ocular and nasal discharge and sneezing (Bannasch and Foley 2005). Chemosis of the conjunctiva is a characteristic feature of *C. felis* infection (Gruffydd-Jones et al. 2009).

Because the clinical signs of feline URTD are often similar, regardless of the infectious agent/s causing them, laboratory tests are required to determine the pathogens involved. Since treatment and management protocols are basically the same for most shelter cats with URTD, it could be argued that spending limited shelter resources on diagnostic testing should be reserved for outbreak situations, when disease symptoms are unusually severe in an individual or population, or for periodic surveillance.

Commercially available real-time polymerase chain reaction (RT-PCR) testing can identify all the major feline URTD pathogens in a single-swab specimen, with excellent sensitivity and fast turnaround times. One shelter-based study reported that an oropharyngeal swab submitted with either an ocular or a nasal swab from each cat was sufficient to detect all infectious agents present (Litster et al. 2015a). Swabs should be submitted in dry sterile tubes, as viral-transport media can contain antibiotics that reduce the yield of bacterial isolates, and bacterial-transport media can contain PCR inhibitors. Plastic-stemmed swabs with synthetic fiber (not cotton, which might have been exposed to bleach during the manufacturing process) tips are ideal.

A positive result does not necessarily identify the causative agent responsible for the clinical signs seen in a particular cat because most of the pathogens can also exist in a subclinical (carrier) state. Additionally, RT-PCR testing merely detects the presence of target sequences of the pathogen genome, and does not denote active infection or provide antimicrobial susceptibility data (Litster et al. 2015a). Vaccination against FHV-1 and/or FCV with intranasal (IN) or modified live (MLV) injectable vaccine can produce positive test results for a few weeks after vaccination (IDEXX 2013). Quantitative RT-PCR is commercially available for FHV-1 and can distinguish active infection from latent (subclinical) infection by determining the amount of virus on the swab specimen.

RT-PCR is a convenient method to identify the presence of bacterial feline URTD pathogens, but specimens should be submitted for bacterial culture and susceptibility if information on antimicrobial susceptibility is required to guide therapeutic choices. Culture of *Mycoplasma* spp. can be challenging, as delays during transport can affect their viability. Specific culture media are usually required, such as peptone-enriched blood agar plates (Foster and Martin 2011). For testing for *B. bronchiseptica*, swabs should be placed into charcoal or regular Amies transport media and selective media such as charcoal or cephalexin agar should be used for culture to reduce the risk of overgrowth by other bacterial URTD agents (Egberink et al. 2009). RT-PCR is the only option available to identify *C. felis* since it is an obligate intracellular organism and there is no established reference standard for its culture in US diagnostic laboratories (Litster et al. 2015a). (See Chapter 4 for more information on diagnostic testing.)

VSFCV infection cannot be distinguished from the more common biotypes of FCV using currently available laboratory methods; therefore, diagnosis is based on the presence of characteristic clinical signs, high mortality rates, and evidence of highly transmissible infection, leading to a presumptive diagnosis in most cases (Pesavento et al. 2008). Molecular testing can be used to confirm the presence of the same FCV biotype from the blood of cats infected by the outbreak (Radford et al. 2009), and necropsy and histopathology of tissue from affected cats that die or are euthanized can confirm hypervirulent infection.

13.8 Treatment

Therapeutic choices for clinically affected animals, including cats with URTD, should be based on a reasonably certain diagnosis and proper administration of medication at the recommended dose rate and frequency, preferably based on the input of a veterinarian familiar with the case/s. Because URTD is so common in shelters and initiating treatment promptly can be important, it can also be acceptable for routine treatment to be directed by a standard written protocol developed by a veterinarian providing regular oversight of the medical program. Unusual cases and those failing to respond to regular treatment should be directly examined by a veterinarian.

13.8.1 Antiviral Agents

Antiviral drugs for feline URTD are directed against FHV-1. However, antiviral agents have not been specifically developed for cats or the treatment of FHV-1, so available drugs are limited to those with activity against closely related human herpesviruses and tested for safety in cats, such as oral famciclovir, topical ophthalmic idoxuridine and cidofovir. Importantly, it should not be assumed that antiviral drugs that are safe and efficacious for human herpesvirus infections are safe for cats or effective against FHV-1. Available drugs cannot clear the infection; they merely reduce viral replication, thereby reducing the severity and/or duration of clinical signs. Because of this, if the decision is made to use antiviral drugs because the infection is severe, persistent or recurrent, the correct dose rate is critical for successful therapy. Clear guidelines for course length have not been developed, but therapy should ideally be continued for a period after the resolution of clinical signs. Since the clinical signs of FHV-1 infection are often self-limiting, clinical trials of antiviral therapies should be placebo-controlled if they are to provide reliable information (Thomasy and Maggs 2016). Table 13.1 provides a summary of information for antiviral drugs for FHV-1 infections.

As stated earlier, there are no approved anti-FCV therapeutic agents at the time of publication of this text. However, there have been sparse but promising reports in the veterinary literature of specific anti-FCV therapeutic agents (Smith et al. 2008; McDonagh et al. 2015a, 2015b), but none are currently approved for clinical use in cats. Supportive therapy to correct dehydration, ensure nutrition, provide analgesia, and treat biotype-specific clinical signs should be provided.

Table 13.1 Anti-viral drugs for the treatment of Feline Herpesvirus (FHV-1) Infection.

Drug	Route of administration	Dose rate	Indication
Famciclovir	Oral	90 mg/kg q8h	FHV-1 infection
Idoxuridine	Topical	0.1% ophthalmic solution or 0.5% ointment, q4-6h	Ocular infection with FHV-1
Cidofovir	Topical	0.1% ophthalmic solution q12h	Ocular infection with FHV-1

q-every.

13.8.1.1 Famciclovir

A randomized, masked, placebo-controlled study of a single oral dose of 500 mg famciclovir administered on intake to adult shelter cats failed to demonstrate any differences between the famciclovir and the placebo groups in clinical signs or viral shedding rates over a seven-day post-dose observation period (Litster et al. 2015b). However, another retrospective case series (uncontrolled) studied 59 client-owned cats and kittens with chronic clinical signs of URTD prior to oral famciclovir treatment and treated with low (approximately 40 mg/kg every [q] 8 hours) or high-dose oral famciclovir (approximately 90 mg/kg q8h), was more promising. Most cat owners and attending veterinarians observed clinical improvement, with higher clinical improvement rates, faster response times and shorter treatment durations noted for the high-dose group compared to the low-dose group. Cat owners reported temporary (n = 8/32, 25%) or permanent (n = 17/32, 53%) improvement of clinical signs. Famciclovir course length was at the discretion of the attending veterinarian; one course was administered in 44/59 (75%) cats and two or three courses in 15/59 (25%) cats. Adverse effects, including diarrhea, vomiting, anorexia and polydipsia were reported in 10 adult cats at 3–36 days after the initiation of treatment (Thomasy et al. 2016).

13.8.1.2 Topical Ophthalmic Antiviral Drugs

Topical ophthalmic preparations for herpetic keratitis include idoxuridine (0.1% ophthalmic solution or 0.5% ointment, q4–6h; available only from compounding pharmacies in the United States) and cidofovir (0.1% ophthalmic solution q12h; commercially available in injectable rather than topical ophthalmic form in the United States) (Thomasy et al. 2016). Idoxuridine is relatively inexpensive and well-tolerated by most cats. A case-series study reported improvement or resolution of clinical signs in three cats and no improvement or worsening in four cats treated with topical ophthalmic idoxuridine (Stiles 1995). A randomized, placebo-controlled study of 0.5% ophthalmic solution of cidofovir compounded in methylcellulose and applied twice daily to cats experimentally infected with FHV-1 reported reduced viral shedding and clinical improvement, but since nasolacrimal stenosis has been reported in humans receiving topical cidofovir, treated cats should be monitored closely for signs of problems with tear drainage (Fontenelle et al. 2008).

13.8.1.3 L-Lysine

Dietary L-lysine supplements have been used extensively for the prevention and treatment of FHV-1 infection in the belief that it lowers plasma and tissue-arginine concentrations by one or more unconfirmed cellular mechanisms, thereby limiting viral replication since FHV-1 requires arginine for protein synthesis. Clinical trials of L-lysine supplementation in cats with FHV-1 have produced conflicting results, but a systematic review of the evidence for L-lysine supplementation concluded that clinical trials with cats had failed to show efficacy and that *in vitro* experiments did not demonstrate that excess L-lysine inhibited viral replication (Bol and Bunnick 2015). Another review concluded that there was some evidence that bolus oral administration of L-lysine might decrease FHV-1 shedding in latently infected cats and reduce clinical signs in cats on their first exposure to the virus. However, it was also noted that the stress of oral bolus administration might negate any beneficial effects of supplementation in shelter cats (Thomasy and Maggs 2016).

The published evidence for the efficacy of oral L-lysine supplementation in cats at risk of FHV-1 exposure or reactivation is conflicting at best. Two studies conducted in shelters failed to show a beneficial effect, including one in which lysine was incorporated into the diet to avoid any stress associated effect of administration (Rees and Lubinski 2008; Drazenovich et al. 2009). In one of these studies, cats that had been pre-treated with lysine developed more severe URTD compared to control cats (Drazenovich et al. 2009). Given these findings, the administration of lysine as a preventative for shelter cats is not recommended.

13.8.2 Antimicrobial Treatment

Protocols for minimizing feline URTD in shelters should be based on effective population management strategies to reduce disease transmission, especially in at-risk groups such as kittens; measures to diminish environmental and behavioral stress; and a robust vaccination on intake protocol. Antimicrobial drugs can be useful in cases where they are clearly indicated by clinical signs of bacterial infection (e.g. mucopurulent ocular or nasal discharge; see Figures 13.1a and 13.3). Prompt initiation of treatment must be balanced against avoiding unnecessary antimicrobial use to minimize the potential development of antimicrobial resistance. Practical issues, such as staffing availability, the required dosing frequency of the antimicrobial chosen, and cat stress due to drug administration, are also important considerations. Additionally, the daily cost of providing shelter care is relevant if LOS is prolonged by illness. Crowding in isolation areas can further increase LOS because of cat stress and poor air quality. In one shelter-based study of 182 kittens with clinical URTD at intake, 19 (10.4%) received antimicrobials within 24 hours of arrival at the shelter; of the remaining 163 kittens, 93 (57.1%) eventually required antimicrobial treatment before they could receive medical approval to move to the adoption area. The kittens that were treated earlier were approved for adoption significantly earlier than those that received delayed treatment (median time to approval = 29 days compared to 39 days) (Litster et al. 2011). This agrees with other studies that report prolonged LOS as a risk factor for feline URTD (Bannasch and Foley 2005; Dinnage et al. 2009; Gourkow et al. 2013). In kittens with clinical signs of bacterial URTD, prompt antimicrobial treatment is also likely to save money and increase lifesaving capacity by reducing time to adoption (Litster et al. 2011).

Minimizing the LOS in isolation is an important component of a successful URTD treatment strategy. To this end, response to therapy should be monitored daily and treatment adjusted accordingly. With the exception of *C. felis*, the bacteria targeted by treatment can also be found in clinically healthy animals, and the aim of treatment is a reduction in pathogen load rather than complete pathogen clearance. Therefore, treatment should continue until resolution of clinical signs rather than to an arbitrary time limit, even if that occurs within a few days of initiating therapy. Lack of response within five to seven days or failure to respond to repeated courses of medications could indicate additional medical or drug-related problems that require further diagnostic workup for specific identification (Lappin et al. 2017).

Doxycycline (5 mg/kg q12h or 10 mg/kg q24h) is a good first choice for acute bacterial URTD in cats because it is well tolerated by most cats and has activity against *M. felis*, *B. bronchiseptica* and *C. felis* (Lappin et al. 2017). Doxycycline formulations approved for use in cats are preferred if available and can be used safely without tooth-enamel discoloration in kittens over four weeks of age. However, doxycycline can also be safely used in kittens under four weeks of age since discoloration is only a cosmetic consideration and is less likely to occur with doxycycline than with other tetracyclines. Compounded doxycycline suspensions can violate prescription regulations in some countries, including the United States (Lappin et al. 2017), and variable loss of drug activity has been reported after seven days with aqueous formulations (Papich et al. 2013) so due attention must be taken to ensure that a safe, effective, and legally permissible product is selected. Orally administered doxycycline hyclate has been associated with esophageal strictures in cats so liquid formulations are preferred for that reason; dosing should be followed by at least 2 ml of water or a small amount of food (German et al. 2005) to reduce the risk of stricture.

If doxycycline is unavailable, minocycline has a similar but slightly broader antimicrobial spectrum (8.8 mg/kg q24h orally; one 50 mg capsule q24h for most cats) (Tynan et al. 2016), though clinical efficacy trials have not yet been performed for feline infections. If *M. felis* and/or *C. felis* infections are not suspected, amoxicillin (22 mg/kg q12h or amoxicillin-clavulanate 12.5 mg/kg q12h) is an acceptable first-line option for the treatment of acute bacterial URTD (Lappin et al. 2017). One randomized, masked, clinical trial of oral doxycycline liquid (10 mg/kg q24h) in *Mycoplasma*-infected adult shelter cats with clinical signs of URTD demonstrated that most of the beneficial clinical effects of treatment were achieved with a seven-day course of treatment. The authors concluded that, if recovery from clinical signs is the primary goal, rather than the complete elimination of *Mycoplasma* spp., a seven-day course of doxycycline is sufficient (Kompare et al. 2013).

There have been several published clinical trials investigating the use of antimicrobials in shelter cats with clinical signs of bacterial URTD as summarized in Table 13.2 (Ruch-Gallie et al. 2008; Litster et al. 2012; Spindel et al. 2013).

Differences in study design and bacterial isolates recovered in each of the study populations probably account for much of the variation in the results reported among the three studies. Importantly, some results were affected by the prevalence of *Mycoplasma* infection in each of the study groups, since penicillin-based drugs (such as amoxicillin or amoxicillin/clavulanic acid) or cephalosporins (such as cefovecin) are ineffective against this organism, and it has variable susceptibility to azithromycin. Of particular relevance to all of these studies is which antimicrobials are typically most effective, based on *in vitro* or ideally *in vivo* data, for the treatment of common feline bacterial URTD pathogens (Table 13.3).

13.8.3 Symptomatic Therapy

While therapy directed at specific pathogens, such as anti-viral or antimicrobial drugs, is sometimes warranted, supportive care to address the clinical signs of disease should be provided whenever possible. Fluid therapy with a balanced electrolyte solution such as lactated Ringer's solution can be administered either subcutaneously or intravenously and is important to correct dehydration resulting from fluid losses in ocular, nasal and oral discharges and lack of fluid intake in anorexic or inappetent cats. Intravenous (IV) fluids should always be administered under the supervision of a veterinarian to reduce the risk of catheter infections, fluid overload or electrolyte disturbances.

Pain relief should be considered on an individual cat basis, especially if there is evidence of oral or corneal ulceration. Appropriate analgesic protocols should be initiated promptly by a veterinarian and cats should be monitored often to ensure that therapeutic efficacy is achieved. Good analgesic choices include opioids such as buprenorphine (0.02–0.04 q 4–8 hours, IM/IV/oral transmucosally), or adjunctive drugs such as gabapentin (5 mg/kg q12h) (Matthews et al. 2014).

Table 13.2 Summary data for published clinical trials of antimicrobials in shelter cats with clinical signs of bacterial URTD.

Reference	Study design	Antimicrobial groups	Outcome measures	Results
Ruch-Gallie et al. (2008)	Case series; Cats failing to respond to the initial antibiotic were then administered the other drug	Amoxicillin (n = 21 initially), Azithromycin (n = 10 initially)	Clinical scores; bacterial culture, virus isolation and PCR results from nasal and oropharyngeal swabs	No differences in clinical scores between groups; 11/31 responded to initial drug; 16/31 switched to alternative drug; 4/31 cats removed from the trial; 8/27 cats failed to respond to either drug
Ruch-Gallie et al. (2008)	Randomized masked clinical trial	Amoxicillin (n = 15), Pradofloxacin (5 mg/kg q24h; n = 13), Pradofloxacin (10 mg/kg q24h; n = 12); 7-day course	Clinical scores and response rates; bacterial culture and PCR results from nasal and oropharyngeal swabs	No differences in clinical scores between groups; Response rates: Amoxicillin – 10/15 cats (67%); Pradofloxacin 5 mg/kg q24h - 11/13 cats (85%); Pradofloxacin (10 mg/kg q24h) - 11/12 cats (92%)
Litster et al. (2012)	Randomized clinical trial	Amoxicillin–clavulanate, Cefovecin, Doxycycline n = 16 cats/group; 14-day course	Clinical scores; bacterial culture and PCR results from nasal and oropharyngeal swabs	Significantly less sneezing in the amoxicillin-clavulanate and doxycycline groups; earlier return to normal food intake and demeanor in the amoxicillin-clavulanate group

q-every.

Table 13.3 Commonly used antimicrobial treatment options for feline bacterial upper respiratory tract disease (Lappin et al. 2017).

Isolate	Amoxicillin/clavulanic acid (12.5 mg/kg q12h PO)	Cefovecin (8 mg/kg SC; 14-day duration of action)	Doxycycline (5 mg/kg q12h PO) Minocycline (8.8 mg/kg q24h PO)	Azithromycin (5–10 mg/kg q12h on Day 1, then q72h PO)	Fluoroquinolones- Marbofloxacin (2.7–5.5 mg/kg q24h PO) Pradofloxacin (5 mg/kg q24h PO for tablets; 7.5 mg/kg q24h PO for oral suspension) Enrofloxacin[a] (5 mg/kg q24h PO)
Bordetella bronchiseptica	First-line option	Ineffective	Likely to be effective	Refer to specific infection susceptibility profiles	Likely to be effective
Chlamydia felis	Inferior to other drugs	Ineffective	Likely to be effective	Unlikely to be effective	Likely to be effective
Mycoplasma spp.	Ineffective	Ineffective	Likely to be effective	Refer to specific infection susceptibility profiles	Likely to be effective
Staphylococcus spp. *Streptococcus* spp.	First-line option	Likely to be effective	Refer to specific infection susceptibility profiles	Refer to specific infection susceptibility profiles	Likely to be effective

PO – Per os or oral.
SC – Subcutaneous.
q-every.
h-hour.
[a] Has been associated with retinal degeneration in cats (Gelatt et al. 2001).

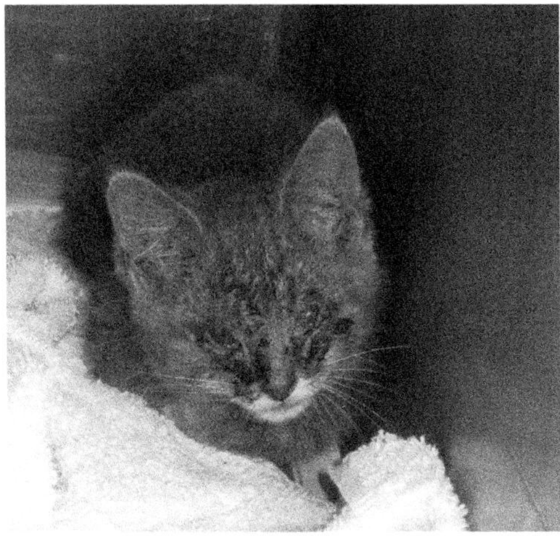

Figure 13.4 Crusted discharges should be cleaned away gently using warm saline and a soft, disposable cloth.

Non-steroidal anti-inflammatory drugs (NSAIDs) can also be used to treat fever and oral or ocular pain (Radford et al. 2009), but caution should be exercised in cats with evidence of clinical or subclinical dehydration, renal, hepatic or gastrointestinal disease (GI) or clotting abnormalities (Griffin et al. 2016). Additionally, cat comfort should be prioritized by the gentle cleaning of crusted ocular and nasal discharges using warm saline and a soft disposable cloth (Figure 13.4). Some cats also benefit from periods of nebulization using 0.9% saline (e.g. 15–20 minutes three to four times a day with the cage door covered in a towel to keep the steam in) to rehydrate upper respiratory tract mucous membranes (Thiry et al. 2009).

Many cats with URTD are inappetent or anorexic because they have lost their sense of smell or because of painful oral ulceration, but the immune system needs to be supported with protein and calories if it is to effectively fight infection. If a cat has not eaten for three days, a feeding tube should be placed by a veterinarian and enteral nutrition commenced (Thiry et al. 2009). Return to normal eating is an important milestone and some cats benefit from appetite stimulants such as mirtazapine (3–4 mg/cat PO q72h) or cyproheptadine (2–4 mg/cat q12–24 hours) (Plumb 2015) to help them commence eating voluntarily once recovery is underway (Radford et al. 2009).

13.8.4 Housing for Cats Undergoing Treatment

Cats and kittens with clinical signs of URTD, such as ocular or nasal discharges or sneezing, should be isolated from the rest of the population. In mild cases, in-cage isolation may be appropriate while leaving the cat available for adoption in the general population. In these cases, the cage should be marked to note that the cat is undergoing medical treatment and biosecurity precautions used before and after handling the cat. For cases that progress in severity to require antibiotic treatment, isolation in a separate housing area is indicated.

Ideally, isolation ward housing should be warm and cozy, with soft bedding and toys and a hiding place in each cage that also allows the cat to be seen, so behavioral and clinical status can be monitored. Sufficiently spacious housing and good air quality are as important here as in other areas of the shelter. Bedding and toys can be disposable or laundered as usual. (See Chapter 8 on Sanitation.) As noted above, daily spot cleaning is acceptable for cats with routine URI as well as healthy cats.

Foster care should be considered a preferred alternative to a shelter isolation unit, depending on the individual care needs of the cat/kitten/litter and the expertise and capacity of available foster homes.

13.8.5 Considerations for Adopters

It is important to alert prospective adopters to the potential of clinical URTD even after the adoption of apparently healthy cats and to educate them about appropriate care and the risk for other cats in the household (Bannasch and Foley 2005). Whenever introducing a new cat into the household, they should make sure that all pet cats already in the home are healthy and current with their vaccinations.

Recovered cats can also be adopted, but adopters should be provided with written copies of their medical history, including all treatment rendered, and advised to provide the records to their own veterinarians. They should also be made aware that some recovered cats may have chronic upper respiratory disease and be subject to recurrent bouts of sneezing and ocular discharges, especially when stressed. These cats may or may not require veterinary care, depending upon the severity of the clinical signs.

Though very uncommon, *B. Bronchiseptica* has also been shown to cause infection and disease in humans. For this reason, feline bordetellosis could potentially be a concern for adoption, but only if the adopter is immunocompromised or already has respiratory disease. In these cases, though the risk is considered minimal, they should be discussed.

13.9 Management and Prevention of URTD

13.9.1 The Role of Stress

Shelter environments are stressful by their very nature, even under ideal conditions. Not only the housing is unfamiliar—animals, people, procedures and routines are completely foreign to new arrivals. While most cats acclimate in two to five weeks (Rochlitz et al. 1998; McCobb et al. 2005), some never adjust to confinement and remain distressed for months. In the shelter environment, the ability to express normal feline coping behaviors is limited, further increasing stress and reducing welfare and potentially, adoptability (McCobb et al. 2005). Stress is also known to reactivate subclinical infections, particularly FHV-1 (Gaskell and Povey 1982). Importantly, this means even perfect biosecurity will not eliminate feline URTD in shelters if stress results in the recrudescence of latent FHV-1 infections. A comprehensive approach to reducing shelter cat stress is essential to managing this disease. Stress management in a shelter requires consideration at a population as well as individual cat level and should include attention to housing and LOS as well as care and handling of each cat. In addition, measures to mitigate stress include gentle and consistent handling practices, minimizing visual and auditory exposure to barking dogs; minimizing noise exposure in general; providing a litter box of sufficient size and positioned to allow normal posturing; limiting disruption through "spot-cleaning" on a day-to-day basis; and provision of a hiding place or other visual protection.

Environmental and social enrichment programs and handling protocols that can offset the negative effects of stress should be implemented as a kind of "first-aid" starting at the time of intake and continuing throughout the shelter stay (Ellis 2009). Placing cats on elevated surfaces and covering carriers with a towel, minimizing the time of confinement in a small carrier before intake processing, gentle handling and examination techniques, and keeping cats and dogs separated during intake can start cats off with less stress. Additionally, there is evidence that cats that display behaviors associated with lower stress levels are more attractive to adopters (Rochlitz et al. 1998.) (See Chapter 2 for more information about wellness). Larger group-housed rooms that are actively and sensitively managed to ensure that crowding does not occur, and negative inter-cat interactions are minimized can also give cats the opportunity and space to exhibit normal behaviors such as playing and running. Wall perches and cat trees allow for jumping and climbing, while hiding places, even simple cardboard boxes or paper bags, facilitate solitude and escape.

Gentle handling remains an important element of stress management throughout the shelter stay. An interesting series of Canadian studies examined the effects of enrichment and handling programs on URTD rates, viral shedding and local mucosal immunity (IgA) in shelter cats classified as contented (Gourkow and Phillips 2015), frustrated (Gourkow and Phillips 2016) or anxious (Gourkow et al. 2014) on arrival at a shelter. Contented cats received human interaction, including petting, playing, and grooming in four 10-minute sessions/day for 10 days. Enrichment was provided for the frustrated cats and consisted of four 10-minute training sessions daily for 10 days where the cat was taught paw-hand contact with a researcher. Anxious cats received gentle stroking and talking for four 10-minute training sessions daily for 10 days. All studies were controlled, and the same person interacted with each cat almost all the time. In each study, lower rates of URTD and higher levels of local mucosal immunity were found in cats in the enrichment groups compared to cats in the control group. Levels of viral shedding by day 10 of the study were also reduced in cats that received enrichment, though, depending on the study, clinical URTD rates varied from 14 to 50% in both treatment and control groups over the study period. These studies demonstrated that simple programs aimed at reducing stress, performed carefully by people who are sensitive to the emotional state of incoming cats, can have tangible benefits for shelter URTD rates. However, while gentled cats were less likely to succumb to URTD, the overall incidence remained relatively high in both groups (cumulative probability of 60% in control and 40% in the gentled groups), suggesting that this strategy alone is unlikely to be sufficient for disease prevention. Biosecurity measures to reduce disease transmission should always be employed when providing enrichment.

In additional to gentle and consistent handling practices, measures to mitigate stress include minimizing visual and auditory exposure to barking dogs; minimizing noise exposure in general; providing a litter box of sufficient size and positioned to allow normal posturing; limiting disruption through "spot-cleaning" on a day to day basis; and provision of a hiding place or visual protection (such as a box placed in the cage). (See Figure 13.5a–c).

13.9.2 Housing and Stress

While hiding boxes, gentle handling and other stress-mitigation strategies are beneficial and should be considered one of the foundations of URTD control, they may not fully offset the effect of cramped or inadequate housing. The Association of Shelter Veterinarians Guidelines for Standards of Care in Animal Shelters identified poor housing as a particularly significant issue for cats (Newbury et al. 2010). Sufficient space is required to provide adequate separation between food and litter; environment choices such as perching, hiding, and stretching; and opportunities to move around, make normal postural adjustments, and thermoregulate by choosing between soft, warm surfaces and firm cool surfaces. For individually housed cats, at least 1.1 m^2 (11 ft^2) of floor space have been recommended (Newbury et al. 2010). A comparison of URTD levels in nine North American shelters found floor space of less than 8 ft^2 and increased movement in and out of the cage were the most significant risk factors for illness. For individually housed cats, sufficient floor space (i.e. >8 ft^2) and double-compartment enclosures that facilitate cleaning and care without removal of the cat or disruption of the environment are recommended.

Multi-cat cage-free housing in group rooms can work for some cats, but behavioral assessment to select appropriate candidates and sensitive, attentive management of inter-cat dynamics is vital if individual cat stress is to be reduced rather than increased. A minimum of 2 m^2 (18 ft^2) of floor space per cat is recommended for group-housed cats along with sufficient resources of food, litter, climbing structures, hiding places, etc.; this is particularly important if the LOS is prolonged (Newbury et al. 2010). Because regrouping of cats has been associated with FHV-1 reactivation, group size should be kept small (ideally five cats or fewer) to limit the number of cats entering and leaving the group daily (Wagner et al. 2018a). See Figure 13.6.

(a)

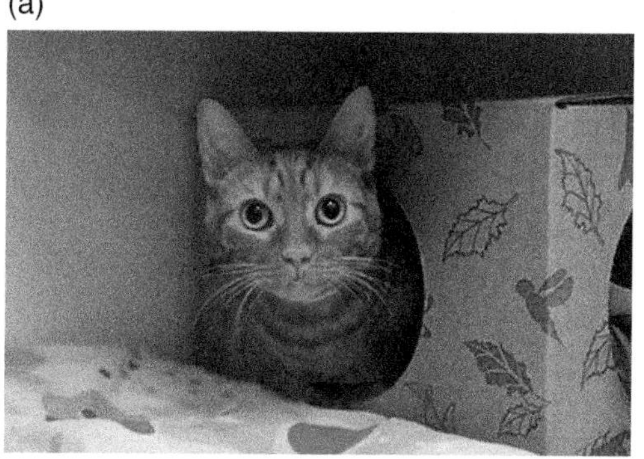

(b)

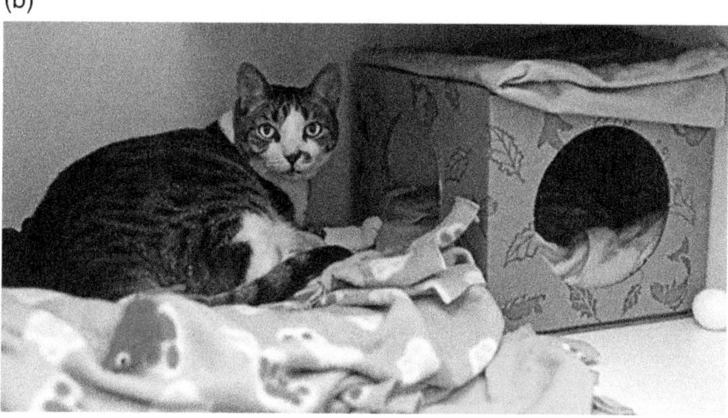

(c)

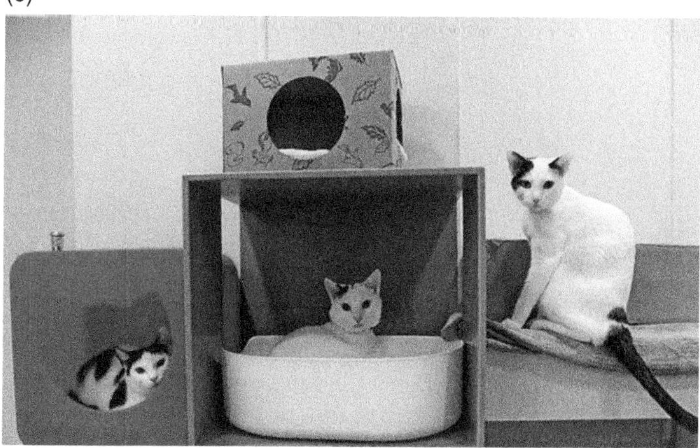

Figure 13.5 (a)–(c) Hiding boxes are an inexpensive and effective way to reduce stress in shelter housed cats.

13.9.3 Length of Stay (LOS)

LOS is frequently reported as the single greatest risk factor for URTD in shelter cats (Edinboro et al. 1999; Bannasch and Foley 2005; Edwards et al. 2008; Dinnage et al. 2009). In addition, LOS has a dramatic effect on the experience and needs of individual animals and directly affects the daily population and staffing requirements at the shelter level (Newbury et al. 2010). While hastening euthanasia should never be used as a population-management strategy, methods to lower LOS to the most appropriate outcome for each cat may be the most effective strategy to reduce feline URTD in shelters.

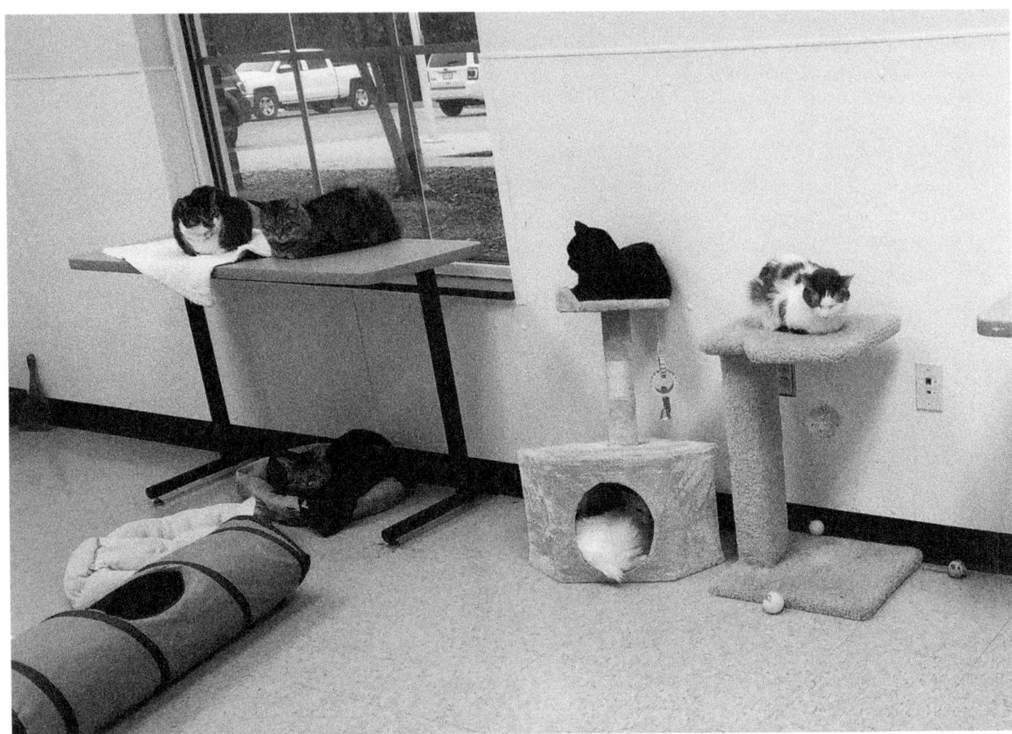

Figure 13.6 Group housing in multi-cat rooms can provide enrichment for some cats, but because individual cats have varying levels of comfort with socialization, group housing must be planned carefully and managed sensitively. In this photo, the tabby and white cat at the far left of the image is showing signs of covert aggression towards the cat sitting beside him - a direct stare, forward whiskers and leaning his weight back; the black cat next to them watches on. Both tabbies (the cat on the table and the one underneath) are possibly feigning sleep, while the white cat is taking advantage of a hiding place; the cat on the right looks more relaxed. Image and caption courtesy of Dr. Sara Bennett, North Carolina State University.

LOS can be reduced by evaluating and eliminating unnecessary holds, ensuring adequate staffing at critical flow-through points such as spay/neuter surgery, active pathway planning and daily rounds, and pro-active promotion of adoptable animals by developing targeted marketing campaigns. Also, formal strategies to reduce the LOS have been described. These include "fast track/slow track" management that prioritizes highly adoptable animals for quick movement through the system, and "open selection" which makes animals available for selection by adopters even during legally required stray holding periods (Newbury and Hurley 2012).

One UK-based year-long longitudinal study of five feline shelters reported that complete separation of incoming cats from the incumbent population and the availability of a separate isolation facility for clinical cases, including separation of staff servicing each section of the shelter, was associated with significantly lower clinical URTD rates. This was despite the fact that this shelter had a far higher intake of cats and housed more cats on-site at any single time than the other shelters and had also experienced substantial and frequent feline URTD outbreaks before the quarantine and isolation units were developed (Edwards et al. 2008). However, it is important to acknowledge that, in this study, a formal assessment of differences in handling practices and other factors between shelters was not performed. Therefore, any potential links between strict quarantine protocols and reduced clinical URTD rates can only be speculative. While quarantine protocols such as those described by Edwards et al. (2008) have potential benefits, they need to be balanced against the costs of housing and equipment, and increased LOS, which is the most important risk factor for the development of clinical URTD (Edinboro et al. 1999; Bannasch and Foley 2005; Edwards et al. 2008; Dinnage et al. 2009).

Housing that meets space requirements as defined by the ASV Guidelines for Standards of Care and strategies to reduce LOS were combined by the British Columbia SPCA in a program termed "Capacity for Care (C4C)." This program resulted in a reported reduction in URTD (the number of cats housed in isolation reportedly went from 12 to 16 at any given time to 10–15 over the course of an entire year) (Canadian Federation of Humane Societies 2012). Capacity for Care was then piloted in an additional six shelters which reported substantial reductions in the number of sick cats, ranging from a decrease of 40–87% (Humane Canada 2018). While strategies such as providing improved housing and reducing cats' LOS often have a profound impact on disease rates in animal shelters, prevention of URTD requires a well-considered assessment of all the factors contributing to disease and a holistic approach to addressing as many of them as possible.

13.9.3.1 Foster-Care Programs

The recurring theme that kittens are at the highest risk of developing clinical URTD and that risk increases with LOS can be addressed by effective and proactive adoption and fostering programs to minimize their shelter-residence time. In addition to reducing stress and exposure to URTD infections for high-risk cats, these programs have distinct advantages because they do not require changes to shelter architecture or equipment and can be instituted quickly. However, they must be carefully monitored and nurtured so that foster caregivers feel appreciated and stay committed to high-quality care and the shelter long-term.

Ideally, all kittens too young to be altered or placed for adoption should be immediately placed in foster homes, completely bypassing the shelter environment. They can return to the shelter for vaccinations and spay/neuter as shelter protocols dictate before being placed for adoption. If kittens must be housed in the shelter, they should be housed in enclosures that facilitate cleaning and daily care with minimal handling (e.g. double-compartment housing). Ideally, healthy kittens and sick kittens would each have housing areas separate from adults and from each other, but, at a minimum, biosecurity precautions should be taken between caring for adults and kittens and between each kitten or litter. However, housing healthy kittens and adults together permits greater flexibility in housing use and is acceptable provided appropriate biosecurity precautions are followed.

If kittens or cats with clinical URTD are housed in foster homes, precautions should be taken to protect resident pet cats and facilitate the recovery of the foster cats. Sick cats should be isolated from other animals in the house in an area that is warm but easy to clean and access frequently, such as a bathroom or laundry. Fomite spread should be minimized by keeping equipment and bedding, etc. separate from the rest of the house, wearing a disposable gown while in the designated "isolation room", and washing hands thoroughly before and after handling sick cats. Resident pet cats should be kept current with vaccinations against FHV-1 and FCV, as well as feline parvovirus (FPV). (Readers are referred to the section in this chapter for further details on environmental decontamination and Chapter 8 for more information on sanitation.)

13.9.4 Minimizing the Risk of Exposure

13.9.4.1 Written Intake Protocols

The foundations of excellent infection control are careful planning to prevent exposure to potential pathogens and effective environmental decontamination. Intake protocols designed to fit shelter capacity and facilities should be decided in advance, preferably with the input of a veterinarian with expertise in shelter medicine. They should be written down and made accessible to all staff and volunteers. Well-designed written protocols are powerful communication and education tools that can facilitate the health of shelter animals; they should be updated regularly to accommodate changes in shelter architecture and facilities, resources, intake type (e.g. age, source, species, health status) and pathogen prevalence.

13.9.4.2 Intake Triage

Cats should be assessed on admission for health status; in nearly all situations, cats and kittens at least four weeks of age should be vaccinated against FPV, FHV-1, FCV at or before intake. Once they have been spayed or neutered, they should be immediately placed into adoption programs if possible. Cats that have an extraordinarily high risk of infection (such as neonatal kittens and some purebred cats) should be housed separately from the main population or ideally, placed directly into foster care. By housing the most vulnerable cats away from the shelter population, the risk of pathogen exposure and transmission is limited.

Quarantine periods that fit the incubation periods of URTD pathogens (up to six days) must be balanced against the increased risk of developing clinical disease with an increased LOS; if implemented as a precaution against URI they are not likely to be practical or effective in most organizations. A shelter rarely has the ability to meet the requirements for a true "all-in, all-out" quarantine, and if this is not met, then holding cats will only result in continual and prolonged exposure. In other words, the risk incurred by longer shelter stays may outweigh any benefit gained by quarantine (Dinnage et al. 2009). However, quarantine of cats that carry an exceptional risk of severe URI, such as sick cats seized as part of a hoarding case, may be helpful. In these cases, the affected group of cats should be housed separately from other incoming and resident cats until their health has been fully evaluated. Shelters that periodically introduce animals into a stable, long-term population (such as in many sanctuary settings) may consider quarantining incoming arrivals for a while as well.

Cats and kittens with clinical signs of URTD, such as ocular or nasal discharges or sneezing, should be isolated from the rest of the population and treated appropriately. (See Chapter 6 for more detailed information on outbreak management.)

13.9.4.3 Shelter Housing, Design and Traffic Patterns

Crowding of adult cats and kittens poses one of the most serious threats to shelter population health. It facilitates the transmission of disease and increases stress, which can reduce the immune response to infectious disease and reactivate latent carrier states of feline URTD pathogens such as FHV-1. Because of this, the provision of adequate space to meet the physical and behavioral needs of every cat and kitten must be absolutely prioritized. See Figure 13.7.

If possible, shelter-traffic patterns for staff, volunteers, potential adopters and visitors should move people from the most susceptible animals, i.e. kittens, to those most resistant to disease (healthy adult cats) to reduce fomite spread. This can also serve the needs of shelter adoption programs by displaying the most highly adoptable cats to potential adopters first (Scarlett 2009). Conversely, some shelters try to feature adult cats by using kittens as an incentive to have visitors move through the entire shelter. Regardless of the flow utilized for adopters in a particular

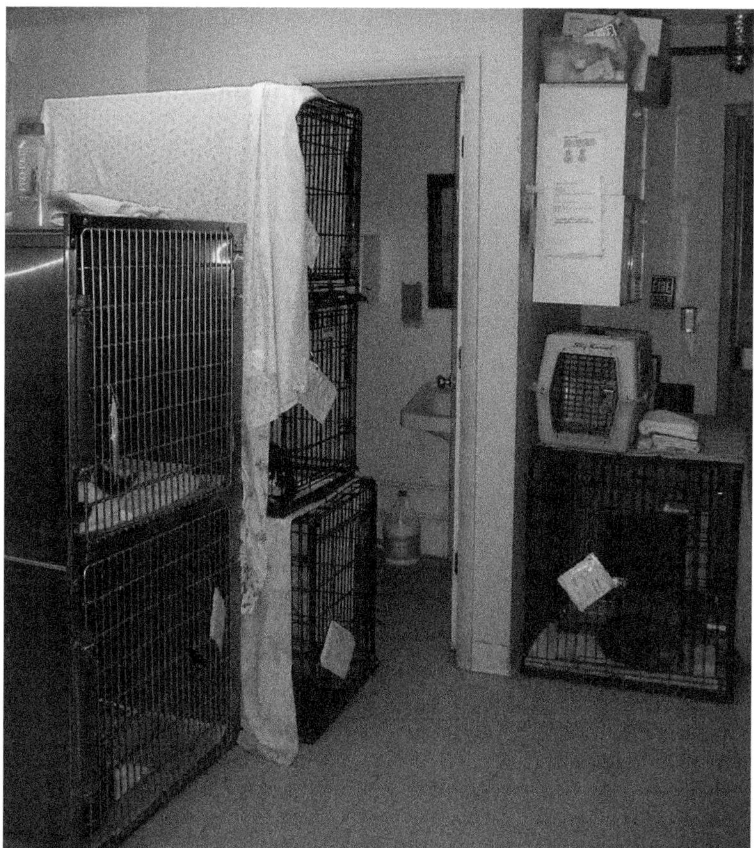

Figure 13.7 Crowding and poor-quality housing poses an important risk to the health of shelter cats and predisposes to the transmission of feline infectious respiratory disease. There is insufficient space to separate eating and eliminating activities from resting, no hiding places, etc.

facility, it is more important to have staff and volunteers follow appropriate biosecurity measures between groups of cats, as adopters generally pose less of a risk for disease transmission because of their relatively lower pathogen load. If possible, cats in quarantine (if applicable) and especially isolation areas should be cared for by dedicated staff and volunteers who do not work in other areas of the shelter. If this is not possible, staff should enter these areas after caring for more susceptible cats and kittens and follow infection control protocols on entering and leaving (Scarlett 2009). (Please see Chapter 2 on wellness and Chapter 6 on outbreak management for more information.)

13.9.4.4 Disease Surveillance

Tracking and documenting the health of the shelter population is an essential tool that alerts shelter management to changes in disease incidence and patterns and allows shelter protocols and interventions to be objectively assessed. Surveillance programs can also demonstrate seasonal disease patterns to inform preventative health programs individualized to the needs of the shelter population. Staff and volunteers need to be trained to recognize the clinical signs of feline URTD promptly and accurately, and appropriate data should be consistently documented using a standardized method that allows for analysis over time (Scarlett 2009).

Ideally, data should be recorded electronically and backed up daily. Relevant data collected should include the number of cats housed, housing type/density, and individual cat data such as identification number, signalment (age, breed and sexual status at intake), intake date, intake examination findings, clinical signs of URTD (plus date of first signs; either at admission or date of occurrence), LOS, specific location(s) within the facility, laboratory data, vaccines administered, surgeries and treatments performed and date of recovery/approval for adoption. Clinical and laboratory information should be interpreted in consultation with a veterinarian if possible, and reporting structures need to be instituted so that management can take appropriate action (Scarlett 2009). Regular reviews of surveillance data should be scheduled so that comparisons can be made over time and ongoing improvements can be individualized to the needs of the shelter population. (See Chapter 3 for more information on data surveillance)

13.9.4.5 Environmental Decontamination

Because of the frequency of subclinical shedding induced by stress, creating an environment that is completely free of the pathogens associated with feline URTD is an unrealistic goal, and even the most vigorous environmental decontamination will be ineffective in preventing disease without concurrent prevention of fomite transmission and meticulous attention to stress management. However, as with any disease, lowering environmental pathogen load is an important component of a comprehensive control plan. Written infection control and sanitation protocols facilitate communication, education and help ensure that quality control is consistent over time.

Hand sanitization, preferably using soap, water and a disposable towel, should be performed after handling each cat and/or the environment where the cat is housed, or disposable gloves should be worn. Hand sanitizers are a convenient alternative where running water is not available, but they are not effective against FPV and have limited efficacy against FCV (Scarlett 2009). Additionally, while many of the pathogens associated with feline URTD are relatively susceptible to decontamination, FCV is not susceptible to quaternary ammonium disinfectants and is only partially inactivated by alcohol. A 1 : 32 solution of 5.25% household bleach, disinfectants containing potassium peroxymonosulfate or accelerated hydrogen peroxide should be used if contamination by FCV is suspected, and wipes containing accelerated hydrogen peroxide will inactivate this virus more reliably than alcohol-based hand sanitizer (ASPCA 2017).

Though *Mycoplasma* is widely thought to be unable to survive outside host cells (Browning et al. 2011), isolates can survive on surfaces and in biofilms for days to months, depending on the species. While routine disinfectants should be effective for *Mycoplasma* spp. infecting cats, one study demonstrated that a quaternary ammonium disinfectant had poor efficacy against the non-feline species of *Mycoplasma* tested (Eterpi et al. 2011).

Cleaning and disinfection themselves are not without risk when it comes to feline URTD. The noise, chemical use, and disruption associated with cleaning can lead to stress and increased opportunities for fomite transmission. Spot cleaning for cats remaining in their housing unit on a day-to-day basis not only saves staff time to attend to more critical needs, but it can also reduce stress and URTD. Spot cleaning is also appropriate for cats under treatment for routine URTD, as cats in residence in a housing unit will immediately recontaminate it anyway after disinfection. When suspected calicivirus outbreak or outbreaks of unknown cause are present, more vigorous cleaning and disinfection may be indicated, especially if cats are being rehoused. Please see Chapter 8 for more detailed information on sanitation.

13.9.5 Vaccination

The clinical outcome of respiratory disease in cats depends on a variety of factors, including the robustness of the immune response, pathogen dose and strain, and the environment the cat is housed in. While vaccination against feline respiratory pathogens such as FHV-1, FCV and *C. felis* helps provide protection against clinical signs of disease, it does not provide complete protection against infection, clinical signs and shedding in all cats on pathogen exposure.

Despite its limitations, FVRCP vaccination against FHV-1 (rhinotracheitis) and FCV (calicivirus) in combination with FPV (feline panleukopenia virus) is recommended for all incoming cats and should be administered at the time of intake, or preferably at least one week before introduction to the shelter by prior arrangement with relinquishing owners or transfer partners. The first dose should be administered subcutaneously (SC) to shelter kittens starting at 4–6 weeks of age and revaccination should be provided every 2–3 weeks until 16–20 weeks of age (Stone et al. 2020). Though inactivated (killed) vaccines may produce more rapid seroconversion for FHV-1, MLV vaccines are strongly recommended for shelters due to the more rapid seroconversion induced by this vaccine against the greater threat of FPV, and because they are more effective at inducing protective antibody titers in the presence of maternally derived antibodies in kittens than inactivated vaccines (DiGangi et al. 2012). However, it is important to note that MLV feline panleukopenia virus vaccines should not be used in kittens under four weeks old or in pregnant queens because of the risk of danger to the developing cerebellum (Truyen et al. 2009).

Vaccine label instructions for storage and handling should be followed carefully for maximal protection, and care should be taken with the route of administration since inadvertent oronasal exposure to the FCV component of the MLV SC vaccine can cause symptoms of URTD. Potential adopters should also be advised regarding requirements for booster vaccinations in the post-adoption period so they can follow up with their veterinarian.

While all shelter cats should receive a three-way FVRCP MLV SC, the evidence for additionally vaccinating against the respiratory viruses by the intranasal (IN) route is less clear. There have been several published studies investigating the effect of the route of vaccine administration for FHV-1 and FCV, but experimental infections administered after vaccines are given under laboratory conditions using purpose-bred initially-uninfected cats might not replicate shelter conditions closely enough for the results to be accurately generalized to shelter cats. However, one shelter-based study divided healthy adult cats into two groups at intake—one group was vaccinated with an inactivated SC FVRCP vaccine alone (single-vaccine group), while the other group was vaccinated concurrently with the same SC vaccine plus a MLV IN vaccine against FHV-1 and FCV (dual vaccine group). During the 30-day post-vaccination observation period (both in the shelter and after adoption), the overall incidence of clinical signs of URTD was much lower in the dual-vaccine group than the single-vaccine group (30.8% vs. 54.8%; a 51.8% reduction) and after statistical adjustment for baseline characteristics, there was a 76% reduction in the overall risk of disease in the dual-vaccine group. A financial analysis demonstrated that the dual-vaccination protocol was more cost-effective because the extra vaccine costs were lower than the cost of treatment for clinical URTD in the single-vaccine group (Edinboro et al. 1999). Because there was no comparison to a MLV SC vaccine alone or in combination with the IN vaccine, it could not be determined whether the benefit came from the route of vaccination or the vaccine type. In contrast to these study results, a more recent study comparing URTD risk between shelters found a higher rate of URTD disease in shelters that used the IN vaccine compared to those that did not (Wagner et al. 2018b). If shelters use an IN vaccine, they should evaluate URTD incidence before and after to evaluate the efficacy and calculate the cost/benefit using a published clinical scoring system.

Foster caregivers should be advised to ensure their own pet cats are properly vaccinated in preparation for disease exposure, especially to at-risk cats such as kittens, and foster cats with clinical URTD. Because protection against the respiratory viruses may not be as long-lived as against FPV, foster caregivers should consult their veterinarians about revaccinating pet cats against FHV and FCV more frequently.

Routine vaccination against *B. bronchiseptica* and *C. felis* is not recommended for shelter cats. However, they can be considered if there is laboratory evidence of widespread infection in cats with clinical URTD. It has also been suggested that vaccination against *B. bronchiseptica* could limit disease transmission in shelters where dogs and cats have direct or indirect contact with each other and the dogs have a recent or current clinical history of canine infectious respiratory disease; however, for many reasons, preventing close contact between these populations is preferred (Stone et al. 2020). See Chapter 9 for more information on vaccinations.

13.9.6 Outbreak Management

The management of outbreaks is described in detail in Chapter 6 and is based on specific pathogen diagnosis, identification and isolation of affected cats, effective environmental decontamination, protection of newly admitted cats, and documentation and communication (Litster 2016). While the broad principles of outbreak management apply, information can be sought from specific resources on VSFCV (Koret Shelter Medicine Program 2017). At the time of writing, Cornell University Maddie's® Shelter Medicine Program and the University of Florida Maddie's Shelter Medicine Program also offered individualized shelter consultations and disease outbreak response assistance (Cornell University Maddie's Shelter Medicine Program 2018; University of Florida Maddie's Shelter Medicine Program 2018).

Fortunately, outbreaks of severe contagious URTD associated with pathogens such as virulent systemic FCV or unusual strains of influenza are uncommon and the vast majority of feline URTD in shelters can be managed with the principles of good population care and stress management described in this chapter. When URTD levels rise, in addition to diagnostic testing, attention should be paid to factors such as crowding, increased stress, and possible compromises in housing, air quality and animal care. Because virtually all pathogens associated with URTD can also be carried by clinically healthy cats, depopulation is very rarely, if ever, useful or indicated in managing an apparent outbreak.

13.10 Conclusion

The control of feline URTD requires a multipronged approach that can be summarized as follows:

- **Prioritize planning**—Time spent on careful management, planning and protocol development is likely to make the most impact on the health of the shelter population
- **Obtain input from a veterinarian**—The input of a veterinarian with expertise in shelter medicine is invaluable for creating scientifically based written protocols for treatment and prevention of URTD
- **Reduce environmental and behavioral stress**—Stress management must be prioritized by avoiding crowding and attending to the behavioral and environmental needs of shelter-housed cats
- **Provide adequate housing at all stages of shelter care**
- **Create a vibrant foster care program**—Foster-home care programs can reduce stress, reduce disease transmission and increase the life-saving capacity of the shelter, but they need to be consistently nurtured and encouraged to be effective and have longevity

- **Utilize active pathway planning to optimize the LOS**—All cats should be triaged immediately on intake, and, based on history, physical examinations and behavioral assessment, routed to an appropriate outcome (such as adoption, foster, or transfer) after appropriate preventative healthcare or treatment has been provided
- **Collect and analyze disease surveillance data**—Daily data collection should be performed for disease surveillance and recorded in a form that can be analyzed and reported so that prompt action can be taken to control outbreaks or address the failure to make improvements to feline URTD rates over time. Data should be reviewed regularly and compared with previous results to inform changes in protocols so that ongoing improvements can be made
- **Perform rounds daily to facilitate data collection, assess the overall health of the general population, identify possible new cases of URTD and monitor treatment**

References

ASPCA (2017). Shelter disinfectant quick reference. ASPCA Professional. https://www.aspcapro.org/resource/shelter-health-disease-management/shelter-disinfectant-quick-reference (accessed 7 August 2020).

Bannasch, M.J. and Foley, J.E. (2005). Epidemiologic evaluation of multiple respiratory pathogens in cats in animal shelters. *Journal of Feline Medicine and Surgery* 7 (2): 109–119.

Belgard, S., Truyen, U., Thibault, J.C. et al. (2010). Relevance of feline calicivirus, feline immunodeficiency virus, feline leukemia virus, feline herpesvirus and *Bartonella henselae* in cats with chronic gingivostomatitis. *Berliner und Münchener Tierärztliche Wochenschrift* 123 (9–10): 369–376.

Binns, S.H., Dawson, S., Speakman, A.J. et al. (2000). A study of feline upper respiratory tract disease with reference to prevalence and risk factors for infection with feline calicivirus and feline herpesvirus. *Journal of Feline Medicine and Surgery* 2 (3): 123–133.

Bol, S. and Bunnick, E.M. (2015). Lysine supplementation is not effective for the prevention or treatment of feline herpesvirus 1 infection in cats: a systematic review. *BMC Veterinary Research* 11: 284.

Browning, G.F., Marenda, M.S., Noormohammadi, A.H. et al. (2011). The central role of lipoproteins in the pathogenesis of mycoplasmoses. *Veterinary Microbiology* 153 (1–2): 44–50.

Canadian Federation of Humane Societies (2012). Cats in Canada: A Comprehensive Report on the Cat Overpopulation Crisis:69

Contreras, E.T., Hodgkins, E., Tynes, V. et al. (2017). Effect of a pheromone on stress-associated reactivation of feline herpesvirus-1 in experimentally inoculated kittens. *Journal of Veterinary Internal Medicine* 32 (1): 406–417.

Cornell Feline Health Center (2016). Influenza outbreak among shelter cats in Manhattan. Cornell University College of Veterinary Medicine. https://www.vet.cornell.edu/departments-centers-and-institutes/cornell-feline-health-center/health-information/cat-health-news/influenza-outbreak-among-shelter-cats-manhattan (accessed 7 August 2020).

Cornell University Maddie's® Shelter Medicine Program (2018) Consultations. Cornell University College of Veterinary Medicine. https://www2.vet.cornell.edu/hospitals/maddies-shelter-medicine-program/services-training/shelters/consultations (accessed 15 April 2018).

Dawson, S., Bennett, D., Carter, S.D. et al. (1994). Acute arthritis of cats associated with feline calicivirus infection. *Research in Veterinary Science* 56 (2): 133–143.

Dawson, S., Gaskell, C.J., McCracken, C.M. et al. (2000). *Bordetella bronchiseptica* infection in cats following contact with infected dogs. *Veterinary Record* 146 (2): 46–48.

DiGangi, B.A., Levy, J.K., Griffin, B. et al. (2012). Effects of maternally derived antibodies on serologic responses to vaccination in kittens. *Journal of Feline Medicine and Surgery* 14 (2): 118–123.

Dinnage, J.D., Scarlett, J.M., and Richards, J.R. (2009). Descriptive epidemiology of feline upper respiratory tract disease in an animal shelter. *Journal of Feline Medicine and Surgery* 11 (10): 816–825.

Drazenovich, T.L., Fascetti, A.J., Westermeyer, H.D. et al. (2009). Effects of dietary lysine supplementation on upper respiratory and ocular disease and detection of infectious organisms in cats within an animal shelter. *American Journal of Veterinary Research* 70 (11): 1391–1400.

Edinboro, C., Dillaman, L., Guptill-Yoran, L. et al. (1999). A clinical trial of intranasal and subcutaneous vaccines to prevent upper respiratory infection in cats at an animal shelter. *Feline Practice* 27 (6): 7–13.

Edwards, D.S., Coyne, K., Dawson, S. et al. (2008). Risk factors for time to diagnosis of feline upper respiratory tract disease in UK animal adoption shelters. *Preventive Veterinary Medicine* 87 (3–4): 327–339.

Egberink, H., Addie, D., Belák, S. et al. (2009). *Bordetella bronchiseptica* infection in cats. ABCD guidelines on prevention and management. *Journal of Feline Medicine and Surgery* 11 (7): 610–614.

Ellis, S. (2009). Environmental enrichment: practical strategies for improving feline welfare. *Journal of Feline Medicine and Surgery* 11 (11): 901–912.

Eterpi, M., McDonnell, G., and Thomas, V. (2011). Decontamination efficacy against *Mycoplasma*. *Letters in Applied Microbiology* 52 (2): 150–155.

Foley, J.E., Rand, C., Bannasch, M.J. et al. (2002). Molecular epidemiology of feline bordetellosis in two animal shelters in California, USA. *Preventive Veterinary Medicine* 54 (2): 141–156.

Fontenelle, J.P., Powell, C.C., Veir, J.K. et al. (2008). Effect of topical ophthalmic application of cidofovir on experimentally induced primary ocular feline herpesvirus-1 infection in cats. *American Journal of Veterinary Research* 69 (2): 289–293.

Foster, S. and Martin, P. (2011). Lower respiratory tract infections in cats reaching beyond empirical therapy. *Journal of Feline Medicine and Surgery* 13 (5): 313–332.

Gaskell, R.M. and Povey, R.C. (1982). Transmission of feline viral rhinotracheitis. *The Veterinary Record* 111 (16): 359–362.

Gaskell, R.M., Dawson, S., and Radford, A. (2012). Feline respiratory disease. In: *Infectious Diseases of the Dog and Cat* (ed. C.E. Greene), 151–162. St. Louis: Elsevier Saunders.

Gelatt, K.N., van der Woerdt, A., Ketring, K.L. et al. (2001). Enrofloxacin-associated retinal degeneration in cats. *Veterinary Ophthalmology* 4 (2): 99–106.

German, A.J., Cannon, M.J., and Dye, C. (2005). Oesophageal strictures in cats associated with doxycycline therapy. *Journal of Feline Medicine and Surgery* 7 (1): 33–41.

Gould, D. (2011). Feline herpesvirus-1 ocular manifestations, diagnosis and treatment options. *Journal of Feline Medicine and Surgery* 13 (5): 333–346.

Gourkow, N. and Phillips, C.J. (2015). Effect of interactions with humans on behaviour, mucosal immunity and upper respiratory disease of shelter cats rated as contented on arrival. *Preventive Veterinary Medicine* 121 (3–4): 288–296.

Gourkow, N. and Phillips, C.J. (2016). Effect of cognitive enrichment on behavior, mucosal immunity and upper respiratory disease of shelter cats rated as frustrated on arrival. *Preventive Veterinary Medicine* 131 (1): 103–110.

Gourkow, N., Lawson, J.H., Hamon, S.C. et al. (2013). Descriptive epidemiology of upper respiratory disease and associated risk factors in cats in an animal shelter in coastal western Canada. *Canadian Veterinary Journal* 54 (2): 132–138.

Gourkow, N., Hamon, S.C., and Phillips, C.J. (2014). Effect of gentle stroking and vocalization on behavior, mucosal immunity and upper respiratory disease in anxious shelter cats. *Preventive Veterinary Medicine* 117 (1): 266–275.

Griffin, B., Bushby, P.A., McCobb, E. et al. (2016). The Association of Shelter Veterinarians' 2016 veterinary medical care guidelines for spay-neuter programs. *Journal of the American Veterinary Medical Association* 249 (2): 165–188.

Gruffydd-Jones, T., Addie, D., Belák, S. et al. (2009). *Chlamydophila felis* infection. ABCD guidelines on prevention and management. *Journal of Feline Medicine and Surgery* 11 (7): 605–609.

Haesebrouck, F., Devriese, L.A., van Rijssen, B. et al. (1991). Incidence and significance of isolation of *Mycoplasma felis* from conjunctival swabs of cats. *Veterinary Microbiology* 26 (1–2): 95–101.

Hartmann, A.D., Helps, C.R., Lappin, M.R. et al. (2008). Efficacy of pradofloxacin in cats with feline upper respiratory tract disease due to *Chlamydophila felis* or *Mycoplasma* infection. *Journal of Veterinary Internal Medicine* 21 (1): 44–52.

Hartmann, A.D., Hawley, J., Werckenthin, C. et al. (2010). Detection of bacterial and viral organisms from the conjunctiva of cats with conjunctivitis and upper respiratory tract disease. *Journal of Feline Medicine and Surgery* 12 (10): 775–782.

Hatta, M., Zhong, G., Gao, Y. et al. (2018). Characterization of a Feline Influenza A(H7N2) virus. *Emerging Infectious Diseases* 24 (1): 75–86.

Helps, C.R., Lait, P., Damhuis, A. et al. (2005). Factors associated with upper respiratory tract disease caused by feline herpesvirus, feline calicivirus, *Chlamydophila felis* and *Bordetella bronchiseptica* in cats: experience from 218 European catteries. *Veterinary Record* 156 (21): 669–673.

Humane Canada (2018) Capacity For Care (C4C) Case Studies. https://humanecanada.ca/wp-content/uploads/2020/03/Capacity-For-Care-English.pdf (Accessed 11 February 2020)

Hurley, K.E., Pesavento, P.A., Pedersen, N.C. et al. (2004). An outbreak of virulent systemic feline calicivirus disease. *Journal of the American Veterinary Medical Association* 224 (2): 241–249.

IDEXX (2013). Quantitative feline herpesvirus PCR. IDEXX Laboratories. https://www.idexx.eu/globalassets/documents/diagnostic-updates/nordic/2013-10-diu-en-quantitative-feline-herpesvirus-pcrnordic380_du-quant-feline-herpesvirus.pdf (accessed 21 February 2017).

Kompare, B., Litster, A.L., Leutenegger, C.M. et al. (2013). Randomized masked controlled clinical trial to compare 7-day and 14-day course length of doxycycline in the treatment of *Mycoplasma* felis infection in shelter cats. *Comparative Immunology, Microbiology and Infectious Diseases* 36 (2): 129–135.

Koret Shelter Medicine Program (2017). Feline calicivirus and virulent systemic feline calicivirus. UC Davis School of Veterinary Medicine. http://www.sheltermedicine.com/library/resources/feline-calicivirus-virulent-systemic-feline-calicivirus-vs-fcv (accessed 3 March 2017).

Lappin, M.R., Blondeau, J., Booth, D. et al. (2017). Antimicrobial use guidelines for treatment of respiratory tract disease in dogs and cats: Antimicrobial Guidelines Working Group of the International Society for Companion Animal Infectious Diseases. *Journal of Veterinary Internal Medicine* 31 (2): 279–294.

Le Boedec, K. (2017). A systematic review and meta-analysis of the association between Mycoplasma spp and upper and lower respiratory tract disease in cats. *Journal of the American Veterinary Medical Association* 250 (4): 397–407.

Litster, A.L. (2015). Feline calicivirus. Clinician's Brief. http://www.cliniciansbrief.com/article/feline-calicivirus (accessed 22 February 2017).

Litster, A.L. (2016). Top 5 strategies for managing shelter infectious disease outbreaks. Clinician's Brief. http://www.cliniciansbrief.com/article/top-5-strategies-managing-shelter-infectious-disease-outbreaks (accessed 3 March 2017).

Litster, A.L., Allen, J., Mohamed, A. et al. (2011). Risk factors for delays between intake and veterinary approval for adoption on medical grounds in shelter puppies and kittens. *Preventive Veterinary Medicine* 101 (1–2): 107–112.

Litster, A.L., Wu, C.C. et al. (2012). Comparison of the efficacy of amoxicillin-clavulanic acid, cefovecin, and doxycycline in the treatment of upper respiratory tract disease in cats housed in an animal shelter. *Journal of the American Veterinary Medical Association* 241 (2): 218–226.

Litster, A.L., Wu, C.C., and Leutenegger, C.M. (2015a). Detection of feline upper respiratory tract disease pathogens using a commercially available real-time PCR test. *The Veterinary Journal* 206 (2): 149–153.

Litster, A.L., Lohr, B.R., Bukowy, R.A. et al. (2015b). Clinical and antiviral effect of a single oral dose of famciclovir administered to cats at intake to a shelter. *The Veterinary Journal* 203 (2): 199–204.

Matthews, K., Kronen, P.W., Lascelles, D. et al. (2014). Guidelines for recognition, assessment and treatment of pain. *Journal of Small Animal Practice* 55 (6): E10–E68.

McCobb, E.C., Patronek, G.J., Marder, A. et al. (2005). Assessment of stress levels among cats in four animal shelters. *Journal of the American Veterinary Medical Association* 226 (4): 548–555.

McDonagh, P., Sheehy, P.A., Fawcett, A. et al. (2015a). Antiviral effect of mefloquine on feline calicivirus in vitro. *Veterinary Microbiology* 176 (3–4): 370–377.

McDonagh, P., Sheehy, P.A., Fawcett, A. et al. (2015b). in vitro inhibition of field isolates of feline calicivirus with short interfering RNAs (siRNAs). *Veterinary Microbiology* 177 (102): 78–86.

McManus, C.M., Levy, J.K., Andersen, L.A. et al. (2014). Prevalence of upper respiratory pathogens in four management models for unowned cats in the Southeast United States. *The Veterinary Journal* 201 (2): 196–201.

Newbury, S. and Hurley, K. (2012). Population management. In: *Shelter Medicine for Veterinarians and Staff* (eds. L. Miller and S. Zawistowski), 93–114. Ames: Blackwell Publishing.

Newbury, S., Blinn, M.K., Bushby, P.A. et al. (2010). Guidelines for Standards of Care in Animal Shelters. Association of Shelter Veterinarians. http://www.sheltervet.org/assets/docs/shelter-standards-oct2011-wforward.pdf (accessed 22 February 2017).

NYC Health (2016). Health Department investigation of H7N2 influenza in shelter cats confirms risk to humans is low. https://www1.nyc.gov/assets/doh/downloads/pdf/han/alert/avian-influenza.pdf (accessed 13 June 2020).

Papich, M.G., Davidson, G.S., and Fortier, L.A. (2013). Doxycycline concentration over time after storage in a compounded veterinary preparation. *Journal of the American Veterinary Medical Association* 242 (912): 1674–1678.

Pedersen, N.C., Elliott, J.B., Glasgow, A. et al. (2000). An isolated epizootic of hemorrhagic-like fever in cats caused by a novel and highly virulent strain of feline calicivirus. *Veterinary Microbiology* 73 (4): 281–300.

Pedersen, N.C., Sato, R., Foley, J.E. et al. (2004). Common virus infections in cats, before and after being placed in shelters, with emphasis on feline enteric coronavirus. *Journal of Feline Medicine and Surgery* 6 (2): 83–88.

Persico, P., Roccabianca, P., Corona, A. et al. (2011). Detection of feline herpes virus 1 via polymerase chain reaction and immunohistochemistry in cats with ulcerative facial dermatitis, eosinophilic granuloma complex reaction patterns and mosquito bite hypersensitivity. *Veterinary Dermatology* 22 (6): 521–527.

Pesavento, P.A., Bannasch, M.J., Bachmann, R. et al. (2007). Fatal *Streptococcus canis* infections in intensively housed shelter cats. *Veterinary Pathology* 44 (2): 218–221.

Pesavento, P.A., Chang, K.O., and Parker, J.S. (2008). Molecular virology of feline calicivirus. *Veterinary Clinics of North America: Small Animal Practice* 38 (4): 775–786.

Plumb, D.C. (2015). *Plumb's Veterinary Drug Handbook*, 8e. Hoboken, NJ: Wiley-Blackwell.

Polak, K.C., Levy, J.K., Crawford, P.C. et al. (2014). Infectious diseases in large-scale cat hoarding investigations. *The Veterinary Journal* 201 (2): 189–195.

Priestnall, S. and Erles, K. (2011). *Streptococcus zooepidemicus*: an emerging canine pathogen. *The Veterinary Journal* 188 (2): 142–148.

Radford, A.D., Dawson, S., Coyne, K.P. et al. (2006). The challenge for the next generation of feline calicivirus vaccines. *Veterinary Microbiology* 117 (1): 14–18.

Radford, A.D., Addie, D., Belák, S. et al. (2009). Feline calicivirus infection. ABCD guidelines on prevention and management. *Journal of Feline Medicine and Surgery* 11 (7): 556–564.

Rees, T.M. and Lubinski, J.L. (2008). Oral supplementation with L-lysine did not prevent upper respiratory infection in a shelter population of cats. *Journal of Feline Medicine and Surgery* 10 (5): 510–513.

Reubel, G.H., George, J.W., Barlough, J.E. et al. (1992). Interaction of acute feline herpesvirus-1 and chronic feline immunodeficiency virus infections in experimentally infected specific pathogen free cats. *Veterinary Immunology and Immunopathology* 35 (1–2): 95–119.

Rochlitz, I., Podberscek, A.L., and Broom, D.M. (1998). Welfare of cats in a quarantine cattery. *Veterinary Record* 143 (2): 35–39.

Ruch-Gallie, R.A., Veir, J.K., Spindel, M.E. et al. (2008). Efficacy of amoxicillin and azithromycin for the empirical treatment of shelter cats with suspected bacterial upper respiratory infections. *Journal of Feline Medicine and Surgery* 10 (6): 542–550.

Scarlett, J.M. (2009). Feline upper respiratory disease. In: *Infectious Disease Management in Animal Shelters* (eds. L. Miller and K.F. Hurley), 125–146. Ames: Wiley-Blackwell.

Schultz, B.S., Wolf, G., and Hartmann, K. (2006). Bacteriological and antibiotic sensitivity test results in 271 cats with respiratory tract infections. *Veterinary Record* 158 (8): 269–270.

Shelter Medicine (2017) H7N2 influenza in shelter cats in New York; City. School of Veterinary Medicine. University of Wisconsin-Madison. http://www.uwsheltermedicine.com/news/2017/10/h7n2-influenza-in-shelter-cats-in-new-york-city (accessed 15 April 2018).

Smith, A.W., Iversen, P.L., O'Hanley, P.D. et al. (2008). Virus-specific antiviral treatment for controlling severe and fatal outbreaks of feline calicivirus infection. *American Journal of Veterinary Research* 69 (1): 23–32.

Song, D.S., An, D.J., Moon, H.J. et al. (2011). Interspecies transmission of the canine influenza H3N2 virus to domestic cats in South Korea, 2010. *Journal of General Virology* 92 (10): 2350–2355.

Spindel, M.E., Slater, M.R., and Boothe, D. (2013). A survey of North American shelter practices relating to feline upper respiratory management. *Journal of Feline Medicine and Surgery* 15 (4): 323–327.

Stiles, J. (1995). Treatment of cats with ocular disease attributable to herpesvirus infection: 17 cases (1983–1993). *Journal of the American Veterinary Medical Association* 207 (5): 599–603.

Stone, A.E., Brummet, G.O., Carozza, E.M. et al. (2020) 2020 AAHA/AAFP feline vaccination guidelines. *Journal of the American Animal Hospital Association* 56: 249–265.

Tan, R.J.S. and Miles, J.A.R. (1974). Incidence and significance of Mycoplasmas in sick cats. *Research in Veterinary Science* 16 (1): 27–34.

Thiry, E., Addie, D., Belák, S. et al. (2009). Feline herpesvirus infection. ABCD guidelines on prevention and management. *Journal of Feline Medicine and Surgery* 11 (7): 547–555.

Thomasy, S.M. and Maggs, D.J. (2016). A review of antiviral drugs and other compounds with activity against feline herpesvirus type 1. *Veterinary Ophthalmology* 9 (Suppl. 1): 119–130.

Thomasy, S.M., Shull, O., Outerbridge, C.A. et al. (2016). Oral administration of famciclovir for the treatment of spontaneous ocular, respiratory, or dermatologic disease attributed to feline herpesvirus type 1: 59 cases (2006–2013). *Journal of the American Veterinary Medical Association* 249 (5): 526–538.

Truyen, U., Addie, D., Belák, S. et al. (2009). Feline panleukopenia. ABCD guidelines on prevention and management. *Journal of Feline Medicine and Surgery* 11 (7): 538–546.

Tynan, B.E., Papich, M.G., Kerl, M.E. et al. (2016). Pharmacokinetics of minocycline in domestic cats. *Journal of Feline Medicine and Surgery* 18 (4): 257–263.

University of Florida Maddie's® Shelter Medicine Program (2018). For Shelters: Maddie's® Shelter Medicine Program. College of Veterinary Medicine. University of Florida. https://sheltermedicine.vetmed.ufl.edu/shelter-services (accessed 15 April 2018).

Wagner, D.C., Hurley, K.F., and Stavisky, J. (2018a). Shelter housing for cats: principles of design for health, welfare and rehoming. *Journal of Feline Medicine and Surgery* 20 (7): 635–642.

Wagner, D.C., Kass, P.H., and Hurley, K.F. (2018b). Cage size, movement in and out of housing during daily care, and other environmental and population health risk factors for feline upper respiratory disease in nine North American animal shelters. *PLoS One* 13 (1): e0190140.

Waites, K.B., Balish, M.F., and Atkinson, T.P. (2008). New insights into the pathogenesis and detection of *Mycoplasma pneumoniae* infections. *Future Microbiology* 3 (6): 635–648.

Wardley, R.C. and Povey, R.C. (1977). Aerosol transmission of feline caliciviruses. An assessment of its epidemiological importance. *British Veterinary Journal* 133 (5): 504–508.

Weiss, E., Miller, K., Mohan-Gibbons, H. et al. (2012). Why did you choose this pet? Adopters and pet selection preferences in five animal shelters in the United States. *Animals* 2 (2): 144–159.

14

Canine Parvovirus and Other Canine Enteropathogens

Erin Doyle

American Society for the Prevention of Cruelty to Animals (ASPCA), Needham, MA, USA

14.1 Introduction

Gastrointestinal signs are one of the most common clinical presentations of disease in shelter dogs. Gastrointestinal disease can result from a multitude of causes and in many cases is multifactorial. However, common etiologies for gastrointestinal disease in shelter dogs are infectious agents or enteropathogens. Canine Parvovirus-2 is one of the most common and significant enteropathogens in dogs. Its epidemiology, diagnosis, management and prevention in shelters will be reviewed in-depth in this chapter. Other commonly encountered enteropathogens not covered elsewhere in this text will also be discussed.

14.2 Canine Parvovirus-2

Canine parvovirus-2 (CPV) continues to be one of the most significant infectious diseases in shelters. The growth of animal relocation programs has necessitated an increased vigilance for CPV in shelters for which local cases are relatively less common. The virus' ability to survive long-term in the environment contributes to its high morbidity among vulnerable, exposed dogs. While most dogs will survive infection with appropriate treatment, the resources necessary for isolation and treatment are significant and beyond the capacity of many shelters. Thankfully, there are effective strategies to prevent CPV outbreaks in shelters.

14.2.1 Etiology and Epidemiology

CPV strains cause the infectious enteritis commonly known as canine parvovirus and were first identified during pandemic spread among dogs in 1978 (Greene and Decaro 2012; Schoeman et al. 2013). However, the presence of positive antibody titers in Europe in 1974 and 1976 indicates that the disease was slowly emerging even prior to this pandemic (Miranda and Thompson 2016a). The designation of Canine Parvovirus-2 was made given that Canine Parvovirus-1, commonly known as the minute virus of canines, had been previously identified in 1967 (Schoeman et al. 2013). This virus will be discussed in more detail later in the chapter.

CPV belongs to the genus *Protoparvovirus* and is a member of the *Parvoviridae* family. The virus is a small, nonenveloped single-stranded DNA virus. Phylogenetic analysis has demonstrated a common ancestor between CPV and viruses in cats, mink, raccoons, raccoon dogs and blue foxes. CPV and feline panleukopenia virus are over 98% identical in their DNA sequences (Miranda and Thompson 2016a).

Infectious Disease Management in Animal Shelters, Second Edition.
Edited by Lila Miller, Stephanie Janeczko, and Kate F. Hurley.

It is likely that CPV crossed species into canines from one of these other viruses and slowly mutated to enable replication in the canine host (Greene and Decaro 2012).

CPV retained a propensity for mutation and two years after the original discovery of the virus a new strain designated as CPV-2a emerged. This was followed by the identification of CPV-2b in 1984 and CPV-2c in 2000 (Greene and Decaro 2012; Schoeman et al. 2013). All three strains are major pathogens worldwide (Decaro et al. 2007; Wang et al. 2016; Miranda et al. 2016b; Duque-García et al. 2017) and as previously identified strains spread, new variants continue to emerge (Wang et al. 2016; Duque-García et al. 2017; Mira et al. 2018). As the virus has mutated from the original form of CPV, it has developed or regained an ability to replicate in cats (Miranda and Thompson 2016a). Clinical disease in cats caused by CPV-2a and CPV-2b is mild or unapparent relative to feline panleukopenia virus. However, cats infected with CPV-2c have developed significant leukopenia and diarrhea (Greene and Decaro 2012).

The clinical significance in dogs of the emergence of new strains and variants remains uncertain. Currently, it appears reasonable to group all strains and variants together when considering the epidemiology, pathophysiology, and clinical characteristics of CPV infection in dogs.

Prevalence studies for CPV support its ongoing clinical significance. Recent data in a population of dogs with significant diarrhea indicated a prevalence of 58% as determined by fecal polymerase chain reaction (PCR) testing (Godsall et al. 2010). Similar data gathered from a population of dogs presenting with diarrhea and depression indicated a prevalence of 77.5%, also as determined by fecal PCR (Miranda et al. 2015). While exact prevalence data varies based on circumstances, evidence suggests that CPV remains a common pathogen in dogs.

Consistently identified risk factors for the development of parvoviral enteritis include a lack of prior vaccination against CPV and an age less than 6–12 months (Godsall et al. 2010; Kalli et al. 2010; Miranda et al. 2015; Zourkas et al. 2015). Previous literature has suggested breed as a risk factor, with Rottweilers, Doberman pinschers, Labrador retrievers, American Staffordshire terriers, German shepherds and Alaskan sled dogs at increased risk. However, more recent research has not supported breed as a risk factor for the development of parvoviral enteritis (Godsall et al. 2010; Kalli et al. 2010). Ultimately, CPV can cause clinical disease in dogs of any age, breed, or gender. Shelter-related risk factors for the development of CPV outbreaks include overcrowding, insufficient isolation of infected dogs, poor biosecurity/sanitation, and an inadequate vaccination protocol.

14.2.2 Pathophysiology

CPV is spread between dogs via direct contact and indirect contact (fomite). The virus enters the host through the oronasal route after exposure to contaminated feces. Viral replication starts in the lymphoid tissue of the oropharynx and then progresses to the mesenteric lymph nodes, thymus and small intestine. The incubation period between exposure and development of clinical disease ranges from 4 to 14 days.

CPV has a tropism for rapidly dividing cells. The virus replicates in the germinal epithelium of the small intestinal crypts. The germinal epithelium normally matures and then migrates from the intestinal crypts to the villi where absorption of nutrients occurs. The destruction of the germinal epithelium blunts the villi thus impairing intestinal function (Greene and Decaro 2012). Factors that increase the mitotic rate of germinal epithelium such as weaning and intestinal parasite infection can increase viral replication and the severity of infection (Goddard and Leisewitz 2010). Lymphoid destruction by CPV is particularly severe in the thymus, resulting in especially significant lymphopenia in juvenile cases (Schoeman et al. 2013).

Intestinal and lymphoid damage can lead to secondary bacterial infections from gastrointestinal microflora, potentially resulting in bacteremia and endotoxemia. Oxidative stress has been shown to be present in parvoviral enteritis more than other causes of enteritis and may contribute to viral pathogenesis (Panda et al. 2009).

Viremia begins one to five days after infection. Viral shedding in the feces begins approximately four to five days after infection, often before the development of clinical signs. Shedding typically occurs for 7–10 days but has been documented for up to several weeks. A reduction in viral shedding often coincides with the resolution of clinical signs, particularly the resolution of diarrhea. Viral antibody titers can be detected three to four days after infection and can remain positive long-term (Greene and Decaro 2012). CPV has no known zoonotic potential.

14.2.3 Clinical Signs

The most common clinical signs of CPV are related to acute enteritis and can include vomiting and/or diarrhea, both often severe. The diarrhea may or may not be hemorrhagic and can vary in character based on the individual case. Infected animals are often depressed and can rapidly develop severe dehydration. In one study, dogs with diarrhea who also displayed depression, lethargy or vomiting on presentation were more likely to be infected with CPV compared to other etiologic agents (Godsall et al. 2010).

Infected dogs often display marked abdominal pain. Pyrexia is another common finding on presentation, particularly for more severe cases. Panhypoproteinemia due to gastrointestinal protein loss may develop with resulting secondary clinical signs. Secondary effects of severe leukopenia such as bacteriuria may also develop (Greene and Decaro 2012). Clinical signs can be exacerbated by the presence of concurrent disease such as infection with intestinal parasites, coronavirus, canine distemper virus, or other enteropathogens. Intestinal intussusception is a potential secondary complication and can also exacerbate clinical signs. No difference in the typical clinical presentation based on CPV strain has been identified (Markovich et al. 2012).

Secondary clinical concerns may develop related to bacterial translocation through the damaged intestinal tract and endotoxemia. Endotoxemia can develop even in the absence of septicemia with the release of pro-inflammatory cytokines and tumor necrosis factor into the bloodstream (Prittie 2004). This pro-inflammatory cascade can result in systemic inflammatory response syndrome as well as disseminated intravascular coagulation (DIC) (Goddard and Leisewitz 2010; Greene and Decaro 2012). *Escherichia coli* has been identified in the liver and lungs of infected dogs (Schoeman et al. 2013). Neurologic signs may occur due to severe hypoglycemia or DIC related hemorrhage. Primary viral damage to the brain occurs in kittens exposed to feline panleukopenia in utero, but is poorly defined in dogs infected by CPV and appears rare (Greene and Decaro 2012).

Another clinical manifestation of CPV is acute myocarditis. Myocarditis can occur if puppies are infected during the period of rapid myocardial cell proliferation, which occurs in utero and within the first two weeks of life (Prittie 2004). Clinical signs related to myocarditis can vary from acute clinical signs of dyspnea, crying, and retching followed shortly by death, to more mild initial symptoms followed by congestive heart failure and death as an older puppy. Enteritis may or may not be present in cases of myocarditis. Parvoviral myocarditis in dogs has become rare as most dams have been vaccinated or naturally exposed to the virus, resulting in high maternally derived antibody titers (Greene and Decaro 2012). However, CPV associated myocarditis is still an important differential for puppies with acute respiratory distress, as evidenced by a recent case report of parvoviral myocarditis in a five-week-old puppy (Sime et al. 2015).

14.2.4 Diagnosis

A prompt and accurate diagnosis of CPV infection is important both for the infected dog as well as for the health of the exposed shelter population. While a presumptive diagnosis is often made based on clinical signs and the signalment of the infected dog, determining a definitive diagnosis of CPV is important to guide treatment and management decisions. Differential diagnoses for CPV infection include parasitic, bacterial or other viral enteropathogens in addition to non-infectious etiologies such as stress-related gastrointestinal concerns, dietary indiscretion, inflammatory bowel disease, or hemorrhagic gastroenteritis.

Point-of-care fecal enzyme-linked immunosorbent assay (ELISA) antigen testing remains the diagnostic test of choice for CPV in the shelter setting. The fecal antigen ELISA test is highly specific, but sensitivity data is variable. ELISA testing has been shown to reliably detect all three circulating strains of CPV (Markovich et al. 2012). However, factors such as low fecal viral load, mild clinical signs, and high fecal CPV antibodies (as can occur with transluminal secretion) can increase the likelihood of a false negative fecal ELISA test (Proksch et al. 2015). Fecal PCR testing has higher sensitivity when compared to ELISA testing or other testing methods such as hemagglutination (Decaro et al. 2005; Silva et al. 2013). Despite this greater sensitivity, the practicality of ELISA testing still makes it the ideal initial diagnostic choice as compared to PCR testing. Nevertheless, negative ELISA results in the face of highly suspicious clinical signs should warrant retesting or follow-up testing with a different modality.

Positive fecal CPV ELISA results are a reliable indicator of CPV infection when associated with consistent clinical signs. Positive ELISA test results because of modified-live vaccination were first shown to occur at a very low rate in kittens vaccinated against feline panleukopenia virus (Patterson et al. 2007). In similar research with dogs vaccinated with a modified-live CPV vaccine, viral material was detected via PCR up to 28 days after vaccination, but no virus was detectable via ELISA or hemagglutination testing (Decaro, Crescenzo et al. 2014; Freisl et al. 2017).

As described later in this chapter, serology to assess CPV exposure is an important tool in outbreak response. However, CPV serology is not a useful test for establishing a diagnosis of CPV infection due to the high rate of vaccination and viral exposure in the canine population.

While not necessary to confirm the diagnosis, additional lab work can be performed to better assess the overall clinical picture of an infected dog. Leukopenia is a common finding in dogs with CPV infection, though is not present in all infected dogs. The severity of the leukopenia and a failure of leukocytes to increase within the first 48 hours of treatment are both negative prognostic indicators during CPV infection (Goddard et al. 2008). Other clinicopathologic findings that can occur with CPV infection include anemia, coagulopathies, electrolyte imbalances, and hypoalbuminemia.

If a shelter dog is found deceased, fecal CPV testing is recommended unless another cause of death is evident. Necropsy can also help to diagnose CPV infection. Gross pathologic findings include thickened and discolored intestinal walls with rough serosal surfaces. These changes are typically worst in the distal duodenum for dogs in the early stage of disease while findings are more pronounced in the jejunum for more severely infected dogs (Greene and Decaro 2012). Confirmation of the diagnosis via necropsy can be made using histopathology to identify characteristic lesions or via immunofluorescence tissue testing (Greene and Decaro 2012).

14.2.5 Treatment

The prognosis for infected dogs with proper treatment is generally good. However, the decision to treat CPV cases in the shelter environment must be made in the context of available resources and the ability to avoid transmission to the remainder of the shelter population. It is vital that an isolation plan is in place before proceeding with the treatment of dogs infected with CPV. Isolation strategies such as treatment in foster care or at a local veterinary hospital may be viable options if the lack of an adequate isolation facility or available staff time makes treatment in the shelter impractical. Regardless of the isolation method chosen, physical isolation must be accompanied by appropriate biosecurity measures including the use of personal protective equipment (PPE) and proper sanitation protocols.

Research suggests that survival rates of outpatient treatment protocols, often more practical in the shelter setting, near those of inpatient treatment protocols. Success rates of 75–80% have been demonstrated with outpatient treatment in recent studies (Sarpong et al. 2017; Venn et al. 2017). However, even outpatient treatment protocols require conscientious patient monitoring and a plan for how to assess selection and respond to treatment failure. It is vital that treatment protocols are directed by a veterinarian, either via individual veterinary case management or through the establishment of a detailed treatment, monitoring, and decision-making protocol. Protocols must be developed by a shelter veterinarian familiar with the individual shelter in accordance with local veterinary practice regulations.

A specific anti-viral treatment for CPV is not available. As such, CPV treatment is focused on supportive care and treatment of the sequelae of infection. Fluid therapy to address gastrointestinal loss and maintain hydration is a cornerstone of treatment. The ideal mode of fluid therapy is intravenous to provide rapid fluid replacement and support. When utilized, the intravenous catheter must be placed in a strictly aseptic manner due to potential immune system impairment and increased susceptibility to disease (Goddard and Leisewitz 2010).

For many shelters, the responsible use of intravenous fluid therapy is not feasible. In this case, the combination of an initial bolus of intravenous fluid followed by ongoing subcutaneous (SQ) fluid support or SQ fluid support alone are reasonable alternatives. Unless clinical signs are very mild, SQ fluids should be administered at least three to four times daily to achieve an adequate total daily volume (Colorado State University, n.d.). The volume of fluid administered should be calculated based on percent dehydration at presentation and ongoing maintenance fluid needs. Dosage charts for SQ fluids are a helpful component of a written CPV treatment protocol, but flexibility in the protocol is necessary to adjust the treatment plan if fluids are not fully absorbed prior to the next treatment.

Crystalloid fluids are the standard fluid choice. However, colloid fluid support, such as with hydroxyethyl starch, may be indicated in cases of significant hypoalbuminemia or with signs associated with third space loss (Leisewitz 2017). Colloid fluid support requires intravenous access.

Nutritional support is another cornerstone of CPV treatment. Early enteral nutrition has been shown to reduce the duration of clinical signs and encourage weight gain during treatment (Mohr et al. 2003). Administration of nutritional support via nasoesophageal tube is ideal when possible, but treatment protocols using syringe feeding of a high caloric diet can also be successful and are more realistic in most shelter settings.

The administration of enteral nutrition is best accompanied by antiemetics to reduce nausea and vomiting. Maropitant is an ideal first-line choice for antiemetic therapy based on its efficacy, ability to be administered subcutaneously and once-daily dosing (Colorado State University, n.d.). Ondansetron can be added into the treatment regimen subcutaneously up to three times daily in dogs with refractory vomiting (Colorado State University, n.d.; Venn et al. 2017). Antiemetics are often not successful in eliminating vomiting in highly symptomatic dogs but can reduce the severity.

Broad spectrum antibiotic administration is indicated in CPV cases given the potential for bacterial translocation and reduced immune function. Cefovicin is ideal because of its broad spectrum of efficacy and its ease of administration as a single-dose SQ injection. Intravenous antibiotics such as ampicillin and amikacin (after fluid replenishment) are effective choices when intravenous access is present (Leisewitz 2017). Oral antibiotics that are commonly used include amoxicillin and metronidazole. However, oral medication is often best postponed until vomiting has ceased to ensure adequate absorption.

Though commonly utilized, metronidazole's efficacy against *E. coli* in an anaerobic environment may be limited (Pendland et al. 2002). As such, metronidazole would not be an appropriate single-agent antibiotic choice and may be better utilized when co-infection with flagellate parasites is diagnosed or suspected. Broad-spectrum treatment for intestinal helminths, if not previously administered, is an important adjunct treatment in all cases to reduce comorbidities.

Analgesia is also an important consideration during CPV treatment as abdominal discomfort can be severe. Opioid therapy is the best choice for analgesia in CPV cases due to its safety profile and efficacy. Because opioids are a controlled substance, their use must be directed by a veterinarian.

Numerous other treatments have been explored with variable success in the treatment of CPV infection. The use of blood products has proven controversial, and recent evidence suggests that a single dose of immune plasma has no clinical benefit in the treatment of CPV infection (Bragg et al. 2012). Administration of recombinant canine granulocyte-colony stimulating factor increased neutrophil levels and reduced the duration of hospitalization in one recent study, but treated dogs had a decrease in survival time compared to the control group (Bragg et al. 2012). As such, caution with its use is warranted pending further investigation. Oseltamivir has been shown to reduce the risk of weight loss and leukopenia in hospitalized dogs undergoing treatment for CPV (Savigny and Macintire 2010). However, these potential benefits must be weighed against the public health risk of widespread use of anti-viral treatment that is the mainstay of influenza treatment in humans.

Ultimately, the core components of a CPV treatment plan include isolation, fluid support, enteral nutrition, antiemetics, antibiotics, deworming, and analgesia. Close monitoring of infected dogs is vital to promptly adjust the treatment plan when needed. Even when protocols are used to initiate treatment by shelter staff, veterinary involvement is vital in developing these protocols and guiding individual patient decisions when necessary. Euthanasia decisions are indicated for dogs that fail to respond to treatment or for shelters without the resources or transfer options to provide safe and humane treatment.

Canine parvovirus is a reportable companion animal disease in some jurisdictions. It is important to follow the appropriate reporting procedure to comply with local regulations. Another important consideration when managing CPV in the shelter setting is determining when to reintroduce a recovered animal into the shelter population and when to proceed with adoption. Dogs recovering from CPV infection can shed viral material in their stools for many weeks as detected by PCR. However, the clinical relevance of this shedding is unknown as detectable viral material via ELISA is typically absent by four to five days after the onset of illness.

If CPV infected dogs are being treated in foster care, the risk to the shelter population can be eliminated by arranging placement directly from the foster home, without the dog returning to the shelter environment. However, this strategy is not feasible for all shelters or foster caregivers. A reasonable alternative is to perform a fecal ELISA test once clinical signs have resolved. A serial test approximately 24–48 hours after the initial post-treatment

ELISA can be added to provide further assurance. Once clinical signs have resolved and negative test result(s) have been obtained, the dog should be bathed to remove viral contamination of the fur coat and paws. Return to the general shelter population can be performed at this point with minimal risk. However, it is still prudent to avoid exposure of recovered dogs to highly vulnerable populations, such as puppies.

Adopters must be notified of the dog's medical history. Consultation with the adopter's regular veterinarian should be recommended if there are concerns about the vulnerability of resident animals to the recovered dog. Recovered dogs typically develop life-long immunity to CPV (Schultz et al. 2010) but routine vaccination is still recommended to protect against other vaccine preventable diseases.

14.2.6 Outbreak Response

Management of canine parvovirus infection in the shelter extends beyond individual animal treatment to the management of the entire susceptible shelter population. After one or more cases of CPV are diagnosed in the shelter, dogs should be categorized as infected, exposed and unexposed. (See Figure 14.1) Infected dogs should be promptly isolated if proceeding with treatment or euthanized if resources necessitate. Unexposed dogs can continue to be placed as per normal. Care must be taken to avoid any subsequent exposure. Depending on the number of dogs infected, this can be accomplished by housing unexposed dogs in a separate "clean" area in the shelter or utilizing off-site resources such as foster care. If unexposed dogs remain in the shelter, strict biosecurity measures are necessary to ensure that exposure does not occur.

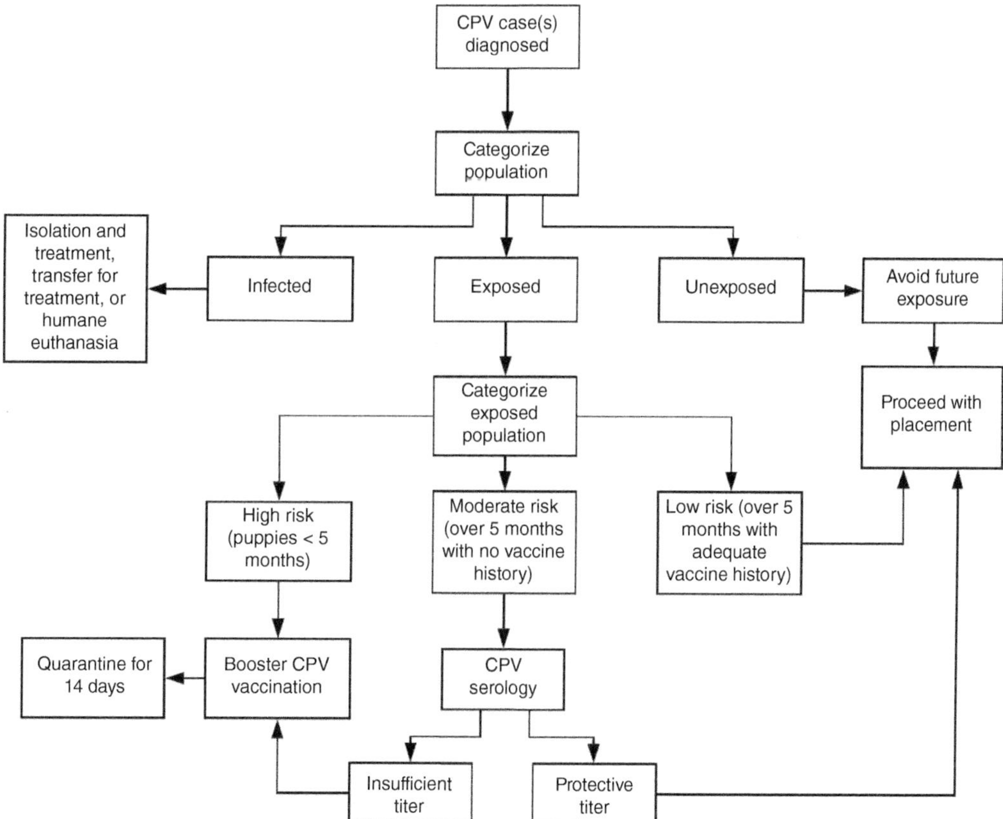

Figure 14.1 CPV outbreak response flow chart.

The designation of which dogs are considered exposed will vary based on shelter operations. All dogs housed with the infected dog(s) or with a history of direct contact with an infected dog (i.e. via playgroups) should be considered exposed. Dogs in the same housing ward will typically need to be considered exposed unless strict biosecurity measures are in place in between individual dogs. The entire canine population in the shelter may be designated as exposed if inadequate biosecurity protocols are practiced or if the infected dog(s) was moved to multiple different housing areas. Because infected dogs can shed virus for up to three to four days prior to the development of clinical signs, the timeframe of exposure risk should start at this point and extend to the time of diagnosis/isolation.

Exposed dogs should then be categorized based on their relative risk of disease. Dogs over five months of age that have been vaccinated with a modified-live CPV vaccine at least four days prior to exposure can typically be considered low-risk. Conversely, because of the impact of maternal antibodies on vaccine efficacy, exposed puppies less than five months of age should always be categorized as high risk. Older puppies and adult dogs without an adequate documented vaccine history generally fall into a moderate risk category. Factors such as age and neuter status are not reliable predictors of humoral immunity so they should not be relied upon instead of vaccine documentation (Lechner et al. 2010; Mahon et al. 2017).

Once exposed dogs have been categorized by relative risk levels, a plan for the management strategy for each category can be developed. Low-risk dogs can usually proceed with placement as per normal. High-risk dogs (exposed puppies less than five months of age) should typically be quarantined for 14 days if it is within the shelter's capacity to do so humanely. Quarantining puppies in foster care can be a useful strategy to reduce disease exposure risk and achieve appropriate socialization. Foster caregivers must be well informed of the risk of infection and take appropriate biosecurity precautions. Puppies should always remain in easily disinfected areas during the quarantine period. All quarantined dogs must be monitored closely for any clinical signs. ELISA fecal antigen testing should be performed on any quarantined dogs who develop clinical signs to promptly identify new cases. If quarantine is beyond the shelter's capacity, placement of exposed puppies with appropriate monitoring and disclosure can be considered.

The management strategy for exposed dogs with a moderate risk of developing disease will vary with the individual shelter and population. Quarantine of moderate risk exposed dogs is a viable option if within the shelter's capacity. Alternatively, serology to measure the level of CPV antibodies is a useful tool to further evaluate the risk of disease in exposed dogs. Dogs in the moderate risk category with protective antibody titers can be re-categorized as low risk and managed accordingly. Dogs without protective antibody titers should be re-categorized as high risk and quarantined as described above. If the exposure level was low and resources preclude titer testing or quarantining moderate risk dogs, proceeding with placement along with close monitoring for signs of disease may be a viable option.

Once cleared for placement, all exposed dogs should be bathed before moving into a clean enclosure to remove viral particles from their fur coats and paws. Full disclosure regarding their exposure history must be included in their medical record with appropriate notification provided to the adopter or placement partner. See Chapter 6 for more information on outbreak management.

14.2.7 Prevention

Infection control of CPV in the shelter setting should involve reducing an individual animal's likelihood of exposure to CPV as well as reducing the likelihood that an exposed animal will develop the infection. Because of the ongoing prevalence of CPV in the canine population, all shelters should have a comprehensive and multi-faceted approach to CPV infection control in place. The following strategies to prevent CPV infection in the shelter should be detailed in shelter protocols and effectively carried out by shelter personnel.

14.2.7.1 Vaccination

Modified-live virus (MLV) parenteral vaccination against CPV is a vital component of a shelter intake protocol. Unless valid documentation of prior vaccination is available, dogs should be considered naïve to CPV on intake into the shelter. Immunity after vaccination develops rapidly so vaccination at or prior to intake is critical to establishing early protection. As supported by published vaccine guidelines (American Animal Hospital Association 2017), any dog for which vaccination is feasible must be vaccinated at intake. This includes dogs not legally owned by the shelter due to a stray or legal hold. The benefit of vaccination to prevent infection in the shelter environment justifies vaccine administration as necessary medical care. Evidence suggests that current vaccines provide adequate coverage for all CPV strains due to cross-protection (Wilson et al. 2014; American Animal Hospital Association 2017).

CPV vaccination should begin at four weeks of age to provide immunological support in the face of waning maternal antibodies (De Cramer et al. 2011). Puppies should then be revaccinated every 2 weeks until 20 weeks of age. Early discontinuation of CPV vaccination in puppies is a major risk factor for infection in vaccinated dogs (Altman et al. 2017) so shelter protocols must ensure that puppies in the shelter's care receive regular CPV vaccination until they are of sufficient age. A booster CPV vaccination 2–3 weeks after the initial vaccine is also recommended for dogs over 20 weeks of age. However, there is evidence that a single MLV CPV vaccination can establish life-long immunity in a high percentage of dogs (Schultz et al. 2010). As such, shelters with limited capacity may reasonably elect to forgo booster vaccinations for adult dogs.

14.2.7.2 Sanitation

As a nonenveloped virus, CPV is hardy in the environment. Well-planned and executed sanitation protocols are necessary to prevent environmental contamination with CPV in the shelter. Given the fecal-oral transmission method, prompt and thorough clean-up of any fecal waste is a critical first step in the sanitation plan. This step, utilized even when spot cleaning, is a useful tool to reduce contamination from dogs that may be shedding virus before the development of clinical signs. Degreasing and detergent agents should be used when performing a full cleaning of the enclosure or when needed during spot-cleaning to remove visible organic waste.

Efficacy against CPV should be considered when selecting the shelter's routine disinfectant and outlining its use. Several readily available disinfectant options are effective against CPV when utilized properly. Accelerated hydrogen peroxide at a 1:32 dilution for a 10-minute contact time or a 1:16 dilution for a five-minute contact time is an ideal choice against CPV in shelters. Accelerated hydrogen peroxide retains some efficacy in the face of organic matter and is safe and less noxious than bleach.

Potassium peroxymonosulfate also retains a small degree of efficacy in the face of organic matter and works against CPV when utilized at a 1% dilution for a 10-minute contact time. The solution, while also safe and less noxious than bleach, is only stable for seven days.

Bleach is inexpensive and effective against CPV at a 1:32 dilution with a 10-minute contact time. However, the solution is only stable for 24 hours and has no efficacy in the face of organic debris. Bleach can also be very noxious for staff and animals. Quaternary ammonium disinfectants are not reliably efficacious against CPV.

In addition to having a robust routine sanitation protocol, shelters must include sanitation in the response plan after a diagnosis of CPV occurs. Sanitation supplies should be dedicated to the CPV isolation area to avoid contamination of clean areas. Spot cleaning of the isolation enclosure is reasonable during treatment, but thorough cleaning and disinfection of the contaminated areas are vital after an infected dog has vacated the enclosure. Any exposed common use areas should be similarly cleaned and disinfected. Multiple cleaning and disinfecting cycles can be a prudent strategy in areas of high exposure before resuming their use with other dogs. However, waiting periods before resuming an enclosure's use are unnecessary after proper sanitation.

It is likely that washing dishes in a dishwasher and bedding in a washer/dryer, particularly after two cycles, will effectively remove viral contamination (Ebner et al. 2000; Moriello 2015). However, caution must be taken with this approach to not contaminate unexposed items or surfaces. Cleaning and disinfecting dishes in situ with the remainder of the kennel and disposal of contaminated bedding and toys are typically more practical strategies to minimize exposure risk to CPV.

Foster homes and outdoor areas such as play yards can be challenging to address after exposure. Both areas are best handled through prevention. Foster caregivers should be advised to keep infected or high-risk dogs on easily disinfected surfaces, oftentimes in a bathroom or kitchen. When outside, these dogs can be kept on a cleanable surface such as a tarp or artificial turf. Play-yard usage should be carefully planned to minimize the risk of exposure. Puppies and high-risk dogs in shelters should ideally receive outdoor exercise on an easily cleaned surface such as cement or gravel rather than in a natural grass or dirt play yard. When exposed, even easily cleaned outdoor surfaces are best disinfected with accelerated hydrogen peroxide due to the difficulty with the removal of all organic debris.

If CPV exposure occurs on grass or dirt, it can be very challenging to fully decontaminate the area. CPV can live in an outdoor environment for up to five months, and even longer when protected from sunlight or drying (Gordon and Angrick 1986). The ideal approach to contaminated grass and dirt is to limit future exposure of highly vulnerable dogs, such as puppies, to this area. See Chapter 8 for more information on sanitation.

14.2.7.3 Biosecurity

Given its robust ability to survive outside the host, CPV easily contaminates not just the environment but also exposed fomites. Indirect viral transmission via fomites is a major cause of CPV spread in the shelter. Effective biosecurity protocols can reduce this risk of fomite transmission.

People and clothing are a common shelter fomite. Hand hygiene is important after handling any dog, even those without signs of illness. Hand washing or changing gloves between dogs is preferable to utilizing hand sanitizers when CPV is of concern, as the efficacy of hand sanitizers is unreliable against parvoviruses (Kampf 2018). Certain scenarios such as playgroups make hand hygiene between dogs unrealistic. Close monitoring for signs of illness helps to mitigate the risk of indirect disease transmission in such settings.

Appropriate use of PPE when handling CPV infected dogs is also vital to reduce the risk of disease spread. At a minimum, protective equipment to cover the hands, trunk and sleeves must be worn. Full body protection is ideal, particularly when contamination of the lower half of the body is anticipated due to holding the infected dog in the lap for treatments or due to the dog jumping up on the handler, and/or when kneeling or sitting on a contaminated surface is necessary. Shoe covers or dedicated isolation footwear are critical to prevent spread from contaminated isolation flooring. Foot baths are not an effective strategy to reduce the spread of CPV via the soles of footwear (Hartmann et al. 2013). All PPE must be appropriately removed and disposed of before exiting the isolation area.

14.2.7.4 Population Management

A critical strategy to reduce the risk of CPV transmission in a shelter is effective population management. Shelters with a robust population management system in place maintain a shelter population within their capacity for care and thoughtfully but efficiently move animals through the shelter system toward their outcome. Overcrowding reduces the ability of personnel to effectively monitor and care for the shelter population. In addition, overcrowding and prolonged lengths of stay in the shelter increase an individual dog's likelihood of exposure to disease. Reducing CPV exposure and transmission is one of many reasons that effective population management is critical to ensuring a healthy shelter population. See the Introduction in Chapter 1, Chapter 2 on Wellness and Chapter 6 on Outbreak Management for more information about population management.

14.3 Other Enteropathogens

Numerous other enteropathogens beyond CPV are also important causes of gastrointestinal disease in shelter dogs. While this chapter will not include an exhaustive list of infectious agents affecting the canine gastrointestinal system, several additional pathogens of note will be reviewed. See Chapter 17 on Internal Parasites and Chapter 11 on Canine Distemper Virus for additional information on important canine enteropathogens.

14.3.1 Canine Coronavirus

Canine coronavirus (CCoV) is a common cause of diarrhea in dogs and is particularly implicated as a frequent cause of diarrhea in juveniles. Prevalence data for CCoV in dogs with diarrhea based on recent studies ranges from 7.9% (Godsall et al. 2010) to 42% (Decaro et al. 2010). One study that subcategorized prevalence by age found a prevalence of 66.3% in puppies with diarrhea but only 6.9% for clinical adult dogs (Soma et al. 2011).

CCoV is an enveloped RNA virus with a poor ability to survive outside the host and susceptibility to most common disinfectants. The virus undergoes frequent genetic evolution with numerous genotypes having been identified (Decaro et al. 2010; Soma et al. 2011). Dogs become infected after exposure to contaminated feces. The incubation period is short at one to four days. The virus is typically shed in the feces of infected dogs for three to fourteen days after infection, though viral shedding for up to six months post-infection has been identified via PCR (Greene and Decaro 2012).

CCoV affects the villi of the small intestine and typical clinical signs of infection include vomiting, diarrhea, lethargy and/or inappetence. Asymptomatic infections are also common, particularly in adult dogs. Leukopenia is not routinely identified. A diagnosis of CCoV infection can be difficult to confirm given the possibility of asymptomatic infection and the non-specific clinical signs. Diagnostics to identify CCoV infection are not normally indicated due to the typically mild nature of the clinical infection. However, given the overlap in clinical signs and the potential for co-infection, CPV testing is often advisable for dogs with clinical signs consistent with CCoV infection.

Infection is usually self-limiting with only supportive care indicated for treatment (if warranted based on the severity of clinical signs). Vaccination against CCoV is available but not recommended due to the mild self-limiting nature of the disease (American Animal Hospital Association 2017). In addition, protection provided by vaccination is incomplete (Greene and Decaro 2012). Though CCoV is an important pathogen in shelter dogs because of its prevalence in juveniles with diarrhea, specific precautions against CCoV in shelters are not necessary beyond routine disinfection and disease monitoring programs.

While CCoV infection is generally not cause for significant concern, a pantropic CCoV disease has been identified that is caused by a variant of the CCoV-II strain identified as CB/05 (Decaro and Buonavoglia 2011). Published accounts are present of pantropic CCoV infection in puppies in Italy (Buonavoglia et al. 2006), France and Belgium

(Zicola et al. 2012). Four of these outbreaks were associated with concurrent CPV infection. However, in one outbreak in Belgium, only CCoV-II was identified as a mono-infection in infected puppies (Zicola et al. 2012). In addition, the CCoV strain isolated from the Italian outbreak was utilized to induce pantropic disease experimentally (Buonavoglia et al. 2006). The virus affects multiple organs in pantropic infection and clinical signs include acute lethargy, vomiting, diarrhea, fever, and convulsions. All documented non-experimentally induced infections have been fatal (Decaro and Buonavoglia 2011). While consideration of pantropic CCoV in acutely ill puppies is warranted, at this time its incidence appears very limited. CPV infection is a much more common cause of similar symptoms in neonates.

14.3.2 Canine Circovirus

Canine circovirus (CanineCV) has been recently identified in dogs with hemorrhagic diarrhea and vasculitis. However, its clinical characteristics are still poorly understood. CanineCV was identified as the only pathogen in a puppy with fatal acute enteritis (Decaro, Martella et al. 2014) and in a dog with fatal necrotizing vasculitis and granulomatous lymphadenitis (Li et al. 2013). However, subsequent research into its prevalence in dogs with diarrhea has demonstrated mixed results. One study indicated a higher prevalence of CanineCV infection in dogs with diarrhea (Hsu et al. 2016) while two studies demonstrated no significant association between CanineCV infection and acute diarrhea (Anderson et al. 2017; Dowgier et al. 2017). However, these same two studies suggested a role of CanineCV as a co-pathogen that may increase the severity of enteritis. Ultimately, the clinical significance of CanineCV in dogs with enteritis remains unknown but an awareness of its possibility as a pathogen or co-pathogen in dogs with enteritis is important.

14.3.3 Clostridium spp.

In contrast, *Clostridium perfringens* and *Clostridium difficile* are commonly documented causes of enteritis in dogs (Greene and Decaro 2012). In fact, in one recent study, *C. perfringens* was the only enteropathogen studied that was statistically significantly more common in dogs with diarrhea compared to dogs with normal feces (Tupler et al. 2012). Both species are part of the normal canine gastrointestinal flora. The development of clinical disease in dogs is poorly elucidated and appears to be secondary to either disruption of the normal intestinal biome such as after antibiotic administration or via fecal-oral transmission from infected dogs or contaminated food.

Clinical disease results from the effects of bacteria-produced toxins. While clostridial infections are typically considered to cause colitis, small bowel diarrhea can also be present with clinical infection. Mild disease is typically self-limiting but dogs with more severe symptoms warrant antibiotic therapy. Metronidazole is an effective antibiotic choice, though amoxicillin and tylosin are also appropriate therapies. Tetracycline should be avoided due to the high risk of resistance (Greene and Decaro 2012). Though people are commonly affected by *Clostridium* spp., there is no evidence at this time to suggest that they are zoonotic pathogens.

14.3.4 Canine Parvovirus-1 (Minute Virus)

A final enteropathogen of note is canine parvovirus-1 (CPV-1), also known as the minute virus of canines. CPV-1 has only been identified in dogs and is generally not associated with clinical signs aside from in neonates less than three weeks of age. Clinical signs in neonates can include enteritis, pneumonitis, myocarditis and/or lymphadenitis. Mortality is high in clinical puppies, and CPV-1 is often implicated as one cause of fading puppy syndrome. Treatment consists of supportive care via warmth, nutrition and fluid support. Fetal death and birth defects are also possible due to the ability of the virus to cross the placenta. CPV-2 diagnostic testing and vaccination are not effective for CPV-1.

14.3.5 Diagnostics

In shelters with effective preventive medicine protocols, mild cases of canine gastrointestinal disease can often be managed empirically without necessitating diagnostic testing. Diagnostic testing becomes indicated for individual cases when there is a high index of suspicion for infectious disease such as CPV or severe, chronic and/or atypical clinical signs are present. Population level diagnostic screening is indicated when gastrointestinal disease increases in prevalence or severity and as a baseline screening tool to guide intervention strategies if endemic gastrointestinal disease is present in the population.

Decisions on the appropriate diagnostic testing for individual cases will vary based on signalment, clinical signs and history and may include CPV testing (reviewed above), evaluation for internal parasites, and advanced health screening such as via lab work or diagnostic imaging. Another valuable diagnostic tool both for individual cases and population screening is reference laboratory gastrointestinal PCR panels. These panels are run on fecal samples and include PCR results for many gastrointestinal pathogens. Exact submission and pathogen details will vary and can be determined via reference laboratory test manuals or through direct communication with the laboratory. When indicated, results can often be followed up with culture using the same submitted sample. PCR panel results can guide intervention decisions both for individual case treatment plans as well as population level decision making, particularly if test results warrant an outbreak response or shelter protocol changes.

14.4 Conclusion

Knowledge of the pathophysiology, diagnosis, and treatment of canine gastrointestinal enteropathogens is important for shelter veterinarians and shelter personnel. Thoughtful management of enteropathogen infections in shelter dogs is critical to individual case management as well as to minimize the risk of disease transmission within the population. The need for thoughtful management is particularly acute for dogs infected with CPV due to the clinical manifestations of the virus and the outbreak potential. Advanced planning through the creation of standard operating procedures that proactively address prevention, diagnosis, isolation, treatment, and outbreak response plans for CPV and other canine enteropathogens is vital for any organization sheltering canines.

References

Altman, K.D., Kelman, M., and Ward, M.P. (2017). Are vaccine strain, type or administration protocol risk factors for canine parvovirus vaccine failure? *Veterinary Microbiology* 210 (April): 8–16.

American Animal Hospital Association (2017). AAHA Canine Vaccination Guidelines. https://www.aaha.org/aaha-guidelines/vaccination-canine-configuration/vaccination-canine (accessed 14 June 2020).

Anderson, A., Hartmann, K., Leutenegger, C.M. et al. (2017). Role of canine circovirus in dogs with acute haemorrhagic diarrhoea. *Veterinary Record* 180 (22): 1–5.

Bragg, R.F., Duffy, A.L., DeCecco, F.A. et al. (2012). Clinical evaluation of a single dose of immune plasma for treatment of canine parvovirus infection. *Journal of the American Veterinary Medical Association* 240 (6): 700–704.

Buonavoglia, C., Decaro, N., Martella, V. et al. (2006). Canine coronavirus highly pathogenic for dogs. *Emerging Infectious Diseases* 12 (3): 492–494.

Colorado State University (2013). Frequently asked questions series: What is the outpatient treatment protocol utilized for the treatment of parvoviral enteritis at Colorado State University? http://csu-cvmbs.colostate.edu/documents/parvo-outpatient-protocol-faq-companion-animal-studies.pdf (accessed 14 June 2020).

De Cramer, K.G.M., Stylianides, E., and van Vuuren, M. (2011). Efficacy of vaccination at 4 and 6 weeks in the control of canine parvovirus. *Veterinary Microbiology* 149 (1–2): 126–132.

Decaro, N. and Buonavoglia, C. (2011). Canine coronavirus: not only an enteric pathogen. *Veterinary Clinics of North America: Small Animal Practice* 41 (6): 1121–1132.

Decaro, N., Elia, G., Martella, V. et al. (2005). A real-time PCR assay for rapid detection and quantitation of canine parvovirus type 2 in the feces of dogs. *Veterinary Microbiology* 105 (1): 19–28.

Decaro, N., Desario, C., Addie, D.D. et al. (2007). Molecular epidemiology of canine parvovirus, Europe. *Emerging Infectious Diseases* 13 (8): 1222–1224.

Decaro, N., Mari, V., Elia, G. et al. (2010). Recombinant canine coronaviruses in dogs, Europe. *Emerging Infectious Diseases* 16 (1): 41–47.

Decaro, N., Martella, V., Desario, C. et al. (2014). Genomic characterization of a circovirus associated with fatal hemorrhagic enteritis in dog, Italy. *PLoS One* 9 (8): e105909.

Decaro, N., Crescenzo, G., Desario, C. et al. (2014). Long-term viremia and fecal shedding in pups after modified-live canine parvovirus vaccination. *Vaccine* 32 (30): 3850–3853.

Dowgier, G., Lorusso, E., Decaro, N. et al. (2017). A molecular survey for selected viral enteropathogens revealed a limited role of canine circovirus in the development of canine acute gastroenteritis. *Veterinary Microbiology* 204 (April): 54–58.

Duque-García, Y., Echeverri-Zuluaga, M., Trejos-Suarez, J. et al. (2017). Prevalence and molecular epidemiology of Canine parvovirus 2 in diarrheic dogs in Colombia, South America: a possible new CPV-2a is emerging? *Veterinary Microbiology* 201: 56–61.

Ebner, W., Eitel, A., Scherrer, M. et al. (2000). Can household dishwashers be used to disinfect medical equipment? *Journal of Hospital Infection* 45 (2): 155–159.

Freisl, M., Speck, S., Truyen, U. et al. (2017). Faecal shedding of canine parvovirus after modified-live vaccination in healthy adult dogs. *Veterinary Journal* 219: 15–21.

Goddard, A. and Leisewitz, A.L. (2010). Canine parvovirus. *Veterinary Clinics of North America: Small Animal Practice* 40 (6): 1041–1053.

Goddard, A., Leisewitz, A.L., Christopher, M.M. et al. (2008). Prognostic usefulness of blood leukocyte changes in canine parvoviral enteritis. *Journal of Veterinary Internal Medicine* 22 (2): 309–316.

Godsall, S.A., Clegg, S.R., Stavisky, J.H. et al. (2010). Epidemiology of canine parvovirus and coronavirus in dogs presented with severe diarrhoea to PDSA PetAid hospitals. *Veterinary Record* 167 (6): 196–201.

Gordon, J. and Angrick, E. (1986). Canine parvovirus: environmental effects on infectivity. *American Journal of Veterinary Research* 47 (7): 1464–1467.

Greene, C. and Decaro, N. (2012). Canine viral enteritis. In: Infectious Diseases of the Dog and Cat, 4e (ed. C. Greene), 67–79. St. Louis: Elsevier.

Hartmann, F.A., Dusick, A.F., and Young, K.M. (2013). Impact of disinfectant-filled foot mats on mechanical transmission of bacteria in a veterinary teaching hospital. *Journal of the American Veterinary Medical Association* 242 (5): 682–688.

Hsu, H.S., Lin, T.-H., Wu, H.-Y. et al. (2016). High detection rate of dog circovirus in diarrheal dogs. *BMC Veterinary Research* 12 (1): 8–13.

Kalli, I., Leontides, L.S., Mylonakis, M.E. et al. (2010). Factors affecting the occurrence, duration of hospitalization and final outcome in canine parvovirus infection. *Research in Veterinary Science* 89 (2): 174–178.

Kampf, G. (2018). Efficacy of ethanol against viruses in hand disinfection. *Journal of Hospital Infection* 98 (4): 331–338.

Lechner, E.S., Crawford, P.C., Levy, J.K. et al. (2010). Prevalence of protective antibody titers for canine distemper virus and canine parvovirus in dogs entering a Florida animal shelter. *Journal of the American Veterinary Medical Association* 236 (12): 1317–1321.

Leisewitz, A.L. (2017). Canine and feline parvovirus infection. In: Textbook of Veterinary Internal Medicine, 8e (eds. S.J. Ettinger, E.C. Feldman and E. Cote), 991–995. St. Louis: Elsevier.

Li, L., McGraw, S., Zhu, K. et al. (2013). Circovirus in tissues of dogs with vasculitis and hemorrhage. *Emerging Infectious Diseases* 19 (4): 534–541.

Mahon, J., Rozanski, E., and Paul, A. (2017). Prevalence of serum antibody titers against canine distemper virus and canine parvovirus in dogs hospitalized in an intensive care unit. *Journal of the American Veterinary Medical Association* 250 (12): 1413–1418.

Markovich, J.E., Stucker, K.M., Carr, A.H. et al. (2012). Effects of canine parvovirus strain variations on diagnostic test results and clinical management of enteritis in dogs. *Journal of the American Veterinary Medical Association* 241 (1): 66–72.

Mira, F., Dowgier, G., Pirpari, G. et al. (2018). Molecular typing of a novel canine parvovirus type 2a mutant circulating in Italy. *Infection, Genetics and Evolution* 61 (November 2017): 67–73.

Miranda, C. and Thompson, G. (2016a). Canine parvovirus: the worldwide occurrence of antigenic variants. *Journal of General Virology* 97 (9): 2043–2057.

Miranda, C., Carvalheira, J., Parrish, C.R. et al. (2015). Factors affecting the occurrence of canine parvovirus in dogs. *Veterinary Microbiology* 180 (1–2): 59–64.

Miranda, C., Parrish, C.R., and Thompson, G. (2016b). Epidemiological evolution of canine parvovirus in the Portuguese domestic dog population. *Veterinary Microbiology* 183: 37–42.

Mohr, A.J., Leisewitz, A.L., Jacobson, L.S. et al. (2003). Effect of early enteral nutrition on intestinal permeability, intestinal protein loss, and outcome in dogs with severe parvoviral enteritis. *Journal of Veterinary Internal Medicine* 17 (6): 791–798.

Moriello, K.A. (2015). Decontamination of laundry exposed to Microsporum canis hairs and spores. *Journal of Feline Medicine and Surgery* 18 (6): 457–461.

Panda, D., Patra, R.C., Nandi, S. et al. (2009). Oxidative stress indices in gastroenteritis in dogs with canine parvoviral infection. *Research in Veterinary Science* 86 (1): 36–42.

Patterson, E.V., Reese, M.J., Tucker, S.J. et al. (2007). Parvovirus Antigen Testing in Kittens. *Journal of the American Veterinary Medical Association* 230: 359–363.

Pendland, S.L., Jung, R., Messick, C.R. et al. (2002). in vitro; bactericidal activity of piperacillin, gentamicin, and metronidazole in a mixed model containing Escherichia coli, Enterococcus faecalis, and Bacteroides fragilis. *Diagnostic Microbiology and Infectious Disease* 43 (2): 149–156.

Prittie, J. (2004). Canine parvoviral enteritis: a review of diagnosis, management, and prevention. *Journal of Veterinary Emergency and Critical Care* 14 (3): 167–176.

Proksch, A.L., Unterer, S., Speck, S. et al. (2015). Influence of clinical and laboratory variables on faecal antigen ELISA results in dogs with canine parvovirus infection. *Veterinary Journal* 204 (3): 304–308.

Sarpong, K.J., Lukowski, J.M., and Knapp, C.G. (2017). Evaluation of mortality rate and predictors of outcome in dogs receiving outpatient treatment for parvoviral enteritis. *Journal of the American Veterinary Medical Association* 251 (9): 1035–1041.

Savigny, M.R. and Macintire, D.K. (2010). Use of oseltamivir in the treatment of canine parvoviral enteritis. *Journal of Veterinary Emergency and Critical Care* 20 (1): 132–142.

Schoeman, J.P., Goddard, A., and Leisewitz, A.L. (2013). Biomarkers in canine parvovirus enteritis. *New Zealand Veterinary Journal* 61 (4): 217–222.

Schultz, R.D., Thiel, B., Mukhtar, E. et al. (2010). Age and long-term protective immunity in dogs and cats. *Journal of Comparative Pathology* 142 (Suppl. 1): S102–S108.

Silva, M.M.O., Castro, T.X., Costa, E.M. et al. (2013). Comparison of three laboratorial tests for diagnosis of canine parvovirus infection. *Arquivo Brasileiro de Medicina Veterinaria e Zootecnia* 65 (1): 149–152.

Sime, T.A., Powell, L.J., Schildt, J.C. et al. (2015). Parvoviral myocarditis in a 5-week-old Dachshund. *Journal of Veterinary Emergency and Critical Care* 25 (6): 765–769.

Soma, T., Ohinata, T., Ishii, H. et al. (2011). Detection and genotyping of canine coronavirus RNA in diarrheic dogs in Japan. *Research in Veterinary Science* 90 (2): 205–207.

Tupler, T., Levy, J.K., Sabshin, S.J. et al. (2012). Enteropathogens identified in dogs entering a Florida animal shelter with normal feces or diarrhea. *Journal of the American Veterinary Medical Association* 241 (3): 338–343.

Venn, E.C., Preisner, K., Boscan, P.L. et al. (2017). Evaluation of an outpatient protocol in the treatment of canine parvoviral enteritis. *Journal of Veterinary Emergency and Critical Care* 27 (1): 52–65.

Wang, J., Lin, P., Zhao, H. et al. (2016). Continuing evolution of canine parvovirus in China: isolation of novel variants with an Ala5Gly mutation in the VP2 protein. *Infection, Genetics and Evolution* 38: 73–78.

Wilson, S., Illambas, J., Siedek, E. et al. (2014). Vaccination of dogs with canine parvovirus type 2b (CPV-2b) induces neutralising antibody responses to CPV-2a and CPV-2c. *Vaccine* 32 (42): 5420–5424.

Zicola, A., Jolly, S., Methijs, E. et al. (2012). Fatal outbreaks in dogs associated with pantropic canine coronavirus in France and Belgium. *Journal of Small Animal Practice* 53 (5): 297–300.

Zourkas, E., Ward, M.P., and Kelman, M. (2015). Canine parvovirus in Australia: a comparative study of reported rural and urban cases. *Veterinary Microbiology* 181 (3–4): 198–203.

15

Feline Panleukopenia

Helen Tuzio[1,2]

[1] *Long Island University - College of Veterinary Medicine, Brookville, NY, USA*
[2] *Forest Hills Cat Hospital, Middle Village, NY, USA*

15.1 Introduction

Feline Panleukopenia is a highly contagious, potentially fatal disease of cats. Though well-controlled in pet cats as a result of widespread vaccination, it can still be prevalent in animal shelters due to the continual influx of unprotected and potentially exposed kittens and cats. Fortunately, even in shelters, this disease can be largely prevented with careful vaccination, sanitation, population management and housing practices.

15.2 Epidemiology and Course of Disease

15.2.1 Etiologic Agent

Feline Panleukopenia virus (FPV) is the causative agent of an extremely contagious disease that has been known by a variety of names such as feline distemper, feline infectious enteritis, feline parvoviral enteritis, pseudomembranous enteritis, laryngoenteritis, feline agranulocytosis, and show fever, among others. Though the disease was recognized before 1900, it was not until 1928 that a viral agent was isolated, and the virus itself was not definitively identified until 1962.

The organism is a single-stranded DNA parvovirus. It is a highly infectious, non-enveloped virus that has an affinity for rapidly dividing cells, particularly in bone marrow, lymphoid tissue, intestinal epithelium, and fetal and neonatal cerebellar tissue. It is ubiquitous, can be very virulent in susceptible animals, and may result in infections that are often fatal. It is extremely hardy, being highly resistant to physical factors, including heat, and many chemical disinfectants. It is able to survive for months or even years in the environment, particularly in infected organic matter (Truyen et al. 2009), and has been shown to remain infective (after storage) at 4–25°C (41–77 °F) for 13 months (Pedersen 1988).

Though FPV and canine parvovirus (CPV) are closely related (CPV may have emerged as a mutation of FPV), FPV has different biologic properties and has only one serotype (Scott 1987; Sturgess 2003). CPV type 2, though originally unable to infect cats, has produced several variants (CPV-2a, CPV-2b, and CPV-2c) that can now infect cats and cause clinical

Infectious Disease Management in Animal Shelters, Second Edition.
Edited by Lila Miller, Stephanie Janeczko, and Kate F. Hurley.

disease in them (Nakamura et al. 2001). Mixed infections with both FPV and CPV-2 variants also have been detected in cats (Sykes 2014). Despite the existence of these variants, FPV is by far still the most common cause of panleukopenia in felines (Kennedy and Little 2012).

See Table 15.7 for an overview of the disease.

15.2.2 Susceptibility

FPV affects cats of all ages. The domestic cat is the primary host, but FPV can infect all members of Felidae worldwide including tigers, panthers, and leopards (Neuerer et al. 2008). It also infects species of the families Mustelidae, Procyonidae, and Viveridae that include the raccoon, ring-tailed cat and mink (Scott 1987). The virus is associated with disease in the fox and is known to replicate in ferrets without causing disease (Sykes 2014). In dogs, it replicates in the thymus, spleen, and bone marrow but not in the gut, and is not shed. The epidemiological significance of this is not fully understood (Truyen and Parrish 2013).

FPV does not infect humans, though it has been isolated from a monkey (Sykes 2014). When human bacterial diseases were first discovered, many people believed the disease in cats was similar or identical to typhoid, diphtheria or cholera. Hence the origin of some of the disease's many other names such as cat plague, typhus, typhoid, and colibacillosis (Scott 1987).

15.2.3 Prevalence

Feline parvovirus is widespread in nature, enzootic in all parts of the US, and reported from nearly all countries in the world. However, panleukopenia is much less prevalent in privately owned cats than it was 20 years ago, primarily due to vaccination programs and client education (Greene 2012). Nevertheless, the disease still poses a serious and constant threat in certain environments and populations, including outdoor cats (particularly unvaccinated free-roaming cats) as well as those housed in shelter settings and poorly managed breeding catteries (Addie et al. 1998). Shelters face several unique and significant challenges that increase the risk of infection with FPV, including the constant influx of cats that are often insufficiently vaccinated and thus susceptible, particularly in summer and fall when there is typically an abundance of kittens with inadequate maternal antibodies to help protect them (Truyen et al. 2009). These large numbers of kittens diminish the overall immunity within the population, increasing the likelihood of both individual cases as well as outbreaks of panleukopenia (Litster and Benjanirut 2013).

In addition, as stated before, the virus is exceptionally stable in the environment. Failure to properly sanitize a contaminated facility may result in prolonged disease exposure (Schultz 2009) that places both current and future populations at risk. The addition of new residents (especially those incubating the disease) and the change in the social hierarchy may also result in stress-induced immunosuppression, leading to an increased susceptibility to infection and disease (Scherk et al. 2013).

15.2.4 Modes of Transmission

Feline panleukopenia virus is transmitted by direct contact between infected and susceptible cats, by contact with the virus in the environment, or transplacentally. The fetus is infected via the maternal circulation, as the virus can pass the placental barrier in pregnant queens, with prenatal infection usually occurring mid-gestation. The primary mode of transmission, however, is fecal-oral, either by direct contact or via fomites, which are objects or materials that are likely to carry infection, such as clothing, utensils, and furniture. Infected animals shed large amounts of virus in all body secretions and excretions, and susceptible animals become infected after they ingest it.

Environmental exposure is of special concern in shelters, boarding facilities, and catteries because the virus may remain infective for months or years, especially in organic material, soil, or moist, cool or shady areas. Clothing, hands, animal fur, food, and water dishes, cages, bedding, litter boxes, toys, and grooming supplies, carpet and soil, etc. can all easily serve as fomites that are sources of infection. Even the bottom of a cat's paw can transmit the virus to other fomites.

Though not a primary source of infection, droplet transmission can also occur, particularly if concurrent infection with an upper respiratory virus results in sneezing (Scott 1987). The droplets containing the virus are expelled into the air. They may be inhaled or ingested by neighboring individuals, or land on surfaces, thus contaminating the environment. Flies and fleas can serve as mechanical vectors, transmitting the disease from infected to susceptible cats (Gillespie and Scott 1973; Scott 1987). Transmission by infected prey has also been hypothesized (Allison et al. 2013). It is important to remember that cats may become infected without ever coming into direct contact with an infected cat.

15.2.5 Pathophysiology

Following infection, the virus uses transferrin receptors to enter and replicate in the lymphoid tissue of the oropharynx and the gut during the first 18–24 hours. It then disseminates via the bloodstream and causes an initial viremia in the ensuing two to seven days. Because it requires the S-phase of cell division to replicate, viral growth is restricted to mitotically active tissues – lymph nodes, bone marrow stem cells, rapidly dividing cells of the intestinal crypts of Lieberkühn, and fetal tissues including the thymus, heart, kidney, and cerebellum (Truyen et al. 2009; Greene 2012). Within 48 hours, every tissue has significantly high levels of virus that remain high as long as seven days after infection. During this time the white blood cell (WBC) count plummets.

This early decrease in WBCs is characterized by a generalized leukopenia from a generalized decrease in production from bone marrow suppression – a result of viral replication in early progenitor cells of the bone marrow that affects all myeloid cell populations and results in the panleukopenia that defines this disease (from the Greek "pan" meaning every, "leuk" meaning white, and "penia" meaning reduction in the circulating blood). Neutrophil losses into the gastrointestinal tract worsen the already severe neutropenia. A lymphoid depletion due to tissue necrosis from viral invasion and subsequent destruction of lymphoid follicles of lymph nodes, spleen, thymus, and gastrointestinal tract, as well as a lymphocyte migration into the tissues all result in a functional immunosuppression (Pedersen 1988; Greene 2012). At the nadir, generally four to six days after initial infection, the WBC count is so low that patients are very susceptible to secondary bacterial infections.

Thymic atrophy can be seen in young affected cats. A nonregenerative anemia may be present but is not as common due to the longer half-life of red blood cells compared to WBCs (Truyen et al. 2009; Kennedy and Little 2012).

Gradually, circulating antibodies rise and virus titers begin to fall. Serum antibodies usually appear three to four days after the onset of clinical signs and are followed two to three days later by a dramatic rebound in WBCs. By two weeks post-infection, most tissues are free of virus, though small quantities may remain in some tissues such as the kidney.

Under normal circumstances, there is a continuous turnover of intestinal epithelial cells. New cells form in the intestinal crypts and migrate up the villus to replace the older cells being shed into the intestinal lumen. Parvovirus infects the epithelium of the crypts, destroying any new cells and leading to the blunting of the villus and eventually to the denuding of the lamina propria. This tissue destruction and inflammation, and the associated loss of epithelial surface area, greatly reduce the absorptive and digestive abilities of the small intestines and result in the severe enteric signs usually seen with this disease.

Nearly three-quarters of the small neurons of the feline cerebellum are formed after birth. Intrauterine or perinatal infection leads to either virus replication in the Purkinje cells of the developing cerebellum of the unborn kittens, impairing its development and resulting in cerebellar hypoplasia/aplasia and permanent dysfunction, or to an invasion of all the cells in the fetus leading to fetal death (Truyen et al. 2009).

15.2.6 Incubation Period and Carrier State

The incubation period may range from 2 to 14 days (Litster and Benjanirut 2013) depending on the age of the animal, the dose of infection and concurrent disease (Gillespie and Scott 1973). Clinical signs appear two to seven days after infection in most cases (Day et al. 2016). This long and variable incubation period means exposed cats may not show clinical signs until days after they have arrived at the shelter or their new home.

There is no carrier state for FPV (DiGangi et al. 2011).

15.2.7 Shedding

Viral shedding is usually for five to seven days; it may be for only one to two days, (Greene and Addie 2006) or it may continue for as long as six weeks after recovery (UC Davis 2016). Shedding in urine and feces may occur 24–48 hours post-infection and 2–3 days before clinical signs appear. During this time, large amounts of the virus may be shed, so the environmental viral load can grow exponentially in affected shelters and catteries (Truyen et al. 2009). Fetal infection may produce an immunological tolerance in the pregnant queen, resulting in shedding of the virus for an extended period of time, but persistent infections and persistent viral shedding are rare (Pedersen 1988).

Shedding can result from vaccination using a modified live product and may cause a weak positive on a fecal antigen test for 5–12 days post-vaccination (UC Davis 2016).

15.3 Clinical Signs

Feline panleukopenia virus can produce a wide range of signs depending on the virulence of the infecting strain, the resistance of the host, and the type and severity of other viral and bacterial complications. Because the virus targets rapidly dividing cells, the age of the cat at the time of infection has great bearing on the clinical presentation. There are four recognized forms of the clinical disease: subacute, peracute, acute, and peri-natal. It is important to note that subclinical infections may also occur. See Table 15.1 for a summary of the clinical signs associated with each form of the disease.

Table 15.1 Summary of clinical signs associated with feline panleukopenia.

Form	Clinical signs
Subacute	Fever, mild lethargy and weight loss, leukopenia
Peracute	Sudden death, subnormal temperature, shock, maybe vomiting, severe abdominal pain
Acute	Fever, lethargy, anorexia, vomiting, and watery, fetid and/or hemorrhagic diarrhea, severe leukopenia and dehydration, abdominal pain
Perinatal	Abortion, stillbirth; newborn kittens suffer early neonatal death or ataxia, incoordination (cerebellar hypoplasia) with wide-base stance and intention tremors

15.3.1 Subacute Form

This mild form of infection is characterized by leukopenia, fever, mild lethargy and weight loss due to anorexia. It may be seen in germ-free cats exposed to the virus. They may have no signs of intestinal disease, or they may have gas-filled intestines and diarrhea, but they usually recover completely in one to three days, due to a lower mitotic rate of crypt epithelial cells that leaves fewer cells for the virus to invade (Rohovsky and Griesemer 1967; Ott 1975).

15.3.2 Peracute Form

The peracute form of panleukopenia is the most severe manifestation of infection, characterized by sudden death four to nine days after exposure to the virus. Illness progresses extremely rapidly, from severe lethargy to coma to death in just a few hours. Vomiting may occur, but death usually ensues before diarrhea or dehydration has a chance to develop. Peracute disease is usually seen in kittens under six months of age, particularly in those that have been recently weaned, but it has also been recognized in adult cats. Since a cat may be found extremely ill or dead after having been healthy and active 8–12 hours earlier, it is often presented to the veterinarian as a case of suspected poisoning. In some cases, severe abdominal pain can be elicited on palpation early in the course of the disease. However, in most cases, shock is advanced, and the body temperature is subnormal by the time clinical signs are recognized. Death is usually within 12 hours as a result of septic shock, dehydration and hypothermia.

15.3.3 Acute Form

The acute form of panleukopenia is the most common manifestation of the disease. There is normally a sudden onset of clinical signs. A fever of 40 °C (104 °F) or higher that lasts for 24 hours is common and signals the viremic phase of the illness. Occasionally, cats will die during this first febrile episode, usually due to dehydration, electrolyte imbalance, septicemia, endotoxemia, and/or disseminated intravascular coagulation (DIC).

More often, this phase is followed by a return to normal body temperature for another 24 hours, and then another fever episode when the WBC count drops. This is a crisis stage that often determines the outcome and severity of disease; the more severe the leukopenia, the more severe the disease and the poorer the prognosis. WBC counts below 2 K/μl indicate a very guarded prognosis. Eventually, the body temperature of the cat becomes subnormal, followed in a few hours by coma and death. In these acute cases, illness seldom lasts more than five to seven days.

The second fever episode starts with lethargy and anorexia that progress to vomiting with or without watery and/or hemorrhagic diarrhea. Gastrointestinal (GI) signs generally coincide with ensuing severe leukopenia, though leukopenia is not always present at the time of the initial presentation. Vomiting is the most common sign observed, initially consisting of the last meal eaten and then changing to a white or yellow (bile-tinged) frothy liquid. *Severe fetid watery diarrhea in large volumes is the hallmark sign and usually develops in 24–48 hours.* It often contains blood and string casts of fibrin or shreds of intestinal mucosa – from an ensuing hemorrhagic enteritis – that produce the typical necrotic "parvovirus smell." *Since diarrhea is not generally the earliest sign,* it may not be seen in cases that result in sudden or rapid fatality. The profuse vomiting, persistent anorexia and watery diarrhea quickly progress to severe dehydration and electrolyte imbalances that result in lethargy and death if untreated.

Clinically, lethargy may be profound as a result of bone marrow depletion, anorexia and fever (Truyen et al. 2009). If severe lethargy and complete anorexia take hold during the first fever, they may become even more profound during the second fever. Due to severe dehydration, cats may act as if they want to drink but are reluctant to do so. This apparent desire for water lasts throughout the course of the disease.

Numerous other abnormalities are readily apparent on physical examination of cats with the acute form of the disease. The eyes are sunken and the third eyelids are generally raised. The eyes are often caked with mucous even in the absence of concurrent respiratory disease. Mucous membranes often appear pale. The hair coat is rough, dry, dull and unkempt, and may be soiled with feces. The chin may be wet from vomiting or attempting to drink. There is a loss of skin elasticity due to dehydration. Abdominal palpation is painful; mesenteric nodes are usually enlarged, and intestinal contents consist primarily of gas and liquid. These cats may meow plaintively, especially when handled, due to pain from intestinal inflammation. To help alleviate the pain and fever, they generally prefer to lie with their abdomen on a cool surface or take a crouched position with their head between their paws or hanging over a water dish; cats often will adopt this position just prior to death.

Cats also may display signs attributable to secondary infections due to a severely low WBC count and subsequent reduced disease resistance. Purulent otitis, oral ulcers, mild jaundice and iritis with aqueous flare have been observed. Areas of depigmentation have been reported to occur on the brown masks of Siamese cats. Rarely there is necrosis of the ear tips – possibly due to fibrin thrombi. Panleukopenia is often reported either preceding or following upper respiratory infection in shelter cats.

15.3.4 Perinatal

Perinatal infection via vertical transmission constitutes the fourth form of the disease. Queens with partial immunity from natural exposure or recent vaccination may show mild or no signs, but evidence of infection may be observed in the fetuses depending on the age of the fetus at the time of infection. Infection early in gestation may cause fetal abortion or death with subsequent resorption, mummification, or stillbirth. Kittens infected in late gestation or during the first few days after birth may either die suddenly with no sign of disease (early neonatal death) or develop a "feline ataxia syndrome" at about three weeks of age.

Since the cerebellum continues to develop during the first two weeks after birth, cerebellar hypoplasia can develop in kittens infected shortly after birth as well as in those infected in utero. Ataxia associated with hypermetria, dysmetria, and incoordination becomes noticeable when the kittens start to walk. Affected kittens are symmetrically uncoordinated with exaggerated movements; they usually sway and may roll or tumble over. They have a wide-base stance with tail held high and stiff for balance. Despite the ataxia, kittens are alert and strong, and mental ability is unaffected. The ataxia is nonprogressive but may be more noticeable as kittens mature and their range of activity increases. Given time, most kittens learn to accommodate the irregularity and become good pets. The degree of disability may vary greatly among members of the same litter. Some may be normal, as transplacental transmission may not occur in all the kittens of an infected queen.

15.4 Morbidity/Mortality/Prognosis

Morbidity and mortality rates vary greatly. The risk of infection and subsequent development of disease varies primarily with age, health and vaccination history of the cat, the magnitude of exposure, and the geographic prevalence of infection (Scherk et al. 2013). The pathogenicity of the strain and the dose of pathogen also play a role in morbidity and mortality, with kitten deaths reported in households of fully vaccinated kittens, possibly due to exposure to large amounts of virus in the environment (Sykes 2014). Even so, the factor having the greatest impact on both morbidity and mortality is the protective antibody titer of the cat at the time of exposure (Lappin et al. 2002a; Litster and Benjanirut 2013), whether due to passive maternal immunity or as a result of vaccination. In unvaccinated populations, panleukopenia is arguably the most devastating disease of cats and may have been the cause of great plagues that are believed to have almost wiped out the cat population in various areas of the world (Scott 1987).

The incidence and severity of panleukopenia tend to decline with the age of the cat. Kittens less than six months of age are most susceptible to infections and typically develop more severe disease than adult cats or older kittens. Morbidity and mortality rates peak in kittens three to five months of age when maternally derived immunity has waned. It is also probably highest in these kittens due to their immature immune system and fast intestinal mucosal cell turnover. Intestinal cell turnover rate is often increased further by mild intestinal pathogens that may predispose young cats to FPV. Mortality rates are frequently over 90% in these kittens (Truyen et al. 2009). Even in the overall population, the disease typically has an explosive short course with high morbidity and high mortality rates; in the peracute form mortality frequently reaches 100% and in the acute form 25–90% (Neuerer et al. 2008; Litster and Benjanirut 2013). Only feline panleukopenia will cause such a high level of mortality (Schultz 2009).

The prognosis is generally dependent on the form of the disease and the speed with which the illness is diagnosed, and supportive care and treatment provided. The peracute form is rapidly fatal. On the other hand, cats with the acute form that survive illness for longer than five days generally recover over the ensuing weeks. Those that do not survive generally die from complications associated with secondary bacterial infections, sepsis, dehydration, electrolyte derangements, and/or DIC.

Neonatally infected kittens who survive the disease may be ataxic when they start walking, but otherwise grow normally if they are coordinated enough to eat (Scott 1987; Pollock and Postorino 1994). Though cerebellar hypoplasia is nonprogressive, signs may become more apparent as kittens age and their range of activities increases. The ataxia may be extremely mild or so severe as to make these cats unsuitable pets.

Hematologic factors associated with a poor prognosis include leukopenia (white blood cell count <2 K/µl, thus depleting the body's immune system), thrombocytopenia, hypoalbuminemia, and hypokalemia. Kruse et al. (2010) determined that serum albumin <30 g/l at presentation was associated with a negative outcome, possibly because the diminished plasma oncotic pressure decreases perfusion at the capillary level, which may lead to DIC, organ failure and death. In this study, a serum potassium of <4 mmol/l at presentation was also associated with a negative outcome. This is not seen in the dog (Kruse et al. 2010).

It is interesting to note that a recent relatively small study of 177 shelter cats with FPV determined that cats without lethargy and with a higher body weight and a higher rectal temperature had a higher survival rate than other cats. It also determined that leukopenia on or after the third day of hospitalization was associated with a poor outcome, suggesting the persistence of leukopenia (rather than the degree of leukopenia) is associated with profound immunosuppression, which increases the chances of secondary infections and death. Leukopenia upon admission was not found to be predictive of the outcome. Due to limitations reported by the authors, additional research is warranted (Porporato et al. 2018).

15.5 Diagnosis

A diagnosis of panleukopenia is based on the history of exposure, clinical signs, detection of viral antigen, and characteristic hemogram changes in an animal. Definitive diagnosis may be made post-mortem via histopathology on tissue specimens. Panleukopenia should be suspected in any case of sudden death in a cat not known to be completely vaccinated.

15.5.1 History

The age and vaccination history of the animal should be evaluated. Panleukopenia is extremely uncommon in fully vaccinated cats over four months of age. However, a history of vaccination is not enough to rule out FPV, particularly in kittens under 20 weeks of age due to interference of maternal antibodies, or in cats of any age that were vaccinated less than 1 week prior to exposure. For more information on evaluating a vaccination history, please see section 15.7.1 on host risk factors in this chapter.

The history should also consider whether the cat may have been exposed to the disease prior to intake; i.e. a stray admitted or transferred from a shelter or an area of high disease prevalence, or exposed after intake into the shelter. This information may be used to help determine the likelihood of the cat being exposed, but possible previous exposure to FPV should **not** be used to determine whether or not to vaccinate.

15.5.2 Antigen Testing

The detection of FPV antigen in feces is one of the most valuable means of diagnosing panleukopenia infection in the shelter setting, primarily because of rapid-assay, point-of-care tests that use commercially available enzyme-linked immunosorbent assay (ELISA), immunochromatographic or latex agglutination technology. Due to the close structural and antigenic properties of CPV and FPV, most tests designed to detect CPV in dog feces (Parvo SNAP Test®: IDEXX Labs, Westbrook, MA; AGEN CPV®: AGEN Biomedical Ltd., Brisbane, QLD, Australia; WITNESS CPV: Synbiotics Corp, San Diego, CA) also have excellent specificity for the detection of FPV, and can be used to detect both canine and feline parvovirus antigens in cat feces (Neuerer et al. 2008; Abd-Eldaim et al. 2009; Truyen et al. 2009).

There are few false positive results because the fecal antigen test has excellent specificity (i.e. ability to identify correctly those *without* the disease), but it has limited sensitivity (i.e. ability to identify correctly those *with* the disease) so false negative results are more likely. Though false positive results are uncommon, they still should be interpreted in light of the vaccination and exposure history. These tests can detect antigen in feces up to two weeks following vaccination with modified live products (MLV) (Truyen et al. 2009). Though this appears to occur relatively infrequently, it is prudent to treat all kittens and cats with positive test results as potentially infectious to others.

On the other hand, the limited sensitivity of this test means there is an increased chance of obtaining false negative results. Therefore, *a negative fecal ELISA does not rule out FPV infection*. Additional testing may be valuable in these cases. Hematology or polymerase chain reaction (PCR) based testing of blood (whole blood should be submitted for cats without diarrhea) or feces can help diagnose FPV in cats that are ELISA negative. However, PCR testing can also yield positive results in recently vaccinated cats (UC Davis 2016). Feces in healthy cats have tested positive for several weeks, but the epidemiologic significance of this is unknown (Schunck et al. 1995; Mostl 2015).

15.5.3 Antibody Testing

Antibodies to FPV can be detected via hemagglutination inhibition (HI), ELISA or indirect immunofluorescence. Because these tests do not differentiate between vaccine-induced and infection-induced antibodies, their use for diagnosing FPV infection in sick animals is limited. However, they are useful for identifying those animals that are protected against panleukopenia. This is discussed in detail later in this chapter in the section on the role of titer testing.

15.5.4 Hematology

A profound panleukopenia (<2000 white blood cells/μl, as determined by complete blood count (CBC) or blood smear, with neutropenia (<2500/μl or 1–2 neutrophils per 40× field) (Greene and Addie 2006) is the hallmark of the disease. Though it is found in almost all infected cats even if they do not show clinical signs, leukopenia may not yet be evident at the time of presentation, so a normal WBC count should not be used to rule out FPV infection.

In general, a decline in the number of circulating WBCs starts on the second or third day after infection (before the onset of clinical signs). The WBC count is usually 4000–8000/μl in subclinical cases and closer to 4000/μl in clinical ones. By four to six days post-infection, there may be fewer than 200 wbc/μl of blood, sometimes making it impossible to do a differential count. Often, the decline is progressive with a precipitous drop at the time of crisis.

- Neutrophils, in particular, are affected – they may disappear as rapidly as up to 4000 cells/day.
- The lymphocytes also decrease, but not as rapidly, so an absolute lymphopenia with a relative lymphocytosis may be seen; the majority of circulating WBCs generally are lymphocytes.
- Monocytes also decrease slowly, resulting in a relative monocytosis, but their numbers are normally much lower than lymphocyte numbers.
- Eosinophil production is decreased, but due to their short life span (two to six days), they may be absent or appear increased in number (Pedersen 1988; Sturgess 2003).
- Erythrocyte production is decreased as well, but the long lifespan of red blood cells (100–200 days) ensures that any anemia from direct viral effects is mild. However, more significant anemia may develop if recovery is prolonged or if there is bleeding into the gastrointestinal tract (Scott 1987). In cases of severe dehydration, there may seem to be an increase in erythrocyte numbers.

Following the crisis (approximately five days after the onset of clinical signs), the leukocytes rapidly return to circulation, usually at the rate of 4000–6000 cells/day. This rebound can result in the total count sometimes reaching 35 000 WBC/μl in three to four days, resulting in a neutrophilia with a left shift.

Serum biochemistry panel results are nonspecific for FPV. Hypoalbuminemia is the most frequent abnormality, probably from decreased protein intake and leakage into the gastrointestinal tract from mucosal lesions (Kruse et al. 2010).

15.5.5 Necropsy

With the exception of peracute cases when changes may not be readily apparent, cats that succumb to FPV are gaunt with sticky, dry tissues and sunken, soft eyes indicative of severe dehydration. Occasionally, the esophagus or mouth is eroded or ulcerated, and there may be sloughing of the palate or inflammation of the larynx. Internally, mild to severe segmental enteritis with or without petechiation is common, particularly in the jejunum and ileum, and occasionally in the duodenum and colon. The intestines are thickened or inelastic. The serosal surface is roughened with a granular appearance that may be covered with fibrinous exudates. The mucosal surface is ragged with mucoid or membranous exudates. Intestinal contents may consist of fluid with mucosal debris and/or blood. Feces are scant, watery, and foul-smelling, often gray or yellow in color. Mesenteric lymph nodes are swollen and edematous, sometimes hyperemic or hemorrhagic. The stomach and esophagus are reddened and bile-stained. Bone marrow may be scarce, gelatinous or liquid and yellow-white in color. (See Chapter 5 on necropsy techniques for more information).

15.5.5.1 Histopathology

Histopathology is the confirmatory test since parvovirus causes the pathognomonic microscopic changes of intestinal crypt necrosis with villus blunting in the jejunum and ileum. Cellular depletion of bone marrow and lymphoid tissues may also be seen. Samples of these four tissues should be submitted for histopathology in any suspect case.

15.5.6 Additional Tests

Other less commonly used methods of diagnosis include viral detection by electron microscopy or hemagglutination, virus isolation from feces, and immunohistochemistry on infected tissues collected postmortem. Problems encountered with virus detection most commonly are false negatives that result from the rapid decline of virus particles in the feces that occurs once an enteric infection is established or a reduction in the number of virus particles by dilution (diarrhea). These tests are all time-consuming, more expensive and less accessible or practical, particularly in a shelter setting.

15.5.7 Differential Diagnoses

Panleukopenia is a deadly disease that can have a major impact on cats in shelters, therefore it is important to rule out more treatable diseases. Diagnostic rule-outs include severe bacterial infections that may result in a toxic leukopenia (particularly *Salmonella* sp., *Clostridium perfringens*, and *Campylobacter* sp.) and other major viral pathogens that can affect the intestinal tract. Infectious causes less likely to be seen affecting multiple individuals include acute toxoplasmosis, feline leukemia virus (FeLV), and to a lesser extent, feline immunodeficiency virus (FIV) and any severe or prolonged diseases that will produce bone marrow suppression and leukopenia. Noninfectious causes include acute poisoning (which may affect individuals or groups), gastrointestinal foreign bodies, and intussusception (especially in kittens).

Cats may be co-infected with more than one pathogen, so the identification of other pathogens does not rule out concurrent infection with panleukopenia. Most of those conditions are less likely in shelter cats, particularly as a cause of outbreaks or an acute cause of death. However, they should be strongly considered as part of a complete workup if well-vaccinated cats are affected and/or diagnostic test results are inconsistent with panleukopenia.

15.6 Treatment

In a shelter environment, panleukopenia should only be treated if strict isolation and biosecurity measures can be maintained and appropriate, skilled nursing care can be offered. The risk of spreading the disease to other cats, the adoptability of the cat, the severity of the disease, and the availability of resources to treat are usually the deciding factors. Because the disease is highly infectious, carries a guarded prognosis, can be both expensive and labor-intensive to treat, requires an isolation area and trained staff to provide appropriate care, and the virus is resistant to disinfection and persists long term in the environment, many shelters choose not to treat clinically ill cats on-site. Other options include to treat them at an off-site location or to euthanize to minimize the suffering of the individual cat and avoid the risk of disease spread throughout the shelter population (Tuzio 2009; DiGangi 2011; Litster and Benjanirut 2013). Ideally, the shelter should have general treatment guidelines or a treatment policy in place ahead of time that reflects all these factors to avoid making hasty, emotional decisions that may have a widespread impact on the entire shelter.

After due consideration, some shelters may decide they have the resources to treat panleukopenia on-site. No specific antiviral drugs are currently available to treat the disease; the goals of treatment are to combat extreme dehydration by restoring and maintaining fluid balance, to minimize continuing losses by resting the gastrointestinal tract and providing nutrients and electrolytes, and to prevent secondary infections. Therefore, supportive care consisting of fluid therapy and antibiotics is the mainstay of treatment and can significantly decrease mortality – particularly if serum FPV antibodies are near protective levels. All medications should be administered parenterally for the first few days since the intestinal lesions, as well as the vomiting and diarrhea, will decrease the absorption of products given orally. Optimum treatment recommendations are offered here, but appropriate adjustments should be made based on the cat's condition, response to therapy and the shelter's resources. See Table 15.2 for a summary of treatment recommendations.

15.6.1 Nursing Care

A cat diagnosed with panleukopenia should be placed in isolation immediately and provided with skilled nursing care by designated staff members who understand the importance of adhering to strict sanitary and isolation protocols. Young kittens require direct contact to stimulate the development of a healthy

Table 15.2 Summary of treatment recommendations.

Goal	Therapy
Restoration of fluid, electrolyte and acid–base balance	IV crystalloids (+/− KCl) @ 2–3 ml/hours
Prevention of bacteremia and sepsis	Ampicillin (20 mg/kg IV every (q) 8 hours) or amoxicillin with clavulanic acid (62.5 mg/cat twice daily [BID] after a meal) AND an aminoglycoside, or fluoroquinolone or cephalosporin[b]; OR piperacillin/tazobactam (40–50 mg/kg IV over 30 minutes q 6 hours).
Prevent vomiting	Maropitant (1 mg/kg SC q24 hours) or ondansetron (0.1–1 mg/kg IV slowly, SC, IM, PO q6–12 hours)
Nutrition	Highly digestible diet or whatever the cat will eat; placement of a feeding tube or central line if necessary. Mirtazapine [1.88–3.75 mg per cat PO q 24–72 hours(a) or Mirataz® (Kindred Bio) 2mg TD q24 hours][a] OR cyproheptadine (1–4 mg/cat PO q12–24 hours)[a] to stimulate the appetite.
Vitamin supplementation	B-complex administered parenterally in a dose sufficient to supply 50–100 mg of thiamine daily in combination with vitamin B_{12}
Pain management	Buprenorphine [Simbadol® (Abbott) 0.24 mg/kg SC once daily for up to 3 days]
Gastric/esophageal mucosal protection	Famotidine (0.5 mg/kg PO q 12–24 hours) or ranitidine (1–2 mg/kg PO, slow IV or SC q12 hours)[b]; sucralfate (0.25–0.3 g PO q6–8 hours), omeprazole (0.7–1 mg PO q12–24 hours)[b]
Immune stimulation/Increase levels of FPV IgG	Good nursing care, handling, direct contact, compassionate care/ Feline recombinant interferon-omega 1 MU/kg SC q24 hours for 3 days[c]
Maintain adequate levels of plasma protein	IV colloids, plasma or whole blood transfusions
Further considerations:	
Eliminate concurrent parasites	Anthelmintics
Maintain glycemic control	Dextrose 2.5–5% PO or IV (Avoid SC)
Protect exposed susceptible cats or colostrum deprived kittens	Hyperimmune serum (2 ml/kitten SC or IP[b]; 2–4 ml/kg cat SC or IP[d])

Dosages courtesy of Plumb (2018), except as noted.
[a] Agnew and Korman (2014).
[b] Marks (2016).
[c] Paltrinieri et al. 2007.
[d] Scott (1987).

immune system and to ensure their behavioral needs are met – particularly during the critical socialization period (one to three months of age). Stress should be minimized, and all patients should be provided compassionate care to encourage their will to live. Closely monitored heating pads, frequent petting, hand feeding, as well as warm, draft-free quarters and scrupulous sanitation are important treatment aids. Because of the real possibility of inadvertent fomite transmission from frequent or careless handling of these animals and the fact that most shelters are not staffed to provide this level of nursing care, young animals that require this degree of care should ideally be treated off-site if possible.

15.6.2 Fluid Therapy

The restoration of fluid, electrolyte and acid–base balance is the most important aspect of treatment. This is best provided via the intravenous (IV) route, paying particular attention to restoring potassium levels. Neonates have significantly higher fluid requirements than adult cats (80–120 ml/kg/day) but need much slower dose rates (2–3 ml/hour) (Sturgess 2003). The subcutaneous (SC) or intraosseous route may be used in kittens if venous access is not possible. When fluids are administered subcutaneously, they should be spread over the body surface to prevent delayed absorption or pooling of fluids in one area. This fluid restoration is critical, as severe dehydration accelerates disease progression. Dextrose may be added to intravenous (*not subcutaneous*) fluids in patients that are hypoglycemic and inappetent.

15.6.3 Colloids, Plasma, or Whole Blood Transfusions

Colloids, plasma, or whole blood transfusions may be indicated if the concentration of the patient's plasma protein is <2.0 g/dl or if the white cell count is <2000/μl (Pedersen 1988; Marks 2016). Whole blood is preferable if there is concurrent anemia. It can be administered at 20 ml/kg body weight per day slowly intravenously, or into the medullary cavity of the femur if a vein cannot be accessed. Platelet count and activated clotting time (ACT) should be monitored for evidence of DIC (Truyen et al. 2009).

15.6.4 Antibiotics

Antimicrobial therapy is necessary to prevent and treat the secondary bacterial infection, sepsis, and bacterial overgrowth that result from the severe leukopenia and tissue destruction caused by FPV infection. *Escherichia coli* is the most serious secondary invader, but other organisms may create complications; therefore, broad-spectrum parenteral (preferably IV) antibiotics effective against both gram-negative and anaerobic bacteria are warranted. Examples include ampicillin 20 mg/kg IV every eight hours or amoxicillin with clavulanic acid in combination with aminoglycosides, fluoroquinolones, or cephalosporins, or piperacillin/tazobactam (Marks 2016). A combination of ampicillin 6.6 mg/kg, intramuscularly (IM), every eight hours given currently with gentamicin 4.4 mg/kg every 12 hours provides protection from gram-positive, gram-negative, aerobic, and anaerobic infections, but can cause renal tubular nephrosis and must be used with caution in dehydrated patients (Pedersen 1988). Antimicrobials should only be administered by mouth if the gastroenteritis has been controlled.

15.6.5 Antiemetics

Anti-emetic drugs such as ondansetron (extra-label) 0.1–1 mg/kg IV (slowly), SC, IM or orally (PO) every 6–12 hours (Plumb 2018) should be considered in cases with persistent vomiting. Maropitant 1 mg/kg SC once a day (SID) may be used up to five consecutive days (per the manufacturer's drug insert, however, it has been used off-label and anecdotally for longer) in kittens older than 16 weeks of age. Metoclopramide is not recommended since the chemoreceptor trigger zone (CTZ) receptors may not play as important a role in emesis in the cat. It is also contraindicated in cases of gastrointestinal hemorrhage (Plumb 2018). If used, its short half-life (90 minutes in dogs) requires administration via constant rate infusion (CRI) at 1 mg/kg every 24 hours (Marks 2016). Phenothiazine derivatives such as chlorpromazine or prochlorpromazine cause hypotension and should not be used in dehydrated animals. Anticholinergics and opiates should also be used with caution as the resultant reduction in gastrointestinal motility may increase the absorption of bacterial toxins and increase penetration of the bowel wall by bacteria and viruses.

15.6.6 Nutrition

Adequate nutrition is an essential component of a successful treatment plan. Food and water restriction to lessen vomiting and slow mitotic activity in the bowel (Truyen et al. 2009) should only be done if vomiting is severe, and only until it can be controlled with parenterally administered medications. Otherwise, enteral feeding should be provided as long as possible or restarted as soon as possible. A highly digestible diet is preferred, but any food that is safe for cats, such as plain meat baby food (with no added onion or garlic that can cause anemia), is better than nothing at all. It may be necessary to start by offering water in small amounts for the first day, followed by a pureed bland diet once vomiting is controlled. If this is tolerated, the normal diet can be gradually introduced.

If vomiting, diarrhea, or anorexia persists despite the use of antiemetics, or if the patient is hypoproteinemic, parenteral nutrition should be initiated, preferably via a central catheter in a jugular or saphenous vein (Marks 2016). This may be beyond the scope of some shelters with limited resources. An esophageal feeding tube may be used in anorectic patients who are no longer vomiting, initially feeding small portions throughout the day, and increased as the cat tolerates it. Appetite stimulants such as mirtazapine ointment [Mirataz® (Kindred Bio) 2 mg TD every 24 hours] or tablet 1.88 mg/cat PO every 12–24 hours to 3.5 mg/cat PO every 72 hours or cyproheptadine 1–4 mg/cat PO every 12–24 hours (Agnew and Korman 2014) may be administered if necessary, only after gastroenteric signs have abated. Mirtazapine and cyproheptadine should not be used concurrently as they may counteract each other, negating the effect of both drugs (Agnew and Korman 2014).

Vitamin supplementation – particularly B-complex administered parenterally – is important to replace losses from diuresis and decreased intake due to inappetence that can lead to thiamine deficiency (Greene and Addie 2006).

The use of nutritional supplements such as Nutri-Cal® or Felovite® once the cat is eating will not hurt, but they do not provide the amount of vitamin B that the cat needs while not eating or only eating small amounts. At this time, intestinal absorption is not yet 100%, so even less will be available to the body. Once the cat is eating normally and on a well-balanced diet, there should be no need for such supplementation.

15.6.7 Pain Management

Given the extent of destruction of gut endothelium, pain management with analgesics such as buprenorphine [Simbadol® (Abbott) 0.24 mg/kg SC once daily for up to three days] (Plumb 2018) should be considered in all cases showing prominent gastrointestinal signs.

15.6.8 Additional Therapeutics

Feline recombinant interferon-omega (Virbagen® Omega, Virbac) has been shown to be effective in the treatment of CPV and is known to inhibit the replication of FPV in cell culture (Martin et al. 2002). Paltrinieri et al. 2007 found that cats administered 1 MU/kg SC SID for three days at the onset of infection produced lower levels of α -1 globulins and higher mean levels of γ globulins. Cats given the same dose also produced higher γ globulin levels and anti-FPV-specific IgG when subsequently vaccinated with MLV vaccine. However, clinical signs and survival rates remained unchanged, so it may not be cost-effective for routine shelter use. Additional *in vivo* studies are needed to better determine interferon-omega's place in the therapeutic protocol for FPV.

Gastric protectants may be helpful if there is secondary esophagitis or gastrointestinal bleeding. These include H2 blockers such as famotidine (0.5–1 mg/kg orally every 12–24 hours) or ranitidine (1–2 mg/kg orally, IV, SC every 12 hours), cytoprotectants such as sucralfate (0.25–0.3 g orally every 6–8 hours), and proton pump inhibitors such as omeprazole (0.7–1 mg/kg orally every 12–24 hours) (Marks 2016).

Treatment with broad-spectrum anthelmintics (when vomiting has ceased) to eliminate concurrent parasites has also been recommended (Marks 2016).

Because parvovirus can remain viable in the environment for months under certain conditions, it is standard to recommend bathing dogs after treatment to remove any virus that may still be on their fur and act as a fomite. However, this is not typically recommended in cats because bathing will increase stress that should be kept to a minimum in these patients. That said, a cat with a dirty perineum should at least be spot-cleaned, and this should be a part of regular nursing care while the cat is too sick to clean itself. Once cats have recovered, they will groom themselves and remove the virus. Ingestion of the virus post recovery will not result in a recurrence of clinical disease.

There are additional treatment considerations for very young kittens. In cases of hypoglycemia, enteral dextrose 2.5–5% may be administered; dextrose should be given parenterally (IV) to hypoglycemic patients with severe vomiting. In the face of an outbreak, anti-FPV serum may be administered to protect exposed susceptible cats and/or colostrum-deprived kittens. Homologous antisera from cats with high titers may be administered at 2 mL per kitten SC or intraperitoneally (IP) (Marks 2016). This passive immunity will last two to four weeks, so subsequent vaccinations will have to be delayed accordingly (Marks 2016).

15.6.9 Immunity after Recovery

Cats that survive clinical or subclinical panleukopenia infection develop lifelong immunity to reinfection. Similarly, kittens that are exposed to FPV when maternally derived antibodies (MDAs) are high may develop an inapparent infection that will also provide lifelong immunity. A strong immune response can also be achieved by both inactivated and MLV vaccine administration (Truyen et al. 2009). This is discussed in more detail in the section 15.7.5 on vaccinations in this chapter.

15.6.10 Euthanasia Decisions

The decision whether to treat or euthanize patients with FPV in a shelter often differs from the decision-making process for patients in a private practice. The shelter's decision must consider the welfare of both the individual patient and population, environmental factors, and the factors discussed earlier in this chapter regarding treatment decisions. Shelter resources, patient comfort, the chance of recovery and adoption, the risk of spreading the disease, and the financial cost of treatment must all be carefully reviewed. Euthanasia should be considered if the cat's condition is poor and/or continues to deteriorate despite treatment, or if pain cannot be adequately managed to provide good quality of life.

15.7 Prevention and Control/Risk Assessment

15.7.1 Risk Assessment

Risk factors for disease are categorized according to the classic epidemiology triad:

1) Host (age, nutritional status, immunity)
2) Environment (population density, cleanliness, animal segregation)
3) Infectious agent (virulence, dose, incubation, stability) (DiGangi 2016)

Host factors are most relevant for clinical decision-making regarding the individual patient (DiGangi 2016), but facility-related factors are more important when assessing risk for transmission of infectious disease in the shelter setting (DiGangi et al. 2012).

The combination of high exposure potential, environmental and social stresses, as well as concurrent diseases commonly found in some shelters often results in severe illness among susceptible cats of any age. In order to minimize the spread of infectious disease, shelters must manage the movement of the population through the facility appropriately to minimize the animal's length of stay (LOS), practice good husbandry and sanitation, administer appropriate and timely vaccinations on intake, test for infectious disease, and reduce stress for the population. (See the Introduction in Chapter 1, Chapter 6 on Outbreak Management, Chapter 8 on Sanitation and Chapter 2 on Wellness for more information.)

15.7.1.1 Host Factors

It is important to recognize that not all exposed cats will become infected, and not all infected cats will develop clinical signs of disease. As with most parvoviruses, healthy adult cats may develop subclinical or mild infections (Gillespie and Scott 1973; Pollock and Postorino 1994). Some host factors that increase risk include young age, stress, poor nutritional status, presence of concurrent disease, and immune status (e.g. lack of vaccination or MDAs). These factors can be determined by physical examination and measurement of antibody titers.

Though the lowest risk of disease is in properly vaccinated adult cats, severe disease may develop in any susceptible animal regardless of age or vaccination status. An incomplete vaccination history is associated with an increased risk of disease. The immunity of some outdoor cats may be naturally boosted by field exposure, while kittens have the highest risk of disease – particularly those who did not have an adequate intake of colostrum or whose maternal antibodies have waned to levels insufficient to protect from infection, but that may still interfere with active immunization. Thus, kittens six to eight weeks of age are considered at greatest risk of developing disease, but the window of susceptibility may routinely extend to 18–20 weeks of age. When the disease is seen in vaccinated cats, they usually did not receive a booster after 12 weeks of age (Sykes 2014).

The risk due to the cat's immune status can be reduced if all cats are vaccinated prior to or immediately upon intake to the shelter. Risk is low in cats over four months old that have been vaccinated with a modified live virus (MLV) FVRCP (feline viral rhinotracheitis, calici, and panleukopenia) vaccine subcutaneously at least one week prior to exposure, and in those with a history of having been vaccinated at or after 18–20 weeks of age and at least two weeks or within three years prior to exposure. (UC Davis 2016). Risk is greater in cats vaccinated less than one week before exposure or those given killed or intranasal (IN) vaccines, and greatest in closely exposed unvaccinated cats (UC Davis 2016). All ages are at risk if unprotected by vaccines. See Table 15.3 for a summary of risk factors.

Table 15.3 Summary of host risk factors (UC Davis 2016).

Risk is very low in cats four months and older that are either

- vaccinated with an MLV SC FVRCP vaccine at least one week prior to exposure
- have a documented history of vaccination at or after 18–20 weeks of age at least 2 weeks and within 3 years prior to exposure.

Risk is greater in

- kittens under four months old even if vaccinated (due to maternal antibody interference)
- cats vaccinated less than a week before exposure
- cats vaccinated with a killed or intranasal vaccine

Risk is greatest in

- closely exposed, unvaccinated cats

All ages should be considered at risk if unprotected by vaccines

Providing passive protection via the administration of hyperimmune serum to kittens and cats deemed to be high risk can substantially reduce risk, but this may not be possible until cats are 20 weeks of age or older. This is discussed in more detail in the section on passive immunity. Administration of feline recombinant interferon-omega (Virbagen® Omega, Virbac) to pregnant queens and neonatal kittens prior to introduction to a potentially contaminated or shelter environment may also enhance antibody production and lower risk of infection (Paltrinieri et al. 2007).

15.7.1.2 Environmental Factors

Environmental factors that affect the risk of infection include population density and the rate of population turnover, number of cats admitted, cleanliness of the environment, availability of isolation wards and biosecurity protocols, and proximity between exposed and infected animals (DiGangi et al. 2012; UC Davis 2016).

Outbreaks tend to be seasonal, coinciding with increases in the number of susceptible kittens. They occur most frequently in multi-cat environments – in catteries and particularly in shelters – where cats are frequently forced to live in unnaturally dense populations, often with high turnover rates, resulting in greater exposure to larger doses of pathogens at a time when the immune system is likely compromised due to the stress of overcrowding and changing hierarchy status (Scherk et al. 2013; Addie et al. 2015). Devastating outbreaks have resulted in the deaths of thousands of cats (Litster and Benjanirut 2013; Sykes 2014); in the case of shelters, this may be due both to the disease itself and/or to management decisions to utilize euthanasia to prevent further disease spread and suffering.

Fortunately, the risk in shelters today can be greatly reduced using sound shelter medicine protocols and population management strategies. Rapid recognition and efficient management of cats at risk is most important. Careful observation and examination of each cat for evidence of illness on arrival and via daily rounds (wherein cats and their enclosures are checked visually during a walk through the facility) are imperative. During an outbreak, all cats should be checked at least twice daily, especially before cage cleaning to prevent spread during the cleaning process (Tuzio 2009; UC Davis 2016). All staff and volunteers should be trained to recognize the signs of FPV and have written instructions regarding the protocol to follow when a potential case is identified (i.e. whom to contact, which tests to perform, what to do with sick or potentially exposed cats). Protocols should be established and staff instructed in proper cleaning and disinfection of cages and all potentially contaminated areas (Litster and Benjanirut 2013).

Because susceptible cats can still become infected even after thorough disinfection of the environment, only fully and properly vaccinated animals should enter an area that may be contaminated with parvovirus (Truyen et al. 2009). Minimally, shelters should be compartmentalized to provide separate areas for healthy adult cats, healthy kittens, new arrivals, a separate ward for pregnant and lactating queens and their kittens, and isolation wards for sick or potentially infectious cats. It should also be able to provide appropriate quarantine areas when needed. Finally, population management plans that reduce the LOS of cats should be prioritized to reduce the incidence of disease in the shelter. See the Introduction in Chapter 1 and Chapter 6 on outbreak management for more information.

15.7.1.3 Infectious Agent Factors

The virulence of the individual strain of the virus, the challenge dose to which the cats are exposed, the particular strain's incubation period and its stability in the environment are all factors that determine the risk for disease (DiGangi 2016).

15.7.2 Quarantine Recommendations

Quarantine of apparently healthy cats is not generally recommended in shelter settings. Unlike other feline population settings such as laboratories and catteries, most shelters have a constant influx of new arrivals and do not have sufficient space or staff to conduct an effective all-in, all-out quarantine. Equally important, quarantines contribute to an increased LOS for the animal, which is a known high-risk factor for increased illness in animal shelters (Edinboro et al. 2004; Dinnage et al. 2009). An increased LOS contributes to crowding, increased stress, potentially suboptimal housing, less staff time for proper care and thus an increased risk of disease exposure and transmission. However, for recently exposed cats, a risk assessment should be performed, and quarantine implemented if indicated.

Vaccination for panleukopenia has the potential to provide cats with rapid and complete protection. Therefore, not all exposed cats will become infected. Cats over five months of age and vaccinated at least five to seven days prior to exposure are at low risk for infection and do not require quarantine. For recently vaccinated cats and for kittens under five months of age, antibody titer testing can be a helpful adjunct to risk assessment. If all cats in a room are exposed and considered at risk, it may be best to close that room to new admissions for a quarantine period. If exposed or at-risk cats are scattered throughout the shelter, they should be brought together in a separate room in a segregated area of the shelter that is easily disinfected and where they can be closely monitored individually. If cats cannot be quarantined in a separate place within the shelter, it may be necessary to stop admitting new cats for the quarantine period or to set up an off-site quarantine facility (UC Davis 2016).

A quarantine of 14 days should be sufficient in the absence of clinical signs or re-exposure to infected cats (DiGangi 2016; UC Davis 2016). If re-exposure occurs, a risk assessment should be repeated, and quarantine restarted unless vaccine protection has been established.

Please see Table 15.4 for basic quarantine recommendations and Chapter 6 on outbreak management for more detailed information.

15.7.3 Isolation Recommendations

The first step in the management of a disease outbreak in a shelter setting is to identify and remove all cats with active disease from the general population. Cats showing any sign of infectious disease should be transferred immediately to an isolation area for evaluation. Those identified with panleukopenia via diagnostic testing, such as a positive fecal FPV antigen test, should be removed from the population immediately and placed in isolation (Abd-Eldaim et al. 2009; Litster and Benjanirut 2013). As previously discussed, treatment and euthanasia decisions should be

Table 15.4 Summary of basic quarantine recommendations.

- Cats who have been meaningfully exposed or determined to be at high risk should be quarantined.
- Cats with signs of infectious disease should be removed from quarantine as soon as possible and placed in an appropriate isolation area for evaluation.
- Kittens should be quarantined only with the queen and their littermates, and not have contact with any other adult cats or kittens.
- Asymptomatic, exposed cats should be titer tested for risk assessment. Cats with inadequate antibody titers should be considered high risk and prioritized for observation.
- Quarantines should be conducted in a segregated area of the shelter. Handling should be minimized to reduce stress, but include socialization, behavioral care, and environmental enrichment.
- Staff should be trained in disease recognition and biosecurity measures and provided with written guidelines and appropriate personal protective equipment (PPE).
- Sanitation supplies should be restricted for use in the quarantine area only and not moved around to other areas of the shelter.
- Footbath use should generally be avoided – shoe covers are preferred.
- Quarantine areas should be made of durable materials that are easily cleaned and disinfected. The use of materials such as carpet, wood, or soil that cannot be effectively disinfected should be avoided.
- If staff clean more than one area, they should clean quarantine areas after cleaning areas with healthy animals, but before cleaning isolation rooms with sick animals.
- Cats and dogs should not be quarantined in the same room.

based on the cat's condition, the ability of the shelter to provide appropriate treatment, the risk to the general population and availability of other treatment options (e.g. transfer to a private hospital).

Isolation areas must be strictly separated from areas for other animals and away from the quarantine area. Ideally, animals in isolation should be located in a separate building or placed off-site in foster care or at a veterinary facility for treatment. Because CPV has been detected in cats and FPV can infect dogs, these two species should not be quarantined or isolated in the same unit.

Cats that are clinically ill should be kept in isolation for a minimum of one week since viral shedding is usually five to seven days. Though cats may potentially shed the virus for six weeks, a six-week isolation period is not feasible or practical in most shelters. Fecal antigen tests in combination with antibody titers can be employed to determine if the shedding has stopped, the cat has mounted an immune response and it is safe to return to the general population. If the cat is clinically normal but still shedding virus, it can be placed in an appropriate foster home or separate area that is not housing any susceptible cats. (Foster caregivers must be advised of the longevity and hardiness of FPV in the environment and the importance of proper disinfection of their premises to prevent its spread to other cats.) Recovered cats should not be kept in the isolation area with clinically ill cats still receiving treatment.

15.7.4 Role of Titer Testing

Antibody titers can be used to determine the level and duration of immunity following vaccination, passive transfer, or recovery from natural infection. Routine testing for FPV of all incoming cats in the absence of clinical signs is not recommended. During an outbreak, however, serology (titers) can be used to make evidence-based management decisions to minimize disease impact. The identification of asymptomatic cats having a high antibody titer and low risk of infection will prevent unnecessary quarantine or euthanasia of animals eligible for adoption (DiGangi 2011; UC Davis 2016). Seronegative cats, on the other hand, are at increased risk for infection and should be quarantined (Lappin et al. 2002a; DiGangi 2016). If identified and quarantined early in the outbreak, it could greatly reduce the risk of transmission to other high-risk individuals.

When measuring titers to determine susceptibility to disease, the numerical value considered protective varies with the lab and/or method of measurement. There is no universal standard for protective titers (DiGangi et al. 2012), except for passively acquired antibodies from the queen or from hyperimmune serum that are protective at HI titers of 80 or higher (Mostl 2015). In cats over 20 weeks of age, the very presence of serum antibody – regardless of titer and whether acquired by immunization or infection – has been correlated with protection against feline panleukopenia (Lappin et al. 2002a), while all kittens under five months of age should be considered at high risk regardless of antibody titer due to waning maternal antibodies (DiGangi 2016).

In some shelter settings, particularly in the face of an outbreak, reference lab titer detection may be impractical due to financial and/or time constraints. (It should be borne in mind, however, that titer testing is often less costly than quarantines that increase the LOS of animals and their risk of infection, in addition to increasing the shelter's labor and resource costs.) Here especially, commercially available, rapid, point-of-care assays for the measurement of serum or plasma antibody titer are crucial for disease management. However, there has been variability in the accuracy of these kits with regard to the detection of FPV antibodies (DiGangi et al. 2011; Mende et al. 2014). Kits designed for the detection of CPV are largely unable to detect antibodies against FPV in cats and should not be used for this purpose (DiGangi et al. 2011; DiGangi 2016). One enzyme-linked immunosorbent assay for dogs (ELISA: *TiterCHEK CDV/CPV*, Synbiotics, San Diego, CA) has been successfully used to evaluate protective antibody titers (PAT) in cats (Day et al. 2016). However, according to one study (DiGangi 2011), it lacks sensitivity for FPV. A more recent feline specific point-of-care ELISA test (*ImmunoComb Feline VacciCheck*, Biogal Galed Laboratories; available in the US as *Feline VacciCheck®*, Nextmune.) is available to determine the level of PAT against FPV, as well as FHV and FCV. After the initial study showed this also lacked sensitivity for FPV, the manufacturer modified the test and recent studies have validated it against the "gold standard" of HI and determined a specificity of 81–89% and sensitivity of 78–87% for FPV antibody, making it suitable for use in practice and shelters (DiGangi 2011; Mende et al. 2014).

15.7.5 Vaccination

Three international panels have produced feline vaccination guidelines (American Association of Feline Practitioners, European Advisory Board on Cat Diseases, World Small Animal Veterinary Association). The recommendations made by these organizations for vaccinating cats in shelters vary from those for individual cats in private practice settings because of the different set of circumstances (heightened stress, increased exposure, unknown vaccination history, etc.) they face. However, without exception, FPV is the most important vaccine a cat receives. Timely vaccination before or upon intake is among the most important factors in preventing panleukopenia in sheltered cats. Ideally, all cats should be protected against FPV at all times, whether by immunity from infection resulting from previous natural infection, vaccination, or passive transfer of maternal antibodies in young kittens. Successful vaccination against FPV results in antibody levels that produce a sterilizing immunity (DiGangi 2016) and prevent viral infection of the host. Acquired immunity is solid and long-lasting whether induced by infection or by inactivated or MLV vaccine. Immunity after recovery from the natural infection is lifelong (Kennedy and Little 2012). Several studies have suggested that immunity following successful vaccination may be at least seven years after the final inoculation (Scott and Geissinger 1999; Lappin et al. 2002b).

15.7.5.1 FPV Vaccine Types

FPV vaccines may be inactivated (killed) or attenuated (modified live) and are usually delivered in trivalent combination products also containing the feline respiratory viruses (i.e. feline viral rhinotracheitis, calicivirus, and panleukopenia – FVRCP). Both inactivated and modified live vaccines produce long-standing immunity. Nevertheless, with few exceptions, MLV vaccines are the standard of care in the shelter setting – mainly because they induce a more rapid immune response and are better able to override MDA than inactivated vaccines.

Parenteral MLV vaccines can provide protection within 72 hours, with full immunity by 5–7 days with one dose in animals over 4 months of age (Brun et al. 1979). Inactivated vaccines generally require two weeks and often a second administration (usually two to four weeks after the first) to be effective, and they are more likely to be blocked by low levels of maternal antibodies (Lappin 2012; DiGangi 2016). This makes them inappropriate for routine use in a shelter setting.

In a shelter where many entering cats may be at high risk and disease exposure is likely to occur early in the course of their stay, vaccination on intake is critical. The faster induction of immunity following MLV administration may protect these cats against illness even if placed in a contaminated environment shortly after vaccination (Scherk et al. 2013; DiGangi 2016).

However, MLV should not be given to kittens under four weeks of age (to avoid the risk of developing cerebellar hypoplasia or clinical panleukopenia), nor to severely immunosuppressed individuals to avoid possible induction of clinical signs. Most recommendations also include avoiding the use of vaccinations – particularly MLV – in pregnant queens due to the risk of transfer of virus to the fetus; however, in some cases, the risk of dying from infection may outweigh the risk of adverse vaccination reactions (Kennedy and Little 2012). Inactivated vaccines should be used in these cases, but the decision to do so must be made in light of the delayed onset of immunity. These particularly vulnerable animals should be protected from disease exposure and their LOS in the shelter minimized, but ideally, especially in shelters where the risk of exposure is known to be high, it is preferable to place them off-site with volunteers or in foster care.

Modified live vaccines for FPV are commercially available for either parenteral or intranasal (IN) administration. The intranasal products produce an immune response against FPV that is comparable to MLV and superior to inactivated parenteral vaccines, but they may not produce a sterilizing immunity quickly enough to provide protection in a high-risk shelter environment (Lappin et al. 2009). Thus, the use of intranasal products in the shelter setting should be limited to providing protection against upper respiratory disease (i.e. feline rhinotracheitis and calicivirus); if a trivalent FVRCP intranasal vaccine is used, it warrants the addition of parenteral MLV FPV vaccine to the protocol (DiGangi 2016).

15.7.5.2 Vaccination Guidelines

If the population is susceptible, the incidence of FPV may be nearly 100%. Therefore, every cat should be vaccinated against FPV. Vaccinating all cats strengthens the immunity of the entire local feline population by producing a type of "herd immunity." Though recent US studies (Fischer et al. 2007; DiGangi et al. 2012) reported seropositivity for FPV in cats entering shelters at 60% and 33% respectively, vaccines can boost immunity and provide much needed protection (Day et al. 2016).

All new shelter arrivals should be assumed to be unvaccinated unless they are accompanied by unambiguous, *written* documentation of having been appropriately vaccinated. It should **not** be assumed that adult cats in shelters (particularly those with an undocumented history of vaccination) are protected from FPV (Litster and Benjanirut 2013). Signs of previous medical care should not be used to determine if a cat needs vaccination at the time of admission to the shelter (DiGangi et al. 2012). Also, in a population setting such as a shelter where the risk of exposure may be high, unknown retroviral status should not be considered a risk or contraindication to vaccination.

Current recommendations for vaccination of sheltered cats against FPV include use of a trivalent FVRCP vaccine administered as follows (Stone et al. 2020):

- All healthy kittens over 4–6 weeks of age (4 weeks in high- risk environments or during an outbreak) should be vaccinated with FVRCP MLV SC at or before admission to the shelter, then revaccinated every two weeks

Table 15.5 Which vaccine to use?

Modified Live Virus (MLV)	**Inactivated or Killed Virus (KV)**
All healthy cats and kittens > 4–6 weeks old	Acutely ill cats if absolutely necessary
Ill cats that are stable	Cats that are FeLV positive
Injured animals	FIV positive cats at high risk of exposure
Cats scheduled for euthanasia	Pregnant queens in a low-risk shelter
Pregnant queens in a high-risk shelter	Severely immune-compromised cats

until 16–20 weeks of age. Kittens whose queens have known high antibody titers (i.e. after recovering from the disease or living in a high-exposure environment, or from being vaccinated just before or during pregnancy) should be vaccinated until 20 weeks of age (Truyen et al. 2009; Day et al. 2016). They should be revaccinated 12 months after the primary vaccine course, then at three-year intervals.

- Cats over 5 months of age that are naïve or with an unknown vaccination history should be given one FVRCP MLV SC at or before admission to the shelter. They should be given a second dose two weeks later. This includes cats that are injured as well as those that are chronically ill but stable. They should be revaccinated 12 months after the primary vaccine course, then at three-year intervals.
- Acutely/severely ill and immunocompromised cats and kittens should not be vaccinated unless absolutely necessary, and then with an inactivated product. The administration of corticosteroids to immunocompromised animals should be avoided at the time of vaccination because they may hamper the cell-mediated immune response. It should be noted, however, that if the cat's immune system is so weakened that a modified live vaccine could induce disease, exposure to the wide variety of infectious pathogens often present in most shelters could very likely be fatal (Scherk et al. 2013, Stone et al. 2020). It would be best to transfer these animals out of the shelter if possible. Animals not vaccinated at admission should be administered MLV FRCPV vaccine as soon as they are sufficiently healthy or stable.
- Cats that are positive for FeLV antigen should be vaccinated against FPV using inactivated products, even though there is no evidence that they are at increased risk of vaccine-induced disease when given MLV products (Mostl 2015). The theoretical risk of deleterious effects resulting from vaccinating with MLV must be balanced against the risk of possible FPV infection. These cats should also be housed in low-stress areas with a low risk of disease exposure. Consideration should be given to vaccinating these cats more frequently since their immune response to each vaccination may not be sufficient to provide full protection.
- FIV-seropositive cats should be vaccinated (Little et al. 2020; Stone et al. 2020). Inactivated vaccines are recommended because one study of MLV administration to FIV-positive cats resulted in vaccine-induced panleukopenia (Buonavoglia et al. 1993), and other studies have suggested that the immunostimulation produced by the vaccine may induce a progression of the FIV infection (Lehmann et al. 1992; Reubel et al. 1994).
- Ideally, pregnant cats expected to carry to term should not be vaccinated with MLV. Pregnant queens should be vaccinated using an inactivated vaccine if housed in a low-risk shelter. In a high-risk environment, it would be preferable to transfer the animal to foster care or to administer passive immunization with hyperimmune FPV serum or anti-CPV-2 canine globulin (Mostl et al. 2013). However, the risk to the queen and the shelter population as a whole, as well as the likely outcome of the pregnancy must be taken into consideration when determining which products to use (DiGangi 2016; UC Davis 2016). The effort to protect the fetuses from the potential adverse effect of MLV vaccination could lead to a deadlier outcome by leaving them vulnerable to FPV.
- Cats scheduled for euthanasia should be vaccinated on intake with MLV FVRCP SC to protect the population from the development of endemic FPV transmission and to reduce the risk of widespread FPV outbreaks (Scherk et al. 2013).

15.7.5.3 Vaccine Efficacy, Side Effects and Safety

Vaccines against FPV are highly effective. If administered correctly to a cat capable of mounting an adequate response, they will induce strong protective immunity. Adult cats receiving the parenteral MLV have an initial immune response almost immediately and can develop immunity in three days (Brun et al. 1979; Schultz 2009), though cats are not considered fully immune until five to seven days post-vaccination. The modified-live components provide complete protection from virulent FPV for at least three years following the second vaccination (Gore et al. 2006). FPV vaccines may even offer protection from the CPV variants (Chalmers 1999; Nakamura et al. 2001). However, no vaccine is 100% effective, so exposure to contaminated areas and infected patients should still be avoided, even for cats that are properly vaccinated.

Vaccine failures have occurred, generally due to immunodeficiencies (genetic, acquired, drug-induced), malnutrition, chronic stress, or concurrent disease. Ideally, in a private practice setting these problems would be corrected before vaccination, but this is unrealistic for most shelters unless foster care or off-site housing is available. In kittens, apparent vaccine failure occurs most commonly when the vaccination course is stopped too early – i.e. while MDAs are still present in sufficient quantity to interfere with the kitten's own immunologic response to the vaccine. If a kitten nurses well, its serum antibody level will likely approach 50% of the queen's. This level gradually decreases in the first few weeks of life (the biological half-life of MDA is approximately 10 days), eventually producing an "immunity gap" (Truyen et al. 2009). At this time, the antibody level is too low to protect from infection but high enough to interfere with an active immune response to vaccination. This gap occurs most frequently between 8 and 12 weeks of age, but studies have demonstrated significant maternal antibody titers even at 12 weeks of age, and some kittens have been reported to have detectable levels at 20 weeks of age. Based on clinical studies, vaccination protocols that end at 16 weeks of age still leave 1/3 of cats unprotected against FPV (Jakel et al. 2012).

Most commercially available vaccines today have an excellent safety record, with the risk of adverse reaction reported to be 0.30–0.52% (Moore et al. 2007; Day et al. 2016). The largest study to date found that most reactions occur in the few days immediately following parenteral vaccination and include lethargy, anorexia, fever and local inflammation at the injection site (Moore et al. 2007). Occasionally, vomiting, facial edema and pruritus have occurred. Rare anaphylaxis (0.01–0.05%) has been observed and exhibited as vomiting, facial edema, generalized pruritus, and respiratory distress. Death occurred in 4/10 000 cats (Moore et al. 2007). The risk of adverse events reported was highest in one-year-old cats and increased with the number of other vaccines administered at the same time.

Feline injection-site sarcomas (FISS) have been identified as a possible rare (<1/10 000) sequella to vaccination as well as other types of injections (Gobar and Kass 2002). Though many factors relative to the specific injection as well as the cat may be involved in FISS formation, one study (Srivastav et al. 2012) found that the occurrence is greater following the use of adjuvanted, inactivated vaccines. Injection site sarcomas frequently recur following surgical removal of the tumors and carry a guarded prognosis, but the risk is outweighed by the benefit of immunity (Mende et al. 2014; Day et al. 2016).

15.7.5.4 Role of Vaccination and Passive Immunity in a Shelter Outbreak

DiGangi's (2016) "Evidence-Based Outbreak Response" to infectious disease in an animal shelter incorporates six core principles: diagnosis and isolation of diseased animals, identification and isolation of ill residents, environmental decontamination, protection of those animals newly admitted, clear documentation, and clear communication with everyone involved (employees, adopters, etc.).

During an outbreak, unvaccinated cats should be kept in an area that is completely separated from exposed and at-risk cats or housed off-site if possible. Susceptible animals should not have contact with each other until they have been properly immunized.

Crucial to the management of at-risk and newly admitted animals is proper and timely vaccination as discussed previously. Shelters that vaccinate against FPV using typical private practice protocols, (i.e. starting at age 6 weeks or older, revaccinating at 3–4 week intervals, and administering the final vaccine at 16–20 weeks of age) must use a shelter vaccination protocol to more effectively control the spread of disease.

In the face of an outbreak:

- Kittens that cannot be housed off-site should be vaccinated with a MLV FVRCP starting at four weeks of age (Greene and Schultz 2006). Booster vaccinations should be administered every 2 weeks and continued until the cats are 20 weeks of age or older (DiGangi 2016). MLV parenteral and intranasal vaccines should not be administered to kittens under four weeks of age.
- All adult cats that have been exposed should be vaccinated with a MLV FRCPV vaccine if they have not received one within the previous 14 days (DiGangi 2016). The administration of MLV causes a viral shedding that helps produce a "herd immunity" in multi-cat environments (Litster and Benjanirut 2013).
- Passive immunization may be considered to protect young kittens with an incomplete vaccination history.

Passive immunization is a means of providing immediate protection to animals that are unvaccinated and cannot avoid entering a high-risk area. Its success depends on the antibody titer of the preparation, volume administered, and the timing of administration with respect to exposure. Hyperimmune serum may be prepared from healthy individuals that have been repeatedly vaccinated. Donors should be blood typed and screened for other diseases (e.g. retroviruses, *Bartonella*, etc.). Ideally, cats should be cross-matched, or only type A donors should be used. The minimum amount required for protection is unknown, but the recommended dose is 2 ml SC or intraperitoneally (IP) per kitten (UC Davis 2016), or 2–4 ml/kg body weight SC or IP per cat (Scott 1987). Serum can be stored in single-dose aliquots at −20 °C (−4 °F) for up to one year if frozen immediately after collection. For an immediate effect, IV administration of citrated plasma (3–10 ml BID depending on the size of the animal) may be used for up to three days (Day et al. 2016).

If anti-FPV serum is not available, hyperimmune serum against CPV may be administered. Protection lasts for two to four weeks (Greene and Addie 2006).

The vaccination of individuals provided with passive immunity should be delayed by three to four weeks to avoid viral neutralization, and vaccinations should continue for two to four weeks longer than usual.

Kittens under one day of age may receive passive immunization by feeding artificial colostrum composed of a 1 : 1 mixture of kitten milk replacer and immune serum from a well-immunized adult cat from the same community (Day et al. 2016). Maximum absorption is at eight hours after birth, then the gut epithelium gradually loses the ability to absorb. If the kitten feeds well, its antibody level will likely approach 50% of the queen's or the donor's level (Truyen et al. 2009).

15.7.6 Environmental Control-Sanitation

One of the most important aspects of FPV control is effective sanitation, which requires thorough cleaning and appropriate disinfection of the facility and all surfaces and equipment that have contact with animals. Of all the viruses that impact shelters, parvovirus is the most difficult to eradicate. If parvovirus is successfully eradicated, most other viruses will be as well (Addie et al. 2015). FPV is environmentally resilient and susceptible to inactivation by only a limited number of disinfectants. It can survive for many years frozen or dried and may persist for over a year in the environment on surfaces and objects such as food and water bowls, litter pans, cage doors and walls, gloves, toys, medical equipment, sponges, etc. with no change in infectivity (Pedersen 1988). Hands and clothing can also serve as fomites. Thus, indirect transmission via fomites is a major concern, particularly in a shelter setting where large numbers of animals are constantly in residence and there is a high turnover rate. (See Chapter 8 for more detailed information about sanitation.)

Proper sanitation requires both cleaning to reduce the number of pathogens on a surface (thereby reducing the potential infective dose and minimizing the risk of infection), and disinfection to inactivate any remaining pathogens. It does not leave the surface sterile, nor completely eliminate the possibility of infection. Chemical disinfection is the most widely used form of disinfection in shelters because it can be applied to most objects found in the facility. (Heat and UV radiation can also be very effective but are considered impractical for use in most shelters.)

The first step in the cleaning process involves the physical removal of all dirt and debris (feces, uneaten kibble, litter, newspaper, etc.) that can serve as contaminants and inactivate disinfectants, followed by thorough scrubbing of all surfaces with a good detergent. The second step is the application of an appropriate disinfectant, allowing for the minimal contact time (usually 10 minutes) and rinsing as recommended by the manufacturer, and drying the surface. Only commercially prepared products that are independently tested for efficacy against non-enveloped viruses should be used. It is important to follow the manufacturer's recommendations for preparation, storage, application and disposal, especially regarding preparation and contact time. The choice of the disinfectant to use must be based primarily on efficacy, but effects on people and toxicity to cats (especially with constant and long-term exposure) must also be considered, with particular consideration given to the fact that cats spend up to 25% of their waking time licking and grooming themselves. Therefore, disinfectants must be safe if ingested or transdermally absorbed, and non-caustic to footpads, tongue tips or esophagus. Also, cats have an innate deficiency of UDP-glucuronyl transferase, thus making phenol-based products such as tea tree and clove oils particularly toxic.

FPV can be inactivated by chlorine compounds such as sodium hypochlorite (household bleach), monopersulfate (potassium peroxymonosulfate) and accelerated hydrogen peroxide. It is resistant to many common disinfectants such as iodophors, quaternary ammonium compounds, alcohol, iodines, and phenols. Other products such as peracetic acid, aldehydes (formaldehyde), or sodium hydroxide will inactivate parvovirus but are not recommended for use in shelters.

When sanitizing isolation and quarantine areas, "spot cleaning" that minimizes stress and handling cats is recommended. Cats should remain in their cages while the cage is tidied and cleaned and litter boxes emptied, but cages must be thoroughly disinfected before another cat is brought in.

See Table 15.6 for a summary of sanitation recommendations and Chapter 8 for more detailed information.

15.7.7 Housing

In order to maintain and promote good physical and behavioral health, housing and animal care should be provided in a manner that reduces stress. This is especially important when caring for animals that are ill. It is important to try to assess the behavior of the cats to accommodate their individual needs and provide them with sufficient space, comfortable, easily disinfected beds and extra bedding, perches, and hiding places, and environmental enrichment. Double-sided housing that separates feeding and resting areas from the litter box, provides a hiding place and perch, and minimizes the need for animal handling during cleaning is ideal. Noise should be kept to a minimum, and environmental temperature should be maintained between 15.5 and 26.6° C (59.9–80° F) (AVMA n.d.). Facial pheromone products may be used to help reduce the feline stress response, though there is insufficient data to determine their efficacy. (See Chapter 2 on Wellness for more information.)

Table 15.6 Sanitation recommendations.

Everything that comes in contact with animals or that can act as a fomite should be discarded or sanitized, including the cage or enclosure, litter boxes, toys, food, and water bowls, transport cages, etc.
Food and water bowls should be cleaned thoroughly each day and returned to the same cat, with complete disinfection occurring before use by another animal.
Each cat should be assigned its own cage and carrier for the duration of its stay.
In these cases, daily spot cleaning is recommended rather than complete disinfection to minimize handling, stress and disease transmission.
Cats may remain in their cages during spot cleaning, but they should be removed whenever a disinfectant is applied.
Cats should never get wet during the cleaning process. If a cage is disinfected, the cat should be removed and returned only after the cage is completely dry.
Shoe covers should be available at the entrance to each area housing animals. Footbaths are not effective and therefore not recommended.
The use of disposable litter boxes and non- tracking litter is recommended.
Bedding and other porous materials that are difficult to disinfect, as well as toys and scratching posts, should be discarded or sent home with the cat.
All transport vehicles, intake areas, common areas, and high contact surfaces such as examination tables should be properly cleaned and disinfected daily or between uses, whichever occurs first.
Laundry should be sorted before washing because viruses can be transferred from contaminated items to uncontaminated ones.
Food and water dishes, litter boxes, tools, and cleaning equipment should be used in the area assigned and not moved between housing areas.
Hand washing stations should be available wherever animals are handled or housed and used by staff, visitors and volunteers. (Though helpful, hand sanitizers will not inactivate FPV and should not be relied upon for this purpose.)
Areas known to be heavily contaminated should be cleaned, then thoroughly disinfected, preferably two to three times before repopulating with cats.
Staff should utilize personal protective equipment (PPE), i.e. protective clothing such as aprons, gloves, eye goggles, and foot covers that are disposable or easily cleaned and disinfected, especially when a contaminated area is being cleaned or a suspect or high-risk animal is being handled.

15.8 Implications for Adoption and Foster Care

Caregiver education is a key factor in dealing with FPV. At the time of adoption, transfer, relocation or placement in foster care, caregivers should always be provided with the cat's complete medical history in writing, including vaccinations, deworming, treatment and any other information pertinent to the animal's health. In an outbreak, if there is a possibility that cats were adopted before the first case of panleukopenia was identified, timely notification by shelter personnel can ensure the cat is observed, receives the necessary care and is kept separate from other animals in an easily cleaned and disinfected area until it is determined to be disease-free. Caregivers should be educated about the symptoms of the disease; if they observe any signs of illness, they should be advised to contact their veterinarian and the shelter immediately and to isolate the animal to keep it from spreading the disease to other unvaccinated or at-risk animals that may be in the household. Caregivers should also be informed of the shelter's policy if the animal develops signs or becomes ill with panleukopenia (i.e. whom to call, who will pay for treatment, etc.).

Those who adopt or provide foster care for an animal that later becomes ill with panleukopenia should be provided with complete written instructions on how to clean and disinfect their home. Ideally, they should not bring a new unvaccinated kitten or cat into the home for at least a year since the virus can persist on furniture, carpets and other objects that may be difficult or impossible to disinfect. An adult cat (over five months of age) that has been fully vaccinated may be safely brought into the home. A consultation with the shelter or their local veterinarian may help provide ideas to prepare the home for a new pet.

It is important to stress the ubiquitous nature of FPV so caregivers can understand that even strictly indoor cats may be at risk and should be vaccinated according to current recommendations for pet cats. In fact, indoor-only cats may be *more* susceptible to disease because their immune system is not stimulated by the constant exposure experienced by outdoor cats. Therefore, it is generally recommended that cats living strictly indoors be revaccinated for FPV one year after the initial series and then every three years thereafter. However, individual cats should have their risk assessed by a veterinarian every year and the vaccination protocol adjusted accordingly.

15.9 Conclusion

Feline panleukopenia virus is a highly pathogenic, highly resistant organism that poses a particular challenge in multi-cat environments such as an animal shelter. However, a proactive approach toward prevention, rapid identification and isolation, proper and timely treatment, and staff and client education, can greatly reduce this ubiquitous threat. See Table 15.7 for an overview of the characteristics of the virus and disease.

Table 15.7 Overview of characteristics of feline panleukopenia.

Agent	Feline parvovirus (FPV)
Susceptible Species	All Felidae
Prevalence	Worldwide; particularly shelters and multi-cat households
Morbidity/Mortality	Highest frequency in kittens 6–20 weeks of age; Seasonal increase in incidence; 50% of susceptible cats <1 year of age die
Transmission	Primarily fecal-oral, by direct contact or via fomites; less so via inhalation of droplets or transplacentally
Incubation period	2–14 days
Diagnosis	Profound leukopenia; positive FPV fecal antigen test, segmental enteritis with intestinal crypt necrosis and villus blunting on histopathology
Main Differential Diagnoses	*Salmonella* sp., *C. perfringens, Campylobacter*
Treatment	See text and Table 15.2
Prognosis	Dependent on the form of disease and speed of recognition and treatment. Can vary from sudden death to complete recovery with life-long immunity
Prevention/Control	Vaccination of all cats on intake Proper husbandry/stress reduction Proper quarantine and isolation procedures Titer testing Appropriate sanitation Employee education and hygiene Population control (avoid crowding and minimize the length of stay) Client education

References

Abd-Eldaim, M., Beall, M.J., and Kennedy, M.A. (2009). Detection of feline panleukopenia virus using a commercial ELISA for canine parvovirus. *Veterinary Therapeutics: Research in Applied Veterinary Medicine* 10: E1–E6.

Addie, D.D., Toth, S., Thompson, H. et al. (1998). Detection of feline parvovirus in dying pedigree kittens. *Veterinary Record* 142: 353–356.

Addie, D.D., Boucraut-Baralon, C., Egberink, H. et al. (2015). Disinfectant choices in veterinary practices, shelters and households. *Journal of Feline Medicine and Surgery* 17 (7): 594–605. https://doi.org/10.1177/1098612x15588450.

Agnew, W. and Korman, R. (2014). Pharmacological appetite stimulation: rational choices in the inappetent cat. *Journal of Feline Medicine and Surgery* 16: 749–756.

Allison, A.B., Kohler, D.J., Fox, K.A. et al. (2013). Frequent cross-species transmission of parvoviruses among diverse carnivore hosts. *Journal of Virology* 87: 2342–2347.

American Veterinary Medical Association (2020). Companion animal care guidelines https://www.avma.org/resources-tools/avma-policies/companion-animal-care-guidelines (accessed 15 June 2020).

Brun, A., Chappuis, G., Precausta, P. et al. (1979). Immunisation against panleucopenia: early development of immunity. *Comparative Immunology, Microbiology and Infectious Diseases* 1 (4): 335–339.

Buonavoglia, C., Marsilio, F., Tempesta, M. et al. (1993). Use of a feline panleukopenia modified live virus vaccine in cats in the primary stage of feline immunodeficiency virus infection. *Journal of Veterinary Medicine, Series B* 40 (1–10): 343–346.

Day, M.J., Horzinek, M.C., Schultz, R.D. et al. (2016). WSAVA guidelines for the vaccination of dogs and cats. *Journal of Small Animal Practice* 57 (1): E1–E45. https://onlinelibrary.wiley.com/doi/full/10.1111/jsap.2_12431 (Accessed June 15, 2020).

DiGangi, B.A. (2011). An evidence-based approach to the control of feline panleukopenia, feline herpesvirus-1, and feline calicivirus in shelter cats. Master of Science thesis, University of Florida.

DiGangi, B.A. (2016). Strategies for infectious disease management in shelter cats. In: *August's Consultations in Feline Internal Medicine*, vol. 7 (ed. S. Little), 674–685. Cambridge, MA: Elsevier.

DiGangi, B.A., Gray, L.K., Levy, J.K. et al. (2011). Detection of protective antibody titers against feline panleukopenia virus, feline herpesvirus-1, and feline calicivirus in shelter cats using a point-of-care ELISA. *Journal of Feline Medicine and Surgery* 13 (12): 912–918. http://dx.doi.org/10.1016/j.jfms.2011.07.009. (Accessed June 15, 2020).

DiGangi, B.A., Levy, J.K., Griffin, B. et al. (2012). Prevalence of serum antibody titers against feline panleukopenia virus, feline herpesvirus 1, and feline calicivirus in cats entering a Florida animal shelter. *Journal of the American Veterinary Medical Association* 241 (10): 1320–1325. http://dx.doi.org/10.2460/javma.241.10.1320. (Accessed June 15, 2020).

Dinnage, J., Scarlett, J.M., and Richards, J.R. (2009). Descriptive epidemiology of feline upper respiratory tract disease in an animal shelter. *Journal of Feline Medicine and Surgery* 11: 816–825.

Edinboro, C.H., Ward, M.P., and Glickman, L.T. (2004). A placebo-controlled trial of two intranasal vaccines to prevent tracheobronchitis (kennel cough) in dogs entering a humane shelter. *Preventive Veterinary Medicine* 62: 89–99.

Fischer, S.M., Quest, C.M., Dubovi, E.J. et al. (2007). Response of feral cats to vaccination at the time of neutering. *Journal of the American Veterinary Medical Association* 230: 52–58.

Gillespie, J.H. and Scott, F.W. (1973). Feline viral infections. *Advances in Veterinary Science and Comparative Medicine* 17: 163.

Gobar, G.M. and Kass, P.H. (2002). World Wide Web-based survey of vaccination practices, postvaccinal reactions, and vaccine site-associated sarcomas in cats. *Journal of the American Veterinary Medical Association* 220 (10): 1477–1482. http://dx.doi.org/10.2460/javma.2002.220.1477 (Accessed June 15, 2020).

Gore, T.C., Lakshmanan, N., Williams, J.R. et al. (2006). Three-year duration of immunity in cats following vaccination against feline rhinotracheitis virus, feline calicivirus, and feline panleukopenia virus. *Veterinary Therapeutics* 7 (3): 213–222.

Greene, C.E. (2012). Feline enteric viral infections. In: *Infectious Diseases of the Dog and Cat*, 4e (ed. C.E. Greene), 80–91. Philadelphia: WB Saunders.

Greene, C.E. and Addie, D.D. (2006). Feline parvovirus infections. In: *Infectious Diseases of the Dog and Cat*, 3e (ed. C.E. Greene), 78–88. Philadelphia: WB Saunders.

Greene, C.E. and Schultz, R.D. (2006). Immunoprophylaxis. In: *Infectious Diseases of the Dog and Cat*, 3e (ed. C.E. Greene), 1069–1119. Philadelphia: WB Saunders.

Jakel, V., Cussler, K., Hanschmann, K.M. et al. (2012). Vaccination against feline panleukopenia: implications from a field study in kittens. *BMC Veterinary Research* 8 (1): 62. http://dx.doi.org/10.1186/1746-6148-8-62. (Accessed June 15, 2020).

Kennedy, M. and Little, S. (2012). Infectious diseases (subsection: viral diseases). In: *The Cat, Clinical Medicine and Management* (ed. S.E. Little), 1036–1038. St. Louis: Elsevier Saunders. http://dx.doi.org/10.1016/b978-1-4377-0660-4.00033-8. (Accessed June 15, 2020).

Kruse, B.D., Unterer, S., Horlacher, K. et al. (2010). Prognostic factors in cats with feline panleukopenia. *Journal of Veterinary Internal Medicine* 24 (6): 1271–1276. https://onlinelibrary.wiley.com/doi/full/10.1111/j.1939-1676.2010.0604.x (Accessed June 15, 2020).

Lappin, M.R. (2012). Feline panleukopenia virus, feline herpesvirus-1 and feline calicivirus antibody responses in seronegative specific pathogen-free kittens after parenteral administration of an inactivated FVRCP vaccine or a modified live FVRCP vaccine. *Journal of Feline Medicine and Surgery* 14 (2): 161–164.

Lappin, M.R., Andrews, J., Simpson, D. et al. (2002a). Use of serologic tests to predict resistance to feline herpesvirus 1, feline calicivirus, and feline parvovirus infection in cats. *Journal of the American Veterinary Medical Association* 220 (1): 38–42.

Lappin, M.R., Sebring, R.W., Porter, M. et al. (2002b). Effects of a single dose of an intranasal feline herpesvirus 1, calicivirus, and panleukopenia vaccine on clinical signs and virus shedding after challenge with virulent feline herpesvirus-1. *Journal of Feline Medicine and Surgery* 8 (3): 158–163.

Lappin, M.R., Veir, J., and Hawley, J. (2009). Feline panleukopenia virus, feline herpesvirus-1, and feline calicivirus antibody responses in seronegative specific pathogen-free cats after a single administration of two different modified live FVRCP vaccines. *Journal of Feline Medicine and Surgery* 11 (2): 159–162. http://dx.doi.org/10.1016/j.jfms.2008.05.004. (Accessed June 14, 2020).

Lehmann, R., Von Beust, B., Niederer, E. et al. (1992). Immunization-induced decrease of the CD4+: CD8+ ratio in cats experimentally infected with feline immunodeficiency virus. *Veterinary Immunology and Immunopathology* 35 (1–2): 199–214.

Litster, A. and Benjanirut, C. (2013). Case series of feline panleukopenia virus in an animal shelter. *Journal of Feline Medicine and Surgery* 16 (4): 346–353. http://dx.doi.org/10.1177/1098612x13497738. (Accessed June 15, 2020).

Little, S., Levy, J., Hartmann, K. et al. (2020) 2020 AAFP feline retrovirus testing and management guidelines. *Journal of Feline Medicine and Surgery* 221: 5–20.

Marks, S.L. (2016). Rational approach to diagnosing and managing infectious causes of diarrhea in kittens. In: *August's Consultations in Feline Internal Medicine*, vol. 7 (ed. S. Little), 1–22. St. Louis: Saunders Elsevier.

http://dx.doi.org/10.1016/b978-0-323-22652-3.00001-3. (Accessed June 15, 2020).

Martin, V., Wojciech, N., Gueguen, S. et al. (2002). Treatment of canine parvoviral enteritis with interferon-omega in a placebo-controlled challenge trial. *Veterinary Microbiology* 89 (2–3): 115–127. http://dx.doi.org/10.1016/s0378-1135(02)00173-6. (Accessed June 15, 2020).

Mende, K., Stuetzer, B., Mende, K. et al. (2014). Evaluation of an in-house dot enzyme-linked immunosorbent assay to detect antibodies against feline panleukopenia virus. *Journal of Feline Medicine and Surgery* 16 (10): 805–811. http://dx.doi.org/10.1177/1098612x14520812. (Accessed June 15, 2020).

Moore, G.E., DeSantis-Kerr, A.C., Guptill, L.F. et al. (2007). Adverse events after vaccine administration in cats: 2,560 cases (2002–2005). *Journal of the American Veterinary Medical Association* 231 (1): 94–100. http://dx.doi.org/10.2460/javma.231.1.94. (Accessed June 15, 2020).

Mostl, K. (2015). Feline Panleukopenia. ABCD Guidelines. http://www.abcdcatsvets.org/abcd-guidelines-on-feline-panleukopenia-2012-edition (accessed 15 June 2020).

Mostl, K., Egberink, H., Addie, D. et al. (2013). Prevention of infectious diseases in cat shelters: ABCD guidelines. *Journal of Feline Medicine and Surgery* 15 (7): 546–554. http://dx.doi.org/10.1177/1098612x13489210. (Accessed June 15, 2020).

Nakamura, K., Ikeda, Y., Miyazawa, T. et al. (2001). Characterisation of cross-reactivity of virus neutralizing antibodies induced by feline panleukopenia virus and canine parvoviruses. *Research in Veterinary Science* 71: 219–222.

Neuerer, F.F., Horlacher, K., Truyen, U. et al. (2008). Comparison of different in-house test systems to detect parvovirus in faeces of cats. *Journal of Feline Medicine and Surgery* 10 (3): 247–251. http://dx.doi.org/10.1016/j.jfms.2007.12.001. (Accessed June 15, 2020).

Ott, R.L. (1975). Viral diseases. In: *Feline Medicine and Surgery*, 2e (ed. E.J. Catcott), 38–47. Santa Barbara: American Veterinary Publication, Inc.

Paltrinieri, S., Crippa, A., Comerio, T. et al. (2007). Evaluation of inflammation and immunity in cats with spontaneous parvovirus infection: consequences of recombinant feline interferon-ω administration. *Veterinary Immunology and Immunopathology* 118 (1–2): 68–74.

Pedersen, N.C. (1988). Feline panleukopenia. In: *Feline Infectious Diseases* (ed. P.W. Pratt), 15–18. Goleta: American Veterinary Publications, Inc.

Plumb, D.C. (2018). *Plumb's Veterinary Drug Handbook*. Ames: PharmaVet Inc.

Pollock, R.V.H. and Postorino, N.C. (1994). Feline panleukopenia and other enteric viral diseases. In: *The Cat: Diseases and Clinical Management* (ed. R.G. Sherding), 479–487. New York;: Churchill Livingstone.

Porporato, F., Horzinek, M.C., Hofmann-Lehmann, R. et al. (2018). Survival estimates and outcome predictors for shelter cats with feline panleukopenia virus infection. *Journal of the American Veterinary Medical Association* 253 (2): 188–195.

Reubel, G.H., Dean, G.A., George, J.W. et al. (1994). Effects of incidental infections and immune activation on disease progression in experimentally feline immunodeficiency virus-infected cats. *Journal of Acquired Immune Deficiency Syndromes* 7 (10): 1003–1015.

Rohovsky, M.W. and Griesemer, R.A. (1967). Experimental feline infectious enteritis in the germfree cat. *Pathologia Veterinaria* 4 (4): 391–410.

Scherk, M.A., Ford, R.B., Gaskell, R.M. et al. (2013). 2013 American Association of Feline Practitioners (AAFP) feline vaccination advisory panel report. *Journal of Feline Medicine and Surgery* 15 (9): 785–808. http://dx.doi.org/10.1177/1098612x13500429. (Accessed June 15, 2020).

Schultz, R.D. (2009). A commentary on parvovirus vaccination. *Journal of Feline Medicine and Surgery* 11 (2): 163–164. http://dx.doi.org/10.1016/j.jfms.2008.05.008. (Accessed June 15, 2020).

Schunck, B., Kraft, W., and Truyen, U. (1995). A simple touch-down polymerase chain reaction for the detection of canine parvovirus and feline panleukopenia virus in feces. *Journal of Virological Methods* 55: 427–433.

Scott, F. (1987). Viral diseases: panleukopenia. In: *Diseases of the Cat: Medicine and Surgery* (ed. J. Holzworth), 182–193. Philadelphia: WB Saunders Co.

Scott, F.W. and Geissinger, C.M. (1999). Long-term immunity in cats vaccinated with an inactivated trivalent vaccine. *American Journal of Veterinary Research* 60: 652–658.

Srivastav, A., Kass, P.H., McGill, L.D. et al. (2012). Comparative vaccine-specific and other injectable-specific risks of injection-site sarcomas in cats. *Journal of the American Veterinary Medical Association* 241 (5): 595–602. http://dx.doi.org/10.2460/javma.241.5.595. (Accessed June 15, 2020).

Stone, A.E., Brummet, G.O., Carozza, E.M. et al. (2020). 2020 AAHA/AAFP Feline Vaccination Guidelines. *Journal of the American Animal Hospital Association* 56: 249–265.

Sturgess, K. (2003). Infectious disease. In: *Notes on Feline Internal Medicine* (ed. K. Sturgess), 287–290. Oxford: Blackwell Science Ltd.

Sykes, J.E. (2014). Chapter 19-feline panleukopenia virus infection and other viral enteritides. In: *Canine and Feline Infectious Diseases* (ed. J.E. Sykes), 187–194. St. Louis: Elsevier. http://dx.doi.org/10.1016/b978-1-4377-0795-3.00019-3. (Accessed June 15, 2020).

Truyen, U. and Parrish, C.R. (2013). Feline panleukopenia virus: its interesting evolution and current problems in immunoprophylaxis against a serious pathogen. *Veterinary Microbiology* 165 (1–2): 29–32.

Truyen, U., Addie, D., Belák, S. et al. (2009). Feline panleukopenia. ABCD guidelines on prevention and management. *Journal of Feline Medicine and Surgery* 11 (7): 538–546. http://dx.doi.org/10.1016/j.jfms.2009.05.002. (Accessed June 15, 2020).

Tuzio, H. (2009). Panleukopenia. In: *Infectious Disease Management in Animal Shelters* (eds. L. Miller and K. Hurley), 183–196. Ames: Wiley Blackwell.

UC Davis Koret Shelter Medicine Program (2016). Information sheet: feline panleukopenia. http://www.sheltermedicine.com/library/resources/feline-panleukopenia (accessed 15 June 2020).

16

Feline Coronavirus and Feline Infectious Peritonitis

Elizabeth A. Berliner

Maddie's Shelter Medicine Program, Cornell University College of Veterinary Medicine, Ithaca, NY, USA

16.1 Introduction

While feline coronaviruses (FCoV) are ubiquitous in cat populations, the incidence of feline infectious peritonitis (FIP) remains low; nonetheless, the disease can be devastating for cat owners and shelter personnel. FIP is often challenging to diagnose, affects highly adoptable kittens and young cats, and creates prognostic uncertainty for healthy siblings of affected cats. Furthermore, the endemic nature of FCoV in feline populations complicates management in the shelter environment, where exposure to the virus is common. Recent developments in diagnosis and treatment rely on some understanding of the biology of the virus in order to provide stakeholders with clear communication around expectations, options, and prognostic indicators for cats in higher risk categories. Management and prevention measures in animal shelters involve a few approaches specific to the disease agent, but primarily center around best practices that strengthen the host and mitigate environmental conditions: i.e. managing at capacity for care, employing pathway planning and other tools to reduce the length of stay (LOS), and providing a low-stress and enriched environment for cats.

16.2 Etiology

FCoV is an enteric pathogen of cats that is often endemic in shelters and other multi-cat environments. FCoV is a large, spherical enveloped RNA *Alphacoronavirus*. It is closely related to other gastrointestinal (GI) pathogens, including canine coronavirus (CCoV) and transmissible gastroenteritis virus of swine (TGEV). FCoV is in a different family than the *Betacoronaviruses*, which are respiratory in nature (e.g. Middle East Respiratory Syndrome [MERS], Severe Acute Respiratory Syndrome [SARS], and canine respiratory coronavirus [CRCoV]). RNA viruses are highly prone to genetic mutations, and coronaviruses in particular are known for their propensity for mutation and recombination events during replication. This is clinically significant in terms of how viral load and mutability contribute to the pathogenesis of FIP and the ongoing development of more sensitive and specific diagnostic tests for FIPV.

Traditionally, the generic term FCoV has been applied to all serotypes and biotypes of coronavirus in cats. However, more recent work distinguishes two biotypes with specific nomenclature: feline enteric coronavirus (FECV) and feline infectious peritonitis virus (FIPV) (see Table 16.1). To date, FECV and

Infectious Disease Management in Animal Shelters, Second Edition.
Edited by Lila Miller, Stephanie Janeczko, and Kate F. Hurley.

Table 16.1 Common nomenclature for feline coronavirus biotypes.

FCoV	General reference to all types of feline coronavirus
FECV	Most commonly applied to the ubiquitous enteric biotype of FCoV present in the intestinal tract and feces of cats that replicates in enterocytes
FIPV	Applied to the biotype of FCoV that replicates at high rates in macrophages, resulting in effusions and/or pyogranulomas in tissues in cats with feline infectious peritonitis (FIP)

FIPV are morphologically and antigenically indistinguishable, though recent technological advances in genetic sequencing have provided insight into how specific site mutations likely play a role in their remarkably different clinical courses. The biologic behavior of the two biotypes is markedly different: one most commonly causing mild, self-limiting diarrhea, and the other, death.

In general, coronaviruses have a marked tropism for epithelial cells, typically infecting cells lining the lungs or intestines. Antigens on the surface of the virus are engaged in primary attachment and entrance into cells. These structural spike (S) proteins give coronaviruses their characteristic shape and are considered essential players in the complex relationship between the relatively harmless FCoV and its fatal form, FIPV. The precise explanation for what prompts the FECV to FIPV transformation remains unclear. The most commonly implicated site of mutation is the gene for the S protein, but other genes under investigation encode the accessory proteins 3c, 7a, and 7b (Chang et al. 2010; Pedersen 2009).

FCoV's primary trophism is for epithelial cells, where FECV normally replicates and may cause intestinal disease. However, in a subset of cases, FECV moves into macrophages and then into the systemic circulation. It was previously thought that this movement into circulation was the signal for FIPV transformation; however, more recent work has demonstrated that FECVs circulate in monocytes and spread to extra-intestinal sites at low levels in cats without FIP (Porter et al. 2014). In contrast, mutations resulting in FIPV enable viral replication at very high levels in macrophages, resulting in profound inflammation and the syndrome of clinical signs comprising the disease FIP (Felten and Hartmann 2019; Kipar and Meli 2014). More importantly for the clinician, this new information that FECVs also circulate systemically complicates the interpretation of available diagnostic testing methods that have traditionally depended on location (intra-intestinal vs. extra-intestinal) to distinguish FECV from FIPV.

In addition to two biotypes, FCoVs also are described as two serotypes: Type I and Type II. Type I serotypes are unique to the cat and dominate in the cat population worldwide, comprising 80–95% of natural infections in North America and Europe (Addie 2012; Benetka et al. 2004). The less common Type II FCoVs have evolved from a recombination between Type I FCoV and CCoV, and certain geographic regions, particularly in Asia, see a higher prevalence of Type II (Kipar and Meli 2014). Because Type II is more readily maintained in cell culture, the majority of FCoV laboratory research has traditionally utilized Type II viruses; however, wild-type viruses, at least in North America and Europe, are primarily Type I.

FIPVs can arise from either Type I or Type II FECVs. In a 2004 study of 154 cats with FIP, 74 cats had viruses that were able to be typed: 64 (86%) had Type I, 5 (7%) had Type II, and 5 (7%) were positive for both types (Benetka et al. 2004). This is consistent with other studies that have also found a double infection of Type I and Type II confirming cats can be infected with both Type I and Type II serotypes simultaneously. The question remains whether genetic point mutations resulting in FIP are the same for Type I and Type II FECVs (Thiel et al. 2014).

16.3 Epidemiology

16.3.1 FECV

FECV is widespread in cat populations. FECV has high infectivity via the oro-nasal route and is considered endemic in multi-cat households, catteries, dense free-roaming colonies, and shelters/rescues. Several studies have demonstrated that cats from multi-cat households and those spending time in shelters are much more likely to be positive on serology and to shed virus in their feces (Drechsler et al. 2011; Foley et al. 1997b; Pedersen et al. 2004). A study of cats relinquished to shelters in the United Kingdom reported that cats from multi-cat households were twice as likely to be FCoV seropositive when compared to cats from single-cat households (Cave et al. 2004). In catteries, seroprevalence rates as high as 87–90% have been reported (Addie et al. 2000; Pedersen et al. 2004). Stray cats have been reported to have lower seroprevalence, likely due to outdoor defecation and less exposure to infected fecal material; in one study sero-prevalence for FCoV in stray and feral cats was only 12% (Luria et al. 2004).

Long-term studies in cats suggest that most cats undergo cycles of shedding, recovery, and reinfection. There is no protective immunity to FECV following initial infection: cats re-exposed to FECV will demonstrate an increase in antibody titers, a recurrence of shedding, and may demonstrate a recurrence of clinical signs. Because these are mild, they can be overlooked (Foley et al. 1997a).

16.3.2 FIP

FIP was first described in 1963 and appears not to have existed prior to the 1950s (Holzworth 1963; Pedersen 2014a). The apparent increase in the incidence of FIP in cats over that last 60 years is attributed at least in part to changes in feline husbandry and lifestyle. The first commercial cat litter, a clay product made of fuller's earth in 1947 and called "Kitty Litter," played an important role in supporting the trend of the indoor cat in the United States (Gross 2015). As cats moved indoors—into homes and shelters—shared litterboxes inadvertently increased dose exposure to FCoV and other pathogens among cats living together. As the popularity of pet cats increased, so did breeding catteries, with subsequent increase in particular genetic lines, high-density housing, and opportunities for FCoV amplification, FECV enteritis, and mutation to FIPV.

FIP is typically thought of as a disease of young cats, with cats at greatest risk up to three years of age, but especially between 4 and 16 months of age (Pedersen 2009). A study in Australia found that 80% of cases of FIP occurred in cats under two years of age, and 50% occurred in kitten under seven months (Worthing et al. 2012). Purebred cats are at greater risk; there are several theories for this, including loss of genetic diversity, less robust immunity, increased risk of viral mutation due to high viral loads, and increased environmental exposure in catteries and other densely housed cat populations. Support for a genetic predisposition comes from studies revealing a higher incidence of disease in purebred cats, including lines of related cats, and wildcats (Foley et al. 1997b; Potkay et al. 1974; Watt et al. 1993).

Overall, the risk of developing FIP is low: fewer than 3% of FCoV seropositive cats will develop FIP (Addie 2012). Risk factors for the individual cat include the following characteristics: under three years of age; a purebred cat (Addie and Jarrett 1992; Cave et al. 2004; Tekes and Thiel 2016); housed in a multi-cat facility (Foley et al. 1997a); and housed under less-than-ideal husbandry conditions (Pedersen et al. 2014). Cats are most likely to develop FIP following their first infection with FECV (Pedersen et al. 2014). Studies considering sex as a risk factor have been contradictory, with some finding higher rates in males, and others in females. Finally, cats exposed to FCoV that had immunosuppressive conditions, including clinical feline leukemia virus (FeLV) or feline immunodeficiency virus (FIV) infections, are more likely to develop FIP and have higher levels of FECV shedding (Foley et al. 1997b; Poland et al. 1996).

Some cats demonstrate resistance to FIPV. Experimentally, 36% of cats (40/111) survived an initial challenge of a Type I FIPV, with only six of the survivors succumbing to a second or third challenge, suggesting this resistance was not always sustained (Pedersen et al. 2014).

Even in high-risk environments such as hoarder homes where FCoV is endemic, the incidence of FIP ranges between 5 and 10% (Addie et al. 1995; Foley et al. 1997b). An outbreak of FIP in a cattery has been defined as greater than 10% incidence (Foley et al. 1997b). Given that cats in animal shelters are not generally genetically related, a greater than 1% incidence of FIP in a shelter population is commonly used as the breakpoint for concern, prompting population level investigation.

Outbreaks are associated with several risk factors, all of which are relevant within a shelter setting as in any other group-housed cats: (i) host-related factors, including age, breed, immune competence, and co-morbidities; (ii) pathogen-related factors, including strain, virulence, and mutability; and (iii) environmental factors, including dose and frequency of exposure, environmental load, overcrowding, and stressors (see Figure 16.1). Prevention and management interventions that can reduce these risk factors in populations are the key to minimizing the risk of developing FIP for individual cats.

16.4 Pathogenesis

16.4.1 FECV Enteritis

The main route of infection with FCoV is oronasal inoculation from contact with infected feces. After inoculation, the virus replicates in oropharyngeal tissues and then moves on to enterocytes of the intestinal villi, where it is considered FECV. Viral shedding occurs within one week and occurs from the ileum, colon, and rectum. Shedding can persist for months to even years but is often intermittent over time. Sub-clinical infections are common.

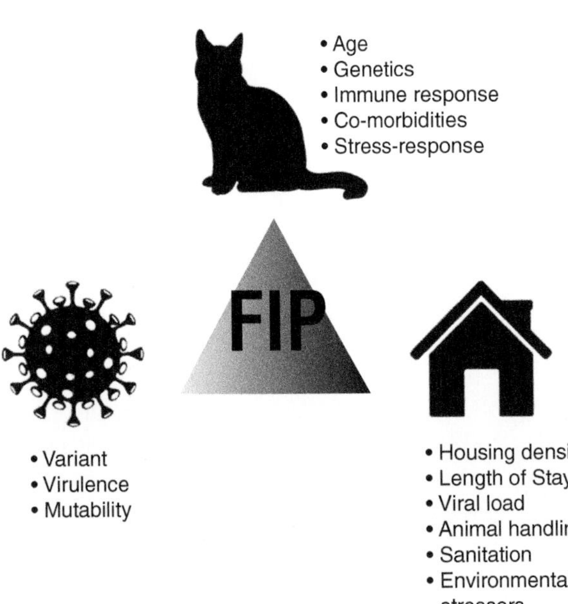

Figure 16.1 Epidemiologic triangle representation of FIP.

16.4.2 FIPV

FIPV is not considered infectious via the fecal-oral route because it cannot replicate in epithelial cells. Since that is the most common mode of transmission of FCoVs in natural infections, FIPV is not thought to be horizontally transmitted, with rare exceptions. Instead, a subset of cats infected with FECV become infected with FIPV on an individual basis. The most common explanation for this transformation is the "internal mutation theory." This theory states that one or more highly specific point mutations in the viral genome of particularly mutable FECV variants occur within an individual cat. This cat may have increased risk factors supporting the genetic mutation. A second version of this theory is that any FECV can mutate to FIPV within the cat, the choice of pathway determined by the intersection of viral load and the host's immune response (Kipar and Meli 2014; Poland et al. 1996). These two theories are not mutually exclusive; all of these factors likely play a role. For a general overview of the hypothesized pathogenesis of FIP, see Figure 16.2. (Felten and Hartmann 2019; Kipar and Meli 2014).

The "internal mutation theory" is supported by work demonstrating high genetic similarity between the FECVs and FIPVs of particular populations of cats (Vennema et al. 1998). This theory continues to be supported by a plethora of investigations using genetic sequencing, as well as the general epidemiology of FIP that has revealed few and isolated outbreaks of the disease.

Factors thought to favor increased viral replication (which is believed to increase the risk of developing FIP for individual cats) include the dose and virulence of a particular FCoV variant; the age, immune status, and co-morbidities of the affected cat, and a genetic pre-disposition of particular cats to FIP development.

16.5 Transmission

16.5.1 FECV

FCoV has high infectivity, resulting in a high rate of seroconversion in exposed cats. Cats exposed to FCoV will begin to shed virus quickly post-infection, usually within two to

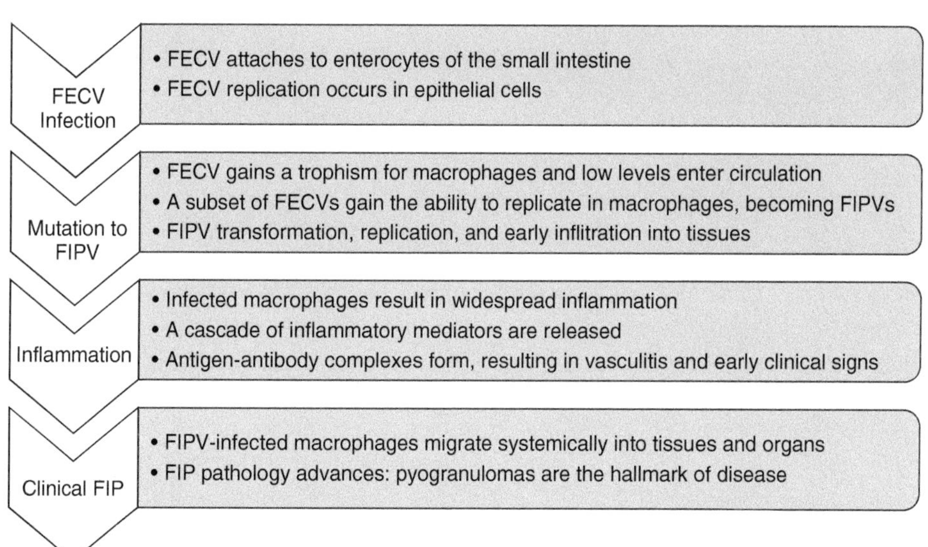

Figure 16.2 Current theory of the pathogenesis of FIP. *Source:* Felten, S. and Hartmann, K. (2019) and Kipar, A. and Meli, M.L. (2014).

seven days following infection. Kittens demonstrate higher rates of shedding than adult cats. Early studies suggested that kittens did not appear to shed virus until at least 8–10 weeks of age (Foley et al. 1997a; Pedersen et al. 2008). However, modern, more sensitive reverse transcriptase polymerase chain reaction (RT-PCR) tests have detected viral shedding in kittens as early as two weeks of age (Hartmann 2016). In one study of cats and kittens entering shelters, shedding of FECV increased by 10^1 to 10^6 after one week in the facility; for kittens between 8 and 16 weeks of age, the mean of primary shedding was 10 000 times higher than adult cats (Pedersen et al. 2004) In one study, stress associated with pregnancy and/or lactation did not increase shedding in infected cats (Foley et al. 1997a).

As previously stated, infection with FCoV generally occurs through fecal-oronasal transmission, most commonly through shared litterboxes contaminated with the virus. However, the virus is also secondarily transmitted by fomites, including hands and equipment, and from cat-to-cat in close contact via viral particles on fur. Viral loads in shelters are reduced through population management and good husbandry practices, including avoiding overcrowding and providing for sanitation and disinfection of litterboxes and tools. Additionally, risk-based management of individual cats based on age and clinical signs, such as not group housing kittens in mixed litters, likely reduces the risk of FECV enteritis.

FECV can produce persistent and chronic infections. Asymptomatic cats can shed virus for months to years, and shedding can be persistent or intermittent. Asymptomatic carriers and shedders act as reservoirs and create a particular challenge in animal shelters with the continuous influx and wide-scale use of communal housing models.

16.5.2 FIPV

FIPV has long been considered to not be transmitted horizontally between cats. In cats with FIP, the majority will shed low levels of FIPV in their feces, as well as in bodily fluids such as urine and saliva. However, the FIPV biotype appears to fail to replicate in the epithelial cells of cats infected in natural infections and is therefore not infectious between cats. In a longitudinal study of 820 cats in 73 households, cats introduced to households where FIP had recently been diagnosed were NOT more likely to develop FIP than cats from households with no FIP (Addie et al. 1995). Furthermore, the remarkably low risk for FIPV transmission between cats is supported by multiple factors: the sporadic incidence of FIP, the fact that a single cat in a multi-cat setting can be affected, the internal mutation theory which specifies mutation of FECV occurs in the individual cat, and the variety of FIPV mutations that have been sequenced in cases of FIP.

Nonetheless, over the years anecdotal and case reports of outbreaks in non-related, co-housed cats have been reported. In very rare instances, it appears particular genetic point mutations may result in a variant of FIPV which can be transmitted between multiple unrelated cats. An investigation of an outbreak in a Taiwanese shelter in 2011 demonstrated that 8 of 13 cats with FIP were all found to be infected with the same type II FIPV with an identical recombination site in the S gene (Wang et al. 2013). This discovery, enabled by newer genetic sequencing techniques, contradicted standard thinking regarding the pathogenesis of FIPV. The theory in this case is that if a specific mutation allowed FIPV to actually replicate in the intestine following ingestion (i.e. it regained the epithelial tropism of FCoV), it would follow that this mutant virus could allow cat-to-cat transmission of FIPV. However, it is important to note that this transformation appears to be extraordinarily rare.

Transmission of particularly mutable variants of FCoVs may play a role in shelter outbreaks, but fortunately, these are also rare. Often what appears to be an outbreak of FIP in a shelter is not a particularly novel virus or viral mutation, but the result of housing and husbandry practices that contribute to opportunities for high FCoV loads and transmission, as well as an amplification of risk factors in the population. However, discrete outbreaks of FIP in unrelated group-housed cats warrants an investigation, to include epidemiologic risk factors and management practices, supplemented by genetic sequencing when available and/or applicable. If a shelter is experiencing what they think is an outbreak of FIP, they are advised to contact a shelter medicine specialist for guidance and/or veterinary diagnostic laboratory for information on the latest testing methodologies, which may include genetic sequencing of outbreak variants. While this is not commercially available (and may be difficult for shelters to obtain at the time of publication), information is rapidly changing, and updates are available through research laboratories engaged in these investigations.

16.6 Immune Response

16.6.1 FECV

Though immune-competent cats generally mount a substantial humoral response to FCoV, as demonstrated by antibody titer testing, the presence of antibodies to FCoV does not reliably protect against disease. This is likely due to the high variation and mutability of coronaviruses. In some cases, more virulent strains of FCoV result in more severe FECV-related disease or an increased likelihood of mutation to FIPV. In others, the stress or immune status of the host plays a role in both decreased immune response and increased levels of shedding.

Natural reinfection with FECV appears to occur with subsequent exposures to the virus, as demonstrated by antibody titer testing in a longitudinal study (Addie et al. 1995) and recurrence of clinical signs in re-exposed cats in a challenge study (Pedersen et al. 2008). Note that many cats with natural infections will have a subclinical infection and no clinical signs.

16.6.2 FIPV

It has been hypothesized that while immunity to FIPV infection engages both humoral and cell-mediated responses, humoral immunity is less important for protection, and actually participates in the development of FIP. Clinical presentations of FIP are considered a direct result of the immune response to the virus. This theory further states that the type and strength of immune response determine the form that FIPV infection will take in the individual cat. A strong humoral immunity with very weak or non-existent cellular immunity will result in a primarily effusive FIP following a Type III hypersensitivity reaction and deposition of immune complexes around blood vessels. An intermediate humoral immunity and cellular immunity will result in a primarily non-effusive FIP comprised of pyogranulomas. A strong cell-mediated response may prevent the development of disease entirely (Pedersen 2009).

Experimental challenge studies of laboratory cats inoculated intraperitoneally with FIPV as well as genome-wide association studies of pedigreed cats have revealed that some cats appear to have natural resistance to developing FIP (Pedersen et al. 2014, 2016). FIPV in macrophages evades antibody responses. Therefore, a strong cell-mediated response has been posited to play a significant role in protection against the development of FIP by acting to restrict the virus to the intestinal mucosa and mesenteric lymph nodes, resulting in eventual elimination (Pedersen 2009).

16.7 Clinical Signs

16.7.1 FECV

Most FECV infections are subclinical. In exposed cats, acute infection may result in mild diarrhea. In challenge studies, FECV-infected specific pathogen-free (SPF) cats demonstrated diarrhea and sometimes vomiting. Kittens with FECV have been reported to have more persistent diarrhea (weeks), accompanied by stunted growth and overall unthriftiness (Addie and Jarrett 1992).

16.7.2 FIP

Though traditionally FIP has been described in two forms—effusive ("wet") and non-effusive ("dry") —it is more accurate to think of FIP as a spectrum of clinical presentations resulting in varying degrees of effusion. In a 2004 study of 154 cats with histopathology consistent with FIP, cats with Type I feline coronavirus showed a spectrum of clinical signs: 58% demonstrated both effusive and non-effusive disease; 28% had non-effusive disease and 14% had effusive disease (Benetka et al. 2004). In this same study, cats infected with Type II also demonstrated a continuum of pathologic disease. Though feline Type I predominates in healthy and FIP-infected cats, both Type I and Type II can result in FIP.

Early clinical signs of FIP include a fever that may wax and wane, inappetence, and lethargy. Particularly in kittens, early signs can be confused with upper respiratory disease or panleukopenia. The development of ascites in a kitten or young cat, however, is highly suggestive of FIP. Kittens or cats with primarily effusive disease will often develop tachypnea or dyspnea, abdominal distention, icterus, and/or pallor. Ocular pathology can occur with both effusive and non-effusive disease: uveitis, iritis, retinitis, and keratic precipitates are common. Neurologic abnormalities occur primarily with non-effusive forms and may be accompanied by thoracic or abdominal masses that are granulomas.

Differentials for the primarily effusive form of the disease include cardiac failure, neoplasia (particularly lymphoma), and other causes of pleuritis and peritonitis. Differentials for less effusive forms include toxoplasmosis, systemic mycoses, feline retroviruses (FeLV or FIV), pancreatitis, and neoplasia (primarily lymphosarcoma and adenocarcinoma).

Mortality in cases of untreated FIP is virtually 100% and rapid once clinical signs are present. However, rare cases have demonstrated a prolonged course of disease for months to years without treatment; these tend to be more non-effusive forms on the spectrum of disease.

16.8 Diagnosis

16.8.1 FECV Enteritis

16.8.1.1 FCoV Serology

No test is diagnostic for FECV enteritis. Positive serology for antibodies to FCoV demonstrates prior exposure to the virus but does not confirm FCoV as a cause for clinical signs given the ubiquitous nature of FCoVs in cats. Only approximately 33% of seropositive cats shed virus (Addie and Jarrett 1992). Therefore, serologic testing for antibodies to FCoV does not aid in identifying viral shedders. Furthermore, a positive FCoV antibody titer does not diagnose FIP, nor indicate protection against disease.

Seronegative cats do not appear to shed virus, and so FCoV titers may be useful as a means to identify cats that have not been exposed to FCoV and are not actively shedding. This is most useful in closed, stable cat populations such as catteries, and not particularly applicable to shelter populations.

16.8.1.2 Reverse Transcriptase-Polymerase Chain Reaction (RT-PCR) for FCoV

PCR is a highly sensitive testing method that amplifies and detects small amounts of DNA. In the case of RNA viruses, a DNA copy of the virus is first generated by the use of the enzyme reverse transcriptase. FCoV antigen can be detected on RT-PCR in feces. A positive result on RT-PCR on feces confirms shedding of FCoV, but again, given the ubiquitous nature of FCoVs, the agent may not be causing the clinical signs. Other infectious, inflammatory, and nutritional etiologies should still be investigated as a cause for the diarrhea.

A negative RT-PCR on feces makes FCoV a highly unlikely cause of clinical signs, which could be useful in addressing an outbreak scenario in a shelter or cattery. RT-PCR testing for FCoV can be useful in identifying shedders, but shedding can also be intermittent and therefore not representative of the cat's true status.

16.8.2 FIP

16.8.2.1 FCoV Serology

FCoV, FECV, and FIPV cannot be distinguished by serologic antibody testing. A positive serology for antibody to FCoV does not diagnose FIPV, nor can it predict whether a cat will develop FIP; it simply confirms that, at some point, the cat was infected with FCoV. Additionally, cats with advanced FIP may test negative for antibodies on serology for several reasons: rapidly progressing disease with a delayed immune response; terminal disease with the exhaustion of antibody; and/or immune complex formation interfering with testing (Addie 2012).

16.8.2.2 Hematology and Serum Chemistry

Hematology and blood chemistry can contribute to the overall clinical suspicion of FIP. Findings commonly include a non-regenerative anemia due to chronic inflammation, accompanied by lymphopenia and thrombocytopenia.

On serum chemistry, common abnormalities include hyperproteinemia with a low albumin: globulin (A : G) ratio. Protein electrophoresis can reveal a polyclonal gammopathy, particularly with the non-effusive form of FIP. Elevation in serum gamma-globulin is more predictive than the A:G ratio or total protein (Addie 2012). Hyperbilirubinemia is also common, likely due to red blood cell destruction rather than cholestasis or other liver diseases (Pedersen 2014b). Liver enzymes may be elevated.

16.8.2.3 Imaging

In effusive disease, radiographs and/or ultrasound will reveal pleural or peritoneal effusion; this can be profound (see Figure 16.3a). Imaging can be important in distinguishing ascites from other causes of abdominal distention, including parasites, intestinal diseases, and urinary obstruction; likewise, imaging can help distinguish pleural effusion from pneumonia and other conditions resulting in dyspnea. In non-effusive FIP, imaging is non-specific but may reveal single to multiple nodules throughout abdominal viscera, most notably in mesenteric lymph nodes. When available, ultrasound-guided centesis can be useful in safely gaining adequate samples of effusion for analysis or fine-needle aspirates for additional testing modalities (see Figure 16.3b). When ultrasound is not available, thoraco- and abdomino-centesis can be safely performed without it, particularly when effusive disease is severe.

16.8.2.4 Effusion Analysis

Overall, analysis of effusions, when present, contributes much more to diagnosis than routine bloodwork. Effusions should be collected sterilely via thoraco- or abdomino-centesis and stored in an Ethylenediaminetetraacetic acid (EDTA) (purple top) tube and a sterile clot tube (red or tiger top) for cytologic and potential chemical analysis, respectively. Color and turbidity of the fluid should be read first. Classically, FIP effusions are described as having a clear to straw-yellow color and a viscous, sticky consistency (see Figure 16.4a–b). They may froth when shaken due to their high protein content. FIP effusions, historically, have been classified as modified transudates with a high total solid count: they are relatively low in cellularity (<500–5000/ul) with a total protein of greater than 3.5 g/dl. As of late, there has been some effort to consider them non-septic exudates, based on the higher protein level; both terms appear in the literature (Center 2012; Pedersen 2014b; Zoia et al. 2009).

An anti-coagulated EDTA sample can be used to make slides to estimate total cellularity and perform cytology; a portion of the effusion should be centrifuged to concentrate the cells for better morphologic assessment.

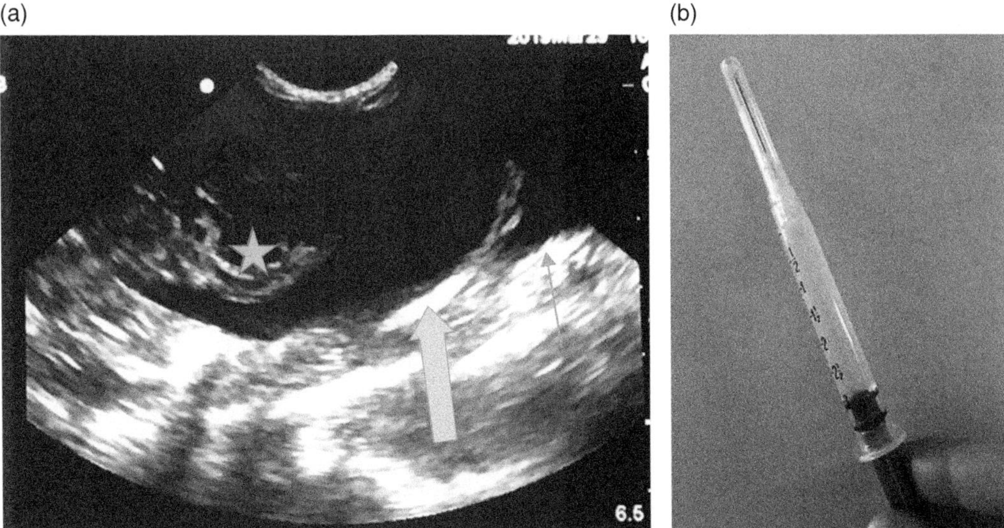

Figure 16.3 (a) Ultrasound image of profound effusion in a young cat with FIP with bi-cavitary effusion: the large arrow indicates pleural effusion surrounding the heart, indicated by the star; at the far right, indicated by the thin arrow, is peritoneal fluid in the cranial portion of the abdominal cavity. (b) Syringe of straw-colored effusion drawn from the peritoneal cavity of a cat with FIP. *Source:* Photo courtesy of Dr. Elizabeth Berliner.

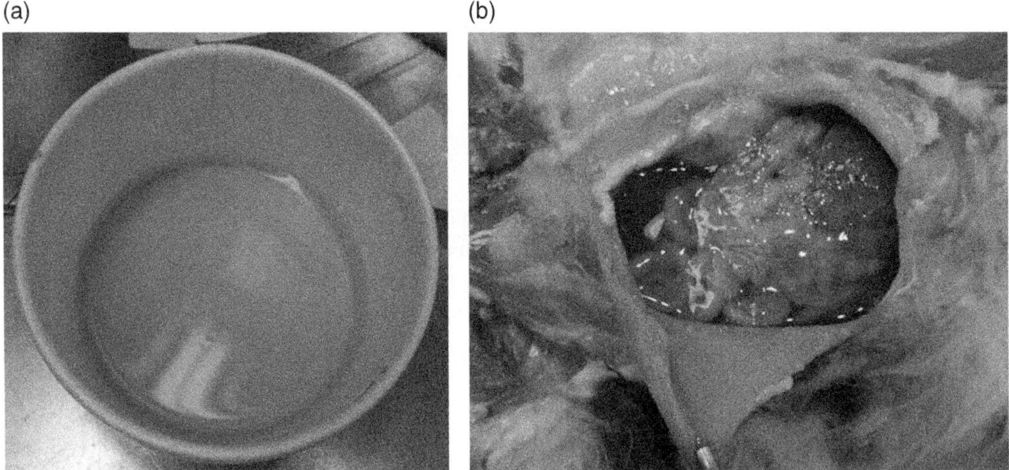

Figure 16.4 (a) Effusion from a cat with FIP. *Source:* Photo courtesy of Dr. Gerald Duhamel. Used with permission. (b) Peritoneal effusion in situ. *Source:* Photo courtesy of Dr. Gerald Duhamel. Used with permission.

The total protein of the fluid should be determined on the supernatant from the centrifuged portion before decanting to make additional slides for cytologic examination from the sediment. The total protein of the supernatant can be read with a standard refractometer. Smears made from the spun-down sediment should be dried and stained with standard rapid stains for cytologic analysis (Center 2012). Differentials for effusive disease such as sepsis and neoplasia tend to produce representative cellularity in a cytologic examination; in contrast, FIP effusion is relatively acellular.

Protein electrophoresis of effusion samples provides additional information when working toward a diagnosis of FIP. An A : G ratio of less than 0.8 is consistent with a diagnosis of FIP, and an A : G ratio of less than 0.5 has a positive predictive value of 89%, which means there is an 89% chance that the patient has FIP (Hartmann et al. 2003). For effusions, an A : G ratio greater than one has a negative predictive value of 91%, which means that there is a 91% chance that the patient does NOT have FIP.

16.8.2.5 Rivalta's Test

Performing a Rivalta's test on effusion provides additional evidence to differentiate FIP from other causes of effusive disease. In particular, Rivalta's test identifies effusions that are high in protein, fibrin, and other inflammatory mediators; not all of these will be FIP. The method is simple: one drop of 98% acetic acid is added to 5 ml of distilled water in a clear collection tube. A drop of the effusion is added to the top. If the drop disappears, the test is negative for FIP; if the drop retains its shape, and floats or falls slowly, the test is positive for FIP.

The sensitivity is of this test is high (91–98%), which means a false negative result in a case of FIP is unlikely; therefore, a negative test reliably decreases the index of suspicion for FIP. However, the specificity of the test is relatively low (66–80%) so the probability of false positive results is relatively high (Hartmann et al. 2003; Fischer et al. 2012). A positive result on Rivalta's test can occur in septic or neoplastic disease. Because positive and negative predictive values are dependent on prevalence in the test population, the predictive value of Rivalta's test increases when the analysis is done only on effusions from cats more representative of the population at high risk for FIP, such as cats under three years of age with effusions. Rivalta's test is less useful in distinguishing FIP from other causes when test subjects include older cats more prone to these conditions, such as bacterial peritonitis and lymphoma (Fischer et al. 2012; Hartmann et al. 2003).

16.8.2.6 Molecular Diagnostics

FCoV's large RNA viral genome encodes four structural proteins (spike [S], matrix [M], nucleocapsid [N], and envelope [E]). Spike proteins are particularly significant because they determine viral entrance into and exit from cells. Mutations significant to the FECV to FIPV transformation are thought to most commonly occur in the genes for the spike (S) protein; the accessory genes identified as 3c, 7a, and 7b; some combination of the above; or others not yet recognized (Chang et al. 2010; Pedersen et al. 2012; Porter et al. 2014). These point mutations are all active areas of research as to their role in infectivity and mutability and sites of interest for diagnostic test development. The sheer size of the RNA genome contributes to the difficulty in pinpointing relevant mutations and the availability of genetic sequencing in a clinical context.

Molecular diagnostics have also contributed to a more thorough understanding of how FECVs and FIPVs can both be found in effusions and affected tissues, complicating diagnostic test interpretation that historically relied on finding any FCoV in tissue samples using immunohistochemistry. A key difference in making the diagnosis using molecular diagnostics is to quantify the viral copy number present in samples in combination with the capture of viral DNA bearing FIPV-associated point mutations. In general, FECVs are known to be present in low levels in tissues, while FIPVs tend to be present at higher levels; these viral copy numbers can be measured by modern molecular diagnostic techniques (Felten and Hartmann 2019).

16.8.2.6.1 RT-PCR for FCoV The same RT-PCR for FCoV used to identify FCoV in feces has been used historically to test effusions or tissues for the presence of FCoV; however, the test does not reliably distinguish FECV from FIPV and is not useful for diagnosing FIP.

16.8.2.6.2 RT-PCR plus S Gene Mutation Detection An enhanced RT-PCR for FIP is commercially available for use on effusions or tissue samples. This test combines the detection of Type I FCoV antigen with genetic sequencing for point mutations in the spike (S) protein; these two elements are consistent with a diagnosis of FIP. While the specificity of this commercial test on tissue samples and effusions is relatively high, sensitivity is relatively low due to the low levels of viral particles in effusions as compared to tissues. Therefore, a positive result on this test can be useful in confirmation of FIP, but negative results or indeterminate results are not helpful. Also, note that this test does not capture Type II FCoVs and other point mutations associated with a subset of FIP cases.

In general, tissue biopsies are more reliably used for confirmation by molecular diagnostics than effusions; however, effusion analysis contributes significant information to making a diagnosis. In non-effusive disease, fine needle aspirate (FNA) samples of mesenteric lymph nodes can be submitted for RT-PCR with S gene mutation detection and have demonstrated utility in contributing to the ante-mortem diagnosis of FIP without more invasive procedures such as surgical biopsies (Dunbar et al. 2019; Felten and Hartmann 2019).

RT-PCR is not recommended to be performed on whole blood samples because viremia is often too low to permit bio-typing and confirmation of FIPV-associated mutations. This test is also not useful on feces since cats with FIP are often concurrently shedding FECV, which can confound results.

16.8.2.7 Biopsy and Other Ante-Mortem Ancillary Tests

An additional diagnostic option, particularly for cases suspected of having primarily non-effusive FIP, is biopsy sampling of commonly affected tissues (lymph nodes, liver, kidney) followed by histopathology and immunohistochemistry (IHC). This requires open laparotomy or ultrasound-guided sampling techniques. Collecting adequate samples using closed abdominal techniques such as needle biopsy or FNA will often fail to yield the diagnosis with IHC. On a study of 25 cats with known FIP, analysis of 16g liver biopsies demonstrated low sensitivity (64%) on diagnostic samples, meaning that even though cats were known to have FIP, the test was incorrectly negative 36% of the time. FNAs were slightly more sensitive at 82% (they were only falsely negative 18% of the time), but only 40% of FNA samples were of adequate quality to be diagnostic in this study. Combining needle biopsies with FNA cytology resulted in higher overall diagnostic sensitivity (86%). Immunohistochemistry sensitivity was very low (11–38%) on these samples which makes it a poor supplemental test for needle biopsies (Giordano et al. 2005).

IHC on tissue biopsies or imprints attained at surgery or necropsy has been the gold standard for FIP diagnosis. This method identifies high levels of FCoV antigen inside of macrophages in lesions, which was long considered pathognomonic for FIP. However, its utility is limited in that IHC is generally performed at specialized diagnostic laboratories, and best performed on surgically attained biopsies of gross lesions (or at necropsy). Attempts to use this technology on effusions are unreliable due to low levels of macrophages in those effusions. The use of IHC of tissue samples as the gold standard has also been confounded by recent recognition that a low level of FECVs also make their way into tissue.

Direct immunofluorescence testing (DIF) is commonly used in Europe and Australia on ante-mortem effusion samples in suspect cases of FIP, with reported 100% specificity and 57–95% sensitivity; a follow-up study found 71.4% specificity and 100% sensitivity (Litster et al. 2013). This test is not commercially available in the United States.

In clinical practice, an ante-mortem diagnosis of FIP relies on formulating an entire clinical picture, including a thorough physical exam and ancillary diagnostic testing, to create a diagnosis of reasonable certainty. (See Table 16.2). A high index of suspicion for FIP is raised in a kitten or young cat with waxing and waning signs of malaise, fever, and ill-thrift, often with a history of diarrhea. Abdominal distention, tachypnea, and/or dyspnea may be

Table 16.2 Findings that aid in the ante-mortem diagnosis of FIP.

Signalment and history	Less than 3 years old Diarrhea Unthrifty kittens, slow growth	
Physical exam	Anorexia, weight loss Fever Uveitis, iritis Retinal hemorrhages Neurologic signs Lethargy	Icterus Abdominal distention Tachypnea Dyspnea Ascites or pleural fluid Abdominal masses
Hematology and blood chemistry	Non-regenerative anemia and lymphopenia consistent with chronic inflammation Hyperglobulinemia Serum gamma-globulin—more predictive than A : G ratio on serum, or total protein. Hyperbilirubinemia and bilirubinuria Mildly increased ALP and ALT	
Imaging: radiographs or ultrasound	Non-specific Effusive disease: will demonstrate fluid in the pleural and/or peritoneal cavities Non-effusive disease: hepato/spleno/reno-megaly, mass lesions associated with mesenteric lymph nodes or the GI tract	
Analysis of effusion (when present)	Clear, straw-colored, viscous; froths when shaken Typically has total solid concentration >3.5 g/dl and a low cell count <5000 nucleated cells /ul (primarily neutrophils and macrophages) A : G ratio <0.8	
RT-PCR for FIP with S point mutation identification	On effusions and/or on FNA samples of affected tissues, such as mesenteric lymph nodes Positive results are highly specific for a subset of FIPVs; however, the test is not very sensitive (i.e. negative results should not be used to rule out a FIP diagnosis); low levels of antigen lead to false negatives. Not for use on blood or feces (low sensitivity due to low viral load)	

present. In such a patient, the presence of a viscous, straw-yellow thoracic or abdominal effusion that is of low cellularity and high total protein (greater than 3.5 g/dl) as read by refractometer is enough to warrant a reasonable presumptive diagnosis of FIP. Additional factors such as hyperbilirubinemia and/or elevations in serum globulin are also consistent with FIPV. Non-effusive disease can be much more difficult to diagnose, as masses may be diffuse and small, or even confined to the central nervous system (CNS). In young cats without effusions, top differentials include systemic toxoplasmosis or sepsis. In older cats, top differentials include pancreatitis, neoplasia, cardiac disease, sepsis, or hepatic disease.

16.8.2.8 Necropsy

The hallmark of FIP is the pyogranuloma. Gross necropsy findings of diffuse, pyogranulomatous lesions on thoracic and abdominal tissues are highly supportive of the diagnosis of FIP. Few differential diseases have similar lesions, though lymphoma or systemic mycoses are primary rule-outs. In cases of FIP, vasculitis is often grossly demonstrable.

Classic lesions of effusive disease include a modified transudate present in thoracic and or abdominal cavities; diffuse miliary pyogranulomas on serosal surfaces of organs; and pyogranulomas surrounding blood vessels, including throughout the mesentery. In non-effusive disease, pyogranulomas are also present, and can usually be found throughout abdominal organs, particularly in the cortex of the kidney. See Figure 16.5a–d for representations of common gross pathology findings in cases of FIP.

Though the gross pathology of FIP is fairly obvious on necropsy, the gold standard for FIP diagnosis has been histopathology demonstrating pathognomonic vasculitis combined with either immunohistochemistry identifying coronavirus antigen inside of macrophages or RT-PCR with S site mutations consistent with FIPV. This is generally best achieved on widespread postmortem sampling and testing of affected tissues, which is only helpful in confirming a presumptive diagnosis after death or euthanasia. In a shelter setting, a presumptive postmortem diagnosis based on classic lesions on necropsy is generally all that is required.

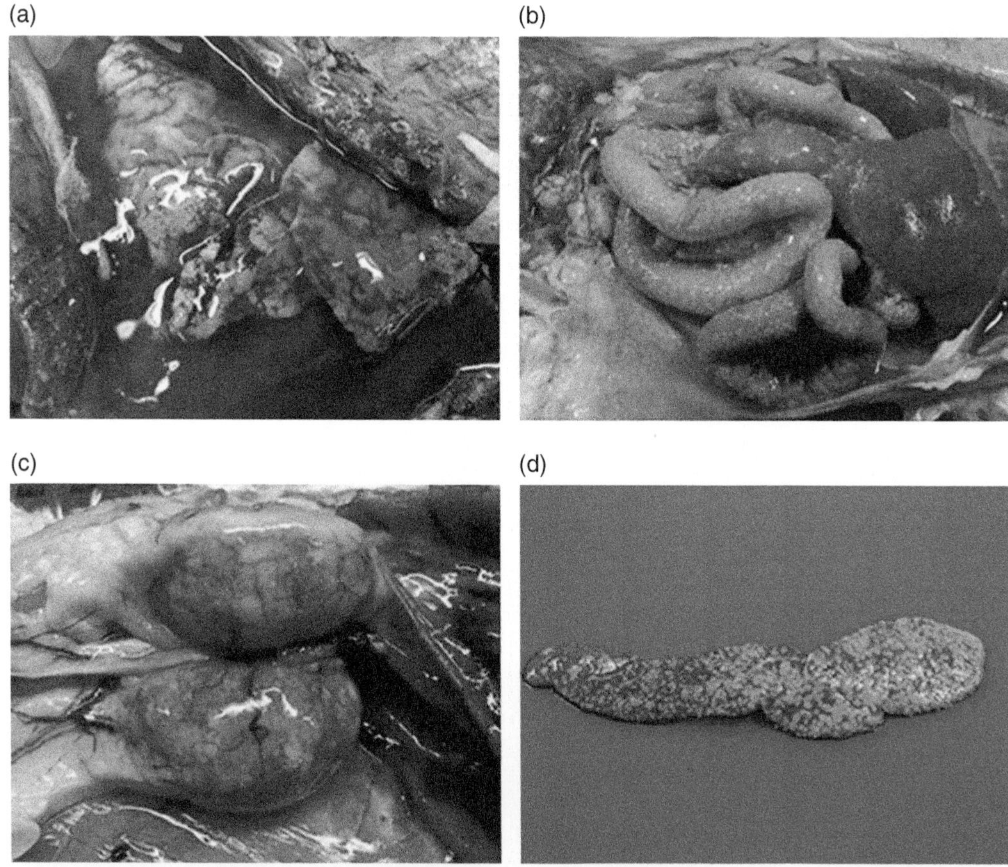

Figure 16.5 (a) Feline lung with multifocal to diffuse pyogranulomas surrounded by classic viscous, straw-colored effusion. (b) Feline intestine, liver, and peritoneum with multifocal to diffuse pyogranulomas on serosal surfaces and mesentery. (c) Feline kidney demonstrating pyogranulomatous lesions visible even with capsule intact. When sectioned, pyogranulomas will be found in the cortex. (d) Feline spleen with classic multi-focal to diffuse pyogranulomas. (a), (b), (c) and (d) *Source:* Courtesy of Dr. Gerald Duhamel. Used with permission.

16.9 Treatment

16.9.1 FECV

FECV rarely requires treatment. When diarrhea is severe, treatment involves basic supportive care to maintain hydration and nutritional support. Kittens in particular may be more likely to develop persistent diarrhea, slow growth, dehydration, and nutritional compromise. Efforts should be made to rule out all common co-morbidities in shelter populations such as parasites and to closely monitor and treat all other conditions that could compromise host response to infection.

16.9.2 FIP

Currently, there is no commercially available treatment specifically for FIP that is approved for use in the United States. Without treatment, FIP has long been considered 100% fatal upon diagnosis; life expectancy is typically days to weeks, especially for the effusive form in young cats. Commonly, these cats are dyspneic due to fluid accumulation in the pleural and peritoneal spaces. In a shelter environment, humane euthanasia is appropriate as a means of preventing suffering as clinical signs progress.

Palliative care has been employed in general veterinary practice to attempt to provide owners with more time with their pets while minimizing patient discomfort with advancing signs. Traditional approaches have included immunosuppressive therapies, including prednisolone or cyclophosphamide, to potentially slow the clinical progression of the disease; however, these do not alter the outcome of the disease. Immune modulators such as interferon have also been used to inhibit key aspects of the inflammatory cascade; however, there is very limited evidence for their efficacy. A third class of drugs called immune stimulants have been used to attempt to enhance the cat's immune response in hopes of overcoming the disease; at least one of these—Polyprenyl Immunostimulant (PI)—is licensed in the United States for reduction of clinical signs due to feline herpesvirus. To date, there are anecdotal reports of successful treatment for individual cats with FIP using all of the above, but overall, none of the treatments appear to be reliably efficacious.

Effective treatment intervention for coronavirus infections with an immune-pathological component—which include SARS, MERS, and FIP—is thought to require a combination of immunomodulatory agents and anti-viral drugs. The goal is twofold: to minimize pathologic immune responses while enhancing protective host immunity and to utilize antiviral drugs to directly inhibit viral replication.

Recent clinical trials have shown very promising results for two classes of anti-viral pharmaceuticals: a nucleoside analog known as GS-441524 and a protease inhibitor known as GC376. Of all the laboratory and clinical trials, these have shown the most promise in reversing the clinical signs of FIP and prolonging survival times. Safety and efficacy trials of GS-441524 have demonstrated prolonged remission of clinical signs of FIP in both effusive and non-effusive disease in both experimentally-induced and naturally occurring infections (Murphy et al. 2018; Pedersen et al. 2019). Likewise, in two trials of GC376 (one laboratory, the other in client-owned cats) a majority of cats demonstrated some reversal of clinical signs and a significant subset achieved prolonged remission (Kim et al. 2016; Pedersen et al. 2018). Both drugs have been trialed in treating deadly diseases in humans, including outbreaks of SARS and Ebola, and so there is reluctance to apply them widely in veterinary patients before knowing their utility for deadly diseases in people. Legal and regulatory restrictions have prevented their official use in cats in the United States.

Several investigations of potential treatments are detailed in Table 16.3. In particular, although not commercially available for cats in the US, the pharmaceutical remdesivir, utilized on an emergency basis for humans with SARS-CoV-2, has significant potential to be a successful therapeutic agent for cats infected with FIP.

Table 16.3 Experimental treatments for FIP.

Drug/Drug Class	Study design	Sample size	Comments	References
GS-441524 Nucleoside analog (a pro-drug of GS-5734 otherwise known as Remdesivir)	Clinical trial in client-owned cats with clinical signs of FIP	31 cats: 26 with effusive disease, 6 with non-effusive disease	6 died/were euthanized; 18/25 went into long-term remission with a single treatment course; 7/25 required a repeat course or higher dosage	Pedersen et al. (2019)
GS-441524 Nucleoside analog (a pro-drug of GS-5734 otherwise known as Remdesivir)	*In vitro* testing in feline cells and clinical trial in laboratory housed cats	10 cats with FIP following FIPV inoculation	10/10 had remission of signs; 2/10 required a second treatment to maintain remission	Murphy et al. (2018)
GC376 3CL-pro protease inhibitor	Clinical trial in client- owned cats with clinical signs of FIP	20 cats: 14 with effusive FIP, 6 with non-effusive FIP	19/20 had short term improvement (2 weeks)	Pedersen et al. (2018, 2019)
GC376 3CL-pro protease inhibitor	Experimental trial in laboratory housed cats	8 cats with FIP following FIPV inoculation	6 showed a temporary response to treatment with improvement in clinical signs; 2 were euthanized due to the severity of the disease	Kim et al. (2016)
PI Polyprenyl Immunostimulant	Clinical trial of owned cats	60 cats with non-effusive FIP; no control group	Prolonged survival times compared to cats not treated, or cats treated with PI and steroids	Legendre et al. (2017)
Anti-feline TNF-alpha monoclonal antibody	Experimental trial in laboratory housed cats	6 FIPV inoculated cats; 3 treated	2 of 3 treated cats had a temporary lessening of clinical signs, inflammatory mediators, and recovery of lymphocyte counts	Doki et al. (2016)
Feline interferon-omega	Randomized placebo-controlled double-blind trial in owned cats	37 cats with confirmed FIP	All received corticosteroid and either placebo or interferon-ω. No statistically significant difference in survival time with treatment vs. placebo	Ritz et al. (2007)

16.10 Prevention and Control

If controlling FECV surpassed all other welfare and enrichment concerns in the shelter, individual caged housing with strict biosecurity measures and minimal handling would be the best control. However, given the importance of enrichment, the demonstrated benefits of managed communal housing for cats, and the ever-constant, ever-changing flow of cats into shelters, "lockdown" of individual cats is not the best overall approach to the management of this agent.

Due to its endemic nature, it is nearly impossible to eliminate FECV in cat populations. While breeding catteries affected by high rates of FIP have developed guidelines for how to eliminate FECV from their facilities, most of these rely on meticulous viral testing and queen selection, separation and early weaning of kittens, and clean breaks in breeding stock. Shelters obviously play a very different role for a very different population. However, this does not imply that shelter professionals should merely accept high rates of FECV and/or FIP in their populations. Other recommendations for catteries focus on reducing colony size, minimizing fecal contamination of the environment, and improving litterbox husbandry. These are particularly useful when thinking about preventive measures in shelters.

Given that it is not possible to distinguish more virulent and mutable strains of FECV from more innocuous and endemic forms, control measures in shelters are primarily aimed at reducing the overall level of virus and co-morbidities, including stress, in the population. These measures include following best practices in capacity for care management, sanitation and disinfection, housing and husbandry, and prevention and treatment of co-morbidities in the population.

16.10.1 Capacity for Care

Capacity for care is a shelter management method encompassing proactive population management through the prevention of relinquishment, accompanied by managed intake, efficient pathway planning, and preventive medicine (Karsten et al. 2017). These steps aim to reduce the LOS for individual animals in the shelter, which in turn, prevents crowding, substandard care, and subsequent disease. In order to control FECV on a population level, avoidance of crowding and amelioration of physiological and mental stress in the shelter supports the reduction of viral load in the shelter; in turn, reducing the LOS for an individual cat reduces its exposure and contributes to a reduction in risk for that cat. See Chapter 1 for more information about capacity for care.

16.10.2 Sanitation and Disinfection

FCoV can survive for up to seven weeks in a dry environment. An enveloped virus, FCoV is generally inactivated by standard detergents and disinfectants used in animal shelters. Viral dose undoubtedly plays as important a role in terms of whether or not disease develops in an individual cat. Minimizing the virus in the shelter environment is a reasonable goal that can be accomplished through standard cleaning and disinfection. General best sanitation practices can be found in Chapter 8 of this text.

Given the high level of FECV shedding that occurs in cats recently introduced to shelters, litterbox management—especially for shelters practicing group housing of cats—is particularly critical for reducing viral load in the environment. Simple measures that represent standard best practices include frequent scooping of litterboxes and frequent cleaning of scoops—or using individual disposable gloves rather than standard scoops when disease concern is heightened, including any increase in diarrhea or other signs of GI disease. When caring for ill cats, eliminating cross contamination by changing gloves and/or hand-washing is recommended. Because kittens are both more susceptible to the development of FIP and more likely to shed FECV at high levels, particular attention should be paid to segregating kittens from adult cats and minimizing exposure of multiple litters to one another. Given that kittens generally have a short LOS, designating one litter per humane enclosure and providing enrichment within their litter is preferable to creating large group kitten housing.

For individually housed cats, daily spot cleaning is preferred to deep cleaning and disinfecting for many reasons, most commonly for stress reduction and minimization of fomite transmission. Recommendations for the management of FECV are consistent with this process, though this does not imply that litterboxes should go unmonitored. Frequent removal of feces even for the individual cat is important for decreasing viral load, minimizing stress, and maintaining appropriate feline hygiene.

If a cat is diagnosed with FIP, the standard recommendation for owners and foster homes has been to avoid introducing a new cat into that environment for two months (Addie 2012; Drechsler et al. 2011). This highly conservative approach reflects the survival time of FECV in a dry, perfect environment and assumes the risk that (i) the strain of FECV shed into the setting is a high-risk strain or (ii) the rare FIPV that transmits horizontally. In the shelter environment, it is not necessary to close down spaces for any longer than it takes to clean and disinfect them well. This issue is more readily addressed by deep and thorough sanitation of all areas used by the affected cat, along with the disposal of items that cannot be disinfected.

16.10.3 Housing and Husbandry

Because kittens have been shown to shed higher levels of FECV than adult cats, and are more prone to developing FIP, housing large groups of kittens communally is not advised. Instead, kittens should be housed with littermates or in select pairs in the case of singletons, and in enclosures that are easily cleaned and disinfected. Cats exhibiting or recovering from diarrhea should be a priority for individual housing rather than sharing spaces with healthy cats. When possible, kittens and cats exhibiting diarrhea should be given disposable litterboxes, which should be disposed of and replaced when soiled; this aids in preventing the accumulation of virus within the enclosure.

Shelters that have communal housing should avoid introducing cats that have recently recovered from infectious disease to new groups or difficult to clean enclosures. Group-housed cats should be in small, well-adapted groups with sufficient resources and square footage per cat and monitored for signs of stress or disease. Studies recommend enclosures housing individual cats should have greater than nine square feet of floor space per cat (Kessler and Turner 1999; Wagner et al. 2018). Recommendations for group-housed cats cite 18 square feet per cat (Newbury et al. 2010).

Minimizing the unnecessary handling of cats for procedures and cleaning is beneficial by both reducing the potential for handlers to act as fomites and reducing stress to cats.

16.10.4 Management of Co-morbidities

The presence of co-morbidities is a risk factor for increased FECV viral load, shedding, and development of FIP due to compromised immunity. Cats with retroviruses are at greater risk for both higher levels of shedding FECV and development of FIP (Drechsler et al. 2011; Poland et al. 1996).

Practicing preventive medicine for other infectious diseases common in shelters is likely to contribute to some element of control of FECV viral load, in addition to just being a best practice. Physical examination and vaccination at intake with core vaccines (FVRCP most commonly), screening for FeLV and FIV in communally housed cats, and administering prophylactic de-wormers contribute to better host defense mechanisms against endemic viruses such at FCoV. Additionally, cats and kittens with persistent diarrhea should be tested for other common GI pathogens and/or prophylactically treated to minimize damage to intestinal defense mechanisms. Primary rule-outs include panleukopenia, giardiasis, coccidiosis, salmonellosis, and *Trichomonas foetus*, any of which could be contributing to ongoing widespread GI illness in cat populations. Finally, providing consistent, age-appropriate, high-quality, and balanced nutrition supports a healthy GI tract and innate defenses.

16.10.5 Vaccination

Vaccination is not a useful control measure for FECV or FIPV in shelters. Only one vaccine product (Primucell FIP®, Zoetis, USA) has been routinely available and it has demonstrated minimal efficacy at preventing FIP. An IN product, the vaccine is comprised of an attenuated coronavirus that is temperature sensitive and therefore only active in the upper respiratory passages. Theoretically, local immunity at this site of exposure then aids in the prevention of feline coronavirus in the vaccinated patient. The American Animal Hospital Association (AAHA)/American Association of Feline Practitioners (AAFP) Feline Vaccination Guidelines Task Force does not advocate the vaccine's use at this time (Stone et al. 2020).

16.10.6 Diagnostic Testing

Antibody titer testing for FCoV is not useful in the management of shelter populations as a standard practice due to high seroprevalence for antibodies in cats and the likelihood of seroconversion upon entry to the shelter. While it has been demonstrated that seronegative cats do not shed virus, ongoing exposure and influx of new cats into shelters is likely to alter any cat's status at any time. Additionally, only one third of seropositive cats will demonstrate shedding, and so positive serology does not identify chronic shedders of FECV and does not imply anything about the risk of developing FIP (Addie and Jarrett 1992).

16.10.7 Quarantine and Isolation

Quarantine for FECV based on serologic or fecal testing is not an efficacious standard approach in shelters due to several factors: (i) the ubiquitous nature of the virus; (ii) prolonged stays in shelters result in higher rates of many diseases; (iii) the rare incidence of FIPV in FECV infected cats; and (iv) the prolonged incubation period of FIP. Isolation should be reserved for suspected infectious causes of diarrhea. For most shelters, success is best achieved with management and control measures that aim to reduce overall FECV viral load in the shelter, stress on resident cats, and environmental contamination. Management of high-risk animals such as kittens and the immunosuppressed should include efforts to protect them from interactions with high numbers of other cats and to minimize their time in the shelter by fast-tracking (see Chapter 1) them for services, including adoption.

16.11 Outbreak Management

16.11.1 FECV

It is crucial to remember that identification of viral antigen does not definitively diagnose FECV as the causative agent for an outbreak of diarrhea, nor does it suggest anything regarding the probability of a shedder developing FIP. If a shelter is having an endemic issue or outbreak of diarrhea in cats for which other causes have been ruled out (including parasitic, bacterial and other viral causes such as panleukopenia), RT-PCR for FECV can be performed on feces. Most cats who are shedding will cease shedding within weeks to months, and fewer than 5% will develop FIP (Addie 2012; Addie and Jarrett 1992).

In the event of an outbreak of diarrheal disease, management of cats based on clinical signs—while enhancing preventive care strategies, minimizing stress and decreasing pathogen load in the environment—are likely to be more successful than conducting RT-PCR tests on feces. In some specialized settings, particularly sanctuaries or shelters with long-term stays, identification of chronic FECV shedders may play a role in husbandry, housing, or management decisions for particular cases or groups of cats. Elimination of the virus from the animal shelter is not an attainable goal due to the ubiquitous nature of the virus, but the reduction of viral loads and minimizing opportunities for exposure are very much in the realm of shelter practice.

16.11.2 FIPV

Outbreaks of FIPV can be associated with several risk factors within a shelter setting: (i) host-related factors, including age, breed, immune competence, and co-morbidities; (ii) pathogen-related factors, including strain, virulence, and mutability; and (iii) environmental factors, including dose and frequency of exposure, environmental load, overcrowding, and stressors. An outbreak of FIP has been defined as greater than a 10% incidence of FIP in a cattery (Foley et al. 1997b). Even in high-risk environments such as hoarder homes where FCoV is endemic, the incidence of FIP ranges between 5 and 10% (Addie et al. 1995; Foley et al. 1997b). Given that cats in animal shelters are generally not genetically related, a greater than 1% incidence of FIP in a shelter population is commonly used as the breakpoint for concern prompting population level investigation.

FIP outbreaks are more likely to occur in groups of related cats or under conditions in which a particular variant of FCoV prone to FIPV mutation is allowed to reach high viral loads in an already stressed population. An experimentally induced outbreak performed as part of a FIP vaccine trial is very informative regarding FIP outbreaks in shelter populations. Ten FCoV seropositive cats from a shelter were added to a colony of 40 specific-pathogen-free (SPF) cats in a densely-housed laboratory setting mimicking an overcrowded animal shelter employing group housing. Social conflicts between cats were severe, and within one week several cats developed upper respiratory signs. This was followed, starting at six weeks, by a series of cats developing FIP, with 45% (23/50) of cats overall succumbing to the disease (Kipar and Meli 2014). The attack rate of FIP in this experiment was much higher than previously reported outbreaks and distinguished by its intensity. However, this experimental epidemic using field virus and methods of natural infection lends support to the principle that outbreaks of FIP are more likely to be severe with conditions of overcrowding, high pathogen loads, co-morbidities, and social stressors. There is some thought that horizontal transmission could have played a role in this scenario, though this was not confirmed (Kipar and Meli 2014). Only one confirmed instance of an outbreak due to horizontal transmission of an identical FIPV (based on sequencing) between unrelated cats has been published (Wang et al. 2013).

Given the complexities of the FECV to FIPV transformation, as well as FIP diagnosis and testing, management of an outbreak in a shelter is not straightforward. However, confronting the outbreak still involves efforts similar to the management of other agents: risk assessment, reduction of the pathogen in the environment, and establishing a clean break between affected and new populations of cats to eliminate the likelihood of transmission of the associated FCoV variant if it is believed to be particularly virulent. Likewise, instituting new practices to reduce risk factors previously described would also be important on a population level. Fortunately, FIP outbreaks tend to be sporadic and self-limiting, especially when general control measures are in place.

In the event of an unusual outbreak of FIP in a shelter, laboratory confirmation of cases and molecular sequencing of the virus can augment other forms of diagnostic testing. Confirmation of horizontal transmission of FIPV relies on finding a significant rate of identical point mutations associated with FIP in commonly exposed cats that cannot be explained by other investigative measures; this is specialty-level testing not commercially available. Shelters are encouraged to contact academic shelter medicine programs and/or veterinary diagnostic laboratories for investigation assistance and current testing advice, especially given the rapidly changing nature of testing with ongoing developments.

16.12 Euthanasia Guidelines

16.12.1 FECV

Neither diagnosis of FCoV exposure via serology nor confirmation of FECV shedding via RT-PCR predicts the development of FIP. Therefore, neither of these tests should be used as a basis for euthanasia. FCoVs are ubiquitous, and FECV tends to be self-limiting. Chronic diarrhea compromising quality of life is likely due to other disease processes rather than FECV and requires further investigation.

16.12.2 FIP

Untreated FIP is still considered uniformly fatal. Since experimental treatments are not readily available and clinical signs and progression of the disease in FIPV-infected cats are usually rapid and severe, shelter cats with FIP are generally humanely euthanized to prevent the suffering that occurs with end-stage disease. Necropsy is advised to confirm the diagnosis, especially when littermates are present for whom diagnostic confirmation is relevant.

16.13 Client Education/ Implications for Adoption, Relocation and Foster Care

Though the incidence of FIP is generally low, statistically speaking, shelters and rescue groups will inadvertently place a small number of apparently healthy kittens that will go on to develop FIP in adoptive homes despite their best efforts. The emotional and financial impact can be traumatic for adopters and may reflect poorly on the shelter if not handled professionally and with transparency. Empathetic and timely communication with the adopter regarding illness and the nature of the disease, the steps taken by the shelter to minimize risks to the cats and kittens in their care, and a willingness to perform confirmatory diagnostics or provide other assistance can go a long way to maintain positive relationships in the community. Additionally, sometimes offering to refund adoption fees, provide some financial assistance with veterinary bills when appropriate, or to provide another kitten at a later date can be gratefully received by adopters.

Based on the fact that FCoV can live up to seven weeks in a dry environment, a conservative recommendation is to wait two months before introducing a new cat to a foster or adoptive environment where a cat with FIP has been housed. However, the virus is also highly susceptible to common cleaners and disinfectants, and so this waiting period may be shorter depending on the surfaces and conditions where the cat was kept and the ability and willingness of the caregiver to diligently sanitize the environment. New litterboxes should be provided, and washable materials laundered.

16.13.1 Management of Littermates of FIP Positive Cats

The most common question that shelter medicine practitioners face regarding FIP concerns outcomes for littermates of kittens with confirmed FIP. Even though the most common presentation of FIP is not thought to be contagious, in rare instances, transmission of FIPV has been documented between cats. Furthermore, genetic predisposition is thought to play an important role in the pathogenesis of FECV to FIP, as well as the immune-mediated response and amplification of the clinical signs. Therefore, it follows that littermates of FIP-affected kittens and young cats are at higher risk for developing FIP. Development of the disease can occur quickly, or months and even years later. Strategies for addressing this risk fall into several categories based on shelter policy, mission, and resources.

16.13.1.1 Adoption with Full Disclosure

Littermates of kittens that have developed FIP are considered at greater risk for developing FIP themselves due to (i) exposure to a higher FCoV viral load, (ii) exposure to a variant that has demonstrated mutations, and/or (iii) potentially a genetic predisposition. However, most siblings will not develop FIP. Adoption of healthy littermates is a reasonable humane outcome for these kittens and messaging to adopters is key.

Shelters adopting out littermates of FIP-affected kittens and cats are advised to disclose the familial history as well as the increased risk for FIP-related illness to potential adopters. In addition, these kittens and cats should be in good health, having been carefully monitored and screened for signs of FECV and/or FIP-related disease. Those demonstrating ongoing medical signs—including diarrhea, slow weight gain, or general un-thriftiness —are not candidates for adoption during the time of their illness except in rare circumstances with full disclosure to a committed adopter assuming full responsibility for their care.

16.13.1.2 Limited Quarantine

Though the incubation period for FIP can be months or years, often in kittens for whom effusive FIP is more common it can be weeks. Therefore, in specific cases, some shelters elect short-term (two to four weeks) quarantine or foster for littermates of kittens that have developed FIP. This quarantine period allows for intense veterinary monitoring for early signs of FIP development and may reduce the risk of adopting out kittens with FIP in the short term. However, the time to disease development can be significantly longer, even years, and so this practice, while providing minimal mitigation of risk, will still result in a sub-set of kittens breaking with FIP after placement.

In risk-averse shelters, long-term foster has been used as a quarantine for kittens and young cats at particular risk; shelters should always keep in mind their capacity for care and humane animal welfare. Given that, in some cases, the incubation time to FIP development is years, there is never a point at which cats can be considered "cleared" of risk and adopted without disclosure. A shelter is likely best served by addressing this challenge early on and placing the animal with full disclosure. Overcrowding the shelter or foster care in order to save these kittens may result in more disease and suffering, rather than less.

16.13.1.3 Euthanasia

In some cases, when the shelter's population, community, and available resources do not support adoption with disclosure, euthanasia of littermates may be necessary to avoid long-term holding under less than humane conditions and/or overcrowding of facilities. If kittens are healthy, shelters are encouraged to provide lifesaving outcomes for these kittens while maintaining the shelter's capacity for care. This can often be accomplished by working with community partners with greater capacity or resources; providing complete information and medical history to adopters, foster homes, and/or rescue groups or other transfer partners is essential.

16.13.2 Management of Non-related (Non-sibling) Kittens

Unless the shelter has experienced one of the rare outbreaks of what may be a highly virulent form of FECV or a transmissible form of FIPV, non-sibling kittens and cats exposed to a cat with FIP are considered to be at no increased risk for developing FIP. Therefore, it is reasonable for shelters to adopt them out via standard procedures.

16.13.3 Management of Large Groups of Cats of with Unknown Genetic Relationships

Cats that are part of hoarding cases and other large groups of intermingled cats can be difficult to assess for the risk of FIP development if there is a high incidence of disease in the population but unknown genetic relationships. Kittens and cats in these scenarios are at greater risk for many diseases due to high viral loads, poor environmental conditions, physiological stressors, compromised immune status, and co-morbidities. Assessing the risk of developing FIP for the individual cat in the affected population can be aided by thorough physical exams, an analysis of age categories and potential sibling relationships, and monitoring during the time of intake and assessment into the shelter for any early signs of FIP-related disease. Additionally, in many cases, these cats will have co-morbidities (both behavioral and medical) that may need to be disclosed to adopters. Language for these disclosures should capture any concerns one might have about ongoing prognoses for these cats based on their history, but should also express gratitude for adopters willing to give these cats the best chance at a long-term humane outcome.

Advances in testing may someday make it possible to more readily type and/or genetically sequence FECVs and determine the likelihood of FIPV development in a particular kitten or cat based on this information. Until then, shelters are, at minimum, advised to disclose to potential adopters whatever concerns they may hold based on the information they have at the time of adoption.

16.13.4 Risk to Other Species

Neither FECV nor FIPV are considered zoonotic diseases. However, of the companion animal species, both dogs and ferrets have their own GI coronaviruses and dogs can share with their feline companions. Canine coronaviruses are frequently transmitted between cats and dogs, with CCoV considered a contributor in the evolution of Type II FCoV. Species separation in shelters, advised for medical and behavioral reasons, should eliminate this risk in shelter populations.

Ferrets have two manifestations of coronavirus: epizootic catarrhal enteritis, and infectious peritonitis. The latter manifestation is very similar to FIP of cats, but as the ferret coronavirus is genetically distinct from FECV, cross-infection is not expected to occur. Nonetheless, due to the mutability of RNA viruses such as coronavirus, theoretically, it could occur. To date, there are no reported cases of transmission of coronavirus between cats and ferrets.

16.14 Conclusion

While grave, the diagnosis of effusive FIP in kittens and young cats in shelters is not typically difficult to make. Given that entrance into a shelter is already a risk factor, the signalment, history, and pertinent clinical signs—particularly when accompanied by a stereotypical abdominal effusion—readily lead to a reasonable presumptive diagnosis. Other aspects are more difficult in a shelter: managing populations at risk, including littermates; communicating with stakeholders; and managing environmental conditions in challenged facilities. Additional challenges exist in the diagnosis of cases on the non-effusive end of the spectrum, which commonly present with a chronic myriad of non-specific signs; these may evade diagnosis for extended periods, only to be determined on necropsy.

Fueled by technological advances, investigational work related to diagnosis and treatment of FIP has accelerated in the last decade, particularly in the areas of genetic sequencing and molecular diagnostics. The ultimate goal is an ante-mortem test on minimally invasive samples (e.g. fecal or blood samples) capable of detecting FIPV and distinguishing it from FECV. A test of this nature would be useful in early identification of disease, though it would not affect the outcome for FIPV-infected cats. The second goal is an accessible and effective treatment for FIP.

Nonetheless, particularly in a shelter environment, the old cliché rings true that an ounce of prevention is worth a pound of cure, and this is where best practices in animal sheltering shine. Elimination of FCoV in a shelter is an unattainable goal, but all of the standard shelter medicine strategies—capacity for care management, low-stress handling and husbandry, sanitation and disinfection, and a comprehensive approach to the medical and behavioral health of shelter animals—are effective means by which to decrease viral load and the overall level of disease, including that caused by FCoV. In the event of an outbreak, shelters are reminded to reach out to programs designed to help them: academic shelter medicine programs and veterinary diagnostic laboratories with access to cutting-edge researchers. Because of the degree of interest in this complex disease, resources are often available to provide both practical steps in shelter management and supplemental testing that aids an individual shelter while advancing the work of the profession. Likewise, ongoing pharmaceutical developments suggest that treatment for FIP may be available in the near future and worth watching for as part of the management of this disease in shelter populations.

References

Addie, D.D. (2012). Feline coronavirus infections. In: *Infectious Diseases of the Dog and Cat*, 4e (ed. C.E. Greene), 92–108. St. Louis: Saunders.

Addie, D.D. and Jarrett, O. (1992). A study on naturally occurring feline coronavirus infections in kittens. *Veterinary Record* 130: 133–137.

Addie, D.D., Toth, S., Murray, G.D. et al. (1995). Risk of feline infectious peritonitis in cats naturally infected with feline coronavirus. *American Journal of Veterinary Research* 56: 429–434.

Addie, D.D. (2000). Clustering of feline coronaviruses in multi-cat households. *Veterinary Journal* 159: 8–9.

Benetka, V., Kübber-Heiss, A., Kolodziejek, J. et al. (2004). Prevalence of feline coronavirus types I and II in cats with histopathologically verified feline infectious peritonitis. *Veterinary Microbiology* 99 (1): 31–42.

Cave, T.A., Golder, M.C., Simpson, J. et al. (2004). Risk factors for feline coronavirus seropositivity in cats relinquished to a UK rescue charity. *Journal of Feline Medicine and Surgery* 6 (2): 53–58.

Center, S.A. (2012). Fluid accumulation disorders. In: *Small Animal Clinical Diagnosis by Laboratory Methods*, 5e (eds. M.D. Willard and H. Tvedten), 232. St. Louis: Elsevier.

Chang, H.W., de Groot, R.J., Egberink, H.F. et al. (2010). Feline infectious peritonitis: insights into feline coronavirus pathobiogenesis and epidemiology based on genetic analysis of the viral 3c gene. *Journal of General Virology* 91 (2): 415–420.

Doki, T., Takano, T., Kawagoe, K. et al. (2016). Therapeutic effect of anti-feline TNF-alpha monoclonal antibody for feline infectious peritonitis. *Research in Veterinary Science* 104: 17–23.

Drechsler, Y., Alcaraz, A., Bossong, F.J. et al. (2011). Feline coronavirus in multi-cat environments. *The Veterinary Clinics of North America. Small Animal Practice* 41 (6): 1133–1169.

Dunbar, D., Kwok, W., Graham, E. et al. (2019). Diagnosis of non-effusive feline infectious peritonitis by reverse transcriptase quantitative PCR from mesenteric lymph node fine needle aspirates. *Journal of Feline Medicine and Surgery* 21 (10): 910–921.

Felten, S. and Hartmann, K. (2019). Diagnosis of feline infectious peritonitis: a review of the current literature. *Viruses* 11: 1068.

Fischer, Y., Sauter-Louis, C., and Hartmann, K. (2012). Diagnostic accuracy of the Rivalta test for feline infectious peritonitis. *Veterinary Clinical Pathology* 41 (4): 558–567.

Foley, J.E., Poland, A., Carlson, J. et al. (1997a). Patterns of feline coronavirus infection and fecal shedding from cats in multiple-cat environments. *Journal of the American*

Veterinary Medical Association 210: 1307–1312.

Foley, J.E., Poland, A., Carlson, J. et al. (1997b). Risk factors for feline infectious peritonitis among cats in multiple-cat environments with endemic feline enteric coronavirus. *Journal of the American Veterinary Medical Association* 210: 1313–1318.

Giordano, A., Paltrinieri, S., Bertazzolo, W. et al. (2005). Sensitivity of Tru-cut and fine-needle aspiration biopsies of liver and kidney for diagnosis of feline infectious peritonitis. *Veterinary Clinical Pathology* 34 (4): 368–374.

Gross, D. (2015). How Kitty Litter went from happy accident to $ 2 billion industry. Washington Post. https://www.washingtonpost.com/national/health-science/you-wont-believe-how-old-that-kitty-litter-is/2015/02/02/9ecac9ea-a1b4-11e4-903f-9f2faf7cd9fe_story.html?utm_term=.5fb19fc9303d (accessed 23 April 2020).

Hartmann, K. (2016). Feline Infectious Peritonitis: New developments in pathogenesis, diagnosis, and management. Fred Scott Feline Health Symposium, Ithaca, NY.

Hartmann, K., Binder, C., Hirschberger, J. et al. (2003). Comparison of different tests to diagnose feline infectious peritonitis. *Journal of Veterinary Internal Medicine / American College of Veterinary Internal Medicine* 17 (6): 781–790.

Holzworth, J.E. (1963). Some important disorders of cats. *The Cornell Veterinarian* 53: 157–160.

Karsten, C., Wagner, D.C., Kass, P.H. et al. (2017). An observational study of the relationship between capacity for care as an animal shelter management model and cat health, adoption and death in three animal shelters. *The Veterinary Journal* 227: 15–22.

Kessler, M.R. and Turner, D.C. (1999). Effects of density and cage size on stress in domestic cats (Felis Silvestris Catus) housed in animal shelters and boarding catteries. *Animal Welfare* 8 (3): 259–269.

Kim, Y., Liu, H., Kankanamalage, A.C.G. et al. (2016). Reversal of the progression of fatal coronavirus infection in cats by a broad-spectrum coronavirus protease inhibitor. *PLoS Pathogens* 12 (3): 1–18.

Kipar, A. and Meli, M.L. (2014). Feline infectious peritonitis: still an enigma? *Veterinary Pathology* 51 (2): 505–526.

Legendre, A.M., Kuritz, T., Galyon, G. et al. (2017). Polyprenyl immunostimulant treatment of cats with presumptive feline infectious peritonitis in a field study. *Frontiers in Veterinary Science* 14: 1–16. https://doi.org/10.3389/fvets.2017.00007.

Litster, A.L., Pogranichniy, R., and Lin, T. (2013). Diagnostic utility of a direct immunofluorescence test to detect feline coronavirus antigen in macrophages in effusive feline infectious peritonitis. *The Veterinary Journal* 198 (2): 362–366.

Luria, B.J., Levy, J.K., Lappin, M.R. et al. (2004). Prevalence of infectious diseases in feral cats in northern Florida. *Journal of Feline Medicine and Surgery* 6 (5): 287–296.

Murphy, B.G., Perron, M., Bauer, K. et al. (2018). The nucleoside analog GS-441524 strongly inhibits feline infectious peritonitis (FIP) virus in tissue culture and experimental cat studies. *Veterinary Microbiology* 219: 226–233.

Newbury, S., Blinn, M.K., Bushby, P.A. et al. (2010). Guidelines for standards of care in animal shelters. *The Association of Shelter Veterinarians.*: 1–45.

Pedersen, N.C. (2009). A review of feline infectious peritonitis virus infection: 1963-2008. *Journal of Feline Medicine and Surgery* 11 (4): 225–258.

Pedersen, N.C. (2014a). An update on feline infectious peritonitis: virology and immunopathogenesis. *The Veterinary Journal* 201 (2): 123–132.

Pedersen, N.C. (2014b). An update on feline infectious peritonitis: diagnostics and therapeutics. *The Veterinary Journal* 201 (2): 133–141.

Pedersen, N.C., Sato, R., Foley, J.E. et al. (2004). Common virus infections in cats, before and after being placed in shelters, with emphasis on feline enteric coronavirus. *Journal of Feline Medicine and Surgery* 6 (2): 83–88.

Pedersen, N.C., Allen, C.E., Lyons, L.A. et al. (2008). Pathogenesis of feline enteric coronavirus infection. *Journal of Feline Medicine and Surgery* 10: 529–541.

Pedersen, N.C., Liu, H., Scarlett, J. et al. (2012). Feline infectious peritonitis: role of the feline coronavirus 3c gene in intestinal tropism and pathogenicity based upon isolates from resident and adopted shelter cats. *Virus Research* 165 (1): 17–28.

Pedersen, N.C., Liu, H., Gandolfi, B. et al. (2014). The influence of age and genetics on natural resistance to experimentally induced feline infectious peritonitis. *Veterinary Immunology and Immunopathology* 162 (1–2): 33–40.

Pedersen, N.C., Liu, H., Durden, M. et al. (2016). Natural resistance to experimental feline infectious peritonitis virus infection is decreased rather than increased by positive genetic selection. *Veterinary Immunology and Immunopathology* 171: 17–20.

Pedersen, N.C., Kim, Y., Liu, H. et al. (2018). Efficacy of a 3c-like protease inhibitor in treating various forms of acquired feline infectious peritonitis. *Journal of Feline Medicine and Surgery* 20 (4): 378–392.

Pedersen, N.C., Perron, M., Bannasch, M. et al. (2019). Efficacy and safety of the nucleoside analog GS-441524 for treatment of cats with naturally occurring feline infectious peritonitis. *Journal of Feline Medicine and Surgery* 21 (4): 271–281.

Poland, A.M., Vennema, H., Foley, J.E. et al. (1996). Two related strains of feline infectious peritonitis virus isolated from immunocompromised cats infected with a feline enteric coronavirus. *Journal of Clinical Microbiology* 34 (12): 3180–3184.

Porter, E., Tasker, S., Day, M.J. et al. (2014). Amino acid changes in the spike protein of feline coronavirus correlate with systemic spread of virus from the intestine and not with feline infectious peritonitis. *Veterinary Research* 45 (1): 1–11.

Potkay, S., Bacher, J.D., and Pitts, T.W. (1974). Feline infectious peritonitis in a closed breeding colony. *Laboratory Animal Science* 24: 279–289.

Ritz, S., Egberink, H., and Hartmann, K. (2007). Effect of feline interferon-omega on the survival time and quality of life of cats with feline infectious peritonitis. *Journal of Veterinary Internal Medicine* 21 (6): 1193–1197.

Stone, A.E.S., Brummet, G.O., Carozza, E.M. et al. (2020). 2020 AAHA/AAFP Feline Vaccination Guideilnes. *Journal of the American Animal Hospital Association* 56 (5): 249–265.

Tekes, G. and Thiel, H.J. (2016). *Feline Coronaviruses*, 1e. Elsevier Inc.

Thiel, V., Thiel, H.J., and Tekes, G. (2014 Nov 2). Tackling feline infectious peritonitis via reverse genetics. *Bioengineered.* 5 (6): 396–400.

Vennema, H., Poland, A., Foley, J. et al. (1998). Feline infectious peritonitis viruses arise by mutation from endemic feline enteric coronaviruses. *Virology* 243 (1): 150–157.

Wagner, D.C., Kass, P.H., and Hurley, K.F. (2018). Cage size, movement in and out of housing during daily care, and other environmental and population health risk factors of feline upper respiratory disease in nine North American animal shelters. *PLoS One* 13 (1): e0190140. https://doi.org/10.1371/journal.pone.0190140.

Wang, Y.T., Su, B.L., Hsieh, L.E. et al. (2013). An outbreak of feline infectious peritonitis in a Taiwanese shelter: epidemiologic and molecular evidence for horizontal transmission of a novel type II feline coronavirus. *Veterinary Research* 44 (1): 1–9.

Watt, N.J., MacIntyre, N.J., and McOrist, S. (1993). An extended outbreak of infectious peritonitis in a closed colony of European wildcats (*Felis silvestris*). *Journal of Comparative Pathology* 108: 73–79.

Worthing, K.A., Wigney, D.I., Dhand, N.K. et al. (2012). Risk factors for feline infectious peritonitis in Australian cats. *Journal of Feline Medicine and Surgery* 14 (6): 405–412.

Zoia, A., Slater, L.A., Heller, J. et al. (2009). A new approach to pleural effusion in cats: markers for distinguishing transudates from exudates. *Journal of Feline Medicine and Surgery* 11 (10): 847–855.

17

Internal Parasites

Dwight D. Bowman[1], *Araceli Lucio-Forster*[1], *and Stephanie Janeczko*[2]

[1] *Cornell University College of Veterinary Medicine, Ithaca, NY, USA*
[2] *Shelter Medicine Services, American Society for the Prevention of Cruelty to Animals (ASPCA), New York, NY, USA*

17.1 Introduction

Many of the animals that enter shelters come from a variety of sources, including stray, neglect and abuse situations, and owner surrenders; therefore, the likelihood of internal parasitism will vary greatly and can be difficult to predict. The number and type of parasites in any given host are influenced by a great number of factors, including the host in question (e.g. cat, dog, human), their age, previous exposures to risk factors such as predation and vector access, and the geographic region where they have resided. While some common internal parasites cause significant clinical signs, are easily transmissible, and have public health significance, many of the more unusual parasites are unlikely to be transmitted between animals in a shelter environment.

The goals for the control and management of parasites in a shelter setting will differ greatly depending on the type of shelter and population in question. For example, the concerns are different for shelters where animals are held long term and shelters where animals have short lengths of stay. The objective may be to make the animal as parasite-free as possible in the short holding time prior to adoption, or it may be to ensure the animal has no parasites that could be detrimental to the health of the other animals housed in the facility.

Animal housing within the shelter may also impact the likelihood of parasite transmission and their potential to become established in the shelter environment. Parasites in animals housed individually in areas that can be easily and routinely sanitized will not usually have the opportunity for further transmission; however, parasites in animals that are group-housed and/or have access to play yards with grass and soil, which are more easily contaminated with excrement, will have much greater potential for transmission and establishment in the environment. Thus, different types of shelters may have different goals and concerns with respect to parasite treatment, control and prevention programs, and a tailored approach is often necessary. It is very difficult to weigh all the different aspects of control and prevention and still provide an all-encompassing programmatic plan.

There are three major concerns of shelters relative to parasites. The first concern is to protect the individual animal's health while preventing the introduction of parasites that will

Infectious Disease Management in Animal Shelters, Second Edition.
Edited by Lila Miller, Stephanie Janeczko, and Kate F. Hurley.

adversely affect the overall health of the shelter population and contaminate the environment. Many parasites of companion animals require time in the environment to mature to the infective stage, or may require additional hosts for such maturation; therefore, proper sanitation and housing that prevents prey or vector access to facilities can greatly reduce transmission in such shelter settings. The second concern is to protect the shelter's staff, visitors, and adopters from potentially zoonotic agents carried by the animals. The third concern is to ensure that untreated parasites in a dog or cat will not reduce the animal's chance of adoption and/or retention in a new home due to post-adoption treatment needs.

The goal of this chapter is to provide some guidance to help alleviate these concerns through the consideration of treatment options and the review of pertinent information regarding the internal parasites of cats and dogs. Due to space constraints and the availability of labeled products and well-established treatment protocols for many of the common parasites of cats and dogs, a detailed treatment discussion for these infections is not included here. For those parasites for which no treatments are approved, some guidance will be provided, but for up-to-date treatment recommendations veterinarians should consult resources such as the Companion Animal Parasite Council (CAPC: www.capcvet.org), the Merck Veterinary Manual (www.merckvetmanual.com), and the latest edition of Blackwell's Five-Minute Veterinary Consult Clinical Companion: Canine and Feline Infectious Diseases and Parasitology. For more information regarding other feline and canine parasites, or for more detailed information on the parasites discussed here, including their biology, specifics for diagnosis, identification, and clinical manifestations of the disease, the reader is directed to the many texts on veterinary and diagnostic parasitology.

17.2 Parasite Transmission and Treatment Considerations in Animal Shelters

As previously mentioned, there are three concurrent goals related to the initial diagnosis and treatment of internal parasitic infections and infestations of shelter animals when they arrive at a facility: preparing the individual animals for adoption, limiting zoonoses, and protecting the other animals within the facility from new infections, which includes preventing environmental contamination. Due to the large and diverse group of parasites that could potentially enter a facility, there is no single recommendation that can be applied to every shelter. Instead, each shelter must consider several factors when determining how to meet the goals. These factors include determining the prevalence of parasites in the region and evaluating the resources available for diagnostics and providing treatment to the shelter's animals. Thus, shelters are left with the conundrums of how much of a diagnostic work-up is sufficient, how much treatment can be afforded, and how much treatment is necessary. There are, unfortunately, no simple or straightforward answers to these questions. One must develop a general scheme of operation with the goal of optimizing prevention and conserving resources for the diagnosis and treatment of sick animals.

There are several prophylactic therapies that shelters can consider to achieve their goals. The most common recommendation and practice for the control of internal parasites in shelter animals is to treat all animals at intake with pyrantel pamoate, as roundworms and hookworms are nearly ubiquitous, both are zoonotic, and roundworm eggs are extremely difficult to remove from the environment. This is a cost-effective approach even for very high-volume shelters. If additional treatments for other intestinal parasites, such as whipworms and tapeworms, are cost-prohibitive, these can be reserved for adoptable animals and/or those for whom diagnostics have been performed. The use of fenbendazole is another option, but because it requires treatment for three consecutive days, it may be infeasible in shelters where the time of intake may be the only opportunity to provide treatment to an individual animal.

In shelters with additional resources that desire broader spectrum coverage, treatment with Drontal® Plus (pyrantel, febantel, and praziquantel) for dogs, or for cats, Drontal® (pyrantel and praziquantel) or Profender® (emodepside and praziquantel) will provide the broadest coverage against internal parasites. These products will treat and remove most intestinal nematodes, tapeworms, and the unusual intestinal trematode. A product with an almost equivalent spectrum of activity is Panacur® (fenbendazole), which will provide treatment for everything except for *Dipylidium* and *Echinococcus* tapeworms; it will also remove a few of the more unusual worms from dogs. Though not approved for cats, fenbendazole at the same dose used for dogs is also excellent for general purpose use. It should be noted that Drontal® Plus adds very substantially to the cost of prophylactic treatment, to the point that its cost becomes prohibitive for many shelters.

The presence of tapeworm segments in an animal's stool can be disconcerting to owners, so some shelters elect to treat these animals if they are being placed for adoption regardless of confirmation of infection. These parasites are often difficult to diagnose because the segments are only shed by dogs and cats sporadically. Treatment with the cestocidal dose of praziquantel also removes most intestinal dwelling trematodes from dogs and cats.

There are many monthly heartworm preventive products that will treat internal parasites as well as provide protection against heartworms. (A comprehensive list of products is at https://capcvet.org/parasite-product-applications/.) Monthly heartworm preventive products all vary slightly as to their ability to control internal parasites, both in spectra of activity and in their ability to kill developing forms of the parasites. Some also provide protection against ectoparasites while providing treatment of intestinal infections. The choice of product will be based largely upon availability, price, and the spectrum of activity required as determined by the attending veterinarian in the shelter. The authors of this chapter are of a very firm conviction that it is inappropriate to use these heartworm preventive products long-term, instead of melarsomine dihydrochloride, for the treatment of adult heartworms in heartworm-positive animals, except under extreme conditions. Resistant strains of heartworm have been documented, and the risk posed by expanding or widespread prevalence of these strains is significant (Kryda et al. 2019; McTier et al. 2019); judicious use of heartworm preventives, adulticidal products, and diagnostics is more important than ever. Further discussion of heartworm disease and preventives can be found in Chapter 18.

The focus of shelter treatment must remain on the parasites that cause disease in the animal, contaminate the shelter's environment, pose a significant risk of zoonosis, or readily spread between animals. Thus, when designing the ideal shelter parasite control protocol in order to prepare an animal for adoption, the plan should include (i) treatment for external parasites (covered in Chapter 19), (ii) administration of antiparasiticides to treat the majority of the common internal parasites, and (iii) for dogs, determination of heartworm status and treatment of adult infection (including microfilarial clearance). Adopters can then be informed about any initial treatment for these parasites and be advised the animal may need additional medications and/or diagnostics to complete treatment. They should be encouraged to set up a post-adoption appointment with a veterinarian to develop a preventive medicine program appropriate for the pet and new owner.

The parasites that may enter shelters are broadly of two types: (i) parasites that have direct transmission (requiring only a single host to complete their life cycle and produce progeny that can then infect others), and (ii) parasites with indirect transmission (requiring at least two different hosts to complete their development). Those with direct life cycles may be capable of immediate infection as soon as they are passed in feces or they may require further maturation to an infective state in the environment. Parasites that require more than one host are less likely to be transmitted or become established within the shelter environment than are those that require a single type of host (i.e. cats or dogs). Precise prevalence estimates for the different parasites are unattainable for stray and homeless animals around the country, but some general estimates will be included below for each parasite as it is discussed.

17.3 Parasites with Direct Transmission

Internal parasites that can enter a shelter in an infected host and be efficiently transmitted between animals in the shelter or to humans are of greatest concern. Because many parasitized animals show no outward clinical signs of disease, shelters must be diligent in creating protocols that aim to prevent internal parasites from perpetuating themselves in the population. *Giardia,* trichomonads, and *Cryptosporidium* spp. are among the few intestinal parasites encountered in the shelter environment that are immediately infectious. Other parasites such as *Toxoplasma gondii*, intestinal coccidia (*Cystoisospora* spp.), *Toxocara* spp., *Ancylostoma* spp., *Strongyloides stercoralis*, and *Trichuris vulpis* are perhaps more commonly encountered in shelter animals but require time outside the host to become infectious. Though these more common parasites are not immediately infective, they can still spread efficiently in several ways: they may have stages that are transmitted to puppies or kittens in utero or in milk, stages that can be ingested if animals have access to prey, or have resistant stages that persist under certain environmental conditions for months to years. Furthermore, some of these parasites have stages that can persist in host tissues, and may, in the case of some nematodes, repopulate the intestines and produce eggs detectable in a fecal examination weeks after a previous exam revealed no eggs of the same parasite. Most of these more common parasites have a very difficult time completing their life cycles in a shelter environment unless there are areas such as grass, soil, dirt, or other materials that are difficult to sanitize. If dogs and cats have access to such areas, a perpetual cycle of infection may be created.

17.3.1 Parasites with Immediate Transmission

17.3.1.1 Protozoa

17.3.1.1.1 Giardia *Giardia* is a common flagellate of the intestine of mammals. There are multiple host-associated species and types. *Giardia* is commonly present in cats, dogs, and humans, but different *Giardia* types, or "Assemblages," are present in each of these hosts. There is discussion, and support from these authors, for reclaiming the original species designations for the *Giardia* in cats and dogs, i.e. *Giardia cati* and *Giardia canis*, respectively (Ryan and Caccio 2013). Zoonotic concern with respect to this parasite is minimal and there has been no conclusive evidence of zoonotic transmission to humans from cats and dogs (Bowman and Lucio-Forster 2010; Tysnes et al. 2014). Infection in cats and dogs is common; prevalence varies by age and between shelter and pet populations but is generally reported to be around 10–15% (Bowman and Lucio-Forster 2010).

Infections are commonly asymptomatic but may also be present in association with diarrhea. Clinical signs are most likely to be present in young animals or those that have been unexposed for long periods and are then reinfected. Cysts shed by infected animals are immediately infective to other cats or dogs, and thus prompt removal of feces from the environment to reduce environmental contamination and the opportunity for coprophagy can help stem transmission.

Eradication of *Giardia* from a shelter population is probably impossible and not necessary, so efforts should be focused on preventing contamination of the environment. Thoroughly drying surfaces is recommended, as cysts are more likely to remain viable in cool, moist environments. Treatment for this parasite should be limited to animals exhibiting clinical signs associated with a diagnosed infection. Treatments that may be of some use are fenbendazole 50 mg/kg orally (PO), once daily (SID) for three to five days (cats and dogs), metronidazole 10–25 mg/kg twice a day (BID) for five to seven days alone or in combination with fenbendazole (cats and dogs), and Drontal® Plus at the labeled treatment dose but given once daily for three days (dogs). Bathing the animal upon completion of treatment is recommended to prevent inadvertent reinfection, particularly in dogs.

Giardia trophozoites may be evidenced in a saline wet mount preparation of fresh, nonrefrigerated diarrheal feces; *Giardia* trophozoites must be differentiated from trichomonad organisms that may be present in such samples. Detection of *Giardia* cysts is best accomplished using fecal centrifugal flotation in a 1.18 specific gravity zinc sulfate solution, though experienced microscopists may also be able to identify them in a sucrose centrifugal flotation. Antigen testing (either point-of-care or reference laboratory) for this parasite is only recommended to rule in this parasitic differential as a cause of diarrhea in a sick animal. Since the treatment of asymptomatic animals is not warranted, antigen tests are not recommended in this population. If clinical signs resolve, further testing in a particular animal is not generally recommended but may be warranted in certain circumstances when managing numerous animals in a shelter population with clinical *Giardia* infection. Because animals treated for *Giardia* that no longer have detectable cyst shedding may still test positive on antigen tests, only centrifugal flotation techniques should be utilized to verify successful treatment in dogs and cats (Janeczko and Griffin 2010, CAPC 2020).

17.3.1.1.2 *Tritrichomonas foetus* (Syn. *T. blagburni*)

Tritrichomonas foetus, sometimes referred to as *Tritrichomonas blagburni,* is a flagellate protozoan of the large bowel of cats and less commonly dogs. It has been associated with large bowel diarrhea in animals exhibiting clinical signs, though asymptomatic infections are commonly present. Diarrhea may be accompanied by mucus and blood and is said to be quite malodorous. Clinical signs do not include systemic manifestations. Purebred cats in cattery situations and those frequenting cat shows are more likely to be infected by this parasite; a prevalence of 31% has been reported in these populations (Gookin et al. 2004). Treatment with ronidazole (30 mg/kg PO SID for 14 days) is the only medication that has been shown to be effective in eliminating *T. foetus* infection, but treatment failures are suspected to be common, with rates reported as high as 20% (Hedgespeth et al. 2020). Because some cats receiving ronidazole develop reversible neurotoxicity, close monitoring is necessary, and treatment should generally be limited to those cats with a confirmed diagnosis of *T. foetus* infection. While clinical signs in untreated cats or those that do not respond to ronidazole may eventually subside, it is unlikely that the infection has resolved and thus these cats may serve as a source of infection for other cats.

An important risk factor for transmission of this parasite is population density, as there are no cysts produced and the trophozoites shed in feces are quite labile in the environment. The main recommendation for prevention and management in a shelter population is the management of population density (Gookin et al. 2004). Though saline wet mounts of fresh fecal material (direct smears) may demonstrate the trophozoites, the sensitivity for this test is quite low; any recovered flagellates would need to be differentiated from other common flagellates, like *Giardia*. Culture of *Tritrichomonas* can increase the chances of detection, but the most sensitive test currently available is PCR. There is no zoonotic risk associated with this infection.

***17.3.1.1.3 Cryptosporidium* spp.** *Cryptosporidium canis* and *Cryptosporidium felis* are the host-adapted species of *Cryptosporidium* present in dogs and cats, respectively. Prevalence of up to 5% for cats (Lucio-Forster and Bowman 2011) in shelter populations and up to 17% for dogs (Uehlinger et al. 2013) have been documented. As with other parasitic infections, these parasites may be present in animals without causing any apparent ill effects, or they may be associated with diarrhea, usually in young or immunosuppressed animals. Infections are self-limiting in immunocompetent hosts, but immunocompromised or immunosuppressed individuals may suffer chronic diarrhea, malnutrition, and potentially death. These two species of parasites have been reported to cause zoonotic infections in people who are immunosuppressed or immunocompromised, but these remain rare events in developed countries (Lucio-Forster et al. 2010; Ryan et al. 2016). Cats and dogs are not hosts for the species typically found in humans, *Cryptosporidium hominis* (the human-associated species) or *Cryptosporidium parvum* (the species in ruminants that routinely causes a number of zoonotic infections in humans). As such, the risk of zoonotic transmission of *Cryptosporidium* from cats and dogs is limited.

Oocysts passed in feces may be demonstrated by fecal smears and staining techniques or sucrose centrifugal flotation with a subsequent examination by experienced personnel, or they may be detected by PCR techniques or fecal-antigen enzyme-linked immunosorbent assay (ELISA). There is no labeled treatment for cryptosporidiosis in cats and dogs and few drugs are consistently effective, but paromomycin (150 mg/kg PO BID for 5 days), tylosin (10–15 mg/kg three times a day [TID] for 14–21 days), and azithromycin (5–10 mg/kg PO BID for 5–7 days (dogs); 7–15 mg/kg PO BID for 5–7 days (cats)) have been used with some success. There is also limited experimental evidence that higher doses of nitazoxanide (75 or 150 mg/kg PO, repeated once in 14 days) may be an effective treatment for cryptosporidiosis in dogs; however, lower doses have not been shown to have similar effects and careful consideration should be given to this treatment option at any dose as it is the only drug approved by the Food and Drug Administration (FDA) for treatment of cryptosporidiosis in humans (Lappin et al. 2008; Moron-Soto et al. 2017). Environmental decontamination through prompt and frequent removal of fecal material should decrease transmission. Unprotected oocysts will dry relatively quickly on solid surfaces but may persist (several months to a year) in cool water or cool and moist environments.

17.3.1.2 Nematodes

There are two nematode genera that have direct life cycles wherein the larvae are infective when they leave the host. One of these, *Ollulanus*, contains small stomach worms that are known to sometimes become problematic in catteries. The other genus, *Filaroides*, parasitizes the respiratory system of dogs and contains two species, one of which, *Filaroides hirthi*, parasitizes the lung parenchyma, and the other, *Filaroides osleri* (synonym = *Oslerus osleri*) occurs within nodules in the trachea and bronchi. If animals are going to remain in the shelter environment for a prolonged period of time, such as in a sanctuary-type setting or if group-housed, attempts should be made to prevent the introduction of these parasites by treating these long-term resident animals with a macrocyclic lactone or, in the case of cats, emodepside/praziquantel (Profender®), followed by quarantine before they are allowed to join the other animals in the facility.

17.3.1.2.1 Ollulanus tricuspis The "cat vomit worm," *O. tricuspis*, is a parasite that is likely to be of limited importance in most cat populations; there is good evidence this worm may be more common in catteries than in the general population (Bell 1984; Caldwell 1984). However, if introduced into a shelter, it could become problematic where cats are housed together for extended periods, as evidenced by the fact that most outbreaks occur in large catteries where animals are housed in groups. Information on general prevalence is lacking as this worm does not have transmission stages passed in feces, and since the adults are only 1 mm in length, they are unlikely to be seen. Transmission seems to be direct through the consumption of infected-cat vomitus containing the infective larvae. Most infected cats do not have clinical signs, but the worms have been shown to cause inflammation along with increased mucus secretion, hemorrhagic gastritis, and hyperplasia of the stomach epithelium. When clinical signs are present, infected cats may present with a history of chronic vomiting that may or may not be associated with wasting, anorexia, and dehydration (Greve 1983). Antemortem diagnosis requires the careful examination of vomitus and stomach irrigation fluids. Though generally not practical in the shelter setting, the diagnosis has also recently been made by gastric biopsy (Cecchi et al. 2006).

Based on one report (Kato et al. 2015), a product containing praziquantel, pyrantel pamoate and febantel with or without ivermectin (150 μg/kg [0.15 mg/kg] subcutaneously [SC] one time) was efficacious in two dogs, and thus might be an appropriate therapy for cats. It is unknown whether cats develop any immunity to the infection. The isolation of known infected animals is recommended to prevent transmission between animals. While it is unlikely to be practical in most shelter situations given the difficulty in establishing an antemortem diagnosis, empirical treatment with a macrocyclic lactone and fenbendazole and isolation may be appropriate when there is strong clinical suspicion of infection in individual cats. Quarantine of incoming animals to observe for signs of this parasite is unlikely to be a successful control strategy. The worms in the vomitus are probably easy to kill with most routine disinfectants. Free larvae on hard surfaces would not survive for more than a few hours and will die rapidly if dehydrated. This parasite is of no zoonotic importance; thus, there are no implications for adoptions or special instructions for adopters.

***17.3.1.2.2 Filaroides* spp.** *F. hirthi* and *F. osleri* are respiratory parasites of dogs. *F. hirthi* is a parasite of the lung parenchyma, while *F. osleri* is found in the trachea and bronchi, and rarely the lungs. Infections with these worms show up periodically in research animal facilities (Vajner et al. 2000; Yao et al. 2011); thus, there is every reason to believe that these pathogens would be of concern in a shelter facility. These worms do not infect humans and there are no implications for adoptions or special instructions for adopters.

Both worms can be difficult to diagnose because the diagnostic stage is the larva that is found in saliva and feces. Thus, cases occur sporadically without any realistic estimate as to what the actual prevalence is in the canine population. Most dogs probably do not show clinical signs of either infection; however, infections with *F. hirthi* can cause dyspnea, nonproductive coughing, exercise intolerance, and other signs of respiratory distress. Fatalities have been described in severely stressed and immunodeficient animals (August et al. 1980; Carrasco et al. 1997). Disease with *F. osleri*, when seen, is characterized by a spasmodic dry cough brought on by exercise. Young dogs tend to be more severely affected and can develop respiratory distress, anorexia, and become emaciated.

Diagnosis of either infection may be accomplished by finding the larvae in the feces using a zinc sulfate centrifugation method flotation or by examination of tracheal wash material. The larvae of *F. hirthi* and *F. osleri* (which are practically indistinguishable from each other) can be differentiated morphologically from other lungworms due to the constriction and a kink just posterior to the end of the tail. Additionally, lung nodules that can be observed by bronchoscope are pathognomonic for infection by *F. osleri*.

Ivermectin (1000 μg/kg [1 mg/kg] once) and albendazole (25 mg/kg BID for five days) are two drugs routinely used to treat infections with *F. hirthi* (Erb and Georgi 1982; Bauer and Bahnemann 1996). Successful treatment with fenbendazole (50 mg/kg SID for 14 days) combined with ivermectin (0.4 mg/kg SC every [q] two weeks for three doses) has also been reported (Cervone et al. 2018). Treated dogs seem to recover very well once the worms are cleared. Anthelmintics used to treat *F. osleri* infections include ivermectin (400 μg/kg [0.4 mg/kg] PO or SC one time) and fenbendazole (50 mg/kg PO, SID, for 10–14 days) (Levitan et al. 1996; Outerbridge and Taylor 1998). Some recommend endoscope-guided debridement of the lesions to the extent possible to improve the success of treatment.

Because the diagnosis is so difficult to make and prevalence is likely to generally be low, quarantine is unlikely to be a workable or desirable means to keep the organism from entering a shelter. If an infection is diagnosed, the affected dog should be isolated, and all exposed dogs should be treated with ivermectin or another effective medication.

When the worms are found in the saliva and feces, they are probably very easy to kill with most routine disinfectants. If the worms are found on a clean surface, they will probably only survive a very few hours or until dry; even in moist soil, they will probably survive only hours to days.

17.3.2 Parasites Requiring some Maturation in the Environment

17.3.2.1 Intestinal Coccidia (*Cystoisospora* spp.)

Intestinal coccidia of the genus *Cystoisospora* are commonly found infecting cats and dogs. These parasites have great host specificity, such that intestinal coccidia of cats (*Cystoisospora felis* and *Cystoisospora rivolta*) do not cause intestinal coccidiosis in other animals (including humans), nor will the intestinal coccidia of dogs (*Cystoisospora canis*, *Cystoisospora ohioensis*, *Cystoisospora neorivolta*, and *Cystoisospora burrowsi*). These protozoans produce oocyst stages that are passed in feces and are not immediately infective (Figure 17.1). They require several hours to days (depending on environmental conditions) to become fully infective to another host. In most situations, daily removal of fecal material will be sufficient to ensure removal of oocysts prior to maturation to infectivity, however, one must consider that under optimal (humid, moist, well-aerated) conditions, oocyst maturation could occur sooner than 24 hours. With daily removal of feces from the environment (and with the absence of vertebrate prey; see below), it is unlikely that transmission can routinely occur in a shelter population. However, oocysts are relatively hardy, and they may persist for several months in moist, contaminated environments.

Coccidia are of most clinical importance in young animals. Crowding, stress, debilitation and/or concurrent infections can increase the

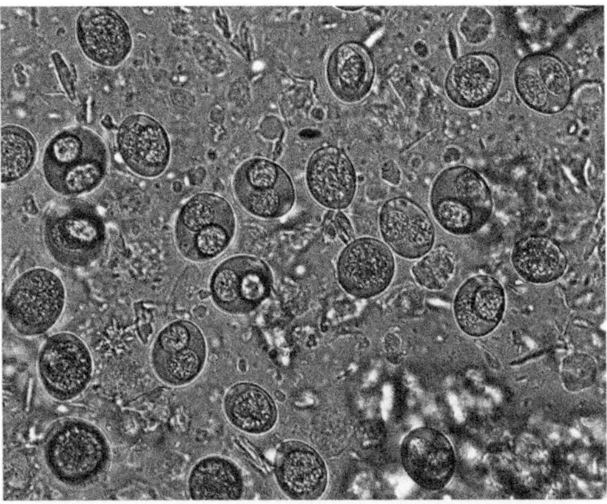

Figure 17.1 *Cystoisospora* spp. oocysts recovered through sucrose centrifugal flotation of a sample submitted for routine fecal examination from a shelter dog.

probability that individuals will have clinical signs associated with infection. Clinical signs may be absent, or include diarrhea, weight loss, anorexia, lethargy, and in extreme cases, death. Coccidial infections are self-limiting and require continuous exposure (i.e. either to infective oocysts from the environment, or the ingestion of rodents that have ingested oocysts and serve to host tissue stages infective to dogs or cats) to maintain infections in an individual. The actual disease of coccidiosis typically occurs in naïve puppies and kittens that are infected through oocyst ingestion. These organisms then greatly amplify their numbers through cycles of replication in intestinal cells, leading to enterocyte destruction and subsequent potential for manifestations of the disease. Eventually, oocysts are produced by the parasite. It is important to recall that the cellular destruction that may lead to disease in the case of many coccidial organisms, including these, occurs before oocyst production, so it is possible for an animal to develop clinical signs before detectable shedding occurs.

No drug is labeled for the treatment or clearance of *Cystoisospora* in cats and dogs. Sulfadimethoxine (50–60 mg/kg PO SID for 14–21 days; after the first dose of 50–60 mg/kg the dose can be halved until the animal is asymptomatic but not to exceed 3 weeks) is labeled for the treatment of bacterial enteritis associated with coccidial infection. Ponazuril, which has coccidiocidal activity, is considered to be the treatment of choice for coccidiosis and is often used at doses ranging from 20 to 50 mg/kg PO SID for one to three days, with or without repeated treatments. Studies have shown that administration of the drug can reduce oocyst numbers, often suppressing them below detectable limits (Charles et al. 2007; Litster et al. 2014). Antimicrobial efficacy is against the stages that contribute to observed initial clinical signs, but these drugs are not always active against later (sexual) stages. Consequently, treatment initiated in animals already having clinical signs may do little to ameliorate symptoms as the later stages continue to proliferate.

In environments where diseased animals will continue to be exposed to oocysts that can compound the damage already caused by initial exposure, anticoccidial treatment is considered to be useful in reducing further injury to enterocytes and may, in these situations of continual exposure, work to reduce oocyst excretion by the affected animal. Anticoccidial therapy is also used in group-housing environments when a member of the cohort exhibits clinical signs of coccidiosis, the illness being an indication that the environment is heavily contaminated and animals housed there will receive large exposure challenges. Thus, such an intervention has the goal of reducing the probability of an outbreak of clinical coccidiosis in that population. In the case of individuals suffering from coccidial illness in a shelter where they can be singly housed for the duration of their illness, and where the environment is such that oocyst accumulation is unlikely, the benefit of anticoccidial treatment may be limited.

17.3.2.2 *Toxoplasma gondii*

T. gondii is one of the most well-studied and widespread parasites of vertebrates. This parasite has well-known zoonotic importance, particularly for pregnant women. (See Chapter 21 for more information.) Cats (domestic and wild) are the definitive host and thus the only source of oocysts, which are passed in the feces of infected felids, most commonly only as a result of acute infection (Elmore et al. 2010; Bowman 2014). These oocysts require several hours to days for maturation into their infective stage. In most situations, daily removal of fecal material will be sufficient to ensure removal of oocysts prior to maturation to infectivity, however, one must consider that oocyst maturation could occur sooner than 24 hours under optimal (humid, moist, well-aerated) conditions. Because oocysts are likely to require more than 24 hours in most environments to become infective, and because cats are only likely to shed oocysts in appreciable numbers for a couple of weeks after the initial exposure to infected prey, there is little risk of acquiring a *Toxoplasma* infection from contact with fresh cat feces. Due to the meticulous grooming nature of cats, contact with cats is not considered a serious risk factor for human transmission. Transmission of *Toxoplasma* for any host, including cats, is through either the ingestion of oocysts that have reached infectivity or from the ingestion of raw (or undercooked) infected meats containing tissue cysts. Oocysts are relatively hardy and may survive for months to years in cool and moist environments (Frenkel et al. 1975), thus if shelters give cats access to outdoor grassy areas, soil transmission of oocysts could occur.

Due to the biology and behavior of cats, there is a high likelihood that cats that have fed on prey will have been infected with this parasite. Thus, the seroprevalence of *Toxoplasma* is likely to be high in free-roaming (including indoor/outdoor pet) cat populations entering and within shelters. Since seropositivity is associated with a decreased risk for shedding oocysts in feces (Bowman 2014), having a serologically positive cat is expected to minimize the risk for human exposure in this setting.

Typically, infections are not clinically apparent, but if cats, and less commonly dogs, become immunosuppressed or severely immunocompromised, the parasite may switch from the dormant or slowly dividing forms to the aggressively replicating stages that may spread throughout the body and lead to signs of disseminated toxoplasmosis (e.g. fever, anorexia, vomiting, diarrhea) (Bowman 2014). Such diseased animals may present with abnormalities often associated with the eyes, lungs, or central nervous system (CNS). There are no labeled treatments for toxoplasmosis in cats and dogs. Disseminated toxoplasmosis is a serious multiorgan disease, and these animals should be hospitalized and treated under the direct care of a veterinarian; underlying causes of immunocompromise should be identified and addressed, where possible. Ponazuril at the same dosages used for *Cystoisospora* may assist in reducing oocyst shedding by cats identified as infected. Both clindamycin (10–12 mg/kg BID for two to four weeks) and pyrimethamine (0.25–0.5 mg/kg) with a sulfonamide (30 mg/kg BID for two to four weeks) can be used for the treatment of disseminated toxoplasmosis.

Oocysts are unlikely to be detected in the feces of infected cats, especially those exhibiting clinical signs of toxoplasmosis, for reasons previously described. Oocysts in feces cannot be definitively differentiated from other feline parasites that produce indistinguishable oocysts (i.e. *Hammondia* and *Besnoitia*) by morphology alone. *Toxoplasma*-like oocysts are generally reported in 1% or fewer cat fecal samples examined (Elmore et al. 2010; Lucio-Forster and Bowman 2011). Cats found to be shedding oocysts can be held in isolation until shedding stops (typically two weeks); daily removal of feces generally precludes the exposure to infective oocysts, but extra preventive care (protective personal equipment and good hygiene) should be taken by shelter personnel to prevent inadvertent ingestion of oocysts.

17.3.2.3 *Neospora caninum*

N. caninum is a protozoan parasite of the dog (and other canids) that is most typically acquired from the ingestion of raw beef or venison, but many mammalian vertebrates, and possibly birds, can serve as intermediate hosts (Bowman 2014). Prevalence in dog populations, based on serology, is generally reported between 0 and 20% (Reichel et al. 2007). The life cycle is much like that of *T. gondii*, but it cycles between dogs and cattle rather than cats and their prey. Dogs pass oocysts in their feces upon initial infection. There are no clinical signs associated with oocyst shedding and thus there is no benefit of instituting treatment at this time. The oocysts resemble those of *Toxoplasma* and are morphologically indistinguishable from other canid parasites that produce similar stages in feces (i.e. *Hammondia* and *Besnoitia*). Though there have been numerous investigations, there is no evidence that *N. caninum* is zoonotic.

Disease due to this parasite in dogs presents as one of two distinct forms. Congenital infection of puppies can result in the classic presentation, typically around three weeks of age, of flaccid posterior limb paralysis (Bowman 2014). In adults, disease presentation is typically associated with neurologic signs, nodular dermatitis, myocarditis, myositis, and other signs (Bowman 2014). Diagnosis is typically presumptive, based on patient history, clinical signs, and serology. There are no labeled treatments for *N. caninum,* but clindamycin (12.5–25 mg/kg PO or IM BID for four weeks) or trimethoprim sulfadiazine (15–20 mg/kg PO BID for four weeks) in combination with pyrimethamine (1 mg/kg PO SID for four weeks) may be used in addition to appropriate supportive care. It is recommended that all littermates of an affected pup be treated, even if they are clinically normal. Dogs suffering from clinical neosporosis should be hospitalized and treated under the direct care of a veterinarian.

17.3.2.4 *Strongyloides stercoralis*

S. stercoralis is a nematode parasite of the small intestine of humans, dogs, and probably other canids. It develops equally well in both dogs and humans. Before the discovery of macrocyclic lactones, *S. stercoralis* would constantly appear in colonies of dogs housed in well-maintained facilities due to transmammary transmission and by the seeming ability of the larvae to develop to the infective stage even in fairly well managed and cleaned facilities. However, with the use of macrocyclic lactones, this infection has become much rarer in large canine facilities; it is believed that dogs maintained on monthly preventives are unlikely to become infected.

Transmission to animals and humans occurs by skin penetration and requires the previous maturation of larvae passed in feces into an infective state. These develop in dirt and debris around pens. Skin-penetrating larvae will also be passed to puppies when the nursing mother acquires an acute infection during lactation (Mansfield and Schad 1995; Shoop et al. 2002). Many dogs are likely to be infected and act as carriers without showing clinical signs. In heavy infections, however, there will be diarrhea (often mucoid) associated with mucosal damage and damage to the lungs and other tissues by migrating larvae (Grove et al. 1983, 1987; Schad et al. 1984). The infection may be difficult to diagnose because larvae are the stage that is passed in feces; thus, individual cases are identified sporadically and unexpectedly. These first-stage larvae can be found in feces of infected animals using the Baermann funnel technique (preferred) or zinc sulfate flotation.

Ivermectin (200 μg/kg [0.2 mg/kg] SC, once and repeated in one week; every four days for three to four doses, or SID for two doses) can be used to treat dogs (Aikens and Schad 1990; Mansfield and Schad 1992; Paradies et al. 2019); while not documented it is expected that other macrocyclic lactones will be similarly effective. Fenbendazole (50 mg/kg PO SID for 5–14 days) has also been reported to be effective in some cases and can be used alone (particularly for ivermectin sensitive breeds) or in combination with ivermectin (Itoh et al. 2009). In five shelter dogs in Italy with strongyloidiasis, three were treated successfully with a combination of fenbendazole and moxidectin/imidacloprid treatment, but two dogs were not cleared of their infections. In a shelter situation, all dogs sharing the same areas should be treated at the same time. Dogs probably do not become immune to reinfection, and they are unlikely to clear an infection spontaneously (Iatta et al. 2019). Dogs do respond very well to therapy. If animals are found to be infected, they should be isolated during treatment and for one to two weeks thereafter.

Larvae in saliva and feces are probably easy to kill with most routine disinfectants. These worms thrive in swampy conditions, so areas of damp soil or damp, heavily soiled cage areas are highly conducive to harboring larvae.

Dogs that are known to be infected should not be allowed to enter new homes until they are treated with a macrocyclic lactone and examined on several occasions a couple of weeks after treatment to make certain they are no longer shedding larvae. There are no special instructions for adopters other than disclosure of the condition and the treatment provided, and guidelines for routine follow-up surveillance for parasites.

17.3.2.5 Roundworms (Ascarids)

There are four roundworm species relevant to dogs and cats in a shelter setting: *Toxascaris leonina*, *Toxocara canis*, *Toxocara cati*, and *Baylisascaris procyonis*. The deadliest zoonotic one of these four (and fortunately the rarest in shelter situations) is *B. procyonis*; the most common cause of zoonosis is *T. canis*; *T. cati* is seemingly less likely to cause disease in humans (visceral larva migrans) than *T. canis*, and *T. leonina* remains an unlikely cause of infection.

All these ascarids can use paratenic hosts (rodents, birds, etc.), but this mode of transmission would be unlikely in most shelters. Relative to the control of these parasites within shelters, the eggs are not immediately infective, so there is no need to quarantine or isolate infected animals. However, after treatment, the feces will contain massive numbers of eggs that can contaminate the environment if prompt and thorough sanitation procedures are not followed. While these eggs are resistant to environmental extremes, when located on hard surfaces, heat and disinfectants such as ammonia or chlorine bleach will effectively kill the eggs by disrupting the outer covering and greatly increasing their susceptibility to dehydration. Aqueous iodine also will kill eggs. Once eggs enter the soil, they become nearly impossible to destroy.

17.3.2.5.1 Toxascaris leonina *T. leonina* adults are found in the intestines of dogs, cats, and various other canids and felids; the prevalence of *T. leonina* in shelter dogs was reported on a national level to be 0.7% (Blagburn et al. 1996; Blagburn 2009) and 1.9% in dogs housed in Canadian animal shelters (Villeneuve et al. 2015). *T. leonina* is capable of causing larval infections in primates, but no human cases of visceral larva migrans have been identified. Dogs and cats become infected with *T. leonina* through the ingestion of embryonated eggs or by ingestion of vertebrate paratenic hosts that contain larvae. There is neither transmammary nor transplacental transmission with this ascarid, and since the infections typically occur in older animals without any extraintestinal migration, these infections tend to occur without any clinical signs.

If infected dogs enter a facility where they would have a long length of stay, this parasite could become problematic, as it is in zoos or laboratory animal facilities. This is due to the very rapid embryonation of the eggs at lower temperatures than the eggs of *T. canis* and *T. cati* (Okoshi and Usui 1968). Thus, sanitation and rodent control measures are recommended to prevent transmission. Many products can be used to treat ascarid infections in dogs and cats, including pyrantel pamoate, fenbendazole, milbemycin oxime and moxidectin.

17.3.2.5.2 Toxocara canis* and *Toxocara cati
T. canis adults are found in the intestines of dogs and other canids. *T. cati* adults are found in the small intestines of cats and other felids. *T. canis* is considered one of the most common infections of humans around the world and is the cause of most cases of visceral and ocular larva migrans. *T. cati* is also very common around the world and is known to be capable of causing visceral larva migrans, but until recently it was not considered as important as *T. canis*.

The prevalence of *T. canis* in shelter dogs was reported on a national level to be 14% in US facilities (Blagburn et al. 1996; Blagburn 2009) and 12.7% in Canadian facilities (Villeneuve et al. 2015). When the data were examined by age, *T. canis* eggs were found in 30% of the samples from dogs less than six months of age (Figure 17.2). A survey of 450 cats in

Connecticut revealed an overall prevalence of *T. cati* of 39.8%, with 67.5% of shelter cats and 30.4% of client-owned cats being infected (Rembiesa and Richardson 2003). A survey of cats less than one year of age in central New York state revealed that 33% were infected with *T. cati*, as were 27% of owned cats, and 37% of sheltered cats (Spain et al. 2001). Another survey of 1322 cats in shelters in New York state revealed that 21% had the eggs of *T. cati* in their feces (Lucio-Forster and Bowman 2011) (Figure 17.3). Using the data presented on the 2011 through 2014 maps of the CAPC, the national prevalence of eggs in

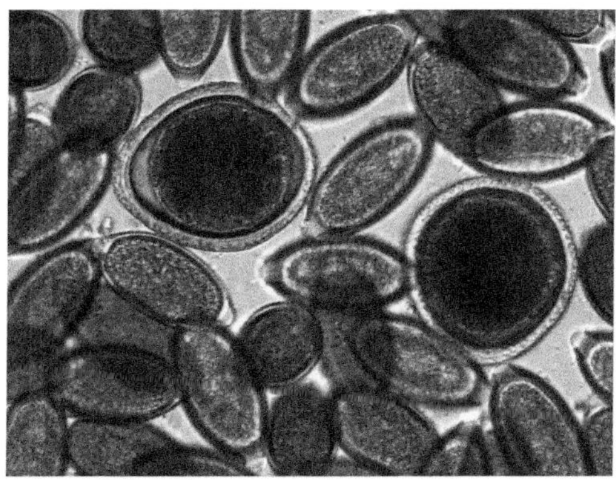

Figure 17.2 Two *Toxocara canis* and numerous *Trichuris vulpis* eggs recovered through sucrose centrifugal flotation of a sample submitted for routine fecal examination from a shelter dog.

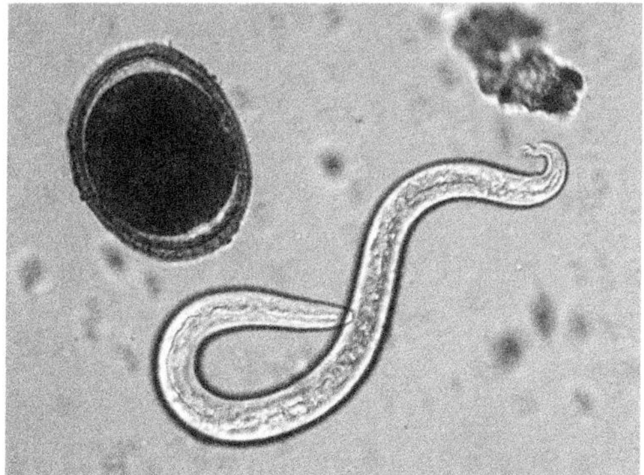

Figure 17.3 *Toxocara cati* egg and *Aelurostrongylus abstrusus* larva recovered through zinc centrifugal flotation of a sample from a shelter cat that was submitted for routine fecal examination.

the feces of pet cats and dogs during this four-year period was 4.6–5.1% and 1.8–2.0%, respectively (Lucio-Forster et al. 2016).

After admission, dogs and cats might become infected in the shelter environment through the ingestion of eggs containing infective larvae. Puppies can be infected in utero with *T. canis*. Kittens can be infected with *T. cati* larvae via nursing from an infected queen if the mother is infected when lactating (Coati et al. 2004). The prepatent period of *T. canis* following egg ingestion is about five weeks, but puppies infected in utero can shed eggs by about three weeks of age. The prepatent period of *T. cati* is six to eight weeks following the ingestion of eggs, and from about six weeks following lactogenic transmission (Coati et al. 2004).

Most dogs with *Toxocara* infections have no clinical signs of infection and are asymptomatic carriers. Cats and kittens infected with *T. cati* typically have no clinical signs, though kittens can sometimes develop thickened bowel walls. Puppies infected prenatally can have clinical signs that include coughing and nasal discharge. Heavy infections in puppies can cause vomiting, anorexia, abdominal distension, mucoid diarrhea, debilitation, reduced growth rate, allergic pruritus, a characteristic foul oral odor, and possibly epileptiform seizures and death due to bile duct blockage or intestinal perforation. Some adult dogs will harbor worms that remain as larvae for extended periods, and these worms may, at some undefined interval (months to years), develop to the adult stage. Thus, untreated dogs that have had negative fecal examinations for extended periods can develop patent infections even though they have been removed from a source of incoming infective eggs or larvae.

The diagnosis can best be made by finding the characteristic eggs in a zinc sulfate centrifugation fecal examination; sometimes the worms can be seen after they are passed in the feces or vomitus, particularly of young pups (Figure 17.4). However, negative fecal flotation

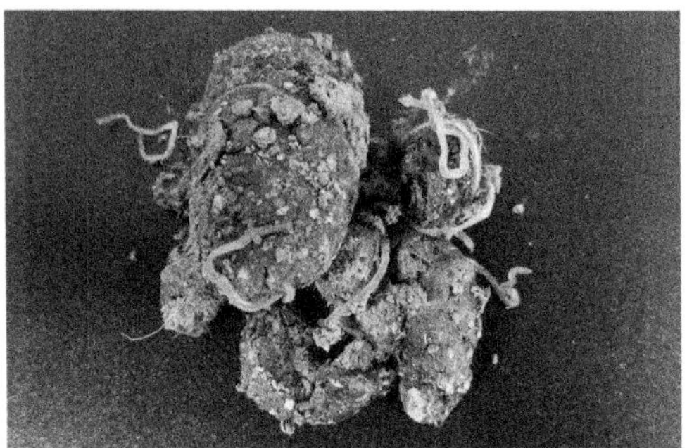

Figure 17.4 *Toxocara cati* adult worms passed in the feces submitted for routine examination for a shelter cat.

results do not rule out infection. It should be expected that most of the dogs and cats that enter a shelter have the larvae of ascarids in their tissues. There is insufficient data about the migration of these larvae back to the intestine to make any firm claims that they do or do not spontaneously begin shedding eggs again; however, one author (Bowman) has observed small developing forms and large adults in dogs that were held for months in raised pens. These worms may be stunted in their development, but the author believes it is much more likely that worms periodically migrate back to the lumen and begin development. Therefore, a dog that has tested negative could spontaneously become positive without ever ingesting another ascarid egg.

Many products can be used to treat ascarid infections in dogs and cats, including pyrantel pamoate, fenbendazole, milbemycin oxime, and moxidectin; numerous products administered for the prevention of heartworm infection are also labeled for the treatment and control of ascarid infections. Intrauterine infection of puppies with *T. canis* can be minimized by administering ivermectin (1 mg/kg) or doramectin (1 mg/kg) to the pregnant bitch 40–50 days after conception (Epe et al. 1995). However, neither treatment prevented all puppies from developing patent infections in either group though there was a very marked decrease in environmental contamination. The Centers for Disease Control and Prevention (CDC) suggests that puppies should be dewormed with a product that covers hookworms and roundworms every other week from week two of life, and kittens beginning at three weeks of life until they are 12 weeks old; typically this would include biweekly administration of a product such as pyrantel to very young puppies and kittens until they are started on regular broad-spectrum parasite prevention. Pregnant and nursing animals should also be treated; guidelines can be found at https://www.cdc.gov/parasites/ascariasis/index.html. The CAPC also has guidelines regarding parasite control that can be found at https://capcvet.org. Dogs and cats seem to become refractory to infection with adult worms as they become older. However, it is still possible for adult dogs and cats to be infected with these worms and regular administration of a broad-spectrum dewormer is recommended; in shelter dogs, 6% of dogs over seven years of age were infected with *T. canis* (Blagburn et al. 1996).

17.3.2.5.3 Baylisascaris procyonis *B. procyonis* is a parasite that is found as an adult in the small intestines of raccoons but can be found on occasion in the small intestines of dogs (Kazacos 2016). *B. procyonis* infected dogs typically have no clinical signs. The ingestion of the eggs of this parasite has caused severe and deadly visceral and neural larva migrans in humans, and the larvae of this parasite have killed more than 120 species of non-human hosts (Kazacos 2016).

A number of dogs have been found naturally infected with *B. procyonis* and shedding the eggs in their feces (Kazacos 2016). This is of considerable concern because of the indiscriminate defecation habits of dogs compared to raccoons, and the fact that some skill is required to distinguish the eggs of this parasite from those of *T. canis* in dog feces.

The life cycle of this parasite in the dog appears to be completed entirely within the GI tract where the worms develop to adults. The prepatent period of *B. procyonis* in dogs is approximately eight weeks (Bowman et al. 2005). It has been suggested that dogs might be infected with this worm prenatally (Kazacos 2016), but this has not been verified by experimentation. Efforts should be made to minimize potential exposure of dogs to raccoons and thus infection with *B. procyonis,* including promptly removing any fecal matter from the yard, limiting opportunities for predation and scavenging activity, and avoiding areas frequented by raccoons. Dogs should also be maintained on a regular broad-spectrum parasite control product with efficacy against ascarids to treat any newly acquired infections.

17.3.2.6 Hookworms

Ancylostoma caninum adults are found in the intestines of dogs and various other canids. *Ancylostoma tubaeforme* adults are found in the intestines of cats and other felids. *Ancylostoma braziliense* adults are found in the intestines of dogs, other canids, cats, and other felids in the coastal areas of the southeastern United States and the Caribbean. *Uncinaria stenocephala* adults are found in the small intestines of dogs, foxes, other canids, and occasionally cats; in Europe, *U. stenocephala* appears to be more common in cats than in the United States, where feline infections are rare (Diba et al. 2004). *A. braziliense* is the species most typically associated with zoonotic disease, causing the majority of cutaneous larva migrans cases in the United States. The larvae of the other species are capable of causing cutaneous larva migrans, but typically these worms do not produce the same type of serpiginous tracks on the skin. This is because *A. braziliense* spends considerably more time in the dermis before seeking deeper muscle tissues in which they will ultimately persist as larvae.

Diagnosis is made by finding the characteristic eggs in a zinc sulfate centrifugation fecal examination. Using fecal examination data, the prevalence of *A. caninum* in shelter dogs in the United States was reported on a national level to be 19% in 1996 and 34% in 2006, but only 3.1% in a 2015 study of Canadian shelters (Villeneuve et al. 2015); the prevalence of *U. stenocephala* was reported to be 1 and 2.4% in 1996 and 2006, respectively (Blagburn et al. 1996; Blagburn 2009). When the data were examined by age, *A. caninum* was found in 15–20% of dogs from all age groups from less than six months to more than seven years of age. For cats, a survey of 450 cats in Connecticut revealed an overall prevalence of hookworm eggs in the feces of 0.4%; the authors cite previous surveys with ranges varying from 0.9 to 84.6% (Rembiesa and Richardson 2003). With care, the eggs of *A. braziliense* can be identified as distinct from the other *Ancylostoma* species found in dogs and cats (Lucio-Forster et al. 2012). In a survey in Rio de Janeiro, Brazil, it was found that of the 135 cats over one year of age that were examined, 66% were infected with *A. braziliense*, and 9% were infected with *A. tubaeforme* (Labarthe et al. 2004).

Infection of dogs and cats with hookworms is most likely to occur through either penetration of the skin by infective-stage larvae or by the ingestion of these larvae that developed in the soil. These larvae are also capable of persisting in the tissues of various paratenic hosts where they can survive for extended periods; thus, the ingestion of rodents or other infected animals is another source of infection. Finally, dogs are capable of becoming infected by the larvae of *A. caninum* found in the milk of the bitch; this does not appear to occur with the other hookworm species that are found in the dog, nor with the species that occur in cats. The prepatent period for hookworms is two weeks; puppies acquiring infections via their mother's milk can begin to shed eggs within two weeks of birth.

Most adult dogs and cats show no clinical signs from hookworm infections and should be considered carriers, but severe disease is possible in young puppies or dogs that are stressed, malnourished, or immunocompromised. It is well known that dogs will become recurrent hookworm egg shedders with the constant migration of larvae from either the intestinal wall or deeper tissues; these larvae develop into adult worms within two weeks after their arrival in the intestinal lumen. This phenomenon of "larval leak" of hookworms back to the intestine has not been as carefully examined in the cat as it has been in the dog.

Anemia is the major clinical sign associated with a hookworm infection. In puppies with *A. caninum* infections, including very young animals infected by transmammary transmission, signs may include mucosal pallor, diarrhea, weakness, progressive emaciation, cardiac failure, and death. Mature, well-nourished animals often have no signs of infection other than a mild hypochromic anemia. Less frequent signs include dermatitis and pruritus due to larval skin penetration in older, sensitized dogs, and coughing and dyspnea due to larval migration in younger dogs. In the case of cats with *A. tubaeforme*, infections result in weight loss and regenerative anemia, while heavy infections may cause death. Infections with *A. braziliense* cause less relative blood loss than the other two *Ancylostoma* species of the dog and cat found in the US. *U. stenocephala* infections are unlikely to cause clinical disease.

Many products can be used to treat hookworm infections in dogs and cats, including pyrantel pamoate, fenbendazole, moxidectin, and milbemycin oxime. The CDC suggests that all puppies should be dewormed with a product that covers hookworms and roundworms every other week from week two of life, and kittens beginning at three weeks of life until they are 12 weeks old and then monthly until 6 months of age. Pregnant and nursing animals should also be treated (http://www.cdc.gov/parasites/ascariasis/index.html).

There does not appear to be a great deal of immunity to infection, and dogs and cats are almost as likely to be infected when they are older as when they are immature (Blagburn et al. 1996). There is no need to quarantine or isolate infected animals.

Hookworm eggs are not as hardy as those of ascarids and are probably destroyed fairly rapidly with dehydration if located on dry surfaces. The eggs start to develop rapidly after deposition onto the ground, and larvae can hatch one to two days after deposition. The worms then molt and grow in the soil and infective-stage larvae can become common a week later. Prevention of infections is far easier and effective than attempting to control environmental contamination and subsequent exposure, and so empirical treatment of all animals on intake and repeat treatment of puppies is advised.

It should be expected that many of the dogs and cats that enter a shelter harbor the larvae of hookworms in their tissues, and it is suspected that dogs that are negative at the time of adoption may begin to shed eggs again later. Thus, adopters should be encouraged to set up a post-adoption appointment with a veterinarian to develop a preventive medicine program appropriate for the pet and new owner.

17.3.2.7 Whipworms

The adults of the canine whipworm, *T. vulpis*, are found in the cecum and colon of dogs and other canids. When animals have only a few whipworms, they are isolated within the cecum; when animals have heavier infections with larger numbers of whipworms, the worms are also found threaded through the colonic mucosa. The prevalence of *T. vulpis* in shelter dogs in the United States was reported in 1996 as 14.3 and 20.5% in 2009 (Blagburn et al. 1996; Blagburn 2009), compared to just 4.4% prevalence reported in Canadian shelter dogs in 2015 (Villeneuve et al. 2015). When the US data were evaluated for age, *T. vulpis* was more common in dogs over six months of age and was found in anywhere from 10% to more than 15% of the animals.

The zoonotic potential for canine whipworms is low. Human whipworm infections are not uncommon, but the human whipworm is a separate species from the canine whipworm. There have been very rare reports of finding *T. vulpis* eggs in the stools of humans (Dunn et al. 2002), but it is thought that eggs of the human whipworm *T. trichiura* can appear similar to those of the canine whipworm and thus confuse the diagnosis (Yoshikawa et al. 1989).

The life cycle of the whipworm is direct. Dogs are infected by ingesting the egg(s) often found in contaminated soil. The eggs can take days to months to reach the infective stage; they are hardy and resistant to many environmental extremes. The prepatent period for whipworms is approximately three months. Most dogs have no clinical signs associated with a whipworm infection unless they have large numbers of worms. Due to the low number of worms, the lack of clinical signs, and the long prepatent period, dogs often serve as carriers of the infection and contaminate the surrounding environment.

When clinical signs are observed in heavily infected dogs, they include weight loss, abdominal pain, and mild to severe diarrhea that sometimes contains blood. The worms live with their anterior ends threaded through the intestinal mucosa, so there are lesions inherently associated with the worms living in the intestinal tissue. The diagnosis is best made by finding the characteristic barrel-shaped egg in a fecal centrifugation sample. Due to the long prepatent period, intermittent nature of shedding, and density of the eggs, it may not always be possible to make an accurate diagnosis from centrifugated fecal samples. In a dog with a compatible history and clinical signs, further testing (i.e. fecal ELISA) and/or empiric treatment may be indicated.

Many commonly used anthelmintics can be used to treat whipworm infections, including fenbendazole, moxidectin, and milbemycin oxime. There does not appear to be a great deal of immunity to infection, and dogs are as likely to be infected when they are older (Blagburn et al. 1996).

There is no need either to quarantine animals or to isolate infected dogs. The eggs are likely hardier than ascarid eggs, but the polar plugs may make these eggs somewhat more susceptible to chlorine bleach than ascarid eggs (Figure 17.2). However, once these eggs contaminate the soil of runs or outdoor kennels, they are almost impossible to eliminate.

If dogs enter the shelter with whipworm infections, the infections may not be patent at the time of arrival due to the three-month-long prepatent period. Therefore, as is recommended for other intestinal parasites, adopters should be advised to seek post-adoption and regular veterinary care to discuss routine diagnostics and preventives for parasites of concern.

17.4 Parasites with Indirect Transmission

17.4.1 Parasites with the Potential for Shelter Transmission

17.4.1.1 *Babesia* spp.

Babesia spp. are red blood cell protozoan parasites. More than 100 species have been described, nine of which infect dogs. This chapter will focus on the two of greatest importance in shelter dogs in the United States: *Babesia canis (vogeli)* and *Babesia gibsoni*. *B. canis* is the most common large *Babesia* species, transmitted by the Brown Dog Tick, *Rhipicephalus sanguineus,* and most frequently diagnosed in the southeastern United States. While *R. sanguineus* is a possible vector for *B. gibsoni*, it is not the primary vector and is only a theoretical means of transmission in the United States, where instead infection typically occurs in association with dogfighting activities (i.e. a fight with or bite from an infected dog, or being born to an infected bitch). At least one study documented a 39% prevalence rate in more than 250 pit bull-type dogs seized in a multi-state dogfighting investigation (Cannon et al. 2016). In other areas of the world, transmission is primarily driven by tick bites from *Haemaphysalis longicornis* and *Haemaphysalis bispinosa*.

The pathogenicity of *Babesia* varies primarily by species, though host factors are also important. For *B. canis*, prevalence rates are reported to be higher in adult dogs compared to puppies, and greyhounds have a notably higher seroprevalence than other breeds. As mentioned earlier, *B. gibsoni* is predominantly seen in association with dogfighting and most infected dogs are pit bulls.

Clinical signs may be absent or mild in many dogs, but acute or chronic signs, including severe or sometimes fatal manifestations of babesiosis (particularly in splenectomized dogs) are possible. When present, non-specific clinical signs such as lethargy, weakness, fever, or anorexia are common. Other signs include hemolytic anemia, icterus, splenomegaly, lymphadenopathy, and death; numerous other symptoms have been reported. Disease caused by *B. canis* is typically less severe and many dogs will have subclinical infections, while disease caused by *B. gibsoni* is believed to often be more severe and frequent. However, the full range of clinical manifestations, ranging from no outwards signs to acute, life-threatening illness, are possible with all *Babesia* species.

The organism is most commonly diagnosed by PCR, with serology and direct examination of a blood smear as other options. *B. canis* piroplasms are often found in pairs, while those of *B. gibsoni* are typically smaller and ring-shaped. Accurate identification is important in selecting an appropriate treatment option.

For *B. canis* infection, treatment is with imidocarb dipropionate (5–6.6 mg/kg, IM or SC, followed two weeks later by a second injection). For *B. gibsoni* infection, a 10-day course of atovaquone (13.3 mg/kg q8 hours) and azithromycin (10 mg/kg SID) is generally considered to be the treatment of choice and may result in apparent clearance in the majority of cases (Birkenheuer et al. 2004), though some strains are resistant to such therapy (Sakuma et al. 2009). This treatment protocol also poses a significant expense, particularly for animal shelters needing to provide treatment for multiple dogs seized as part of a dogfighting case. The use of compounded rather than commercially available preparations of atovaquone was found in one study to be efficacious and can be considered as part of a more economical protocol for the management of *B. gibsoni* infections in dogfighting cases (Kirk et al. 2017). Where treatment with atovaquone and azithromycin is not feasible or has failed, triple antibiotic therapy may be considered. The combination of metronidazole (25–50 mg/kg PO SID), clindamycin (12.5–25 mg/kg PO BID), and doxycycline (10 mg/kg PO BID) for an extended course of treatment has been reported to decrease clinical signs and lead to apparent elimination of the parasite in a small number of dogs (Suzuki et al. 2007).

It is difficult to completely eliminate the parasite, and no treatments have been documented to be fully efficacious in all dogs. Successful treatment, particularly for *B. gibsoni*, can best be characterized as reducing parasitemia (sometimes to levels below the detection threshold) and reducing or eliminating clinical signs, but not actually clearing the infection. Treated dogs should be considered permanent carriers but can be placed for adoption with appropriate counseling about the disease, including the potential for relapsing disease, and the need for routine tick preventive use and other control measures.

Dogs are not likely to serve as a source of infection in the shelter unless there is poor tick control and dogs are housed together or otherwise allowed to interact in a way where bites may occur. Shelters need to ensure all ticks are removed promptly once an animal enters the shelter, and other environmental tick control measures are in place.

17.4.1.2 *Trypanosoma cruzi*

Trypanosoma cruzi is the causative agent of Chagas disease in humans and dogs. Due to the distribution of its vector (triatomine bugs, also known as kissing bugs), infection is of greatest concern in Central and South America and southern US states along the Mexican border. Transmission to a vertebrate host occurs when the insect vector takes a blood meal, defecates near the wound, and the infective stage of the parasite (known as a trypomastigote) present in the bug's feces enters the wound, or if the host ingests the vector carrying *T. cruzi*.

While infection is less common in the United States than in other areas of the world, this parasite has the potential to be transmitted within a shelter if the vector is present in the animals' immediate environment or in areas surrounding the shelter. In Texas, it was found that 20.3% of samples submitted to the state animal health diagnostic lab for *T. cruzi* serology were positive (Kjos et al. 2008), and 8.8% of shelter-housed dogs sampled across the state were seropositive (Tenney et al. 2014). It has also been suggested that domestic dogs appear to be key in the transmission cycle of *T. cruzi* in Texas, given their roles both as blood hosts for the vectors and as potential reservoirs for the parasite; 82% of triatomine bug specimens collected from dog kennels were infected with *T. cruzi* (Kjos et al. 2013). Though little is known about infection in cats in the United States, seroconversion and histologic cardiac lesions have been documented in cats from a South Texas shelter (Zecca et al. 2020). In southeastern Louisiana, in response to a locally acquired human infection, houses were examined and bugs were collected. Houses without air conditioning that had cats (or chickens) were more likely to have peridomestic bugs (Moudy et al. 2014). As with babesiosis, it is likely that *T. cruzi* could be spread between dogs via blood if fighting occurs; transplacental transmission is also possible. This is an organism that can infect both dogs and humans (and potentially cats) with serious long-term complications, so staff in areas where this parasite is present need to take special care when handling blood from animals, including dogs and cats.

Clinical manifestations of *T. cruzi* infection in dogs are characterized by non-specific signs of illness; cardiac abnormalities can be severe and ultimately fatal. Diagnosis is most commonly made through the combination of compatible history (i.e. geographic location or travel), clinical signs and positive serology, but PCR and culture are also available. Trypomastigotes may also be detected in blood smears collected from animals in the parasitemic phase of infection that corresponds with acute disease. Treatment is difficult and the two drugs for treating this infection, benznidazole and nifurtimox, are only available to the veterinary community through the CDC; euthanasia is often elected.

17.4.1.3 *Dipylidium caninum*

Dipylidium caninum tapeworms use fleas as intermediate hosts that become infected by feeding on the egg balls (Figure 17.5) present within the segments that are shed by infected cats and dogs. Therefore, these tapeworms will be very successfully transmitted within a shelter environment that contains fleas. A well-executed flea control program should be capable of controlling *D. caninum* within shelters, including those with outdoor runs. Shelters located in areas where fleas are common should consider treating cats and dogs for fleas with an appropriate product at the time of intake. In regions where fleas are not common, shelters can consider treating only those animals when fleas or flea dirt are noted; they must be diligent about examining for fleas at the time of intake. If tapeworms are diagnosed, either via routine fecal examination or visualization of tapeworm segments around the rectum or in feces, the animal should be treated with praziquantel or epsiprantel. Many shelters

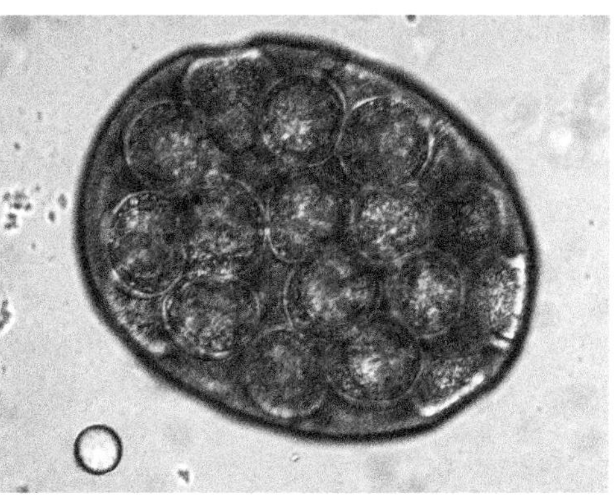

Figure 17.5 *Dipylidium caninum* egg ball recovered through a squash preparation of a proglottid passed in feces of a shelter dog submitted for routine examination.

opt to treat all incoming dogs with praziquantel for tapeworm control, however, if *D. caninum* appears within a shelter it is likely an indication that the facility's flea-control program needs to be reviewed. *D. caninum* is zoonotic, with most infections occurring in young children who have ingested a flea containing the larval tapeworm that undergoes final maturation after the flea has been on a dog or cat for a day or two.

17.4.1.4 *Dirofilaria immitis*

The reader is referred to Chapter 18 for detailed information on heartworm disease.

17.4.2 Parasites Unlikely to be Perpetuated in a Shelter Setting

17.4.2.1 Taeniid Tapeworms

All taeniid tapeworms require a mammalian intermediate host. Thus, unless there are rabbits or rodents within a shelter, these tapeworms are unlikely to be able to complete their life cycle within a facility. For a dog to become infected with *Taenia pisiformis*, it would have to ingest the entrails of a rabbit with cysticerci. For a cat to become infected with *Taenia taeniaeformis*, it would have to ingest the liver of a rat containing strobilocerci.

Disease caused by infection with *Echinococcus* species is of particular concern. Though *Echinococcus multilocularis* is typically a parasite of foxes and rodents, it can make its way into domestic situations through the infection of dogs or cats that enter the fox/rodent ecosystem. *Echinococcus granulosus* (with its canid–ruminant–canid cycle) does not develop well in cats, and cats are also believed to have only minimal importance as a host of *E. multilocularis* in domestic (dog-rodent) cycles, though the parasite can develop to some extent in domestic felids (Thompson et al. 2006). Both species of tapeworm flourish in the domestic dog and other canids.

Adult *Echinococcus* tapeworms are exceedingly small, thus eggs will appear in the feces, but segments will not be grossly visible. In foxes, *E. multilocularis* has been found in the continental United States and has a distribution that extends down from Canada with a southernmost front along the southern border of Wyoming, eastward through central Nebraska and central Illinois into Indiana and Ohio. Thus, in these parts of the United States, it is possible that dogs, especially strays or those housed primarily outdoors, could be infected with this parasite.

The larval stages of the unilocular hydatid of *E. granulosus* and the multilocular hydatid of *E. multilocularis* are major disease agents in their intermediate hosts, and unfortunately, a human, like many other mammals, can serve as an intermediate host. Zoonotic hydatid disease due to the larvae of *E. multilocularis* (the alveolar hydatid) is of significant concern. The larva of this parasite grows typically in the hepatic tissue of the human host much like a cancer and the infection is 100% fatal without treatment (Wilson et al. 1995). The ingestion of one egg can be lethal. The parasite grows slowly and insidiously, so there may be a lag time of months to years from the time of infection until the development of first signs. Thus, it is important to make sure staff in endemic areas are aware of the potential risk of exposure to eggs in canine feces. Staff at shelters in Alaska and Canada need to be especially wary.

The most reliable drug for treatment of these tapeworms, and specifically for *Echinococcus* species, is praziquantel. If this is cost-prohibitive, the other choice is fenbendazole, but this drug will not treat *D. caninum* or *Echinococcus* spp.

17.4.2.2 Trematodes, Nematodes, and Other Cestodes

Trematodes are acquired by animals either through the ingestion of an intermediate host or through the penetration of skin by cercariae (a special case of the Schistosomatidae, e.g. *Heterobilharzia americana* in the southeastern United States). There is a chance that free-roaming animals will have acquired the infection by eating a fish, amphibian, lizard, or crayfish. However, within the shelter, there will neither be the proper snail first intermediate host nor the invertebrate or vertebrate second intermediate host to perpetuate the cycle. Thus, for the parasite, these animals are dead-end hosts in every single scenario. These parasites pose no threat to shelter staff as zoonotic agents.

Similarly, there are a number of nematode and cestode parasites that require intermediate hosts as part of their life cycles and thus will generally pose no risk of further transmission even if they enter the shelter via an infected dog or cat. These include the metastrongyloid lungworms (*Crenosoma vulpis* and *Angiostrongylus vasorum* of the dog, and *Aelurostrongylus abstrusus* of the cat), the spirurid nematodes (*Dracunculus insignis*, *Gnathostoma spinigerum*, *Physaloptera* spp., and *Spirocerca lupi*), some capillarid nematodes (*Aonchotheca putorii*, *Eucoleus aerophilus*, *Eucoleus boehmi*, and *Pearsonema plica*), and various tapeworms (*Dibothriocephalus latus*, *Spirometra mansonoides* and *Mesocestoides lineatus*). *Dibothriocephalus* and *Spirometra* have to go through copepods to infect the host that is then ingested by the dog or cat, and *Mesocestoides* spp. go through some unknown host before they make their way into the host that can infect the dog or cat via ingestion. *Physaloptera* spp. and *S. lupi* require insect intermediate hosts (beetles, cockroaches, crickets, etc.) and most of the capillarids require earthworms as intermediate hosts, so in certain shelter environments transmission of these species may occur if animals are housed and cared for in such a way that allows them ready access to these intermediate hosts. If a shelter has outdoor runs that are not screened to keep out insects, and if snails or earthworms are present, these parasites would be potentially transmissible within the facility.

There is no zoonotic risk to shelter staff posed by any of the trematode or nematode parasites included in this section.

17.4.2.3 *Cuterebra*

There are a number of the fly species *Cuterebra* in North America, and they all require a living host to complete their development after the larva hatches out of the egg. The typical hosts are rodents or rabbits that become infected when they walk past an egg attached to a blade of grass along a game trail, and a maggot hatches out of its eggshell onto the mammal's fur. The maggot will then enter the animal through one of the natural orifices and migrate through the body of the host for several weeks until arriving at the skin and creating a small hole through which they breathe through their posterior spiracles with their mouth pointing inwards. Once in the skin, *Cuterebra* larvae rapidly increase in size before ultimately emerging from the host and dropping to the ground into which they will burrow before metamorphosing into the adult fly.

These *Cuterebra* species can also enter the bodies of other animals, including cats and dogs, which are accidental hosts. In these hosts, they usually act much like they do in the rodent or rabbit and appear as large maggots in boils in the skin. However, aberrant migration may occur and lead to neurologic, ocular, or nasal disease manifestations. Treatment of the skin forms is simple extraction. Those in deeper tissues will require surgical removal. It is very unlikely that *Cuterebra* would perpetuate in a shelter unless there was an outdoor exercise area with rodents and rabbits on the opposite side of a surrounding fence. The reader is directed to Chapter 19 for additional information on *Cuterebra*.

17.5 Conclusion

Animals entering a shelter should receive treatment for the most common internal and external parasites found in that area. Additional therapy will depend on the ability of the shelter to strategically assess the need for diagnostics, treatment, and disease prevention. Prompt removal of feces from the environment and subsequent sanitation with appropriate disinfectants will provide a good first line of defense against the transmission of parasites through mechanical removal of the parasite stages shed in feces. Most parasitic stages left behind on hard surfaces are likely to desiccate within hours and will not persist. Feces that become incorporated into dirt, soil, or yards will provide an environment for the transmission of parasites which, in some cases (e.g. roundworms and whipworms), could have long-lasting consequences. It should not be expected that shelters can be entirely parasite free, but policies should be implemented to minimize the introduction of parasites and to treat and/or control those parasites that are present in the animal population.

Of those intestinal parasites most commonly found in cats and dogs, relatively few have zoonotic importance and good hygiene practices can minimize the risk of human infection. The few parasites capable of immediate infection, and thus the most prone to transmission within a shelter setting, have limited to no zoonotic importance. Regardless, it is always recommended that personnel take appropriate precautions (i.e. good hygiene practices, use of personal protective equipment) when handling animals. If appropriate sanitation procedures are in place and fecal contamination is minimized, zoonotic transmission to shelter personnel who are conscientious regarding handwashing and not eating or drinking with soiled hands will be significantly minimized. (See Chapter 21 for more information on zoonosis.)

References

Aikens, L. and Schad, G.A. (1990). Treatment of chronic active and hyperinfections of *Strongyloides stercoralis* in the dog with ivermectin. *Journal of Veterinary Internal Medicine* 4: 131.

August, J.R., Powers, R.D., Bailey, W.S. et al. (1980). *Filaroides hirthi* in a dog: fatal hyperinfection suggestive of autoinfection. *Journal of the American Veterinary Medical Association* 176: 331–334.

Bauer, C. and Bahnemann, R. (1996). Control of *Filaroides hirthi* infections in beagle dogs by ivermectin. *Veterinary Parasitology* 65: 269–273.

Bell, A.G. (1984). *Ollulanus tricuspis* in a cat colony. *New Zealand Veterinary Journal* 32: 85–87.

Birkenheuer, A.J., Levy, M.G., and Breitschwerdt, E.B. (2004). Efficacy of combined atovaquone and azithromycin for therapy of chronic *Babesia gibsoni* (Asian genotype) infections in dogs. *Journal of Veterinary Internal Medicine* 18 (4): 494–498.

Blagburn, B.L (2009). National parasite prevalence survey: interim report in Small Animal and Exotics. North American Veterinary Conference, Orlando.

Blagburn, B.L., Lindsay, D.S., Vaughan, J.L. et al. (1996). Prevalence of canine parasites based on fecal flotation. *Compendium on Continuing Education for the Practicing Veterinarian* 18: 483–509.

Bowman, D.D. (2020). Georgi's Parasitology for Veterinarians. 11th edition. St. Louis: Elsevier.

Bowman, D.D. and Lucio-Forster, A. (2010). Cryptosporidiosis and giardiasis in dogs and cats: veterinary and public health importance. *Experimental Parasitology* 124: 121–127.

Bowman, D.D., Ulrich, M.A., Gregory, D.E. et al. (2005). Treatment of *Baylisascaris procyonis* infections in dogs with milbemycin oxime. *Veterinary Parasitology* 129: 285–290.

Caldwell, D. (1984). *Ollulanus tricuspis* in an Ontario cattery. *Canadian Veterinary Journal* 25: 314.

Cannon, S.H., Levy, J.K., Kirk, S.K. et al. (2016). Infectious diseases in dogs rescued during dogfighting investigations. *The Veterinary Journal* 211: 64–69.

Carrasco, L., Hervas, J., Gomez-Villamandos, J.C. et al. (1997). Massive *Filaroides hirthi* infestation associated with canine distemper in a puppy. *Veterinary Record* 140: 72–73.

Cecchi, R., Wills, S.J., Dean, R. et al. (2006). Demonstration of *Ollulanus tricuspis* in the stomach of domestic cats by biopsy. *Journal of Comparative Pathology* 134: 374–377.

Cervone, M., Giannelli, A., Rosenberg, D. et al. (2018). Filaroidosis infection in an immunocompetent adult dog from France. *Helminthologia* 55 (1): 77–83.

Charles, S.D., Chopade, H.M., Ciszewski, D.K. et al. (2007). Safety of 5% ponazuril (toltrazuril sulfone) oral suspension and efficacy against naturally acquired Cystoisospora ohioensis-like infection in beagle puppies. *Parasitology Research* 101: 137–144.

Coati, N., Schnieder, T., and Epe, C. (2004). Vertical transmission of *Toxocara cati* Schrank 1788 (Anisakidae) in the cat. *Parasitology Research* 92: 142–146.

Companion Animal Parasite Council (2020). Giardia. https://capcvet.org/guidelines/giardia (accessed 11 August 2020).

Diba, V.C., Whitty, C.J.M., and Green, T. (2004). Cutaneous larva migrans acquired in Britain. *Clinical and Experimental Dermatology* 29: 555–556.

Dunn, J.J., Columbus, S.T., Aldeen, W.E. et al. (2002). *Trichuris vulpis* recovered from a patient with chronic diarrhea and five dogs. *Journal of Clinical Microbiology* 40: 2703–2704.

Elmore, S.A., Jones, J.L., Conrad, P.A. et al. (2010). *Toxoplasma gondii*: epidemiology, feline clinical aspects, and prevention. *Trends in Parasitology* 26: 190–196.

Epe, C., Pankow, W.R., Hackbarth, H. et al. (1995). A study on the prevention of prenatal and galactogenic *Toxocara canis* infections in pups by treatment of infected bitches with ivermectin or doramectin. *Applied Parasitology* 36: 115–123.

Erb, H.N. and Georgi, J.R. (1982). Control of *Filaroides hirthi* in commercially reared beagle dogs. *Laboratory Animal Science* 32: 394–396.

Frenkel, J.K., Ruis, A., and Chinchilla, M. (1975). Soil survival of *Toxoplasma* oocysts in Kansas and Costa Rica. *American Journal of Tropical Medicine and Hygiene* 24: 439–443.

Gookin, J.L., Stebbins, M.E., Hunt, E. et al. (2004). Prevalence of and risk factors for feline *Tritrichomonas foetus* and *Giardia* infection. *Journal of Clinical Microbiology* 42: 2707–2710.

Greve, J.H. (1983). A nematode causing vomiting in cats. *Feline Practice* 11: 17–19.

Grove, D.I., Heenan, P.J., and Northern, C. (1983). Persistent and disseminated infections with *Strongyloides stercoralis* in immunosuppressed dogs. *International Journal for Parasitology* 13: 483–490.

Grove, D.I., Warton, A., Yu, L.L. et al. (1987). Light and electron microscopical studies of the location of *Strongyloides* stercoralis in the jejunum of the immunosuppressed dog. *International Journal for Parasitology* 17: 1257–1265.

Hedgespeth, B.A., Stauffer, S.H., Robertson, J.B. et al. (2020). Association of fecal sample collection technique and treatment history with Tritrichomonas foetus polymerase chain reaction test results in 1717 cats. *Journal of Veterinary Internal Medicine* 34 (2): 734–741.

Iatta, R., Buonfrate, D., Paradies, P. et al. (2019). Occurrence, diagnosis and follow-up of canine strongyloidiosis in naturally infected shelter dogs. *Parasitology* 146 (2): 246–252.

Itoh, N., Kanai, K., Yori, Y. et al. (2009). Fenbendazole treatment of dogs with naturally acquired *Strongyloides stercoralis* infection. *Veterinary Record* 164 (18): 559–560.

Janeczko, S. and Griffin, B. (2010). Giardia infection in cats. *Compendium Continuing Education for Veterinarians* 32 (8): E1–E7.

Kato, D., Oishi, M., Koichi, O. et al. (2015). The first report of the ante-mortem diagnosis of *Ollulanus tricuspis* infection in two dogs.

Journal of Veterinary Medical Science 77: 1499–1502.

Kazacos, K.R. (2016). National Wildlife Health Center. Baylisascaris Larva Migrans. https://pubs.usgs.gov/circ/1412/cir1412.pdf (accessed 27 June 2020).

Kirk, S.K., Levy, J.K., and Crawford, P.C. (2017). Efficacy of azithromycin and compounded Atovaquone for treatment of *Babesia gibsoni* in dogs. *Journal of Veterinary Internal Medicine* 31 (4): 1108–1112.

Kjos, S.A., Snowden, K.F., Craig, T.M. et al. (2008). Distribution and characterization of canine Chagas disease in Texas. *Veterinary Parasitology* 152: 249–256.

Kjos, S.A., Marcet, P., Ybsley, M.J. et al. (2013). Identification of bloodmeal sources and *Trypanosoma cruzi* infection in triatomine bugs (Hemiptera: Reduviidae) from residential settings in Texas, the United States. *Journal of Medical Entomology* 50 (5): 1126–1139.

Kryda, K., Six, R.H., Walsh, K.F. et al. (2019). Laboratory and field studies to investigate the efficacy of a novel, orally administered combination product containing moxidectin, sarolaner and pyrantel for the prevention of heartworm disease (*Dirofilaria immitis*) in dogs. *Parasites & Vectors* 12 (1): 445–456.

Labarthe, N., Serrão, M.L., Ferreira, A.M.R. et al. (2004). A survey of gastrointestinal helminths in cats of the metropolitan region of Rio de Janeiro, Brazil. *Veterinary Parasitology* 123: 133–139.

Lappin, M.R., Clark, M., and Scorza, A. (2008). Treatment of healthy *Giardia* spp. positive dogs with fenbendazole or nitazoxanide. Abstract #257. *Journal of Veterinary Internal Medicine* 22: 778–779.

Levitan, D.M., Matz, M.E., Findlen, C.S. et al. (1996). Treatment of *Oslerus osleri* infestation in a dog: case report and literature review. *Journal of the American Animal Hospital Association* 32: 435–438.

Litster, A.L., Nichols, J., Hall, K. et al. (2014). Use of ponazuril paste to treat coccidiosis in shelter-housed cats and dogs. *Veterinary Parasitology* 202 (3–4): 319–325.

Lucio-Forster, A. and Bowman, D.D. (2011). Prevalence of fecal-borne parasites detected by centrifugal flotation in feline samples from two shelters in upstate New York;. *Journal of Feline Medicine and Surgery* 13: 300–303.

Lucio-Forster, A., Griffiths, J.K., Cama, V.A. et al. (2010). Minimal zoonotic risk of cryptosporidiosis from pet dogs and cats. *Trends in Parasitology* 26: 174–179.

Lucio-Forster, A., Liotta, J.L., Yaros, J.P. et al. (2012). Morphological differentiation of eggs of *Ancylostoma caninum*, *Ancylostoma tubaeforme*, and *Ancylostoma braziliense* from dogs and cats in the United States. *Journal of Parasitology* 98 (5): 1041–1044.

Lucio-Forster, A., Mizhquiri Barvecho, J.S., Mohammed, H.O. et al. (2016). Comparison of the prevalence of *Toxocara* egg shedding by pet cats and dogs in the USA, (2011–2014). *Veterinary Parasitology Regional Studies and Reports* 5: 1–13.

Mansfield, L.S. and Schad, G.A. (1992). Ivermectin treatment of naturally acquired and experimentally induced *Strongyloides stercoralis* infections in dogs. *Journal of the American Veterinary Association* 201: 726–730.

Mansfield, L.S. and Schad, G.A. (1995). Lack of transmammary transmission of *Strongyloides stercoralis* from a previously hyperinfected bitch to her pups. *Journal of the Helminthological Society of Washington* 62: 80–88.

McTier, T.L., Kryda, K., Wachowski, M. et al. (2019). ProHeart® 12, a moxidectin extended-release injectable formulation for prevention of heartworm (*Dirofilaria immitis*) disease in dogs in the USA for 12 months. *Parasites & Vectors* 12: 369–382.

Moron-Soto, M., Gutierrez, L., Sumano, H. et al. (2017). Efficacy of nitazoxanide to treat natural giardia infections in dogs. *Parasites & Vectors* 10: 1–9.

Moudy, R.M., Michaels, S., Jameson, S.D. et al. (2014). Factors associated with peridomestic

Triatoma sanguisuga (Hemiptera Reduviidae) presence in southeastern Louisiana. *Journal of Medical Entomology* 51: 1043–1050.

Okoshi, S. and Usui, M. (1968). Experimental studies on *Toxascaris leonina*. IV. Development of eggs of three ascarids, *T. leonina*, *Toxocara canis*, and *Toxocara cati* in dogs and cats. *Japanese Journal of Veterinary Science* 30: 29–38.

Outerbridge, C.A. and Taylor, S.M. (1998). *Oslerus osleri* tracheobronchitis: treatment with ivermectin in 4 dogs. *Canadian Veterinary Journal* 39: 238–240.

Paradies, P., Buonfrate, D., Iatta, R. et al. (2019). Efficacy of ivermectin to control *Strongyloides stercoralis* infection in sheltered dogs. *Acta Tropica* 190: 204–209.

Reichel, M.P., Ellis, J.T., and Dubey, J.P. (2007). Neosporosis and hammondiosis in dogs. *Journal of Small Animal Practice* 48: 308–312.

Rembiesa, C. and Richardson, D.J. (2003). Helminth parasites of the house cat, *Felis catus*, in Connecticut, USA. *Comparative Parasitology* 70: 115–119.

Ryan, U. and Caccio, S.M. (2013). Zoonotic potential of *Giardia*. *International Journal for Parasitology* 43: 943–956.

Ryan, U., Zahedi, A., and Paparini, A. (2016). Cryptosporidium in humans and animals – a one health approach to prophylaxis. *Parasite Immunology* 38: 535–547.

Sakuma, M., Setoguchi, A., and Endo, Y. (2009). Possible emergence of drug-resistant variants of Babesia gibsoni in clinical cases treated with atovaquone and azithromycin. *Journal of veterinary internal medicine* 23 (3): 493–498.

Schad, G.A., Hellman, M.E., and Muncey, D.W. (1984). *Strongyloides stercoralis*: hyperinfection in immunosuppressed dogs. *Experimental Parasitology* 57: 287–296.

Shoop, W.L., Michael, B.F., Eary, P.H. et al. (2002). Transmammary transmission of *Strongyloides stercoralis* in dogs. *Journal of Parasitology* 88: 536–539.

Spain, C.V., Scarlett, J.M., Wade, S.E. et al. (2001). Prevalence of enteric zoonotic agents in cats less than 1 year old in central New York; State. *Journal of Veterinary Internal Medicine* 15: 33–38.

Suzuki, K., Wakabayashi, H., Takahashi, M. et al. (2007). A possible treatment strategy and clinical factors to estimate the treatment response to *Babesia gibsoni* infection. *Journal of Veterinary Medical Science* 69: 563–568.

Tenney, T.D., Curtis-Robles, R., Snowden, K.F. et al. (2014). Shelter dogs as sentinels for *Trypanosoma cruzi* transmission across Texas. *Emerging Infectious Diseases* 20 (8): 1323–1326.

Thompson, R.C.A., Kapel, C.M.O., Hobbs, R.P. et al. (2006). Comparative development of *Echinococcus multilocularis* in its definitive hosts. *Parasitology* 132: 709–716.

Tysnes, K.R., Skancke, E., and Robertson, L.J. (2014). Subclinical *Giardia* in dogs – a veterinary conundrum relevant to human infection. *Trends in Parasitology* 30: 520–527.

Uehlinger, F.D., Greenwood, S.J., McClure, J.T. et al. (2013). Zoonotic potential of *Giardia duodenalis* and *Cryptosporidium* spp. and prevalence of intestinal parasites in young dogs from different populations on Prince Edward Island, Canada. *Veterinary Parasitology* 196: 509–514.

Vajner, L., Vortel, V., and Brejcha, A. (2000). Lung filaroidosis in the beagle dog breeding colony. *Veterinaria Medicina* 45: 25–30.

Villeneuve, A., Polley, L., Jenkins, E. et al. (2015). Parasite prevalence in fecal samples from shelter dogs and cats across the Canadian provinces. *Parasites & Vectors* 8: 281–290.

Wilson, J.F., Rausch, R.L., and Wilson, F.R. (1995). Alveolar hydatid disease. Review of the surgical experience in 42 cases of active disease among Alaskan Eskimos. *Annals of Surgery* 221: 315–323.

Yao, C.Q., O'Toole, D., Driscoll, M. et al. (2011). *Filaroides osleri* – two case reports and a review of canid infections in North America. *Veterinary Parasitology* 179: 123–129.

Yoshikawa, H., Yamada, M., Matsumoto, Y. et al. (1989). Variations in egg size of *Trichuris trichiura*. *Parasitology Research* 75: 649–654.

Zecca, I.B., Hodo, C.L., Slack, S. et al. (2020). Prevalence of *Trypanosoma cruzi* infection and associated histologic findings in domestic cats (*Felis catus*). *Veterinary Parasitology* 278: 109014–109021.

18

Heartworm Disease

Martha Smith-Blackmore[1,2]

[1] *Cummings School of Veterinary Medicine at Tufts University, North Grafton, MA, USA*
[2] *City of Boston Animal Care and Control, Boston, MA, USA*

18.1 Introduction

Heartworm disease is a serious vector-borne disease that is caused by the mosquito-borne filarial nematode *Dirofilaria immitis*. Though preventable, the disease is a global veterinary healthcare challenge, with *D. immitis* affecting dogs, cats and ferrets throughout the United States, many parts of South America, Europe, Asia, and Australia (Morchón et al. 2012). *D. immitis* is one of the most important parasitic infections of domestic dogs; it is relatively to very common in the United States and is endemic in most areas of the country, including urban areas where approximately 80% of the human population lives. Heartworm disease is also a health concern for wildlife species that serve as reservoirs.

Heartworms pose difficult challenges for shelter veterinarians and managers. Selecting and advocating for protocols regarding testing, prevention and treatment of a condition that is largely clinically invisible, has a long disease course, is expensive to treat and is unlikely to significantly impact the dog or cat during their shelter stay can be difficult. Despite these challenges, it is important for both population and individual health that heartworm disease is addressed in animal shelters, and it is feasible to do so.

It is especially important to maintain the separate concepts of infection versus disease. Heartworm infection is the occupation of the body by the parasite, whereas heartworm disease is the result of the pathophysiology of the worms within the body. The disease response varies depending on the lifestyle and activity of the animal, the worm burden and the individual immune response to the presence of the worms. Many animals can be infected with heartworms for several months before showing any clinical signs of disease.

A leading source of research and education on heartworm disease is the American Heartworm Society (AHS), which was founded in 1974 to "lead the veterinary profession and the public in the understanding of heartworm disease." The AHS convenes a triennial symposium where researchers and veterinarians from around the world meet every three years to present studies and discuss the latest scientific information on heartworm disease. The AHS frequently issues comprehensive guidelines for the diagnosis,

Infectious Disease Management in Animal Shelters, Second Edition.
Edited by Lila Miller, Stephanie Janeczko, and Kate F. Hurley.

prevention, and management of heartworm infection in pets based on the most recent scientific information. The AHS guidelines were developed specifically for individually owned animals and not for those housed in animal shelters, but the guidelines and other AHS resources can be used to help shelter staff, managers and adopters better understand this insidious disease and facilitate the implementation of practical shelter protocols that are medically responsible, provide for good animal welfare, make judicious use of limited resources, and serve as a proper example for adopters to follow for ongoing management and prevention of the disease. The Association of Shelter Veterinarians (ASV) and the AHS collaborated on a Heartworm Disease Resource Task Force to create a series of educational brochures that provide information to adopters about the disease (AHS 2017; ASV 2017). Downloadable, printable brochures help explain the shelter policy with regards to testing for and treating heartworms (i.e. whether or not a facility tests or treats, and which modalities are used) and recommendations for follow-up with a local veterinarian. These brochures offer shelter staff a concise and accurate tool to facilitate communicating about this complex disease.

18.2 Lifecycle of *Dirofilaria immitis*

Knowledge of the lifecycle of *D. immitis* in conjunction with the pharmacology of preventive and adulticidal medications is crucial to understanding prevention and treatment strategies and failures. (See Figure 18.1).

Heartworms have a complicated lifecycle characterized by a relatively long period from the initial introduction of the larval parasite by a mosquito to patent infection with adult worms. In a patent infection, adult female heartworms living in an infected animal produce microfilaria that circulate in the bloodstream. When a mosquito bites and takes a blood meal from this animal, microfilariae are picked up. These microfilariae develop and mature into "infective stage" larvae (L3) within the mosquito over a period of 10–14 days when suitable environmental conditions exist. Then, when the infected mosquito bites another susceptible animal, the infective L3 larvae enter the new host through the mosquito bite wound.

Once the larvae are inside a new host, they undergo continued maturation to the L4 stage and then become immature adults, followed by final maturation to the adult stage. It takes approximately six months for the L3 larval form to mature into adult heartworms. The period of time following infection from a mosquito bite until mature adult worms are present is known as the pre-patent period. When mature, heartworms can live for five to seven years in dogs and up to two or three years in cats. It is not known how long the adult heartworm can live within the ferret. Repeated exposures via bites on the same animal by infected mosquitos can lead to heavier worm burdens, and the presence of multiple life-stages and/or adult worms of various ages is possible in one patient.

While ferrets are considered an aberrant host, laboratory studies have shown the ferret to be highly susceptible to *D. immitis*, with infection and recovery rates similar to those achieved in the dog and higher than those seen in cats (McCall 1998). Microfilaremia is characteristically of low concentration and transient in nature, as seen in heartworm-infected cats.

18.3 Transmission

D. immitis can be transmitted by over 70 species of fresh and saltwater mosquitoes, though certain species (e.g. *Aedes trivittatus*, *Aedes sierrensis* and *Culex quinquefasciatus*) are considered more important vectors (Wang et al. 2014).

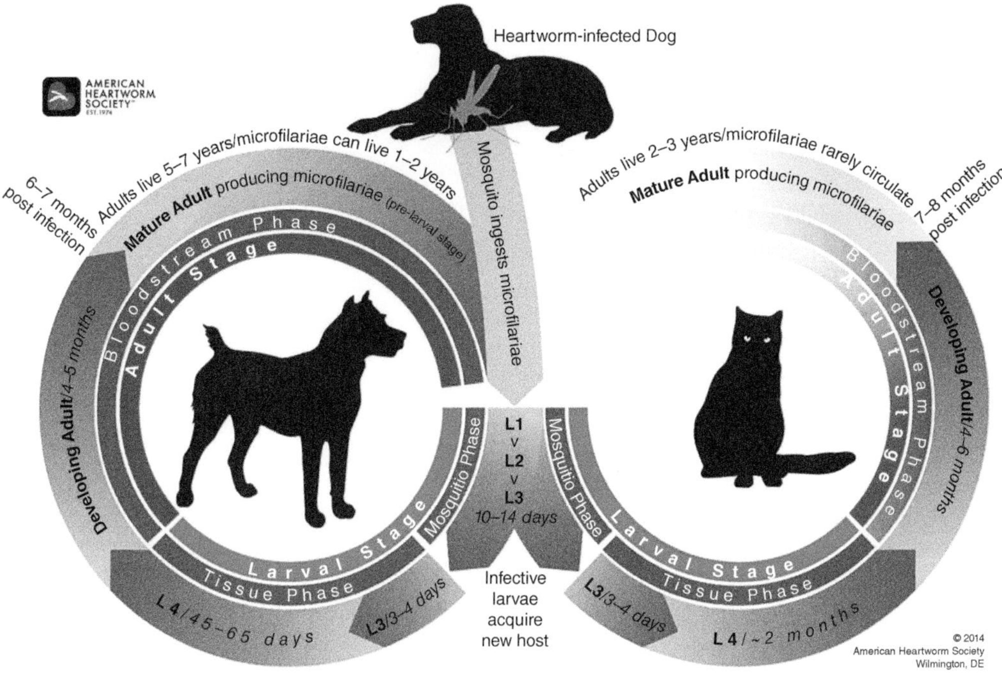

Figure 18.1 Heartworm lifecycle in the dog and cat. *Source:* Illustration courtesy of the American Heartworm Society.

Different species of mosquitoes have widely varying feeding and breeding habits, as well as inherent differences – such as how far they can travel or their ability to survive unfavorable weather – that affect their efficiency as heartworm vectors.

Environmental changes have led to the spread and increased prevalence of heartworms. Urban "heat islands" and artificial irrigation have enabled mosquitos to flourish in geographic areas where they previously did not survive. *Aedes albopictus* (the Asian tiger mosquito) is an invasive mosquito that is adapted to colder weather and lives successfully in urban areas. It does not need wetlands to reproduce; any water that is standing for three days or more (e.g. in puddles, birdbaths, flowerpots, old tires) can support Asian tiger mosquito reproduction (Benedict et al. 2007). In the western United States, the irrigation of lawns and golf courses and planting of trees has expanded the habitat for *A. sierrensis* (western knot hole mosquito), the primary vector for transmission of heartworms in those states. Additionally, relocation of microfilaremic dogs exposes wildlife reservoirs such as coyotes in these areas, ensuring the establishment of enduring endemic heartworm infections in these new geographic areas (Aher et al. 2016).

Mosquito infection rates in the locations immediately surrounding a heartworm positive dog have been shown to be *10 times* higher than mosquito infection rates otherwise detected in that community (Mckay et al. 2013), so rapid identification and intervention with heartworm positive dogs are important as they pose a risk to other animals as well as themselves. A dog can serve as its own reservoir if it is bitten more than once by the same mosquito; the mosquito ingests the microfilaria, incubates them and redeposits the now maturing L3 forms. Similarly, puppies can be born with microfilaremia inherited from their dam with a patent infection, but the microfilariae will not be able to mature to adult heartworms unless a mosquito ingests and then redeposits the maturing larval form into the puppies via a bite.

The *Culex* species mosquito, which is the most common species in many urban areas, feeds on both cats and dogs without preference (Gomes et al. 2007). Thus, microfilaremic dogs in a shelter or community environment are an exposure risk to themselves, other dogs, cats and ferrets. Cats and ferrets do not pose the reservoir risk that dogs do, as the infection rarely becomes patent in cats and ferrets, and when it does, microfilaremia is brief and transient. It should be stressed that, in order for successful transmission of the parasite to occur, there must be a reservoir of infection, a competent mosquito vector and the appropriate climatic conditions (Nelson et al. 2020a).

18.4 Heartworm Disease in Dogs

In the dog, adult worms can reach 30 cm (11.8 in.) in length. Heartworms reside in the pulmonary arteries and may cause severe inflammation, truncation of pulmonary vessels, thickening of the arterial parenchyma, pulmonary arterial occlusion, inflammation, pulmonary hypertension and right-sided heart failure. (See Figure 18.2).

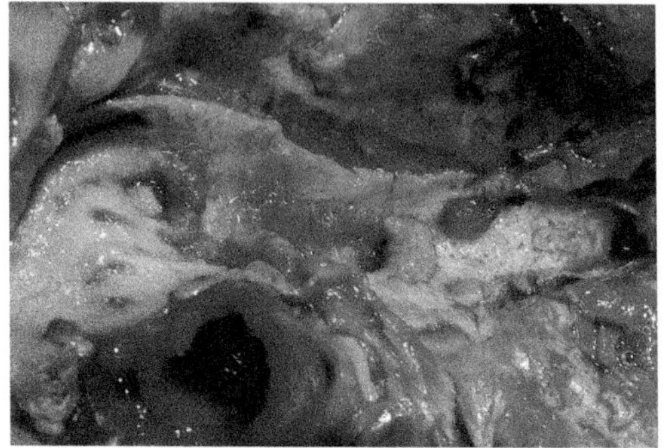

Figure 18.2 Inflammation and thickening of the arterial parenchyma in a dog due to heartworms. *Source:* Image courtesy of Stephen Jones.

Clinical signs of heartworm disease in domestic dogs include exercise intolerance, coughing, dyspnea, jugular distension, hepatomegaly, cachexia, anorexia, epistaxis and ascites. It is important to note, however, that many infected dogs do not show any clinical signs for a prolonged period of time. Because shelters rely heavily on physical examinations to detect infectious disease in their populations, it is easy to understand why the disease may not be suspected. These occult infections will only be detected with appropriate diagnostic testing protocols and/or after enough time has passed that the worms have caused sufficient damage to the cardiovascular system that abnormalities can be readily detected on a physical examination. Numerous differential diagnoses exist for each of the common clinical signs, and mild cases may be mistakenly attributed to other causes. For example, dogs presenting with coughing as the primary or only clinical sign may be erroneously diagnosed with canine infectious respiratory disease (CIRD) or heart disease. (See Chapters 10, 11, and 12 for information about CIRD, Canine Distemper (CDV), and Canine influenza (CIV) respectively.)

18.5 Heartworm Disease in Cats

While cats can be infected with heartworms in a manner similar to dogs, the presentation of heartworm disease in cats is very different from heartworm disease in dogs; the frequency of infection is lower and the heartworm's lifespan is shorter. The cat is an atypical host for heartworms, and most worms in cats do not survive to the adult stage. Cats with adult heartworms typically have just one to three worms, and many cats affected by heartworms have no adult worms present (Biasato et al. 2017).

There are two distinct phases of heartworm disease in the cat. The first phase occurs in the early stages of infection when the immature worms reach the caudal pulmonary arteries and most of them die. The immature dead worms induce a strong vascular and parenchymal inflammatory response in the lung tissue (Browne et al. 2005), which is often referred to as Heartworm Associated Respiratory Disease (HARD).

The second phase occurs later in the course of infection in some cats when adult worms die. Heartworms that reach maturity in the cat seem to have anti-inflammatory properties that minimize some of the pathologic changes, and thus also minimize the types of clinical signs more commonly seen in dogs. A cat with a single or low number of adult worms may be asymptomatic until the death of the adult worm(s). Cats will exhibit acute respiratory distress or sudden death due to embolization of dead worms or worm fragments resulting in pulmonary thromboembolism. See Figure 18.3.

Cats with only a few worms are still considered to be heavily infected in terms of parasite biomass because of the relatively small feline body size. Aberrant migration occurs more frequently in cats than in dogs. Though uncommon, heartworms are found disproportionately in the body cavities, systemic arteries, and central nervous system of cats.

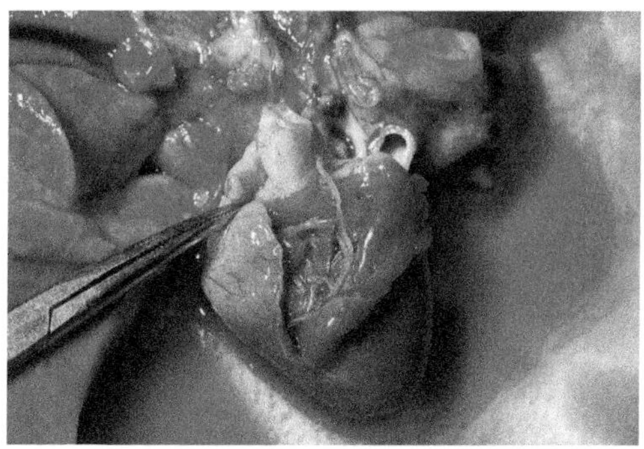

Figure 18.3 A single dead adult heartworm was found at necropsy in a cat's heart after a short illness followed by respiratory distress and death. *Source:* Image courtesy Stephen Jones.

18.6 Heartworm Disease in Ferrets

Clinical signs of heartworm disease in the ferret include lethargy, open-mouth and/or rapid breathing, pale blue or muddy gum color and coughing. While it was hypothesized in earlier literature that heartworm disease in ferrets is similar to the disease presentation in cats, the disease actually bears a mix of features seen in both canine and feline disease.

Clinical signs can develop rapidly with even a single worm because of the relatively small size of the ferret heart and lungs. Severe signs of right-sided heart failure with pleural effusion and ascites can be seen with just one worm in the ferret heart. Acute death may occur without preceding clinical signs, even with very low worm burdens, due to pulmonary artery obstruction. Interestingly though, worm burdens as high as 30 have been recorded in the ferret (Mobley 2010).

18.7 Screening and Diagnostic Testing

18.7.1 Screening and Diagnostic Testing in Dogs

Heartworm infections are most commonly detected through the use of a variety of commercial antigen blood tests and screening tests to detect circulating microfilaria. Currently available antigen tests only detect circulating antigen of adult female worms. Microfilariae are produced when mature adult worms of both sexes are present in the animal. Thus, testing before seven months of age is a waste of resources: if an early-stage of infection is present, the worms will not yet be detectable by any currently available method due to the prepatent period (the period between infection with heartworm and the ability to demonstrate the presence of the parasite in the body).

The commercial antigen blood tests can be performed on individual blood samples or batched, with multiple tests run simultaneously. Heartworm infected dogs tested within the prepatent period will not have detectable antigen, and those dogs that have been on preventive medication may have a false negative antigen test due to antibody–antigen complex formation. Recent studies have shown that heat-treatment of serum samples may lead to positive test results in canine serum samples that had no heartworm antigen previously detected, presumably by breaking antigen–antibody complexes (Little et al. 2014). One method of heat treatment is described as using an aliquot (0.7–1.5 ml) of a serum sample placed in a dry heat block at 103° C (217° F) for 10 minutes, the resultant coagulum centrifuged, and the supernatant used in the assay (Velasquez et al. 2014). Another method described is to place 1 ml of whole blood into a tube, dilute it with 1 ml of saline solution to prevent clotting, place the tube in a cup of water that has been heated to boiling in the microwave and allow the sample to sit in the hot water for 10 minutes (DiGangi 2017). Regular testing procedures can then be followed using this heat-treated sample. Most commercial laboratories are willing to perform a heat-treated heartworm antigen test as an add-on.

Microfilaria may be detected by direct microscopy or by using a variety of concentration tests. Concentration tests increase the likelihood of detecting microfilariae; direct screening of blood smears alone is not recommended due to its inability to detect infections with small numbers of circulating microfilariae. However, circulating microfilariae are seldom found in infected cats or ferrets and therefore routine screening of these species for microfilariae is not recommended because of the low sensitivity. See Table 18.1

In their current guidelines, the AHS recommends (Nelson et al. 2020a) running both a heartworm antigen and microfilaria test to screen all dogs over the age of six months of age. This is sometimes referred to as "tandem testing". The reasons for advocating both the antigen and microfilaria tests is because using just one test modality may miss infections; testing for both antigen and microfilariae may unmask otherwise undetected infections. See Table 18.2.

Discordant results should be interpreted within the context of the patient's circumstances. If an animal is positive by microfilaremia only, a heat-treated antigen test is

Table 18.1 Diagnostic testing methods for microfilariae.

Test	Method
Direct microscopy	A drop of whole blood under a coverslip or a stained blood smear is examined under the microscope for the presence of microfilariae
Hematocrit tube concentration	A blood sample is spun in a hematocrit tube; microfilariae will accumulate at the level of the buffy coat. A drop of buffy coat diluted in a drop of saline or a stained smear of the buffy coat can be examined microscopically.
Filter test	A lysed blood sample is forced through a filter, trapping the microfilariae. The filter is then stained and examined by microscopy to determine the presence of microfilariae.
Modified Knott test	9 ml of 2% formalin is added to 1 ml of whole blood, which lyses the blood cells. The mixture is centrifuged at 1200 × g, the pellet stained with methylene blue and examined by microscopy for microfilariae.

Table 18.2 Diagnostic test limitations.

Testing for antigen only	Can lead to false negatives due to immature infections, male-only infections, low worm burdens, poor technique or antigen–antibody complex interference.
Testing for microfilariae only	May miss single-sex infections, immature life stages, immune responses that eliminate microfilariae, and cases of infection where the patient is on or has received preventive medication. • False negatives are possible due to poor technique • False positives are possible if microfilariae of the parasite *Acanthocheilonema (Dipetalonema) reconditum* are incorrectly identified as *D. immitis*.

recommended. Antigen positive dogs should be retested with a confirmatory laboratory test before starting adulticidal therapy.

18.7.1.1 Additional Diagnostics for Infected Dogs

Thoracic radiographs and/or an echocardiogram may be helpful in confirming disease and staging the dog. Radiography provides the most objective method of assessing the severity of heartworm-associated cardiopulmonary disease. Typical (nearly pathognomonic) signs of heartworm vascular disease in the dog are enlarged, tortuous, and often truncated peripheral intralobar and interlobar branches of the pulmonary arteries, accompanied by variable degrees of pulmonary parenchymal disease. In the worst cases, the right heart eventually enlarges and may appear as a classic “reverse D” shape.

Echocardiography can provide definitive evidence of heartworm infection if worms are visualized; cardiac ultrasound also allows for assessment of cardiac anatomic and functional consequences of the disease. Serial echocardiograms can follow a patient’s recovery from heartworm disease over time. It is not an efficient screening method for diagnosis, particularly in dogs with light worm burdens.

Additional diagnostics, such as a complete blood count, serum biochemical profile, and urinalysis allow for assessment of the patient for coexisting conditions, to better understand the extent of damage from the disease, and to evaluate the patient’s suitability for adulticidal therapy. It is important to note that diagnostic test results are not fully predictive of posttreatment complications or success. Many shelter veterinarians successfully treat heartworm disease based on heartworm screening tests and clinical examination without further laboratory or radiographic pre-treatment evaluation. When a dog is adopted out with or immediately following treatment for heartworm disease and the adopter will be following up with their own veterinarian, they should be advised that their veterinarian may have different pre-treatment evaluation protocols or follow-up care recommendations.

18.7.2 Screening and Diagnostic Testing in Cats

Clinical signs of heartworm disease in cats are often nonspecific and include lethargy, anorexia, vomiting, coughing, dyspnea, and syncope. Clinical signs can be indistinguishable from and are easily mistaken for feline asthma. The reported vomiting may be true vomiting, or an observer may mistakenly identify coughing as vomiting as these are difficult to distinguish in cats, and cats may regurgitate gastrointestinal (GI) contents after coughing.

Diagnosis of heartworm infection can be elusive in cats because clinical signs may be absent or atypical; the first presenting sign may be sudden death. Due to the nature and the pathophysiology of heartworm infection in cats, a multistep diagnostic process is needed. No single ante-mortem diagnostic test can reach a high level of sensitivity for feline heartworm infection.

None of the presently available antigen tests can be relied upon to rule out heartworm infection in cats even when testing is limited to those animals with consistent clinical signs because infections consisting of only male worms, low worm burdens, and/or symptomatic immature infections are more common in cats. Necropsy surveys of shelter cats have shown that 30–50% of infected cats do not have a female worm present and would thus test negative on all antigen tests (Levy et al. 2011). Detectable antigenemia develops at about 5.5 to 8 months post-infection with a female worm in the cat.

Antibody tests for cats have the advantage of being able to detect infection by both male and female worms, as larvae of either sex can stimulate a detectable immune response as early as two months post-infection. Antibody tests do not offer an indication of the continued existence of an infection, however, just that an infection occurred at some point in the past. The different antibody tests vary in their sensitivity to each stage of larval development; thus, discordant results between test methods are common (Nelson et al. 2020b).

The correct interpretation of antibody test results requires thoughtful analysis and additional information, such as evaluation of the cat's history (which may or may not be available in the shelter setting). Since both juvenile and adult worms can cause clinical disease in the cat, both antibody and antigen tests are useful tools and, when used together, increase the probability of making appropriate diagnostic decisions. The performance of both antigen and antibody tests together increases the sensitivity of either single test alone (Berdoulay et al. 2004). As with dogs, heat treatment of feline serum increases antigen test positive results (Gruntmeir et al. 2017).

Because of the limitations of testing in cats and the fact that they do not pose a risk for heartworm transmission to other animals, testing for heartworms in the shelter cat should be reserved for symptomatic cats. Routine screening for heartworm disease is not indicated in asymptomatic shelter cats.

The most efficient approach for the diagnosis of feline heartworm disease in symptomatic cats is based upon the collective interpretation of several tests: thoracic radiography and serum antibody tests for a rising index of suspicion, and echocardiography and serum antigen tests for confirming the infection (Venco et al. 2015). Though it is a logical choice to place all cats in the shelter on heartworm preventive and perform diagnostic testing on symptomatic cats only, many shelters lack the resources and staffing to do so; they should inform adopters of potential heartworm disease concerns, particularly in symptomatic animals.

18.7.3 Screening and Diagnostic Testing in Ferrets

Due to the apparent transient nature of microfilaremia in ferrets, microfilaria detection is more challenging in ferrets than dogs; however, when found, it is diagnostic of heartworm infection. Combining heartworm antigen tests with imaging techniques, such as thoracic radiographs, echocardiography, and angiography (to detect adult heartworms in the heart and associated vessels), appears to yield a relatively high and accurate detection rate. False negative antigen tests are presumed to be due to antigenic loads below detectable levels—when lower worm burdens or single sex male worm infections are present—as in cases of feline and canine infections. Evidence of the accuracy and efficacy of antibody testing in ferrets is lacking (Zaffarano 2015).

Bilirubinuria is the clinicopathologic change detected most consistently in ferrets with heartworm disease and it may prove to be a consistent indicator for the disease (Antinoff 2001). Ferrets with heartworm disease may have radiographic signs of pleural effusion; along with tortuous and dilated pulmonary vasculature, right atrial and ventricular enlargement and dilation, and tricuspid regurgitation (Supakorndej et al. 1995).

Because of the limitations of testing in ferrets and the fact that they do not pose a risk for heartworm transmission to other animals, testing for heartworms in the shelter ferret should be reserved for symptomatic animals. Routine screening for heartworm disease is not indicated in asymptomatic shelter ferrets.

18.7.4 Diagnostic Strategies for Animal Shelters

When designing practical testing protocols for the animal shelter, it is important to consider that heartworm disease is endemic in dogs in the United States and the prevalence of heartworm disease varies by geographic location. The prevalence of heartworm disease in any community can theoretically be predicted based on several factors. The presence of certain species of mosquitos (*A. trivittatus* and *sierrensis*, *C. quinquefasciatus*), ambient temperature, median household income (affecting access to veterinary care), precipitation, elevation, relative humidity, forestation coverage, and surface water coverage all significantly influence *D. immitis* prevalence in dogs. Additional factors thought to be of influence include human population density and the prevalence of reservoir animals (e.g. feral dogs and coyotes) (Wang et al. 2014). Given the distribution mapping of *D. immitis* in the United States by the AHS (www.heartwormsociety.org, 2016) and the Companion Animal Parasite Council (CAPC), it is appropriate to consider all susceptible species to be at risk of heartworm transmission in the continental United States and Hawaii.

Necropsy surveys of shelter cats have placed the prevalence of adult heartworm infections at 5 to 15% of the rate in unprotected dogs in any given location (Venco et al. 2011). Within areas where heartworm infection is considered common, there can be considerable local variation, with prevalence reaching as high as 70% in dogs (Tzipory et al. 2010). In shelter animals, the risk for heartworm infection is thought to be higher than in privately owned pets because stray and surrendered shelter animals are less likely to have received prior veterinary care or preventive medication (Colby et al. 2011).

Though the AHS recommends "tandem testing" in their current guidelines (Nelson et al. 2020a), animal shelters should consider this recommendation in balance with available resources and relative disease risk. Animal shelters that do not routinely test for heartworm disease often cite cost, time and a lack of technical skill among shelter staff (Colby et al. 2011). The benefit of testing at intake identifies and allows for addressing positive dogs that may serve as a reservoir for transmission within the shelter and community. Shelters in areas where prevalence is low or those with scant resources may consider testing for heartworm disease at the point of adoption at the adopter's expense.

In areas of high heartworm prevalence, it may be more cost-effective for shelters to screen dogs for microfilaria first. In cases where preventive is known to have been used, it may be most effective to test for antigen first. Using this logical approach may increase the number of positive cases identified with a single screening test; it should be carefully considered which testing modality to use if shelters do not perform both antigen and microfilariae testing.

If the shelter designs a protocol where only some dogs are tested, the dogs at highest risk and/or most likely to be placed with an adopter or other sheltering organization should be tested; i.e. symptomatic and stray dogs, dogs transported from higher risk regions and those dogs selected for adoption or transfer. Because of the lifecycle of *D. immitis*, testing of puppies under seven months of age is not indicated regardless of other risk factors.

Due to the lag time between exposure to heartworm via the mosquito bite and the point at which an animal may test positive (the prepatent period), adopters should be counseled that an animal is not considered truly heartworm-free until two antigen tests – separated by six months – detect no evidence of infection. The language "no antigen detected" or "below detectable limits" is preferred over "negative" as it more accurately communicates testing as a single-point-in-time or "snapshot" result. Shelters should communicate clearly with adopters, verbally and in writing, what test(s) were used and the results. Similarly, if a dog is not tested for heartworm disease, this should be explained to adopters along with guidance for the next steps.

Cats are at risk for heartworm infection wherever the disease is endemic in dogs (Nelson et al. 2020a) and by extrapolation, so are ferrets. Because diagnosis is more difficult in cats and ferrets and few options are available for effective palliative and curative treatments, screening healthy cats and ferrets housed in shelters is not generally recommended. In contrast to the challenges of diagnosis and treatment, chemoprophylaxis is highly effective, and current AHS guidelines call for preventive medications to be administered to all cats and ferrets in endemic areas (Dunn et al. 2011). It is important to note that AHS guidelines are general guidelines and are not specific for shelters; each organization must carefully balance these recommendations along with the needs of the population and available resources.

18.8 Prevention

One of the most effective preventive measures to minimize the risk of heartworm infection in animal shelters is to avoid keeping heartworm infected dogs in the facility. Maintaining an untreated microfilaremic dog in the shelter combined with a lack of mosquito control poses serious health and welfare risks to the other susceptible animals. Testing, using preventives, addressing mosquito concerns in and around the shelter, and treating infected dogs in low prevalence areas may help prevent the establishment of additional heartworm-endemic areas; on a population level, the impact of treatment is greatest where the prevalence is low.

Multimodal strategies for heartworm prevention incorporate administration of systemic monthly preventives (as well as the use of topical mosquito-repellent ectoparasiticides and other adjunctive measures (e.g. mosquito control, reducing exposure) to prevent in-shelter heartworm transmission (McCall et al. 2008). Mosquito control measures include drainage of standing water, environmental treatment for mosquito larvae, and knowing when mosquito feeding is at its peak so animals may be housed indoors during those times of the day. Because mosquito feeding times may also be the best hours for outdoor enrichment (not in the heat of the day), mosquito control and ectoparasiticides may be of higher priority in some locations.

There are several products available for use on dogs to repel and kill mosquitoes for an entire month; these products contain permethrin at relatively high concentrations (e.g. Effitix® [44.88%; Virbac], K9 Advantix® II [44%; Bayer], Vectra 3D® [36.08%; Ceva]; Activyl Tick Plus [42.5%; Merck]). Recent research indicates that treatment of dogs with a combination of dinotefuran, permethrin and pyriproxyfen (Vectra 3D) inhibits the uptake of heartworm microfilariae from infected dogs and prevents transmission of infective larvae from infected mosquitoes to non-infected dogs (McCall et al. 2016). These spot-on products are not labeled for use in cats, nor should they be used in cats due to severe toxicity. Insect repellents containing DEET (N, N-diethyl-meta-toluamide) are not safe for use in dogs, cats or ferrets. Neurologic signs (tremors, hyperexcitation, ataxia, and seizures), skin irritation, hypersalivation and vomiting can result.

Long-lasting permethrin-impregnated clothing and bedding are available for dogs to repel mosquitoes (McCall et al. 2016). Repellent or barrier systems available at home improvement stores or a mosquito control service from a pest management company can assist in the reduction of mosquito exposure risk in and around the animal shelter.

Although year-round heartworm preventive use is recommended throughout the United States, only about 60% of dogs receive preventive, and most dogs only receive seasonal prevention. Only 5% of cat owners provide heartworm prevention for their cats and use in ferrets is thought to be less. Even within highly endemic regions, preventive use varies based on client compliance, knowledge, or pet owner's demographics (Gates and Nolan 2010). Because preventive medication minimizes the risk of infected dogs acting as reservoirs in the shelter, and many combination products help with the elimination of other parasites, the use of preventive medication is strongly recommended for all puppies and dogs. This will benefit the individual dogs' health as well as that of the dog, cat and ferret populations.

While cats and ferrets are not generally considered to be reservoirs of heartworm disease, kittens and kits should be started on heartworm prevention at eight weeks of age for their own health. The ASV has issued a position statement urging sheltering organizations to maintain all dogs and cats on monthly heartworm preventive medications year-round regardless of geographic location to protect individual animal health and welfare and limit disease transmission within the community. Shelters that do not test for heartworm disease should still consider using monthly heartworm prevention, particularly in communities with high rates of heartworm disease. Shelter staff should be trained to recognize the signs of anaphylaxis from microfilaria die-off and how to respond.

Shelters should maintain accurate, detailed medical records on every animal so that each monthly dose can be administered on time. The medical record or the information in the record should be given to the adopter so they may provide it to their own veterinarian. Some shelters may find it more efficient to administer the first dose of preventive on intake and repeat for all residents on the first of the month. Macrocyclic lactone-containing products approved for heartworm prevention in dogs or cats include the avermectins (ivermectin, selamectin) and the milbemycins (moxidectin, milbemycin oxime). If shelters use ivermectin as a preventive treatment extra-label, they must be aware that toxicity is a concern. To minimize risks of complications, animals should be weighed carefully, the solution should be diluted for more accurate dosing (at 5–6 μ/kg) and a dosing chart should be created to reduce the risk of human error (Polak and Smith-Blackmore 2014). There are many approved commercially available oral, topical and injectable heartworm preventive products. See Table 18.3.

Table 18.3 Heartworm preventives.

Heartworm preventive product	Route of administration	Active ingredient	Species approval
Interceptor®, Interceptor Plus®, Trifexis™ (Elanco); Sentinel®, Sentinel Spectrum (Virbac)	Oral, monthly	Milbemycin oxime	Dogs
Heartgard®, Heartgard Plus (Merial), Tri-Heart® (Merck) IverheartMax® (Virbac)	Oral, monthly	Ivermectin	Dogs (Merial also makes Heartgard® for cats)
Revolution ®(Zoetis)	Topical, monthly	Selamectin	Dogs, cats
Proheart 6® (Zoetis)	Injectable, once every 6 months.	Moxidectin	Dogs
Advantage Multi® (Bayer)	Topical, monthly	Moxidectin	Dogs, cats, ferrets

The licensure and approval of imidacloprid/moxidectin topical (Advantage Multi® for Cats, Bayer) for use in ferrets provides a scientifically proven and licensed product for preventing heartworm transmission to ferrets. If used, this product should be administered monthly at the recommended minimum dose of imidacloprid, 20 mg/kg (9 mg/lb), and moxidectin, 2 mg/kg (0.9 mg/lb), by topical administration, regardless of indoor/outdoor status.

18.9 Heartworm Treatment

18.9.1 General Considerations Regarding Heartworm Treatment

Heartworm disease may be treated by a variety of methods, each with their own challenges of expense and exercise restrictions. In foster-based or sanctuary shelter settings, length of stay (LOS) considerations may be of lesser concern and less expensive, but longer treatment protocols may be chosen (so-called "moxi doxy" protocols). In other settings, a more aggressive treatment modality (two or three injection melarsomine protocols) may be chosen. Melarsomine, administered via deep intramuscular injection into the belly of the epaxial lumbar muscles (between L3 and L5), is the only adulticidal drug approved by the Food and Drug Administration (FDA).

Shelters should inform adopters which treatment protocol was used so their veterinarian can provide appropriate follow-up care. Some shelters will treat the disease and offer the dog for adoption, shifting the exercise restriction responsibility to the adopters. Other shelters will adopt heartworm positive dogs out and the treatment will be provided by the adopter through their own veterinarian or the shelter veterinary services. Different approaches may be appropriate given the variety of available resources in shelter settings, the number of heartworm positive dogs, and the local adopting communities.

18.9.1.1 Cage Rest

Live heartworms can cause endarteritis and arteriolar muscular hypertrophy of the caudal pulmonary arteries primarily, but most of the pathology seen in acute clinical disease is caused by dying heartworms. After worms die from adulticidal treatment, they decompose and fragment. Worm fragments lodge in the distal pulmonary arteries and capillary beds in the caudal lung lobes, blocking blood flow. Increased activity, stress or exercise increases the blood flow to blocked vessels, causing capillary delamination, rupture, and subsequent fibrosis which, in turn, may lead to increased pulmonary vascular resistance, pulmonary thromboembolism, and potential right-sided heart failure.

There is no test (or combination of tests) to accurately determine the number of heartworms present, thus every infected animal must be managed as though a substantial heartworm mass is present and that a severe individual immune reaction to the dead and dying worms could occur. Key factors influencing the probability of post-adulticide thromboembolic complications and outcome of treatment include activity level of the dog (including exercise, excitement, and overheating) and severity of infection (e.g. worm burden). Pathological sequelae can be limited using exercise restriction. The two-dose melarsomine protocol causes a larger worm die-off at one time as compared to the three-dose melarsomine protocol, and therefore the risk of a thromboembolic event may be higher with the shorter protocol. Regardless of the treatment protocol used, exercise restriction starting at the time of diagnosis and particularly during the period of adulticidal therapy through six to eight weeks post-treatment is essential for minimizing cardiopulmonary complications.

Most dogs can be safely leash-walked during the treatment recovery period, provided the dogs are calm and free from strenuous activities (reactive barking or straining against the leash). During cage rest, social interaction with people is crucial and should focus on simple, calming, affiliative interactions (e.g. sitting on the floor and stroking the dog, reading to the dog or gentle grooming). The long history of human-canine coevolution may explain why contact with humans appears to be more beneficial to dogs in terms of decreasing stress, and why providing beneficial social experiences with humans renders dogs more outgoing and tractable than does mere contact with conspecifics (Overall and Dyer 2005). Caregivers should be encouraged to talk to and interact with cage rested dogs. This is also a great opportunity for quiet clicker training. Dogs for whom grooming is non-traumatic are more likely to anticipate grooming positively, and to associate grooming with desirable human interaction. This is another quiet activity that can have a residual positive post-adoption effect.

Dogs on cage rest benefit from visual stimulation. If it is possible to provide them with housing with a window view, this may help to keep them engaged, provided they do not become overstimulated. Dogs who are quiet on car rides can enjoy drives with volunteers to enjoy stimulating sights, sounds and smells without physical exercise. However, dogs who become agitated in the car will not be candidates for this form of enrichment. Food toys that provide mental and physical stimulation may be used as the exclusive feeding method during cage rest. This ensures that the dog is engaged for a longer period during meals. There are many food-dispensing toys and feeding puzzles commercially available to assist with this challenge. Alternatively, cardboard boxes, empty washed polystyrene soda or water bottles can be used in similar ways. Nose-work games help to keep dogs mentally engaged (Center for Shelter Dogs 2016).

18.9.1.2 Timing of Spay/Neuter and Other Elective Surgery

Shelter veterinarians are frequently faced with the decision whether to perform an elective procedure, such as spay or neuter surgery, a dental procedure or a wound treatment on a heartworm-positive dog. It is likely that the risk of hemodynamic complications in the perioperative period is increased compared to heartworm negative patients in similar health. However, the benefits of expedited home placement may outweigh the anesthetic risk (Peterson et al. 2014) and it appears that the complication rate for asymptomatic or mildly affected heartworm positive dogs is not significant. The risk of hemodynamic complications increases significantly following the administration of adulticidal therapy, so surgery should either be performed before treatment or delayed until six months after. Elective surgical procedures should be avoided in dogs exhibiting clinical signs of more advanced disease; treatment to eliminate the heartworm infection should be initiated first. Surgery can then be performed six months after completion of adulticidal treatment.

18.9.1.3 Relocation and Transport Considerations

Relocation of dogs from communities with more dogs than adopters to communities with fewer dogs and more adopters can be a critical lifesaving activity. Because heartworm disease is an infectious disease, precautions must be taken to ensure the activity is legal and done in a manner to reduce the risk of harm to the transported dogs as well as to the animals in the receiving community.

Risks may be reduced by checking with the state veterinarian about regulations regarding the importation of heartworm positive dogs; taking steps to ensure microfilaremic dogs are rendered amicrofilaremic prior to transport and delaying transport for dogs that have been treated with melarsomine dihydrochloride for at least four weeks after an injection to minimize stress and physical exertion that accompany the relocation process.

Some states will not allow entry for heartworm positive dogs but do not mandate testing. In those cases, some organizations will send dogs without first testing them as the health certificate may be issued by a veterinarian stating that the animal is free from signs of infectious disease based on a physical exam (but not laboratory testing). Other states will allow entry to a heartworm positive dog provided they do not have circulating microfilaria.

What is legal or allowed may be different than what is in the best interest of the individual animal as well as the animals in the receiving community. Because of this, the American Veterinary Medical Association (www.avma.org), the Association for Animal Welfare Advancement (www.theaawa.org), the ASV (www.sheltervet.org), and AHS (www.heartwormsociety.org) have issued various guidelines for recommendations on minimizing heartworm transmission risk in transported dogs (AHS and ASV 2017; AAWA 2019; AVMA and ASV 2020). The ASV and AHS have developed a useful algorithm for decision making when selecting dogs for transport. See Figure 18.4.

18.9.2 Pharmacologic Considerations in the Management of Heartworm Infection

The various life-stages of heartworms have varying susceptibility to different drugs. Macrocyclic lactones are preventive drugs labeled to be effective in eliminating microfilaria to L3 forms when the worms have been present in the dog or cat for 30 days or less. These products have some activity on worms that have been in the body for as long as 45 days, but they are not reliable if the dosing period is greater than 30 days. When more than 30 days have elapsed since the last administration of the macrocyclic lactone, it is possible that an animal will develop heartworm infection because of the diminished efficacy of the drug against older immature stages.

Melarsomine is an adulticidal drug that is effective against adult worms aged 120 days

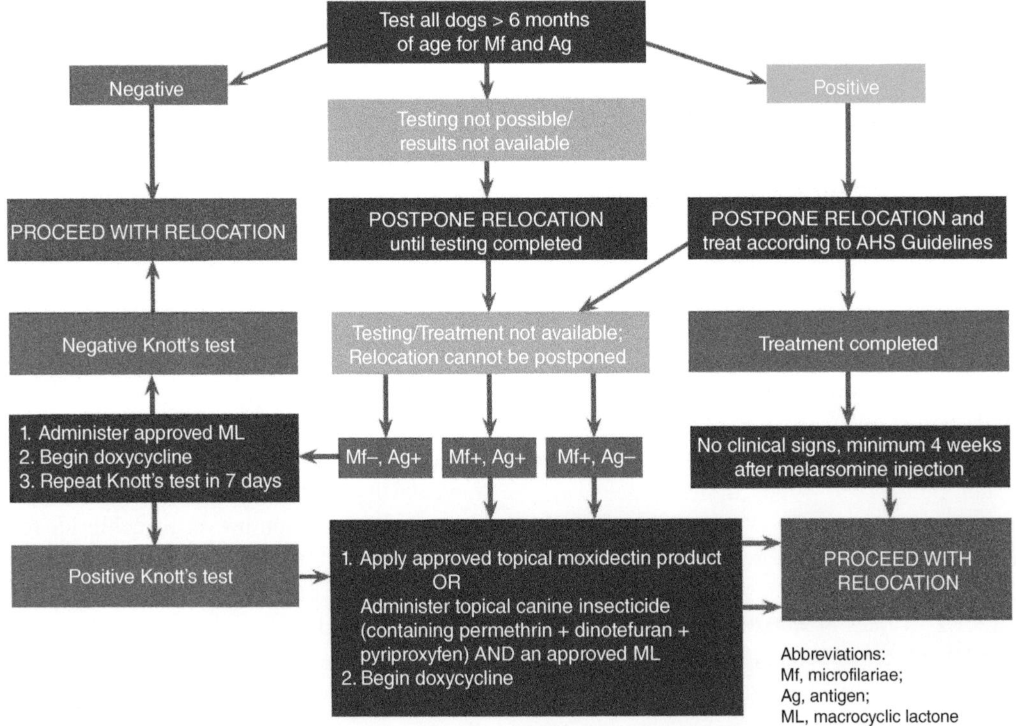

Figure 18.4 Algorithm for minimizing heartworm transmission in relocated dogs. *Source:* Courtesy of American Heartworm Society, www.heartwormsociety.org.

and older and is labeled for such use. The period between 30 and 120 days has been referred to as the "susceptibility gap" where the juvenile worms were thought to be too old to be killed by preventive, but too young to be killed by an adulticide. For this reason, it was recommended to administer preventive doses of macrocyclic lactones and doxycycline 60 days prior to adulticidal therapy, giving the juvenile worm forms enough time to mature so they would be susceptible to the adulticidal therapy. See Figure 18.5 for an image of female and male heartworms.

More recently, it has been suggested that no susceptibility gap exists when the first adulticidal treatment is given at the time of diagnosis, and if a three-dose protocol combined with doxycycline and ongoing administration of a macrocyclic lactone is used. (See the section on adulticidal therapy for additional information.)

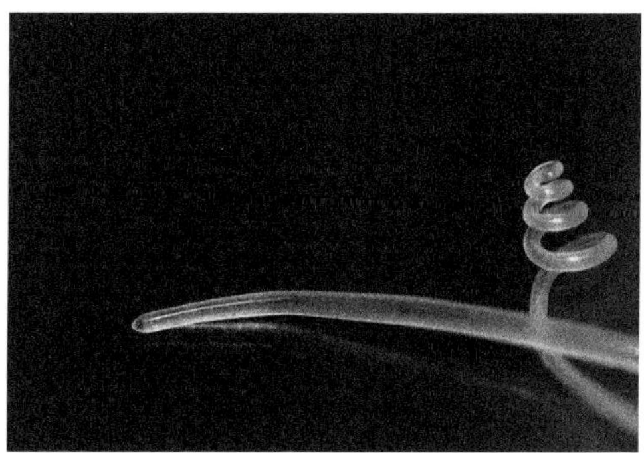

Figure 18.5 Adult female and male heartworms. The female heartworm has a straight tail while the male has a corkscrew tail. *Source:* Image courtesy Stephen Jones.

This protocol will likely be sufficient to eliminate all heartworm stages (including those 120 days and younger) and will protect the dog from subsequent infection (Bowman and Drake 2016). Thus, starting treatment with melarsomine, doxycycline and a macrocyclic lactone at the time of diagnosis appears suitable for maximum worm clearance; delaying treatment does not enhance the efficacy of the protocol and allows for disease progression. (See Figure 18.6 for an illustration of the susceptibility gap).

18.9.3 Principles of Adulticidal Therapy

Melarsomine is an organic arsenical chemotherapeutic agent that is the basis for adulticidal heartworm therapy. There are two commercial manufacturers of melarsomine dihydrochloride (*Immiticide*®, Merial and *Diroban*®, Zoetis). The drug should be given as part of either a two-dose or three-dose protocol. A two-dose treatment protocol reduces worm burden by 90.8% and a three-dose protocol reduces worm burden by 99%. Several treatment protocols are described later in this chapter and are compared in Table 18.4.

More recently, protocols have been developed using doxycycline and moxidectin to render heartworms sterile and attenuate the survival of the worms. These protocols are safer and more efficacious to use than ivermectin only "slow kill" protocols. In the shelter setting, the decision to use a treatment protocol other than that recommended by the AHS may

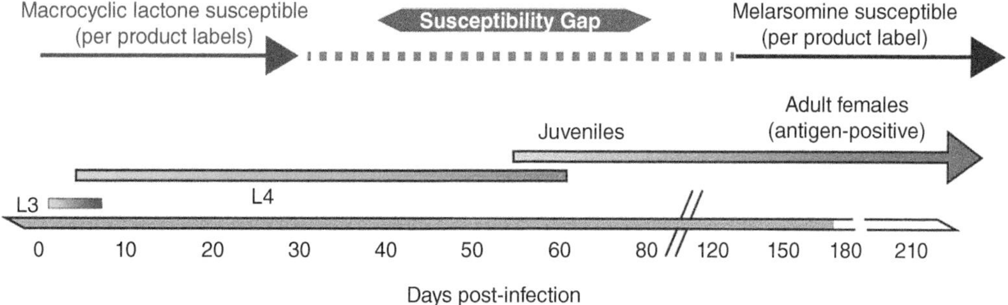

Figure 18.6 The susceptibility gap. *Source:* Illustration provided courtesy of Boehringer Ingelheim.

Table 18.4 Comparison of heartworm treatment protocols.

Treatment protocol	Benefits	Challenges	Consider when
Three-dose (split dosing) protocol with doxycycline and monthly macrocyclic lactone[1]	99% of worms eliminated Rapid decrease in infectivity of microfilaria Maximizes medical benefits for the individual dog	Treatment expense for medication[2] Long duration of cage rest Injection site complications (rare when injected properly)	Financial resources allow Adopter preference is for disease-free Dog is showing clinical signs Appropriate enrichment for the duration of cage rest is available either in the shelter or in foster homes[3]
Two-dose protocols with doxycycline and monthly macrocyclic lactone	Very effective but less efficacious than three-dose protocol, with 90% of worms eliminated Rapid decrease in infectivity of microfilaria Less expensive than three- dose protocol Shorter duration of cage rest	Treatment expense for medication Injection site complications (rare when injected properly) Cage rest duration Possibility of some female and juvenile worms surviving treatment	Financial resources allow Emphasis is on treat and release Adopting population is willing to accept the risk associated with incomplete treatment
Topical moxidectin/ imidacloprid with doxycycline "Moxi Doxy"	No injection Less expensive Rapid decrease in infectivity of microfilaria	Four to six months of cage rest Further research needed to understand the duration of live heartworms causing pathology Not an AHS approved protocol	Financial or other resource restrictions do not allow melarsomine therapy
Oral macrocyclic lactone with doxycycline	No injection Rapid decrease in infectivity of microfilaria	Long duration of heartworms in the dog (1–2 years) with ongoing cardiovascular pathology Not an AHS approved protocol	Not recommended for adulticidal treatment; may be used as an interim treatment until adulticidal methods are pursued

Table 18.4 (Continued)

Treatment protocol	Benefits	Challenges	Consider when
Oral macrocyclic lactone only WITHOUT DOXYCYCLINE "Slow Kill"	Reduces microfilaremia No injection	Long duration of heartworms in the dog (as long as three years), longer duration of infectivity Risk of producing macrocyclic lactone resistant microfilaria Not an AHS approved protocol	Not recommended in any circumstances

1) *Use of doxycycline and macrocyclic lactone at the outset of the treatment period leads to a rapid decrease in infectivity of microfilaria*
2) *Treatment expense may include LOS calculations that can influence choices*
3) *Transfer to a foster home or adoption is an option with any of the treatment protocols available, provided humane cage rest protocols are communicated and used.*

be based upon consideration of the financial resources of the organization, the overall health and needs of the overall population, and/or behavioral needs of the patient. Regardless of the specific approach taken in terms of drugs and dosing schedule, exercise restriction is the cornerstone for mitigating disease progression in the affected animal.

Treating heartworm infections in asymptomatic patients or those exhibiting signs of mild disease is usually not problematic when exercise is curtailed. However, dogs exhibiting moderate to severe clinical signs should be stabilized before an adulticide is administered. Stabilization should include attention to two aspects of pathology: disease induced by inflammation in the lungs and pulmonary vasculature, and signs of right-sided congestive heart failure. This may require administration of glucocorticoids, diuretics, vasodilators, positive inotropic agents, and fluid therapy. Dogs with significant clinical signs may not be candidates for heartworm treatment in the animal shelter setting.

Acute onset or exacerbation of clinical signs in a heartworm-infected animal is likely due to the recent death of one or more adult worms. Worm death results in the release of vasoreactive substances that cause inflammation. Prednisone used in a tapering dose regime for a month has been shown to reduce parenchymal and arterial wall pathology. Some veterinarians will use prednisone prophylactically; however, in the animal shelter setting it may be more prudent to reserve its use for when symptoms arise, given the immune-suppressive properties of prednisone.

In chronic heartworm disease, right-sided congestive heart failure may result from interstitial fibrosis obliterating pulmonary capillary beds or, in acute disease, from thrombosis in small pulmonary arterioles. Right-sided congestive heart failure may be treated with furosemide and angiotensin-converting enzyme inhibitors. (See Figure 18.7).

18.9.3.1 *Wolbachia* and the Use of Doxycycline

Wolbachia is a gram-negative, intracellular bacterium that infects arthropod species, including many insects and some nematodes, including *D. immitis*. This bacterium does not live outside of its host and is transmitted vertically from adult female heartworms to microfilariae. *Wolbachia* infects all stages of the heartworm lifecycle and is believed to be

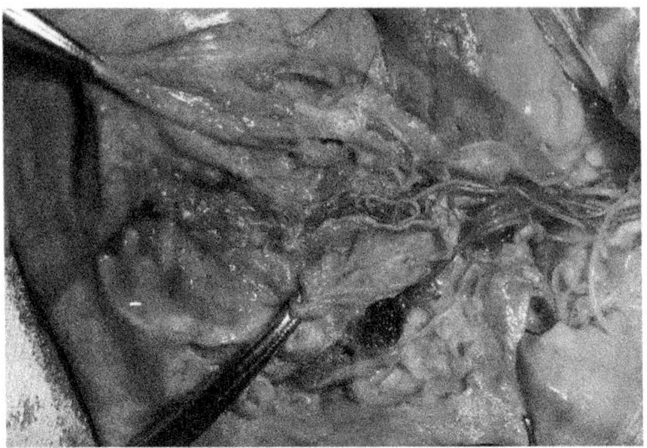

Figure 18.7 Heartworms present in the pulmonary vasculature, and necrotic material from dead worms in the distal pulmonary vasculature. *Source:* Image courtesy of Stephen Jones.

necessary for the development, reproduction, and long-term survival of the parasite.

The concomitant use of doxycycline with macrocyclic lactone preventives has several notable benefits in the management of heartworm infected dogs. Proteins derived from *Wolbachia* are directly associated with the inflammatory response, and innate and adaptive immune responses in filarial infections. Pretreatment of heartworm-positive dogs with preventive and doxycycline (or minocycline in cases of drug shortage) prior to receiving melarsomine injections to kill adult heartworms resulted in less pulmonary pathology associated with worm death in 60% of the dogs, compared to dogs treated with melarsomine alone (Dzimianski et al. 2006).

Doxycycline use decreases the microfilariae count more rapidly than preventives alone due to its ability to suppress the endo-symbiotic bacteria *Wolbachia*. When given daily to heartworm positive microfilaremic dogs for four weeks, tetracycline drugs, particularly doxycycline, are highly effective against the L3 and L4 stages, and at least moderately effective against juvenile heartworms.

Mosquitos fed on blood from dogs treated with doxycycline produce non-infective L3. Thus, the treatment of microfilaremic dogs with doxycycline at 10 mg/kg twice daily for one month blocks further transmission of heartworm infection. Doxycycline treatment should greatly reduce further selection of filarial strains that may carry genes that confer resistance to the macrocyclic lactone heartworm preventives, improve prophylactic efficacy, and subsequently lead to a reduction in cases of treatment failure (McCall et al. 2014). Doxycycline treatment also appears to have a slow-kill effect on adult heartworms, but more research is needed to determine the level of efficacy and length of time needed for all the worms to die.

18.9.4 Heartworm Treatment Protocol Selections for Dogs

18.9.4.1 Three -Dose "3D" (Split Dosing) Protocol

When considering the medical benefit to the individual dog in the typical home setting, the AHS three-dose protocol is the best choice; however, this must be balanced with a shelter's resources and ability to provide adequate behavioral care and cage rest during the treatment period. The split dosing protocol is a single dose of melarsomine administered at the time of diagnosis, followed by two injections on subsequent days one month later. No improvement in efficacy is expected with a delay in initiating therapy with both melarsomine dihydrochloride and macrocyclic lactones, even with the presence of younger heartworms; however, alternative versions of what is otherwise the same protocol may note initiation of melarsomine at day 60.

On day one, one deep intramuscular (IM) injection of melarsomine is administered at 2.5 mg/kg (5 mg/lb) into the belly of the epaxial lumbar muscles between L3 and L5. Melarsomine must not be injected into any other muscles, intravenously (IV) or subcutaneously (SC). This is followed one month later by two IM injections of the same dose 24 hours apart. From a strictly biologic perspective, this split-dosing protocol is preferred due to the increased safety and efficacy compared with the two-dose regimen. The first injection eliminates most of the male worms, which comprise approximately 50% of the adult worm population in the typical dog. Waiting one month before administering two back-to-back melarsomine injections allows the dog to clear the first round of dead worms and recover before the second set of injections, which is necessary to eliminate the hardier female worm. The AHS recommends this protocol for all dogs regardless of clinical disease status, however, dogs with clinically severe signs should be stabilized before the administration of melarsomine.

18.9.4.2 Two-Dose "2D" Protocol

In sheltering agencies, the medical benefits of the three-dose protocols must be weighed against a 50% increase in drug costs and a longer treatment time, which can lead to shelter crowding and reduce the quality of life if dogs are kept in the facility throughout the treatment period (Colby et al. 2011). When a two-dose protocol is used, all adult worms are killed at virtually the same time. Shelters that treat with the two-dose treatment protocol should understand that this protocol is 90% adulticidal, and usually 100% of the male worms are killed. Some female worms may survive treatment and thus treatment with this protocol may result in some dogs requiring repeated treatment. The actual two-dose protocol may be found on the AHS website.

18.9.4.3 Non-Arsenical Protocols

In what has become known as "slow kill" therapy, the ivermectin-based heartworm preventives are used to clear the microfilariae from the blood and reduce the lifespan of immature and adult heartworms. However, older adult worms appear to be more resistant to these effects and it may take more than two years of continuous administration of the preventive for all worms to die off. "Slow kill" is much less effective than adulticide treatment and may not eliminate all the worms, even after 16–36 months of treatment. Cage rest is necessary for the duration of this period, and pathologic changes will continue to accumulate.

"Slow kill" ivermectin-only preventive administration is not recommended by the AHS as a treatment for heartworm disease. However, AHS guidelines do state that if adulticide treatment is contraindicated or unavailable, a macrocyclic lactone may be used long-term with doxycycline (Grandi et al. 2010). The myth that the "slow kill" method is "just as good" as melarsomine therapy may have originated in McCall et al.'s 2001 study. This study demonstrated that 30 months of ivermectin at preventive doses reduced seven-month-old worms by 94% and eight-month-old worms by 56%. However, the older the worms are at the start of "slow kill" therapy, the less efficacious the therapy will be.

It is the author's experience that unfortunately adopters (and the public) are frequently instructed that the worms will "just go away" if monthly heartworm preventive medication is administered. Though "slow kill" protocols usually result in the eventual conversion to a negative heartworm test, dogs must be cage rested for the duration of this treatment (up to two years), and disease pathology will continue to progress during that time. The longer the heartworms are in the dog, the more damage that is occurring, especially to the pulmonary vasculature. Indeed, heartworm-infected dogs administered macrocyclic lactone for one year developed radiographic signs of heartworm disease and severe pulmonary pathology with multiple pathologic changes including enlarged pulmonary arteries, villous proliferation characteristic of heartworm infection, alveolar disease, interstitial lung disease, and parenchymal fibrosis (Rawlings et al. 2001). See Figure 18.8.

Recent research suggests immune complex formation in dogs infected with heartworm and managed with "slow kill" can induce false-negative antigen test results, misleading veterinarians and owners about the efficacy of this approach. Moreover, compliance with monthly preventive administration appears poor, even after a heartworm diagnosis. The presence of persistent microfilaremia reported in at least one dog has implications for resistance selection (Drake et al. 2015).

Doxycycline (or minocycline or azithromycin in cases of shortages) and ivermectin (or

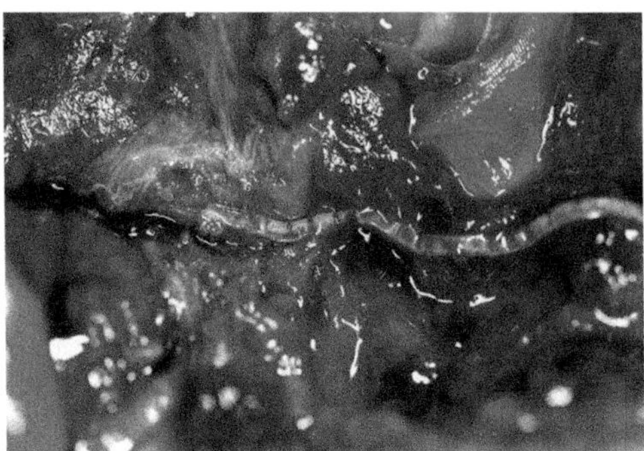

Figure 18.8 A dead worm and endarteritis in a dog treated with "slow-kill" therapy for three years, euthanized after presenting in heart failure. *Source:* Image courtesy of Stephen Jones.

moxidectin/imidacloprid) may be considered for treatment in cases where there are no clinical signs, when the LOS in the facility is less of a concern (e.g. sanctuary or foster, where the dog tolerates cage rest well) and when there is a shortage of melarsomine. In all cases, there should be clear communication with the adopter of what testing, prevention and treatment protocols were used, and what the next steps should be with the adopter's veterinarian.

Topical moxidectin/imidacloprid (Advantage Multi, Bayer) therapy provides higher blood and tissue concentrations that may be maintained longer than other macrocyclic lactones. This decreases macrocyclic-lactone resistance; the product is an approved microfilaricidal agent. In one limited pilot study, topical moxidectin/imidacloprid was administered to five heartworm antigen-positive dogs with or without microfilaremia. All dogs were amicrofilaremic by day 90, antigen clearance was seen as early as day 90 and, in most cases, by day 120. All dogs were antigen-negative by day 210. A subsequent larger study is producing similar data (Ames 2016).

18.9.4.4 Post-Treatment Testing

Follow up for testing (i.e. both antigen testing and screening for microfilariae) is recommended six months after adulticide treatment is completed. If a dog is found to be microfilaremic at this time, it may be due to several possibilities, including incomplete clearance of adult worms, maturation of immature worms (if a preventive was not given during adulticide therapy), or a new infection due to a lapse in chemoprophylaxis. Historically, microfilaricidal treatment was usually administered three to four weeks after adulticidal therapy, with the understanding that several weekly treatments were often required to completely eliminate circulating microfilariae (McCall et al. 2008). Current protocols utilizing doxycycline, in combination with regular preventive doses of macrocyclic lactones, have essentially eliminated the need for post-adulticidal elimination of microfilariae in this manner (Bazzocchi et al. 2008).

If all adult female worms are killed with adulticidal treatment, dogs should be antigen-negative by six months after treatment has been completed. However, adult worms may continue to die for at least a month following adulticidal treatment. Dogs that are still antigenemic at any time less than nine months post-melarsomine treatment should be allowed more time to clear before being considered for retreatment. Dogs that test positive on antigen testing nine months (or longer) post-adulticidal treatment are recommended to undergo a second round of adulticidal treatment.

18.9.4.5 Treatment for Cats and Ferrets

There are no adulticidal therapies available for cats or ferrets, however, a diagnosis of heartworm disease will guide the management of the animal's clinical signs and a more specific prognosis. If a cat can be managed symptomatically for two to three years while continuously on heartworm prevention, the cat may be cleared of heartworms. Additionally, pulse therapy of doxycycline may be considered to reduce *Wolbachia*-related consequences.

Administering doxycycline and either ivermectin or moxidectin (Advantage Multi) should kill adult worms in cats over a month-long period. However, killing worms often causes clinical signs and sudden death in cats. By treating with doxycycline and eliminating *Wolbachia*, it is postulated that the dying worms will be less antigenic and inflammatory, but research is needed to see whether this is true. Transjugular extraction of heartworms has been performed in cats, but this is not a practical approach in most animal shelters.

Previously published ferret heartworm treatment protocols using adulticide therapy with melarsomine have fallen out of favor because of adverse reactions (Morrissey and Kraus 2012). A small study of ferrets treated for heartworm disease that compared administration of ivermectin alone to ivermectin in combination with melarsomine suggested that higher survival rates may be achieved when ivermectin is administered alone (Antinoff 2001). This study's small sample size makes the significance of mortality rates, survival times, and co-morbid conditions difficult to interpret.

Anecdotally, moxidectin (ProHeart®, Zoetis) has been used at 0.17 mg/animal in a small number of heartworm antigen-positive ferrets, with evidence of the potential for higher survivability than traditional treatments with melarsomine or ivermectin (Cottrell 2004). Research is needed to understand the benefit of doxycycline in heartworm infected ferrets.

18.10 Conclusion

Heartworm disease in animals in shelters and resource-scarce communities presents a unique set of challenges. Shelter staffing and budgets vary widely from scant to extensive; this, along with a lack of clear guidance for heartworm disease management in animal shelters, creates significant confusion on the best approach to manage the disease in dogs, cats and ferrets. Without accurate information, animal shelter staff may either ignore heartworm disease or implement compromised management practices that may lead to suboptimal protection of shelter animals, ineffective treatment of infected animals, or adoption of infected animals to unsuspecting adopters.

In the animal shelter setting, resources must be allocated to best serve a variety of competing needs. Decisions should be based on careful consideration of the best use of resources in balance with known risks and with clear information communicated to adopters regarding heartworm post-adoption testing and treatment recommendations. Failure to address heartworm disease in the shelter may lead to an increased risk of disease transmission throughout the shelter, community and wildlife reservoirs. A collaborative effort between shelter management, the shelter veterinarian, adopter and family veterinarian can provide an opportunity to work together to minimize disease transmission and help ensure that once-homeless pets have long and healthy, heartworm-free lives with their new families.

References

Aher, A., Caudill, D., Caudill, G. et al. (2016). Prevalence, genetic analyses, and risk factors associated with heartworm (*Dirofilaria immitis*) in wild coyotes (*Canis latrans*) from Florida, USA. *Journal of Wildlife Diseases* 52 (4): 785–792.

American Heartworm Society (AHS) (2017). Shelter Educational Brochures. https://www.heartwormsociety.org/veterinary-resources/shelter-resources/shelter-resources (accessed 15 November 2020).

American Heartworm Society (AHS) and Association of Shelter Veterinarians (ASV) (2017). Minimizing Heartworm Transmission in Relocated Dogs. https://www.sheltervet.org/assets/Brochures/sko_transport_guidelines_for_web_e.pdf (accessed 15 November 2020).

American Veterinary Medical Association (AVMA) and Association of Shelter Veterinarians (ASV) (2020). Non-emergency Relocation of Dogs and Cats for Adoption

Within the United States Best Practices. https://www.avma.org/KB/Resources/Reference/AnimalWelfare/Documents/AVMA_BestPracticesAdoption_Brochure.pdf (accessed 18 June 2020).

Ames, M. (2016). Nonarsenical Heartworm Adulticidal Therapy. Heartworm Symposium, New Orleans.

Antinoff, N. (2001). Clinical Observations in Ferrets with Naturally Occurring Heartworm Disease, and preliminary evaluation of treatment with ivermectin with and without melarsomine. Heartworm Symposium, San Antonio.

Association for Animal Welfare Advancement (AAWA) (2019). Companion Animal Transport Programs Best Practices. https://cdn.ymaws.com/theaawa.org/resource/resmgr/files/2019/Transport1_Update_March_2019.pdf (accessed 18 June 2020).

Association of Shelter Veterinarians (ASV) (2017). Are You Adopting a Dog From Another Area of the Country? https://www.sheltervet.org/assets/Brochures/ahs_asv_adopt%20fr%20elsewhere%20hi-res.pdf (accessed 15 November 2020).

Association of Shelter Veterinarians (ASV) (2017). Heartworm Disease Resource Task Force. https://www.sheltervet.org/heartworm-disease-resources (accessed 15 November 2020).

Bazzocchi, C., Mortarino, M., Grandi, G. et al. (2008). Combined ivermectin and doxycycline treatment has microfilaricidal and adulticidal activity against *Dirofilaria immitis* in experimentally infected dogs. *International Journal for Parasitology* 38 (12): 1401–1410.

Benedict, M., Levine, R., Hawley, W. et al. (2007). Spread of the tiger: global risk of invasion by the mosquito *Aedes albopictus*. *Vector Borne and Zoonotic Diseases* 7 (1): 76–85.

Berdoulay, P., Levy, J.K., Snyder, P.S. et al. (2004). Comparison of serological tests for the detection of natural heartworm infection in cats. *Journal of the American Animal Hospital Association* 40: 376–384.

Biasato, I., Tursi, M., Zanet, S. et al. (2017). Pulmonary artery dissection causing haemothorax in a cat: potential role of *Dirofilaria immitis* infection and literature review. *Journal of Veterinary Cardiology* 19 (1): 82–87.

Bowman, D. and Drake, J. (2016). Susceptibility Gap and Patent Heartworm Infection Treatment. Heartworm Symposium, New Orleans.

Browne, L., Carter, T., Levy, J. et al. (2005). Pulmonary arterial disease in cats seropositive for *Dirofilaria immitis* but lacking adult heartworms in the heart and lungs. *American Journal of Veterinary Research* 66 (9): 1544–1549.

Center for Shelter Dogs (2016). Cummings School of Veterinary Medicine, Tufts University. Nose Work Games for Dogs. https://centerforshelterdogs.tufts.edu/wp-content/uploads/2016/03/4.0.4d_Nosework-Games.pdf (accessed 18 June 2020).

Colby, K., Levy, J., Dunn, K. et al. (2011). Diagnostic, treatment, and prevention protocols for canine heartworm infection in animal sheltering agencies. *Veterinary Parasitology* 176 (4): 333–341.

Cottrell, D. (2004). Use of Moxidectin (ProHeart 6) as a Heartworm Adulticide in 4 ferrets. *Exotic DVM* 5: 9–12.

DiGangi, B. (2017). Update on Heartworm Disease Management for Animal Shelters. Maddie's Fund webinar. https://www.maddiesfund.org/updates-on-heartworm-disease-management-for-animal-shelters.htm (accessed 18 June 2020).

Drake, J., Gruntmeir, J., Merritt, H. et al. (2015). False negative antigen tests in dogs infected with heartworm and placed on macrocyclic lactone preventives. *Parasites & Vectors* 8 (1): 68.

Dunn, K.F., Levy, J.K., Colby, K.N. et al. (2011). Diagnostic, treatment, and prevention protocols for feline heartworm infection in animal sheltering agencies. *Veterinary Parasitology* 176 (4): 342–349.

Dzimianski, M., McCall, J., Roberts, R. et al. (2006). Effects of ivermectin and doxycycline administered alone, together, or together plus melarsomine against adult *D. immitis* in dogs with induced infections: clinical observations. 51st Annual Meeting American Association of Veterinary Parasitologists, Honolulu.

Gates, M.C. and Nolan, T.J. (2010). Factors influencing heartworm, flea, and tick preventative use in patients presenting to a veterinary teaching hospital. *Preventive Veterinary Medicine* 93 (2): 193–200.

Gomes, L.A., Serrão, M.L., Duarte, R. et al. (2007). Attraction of mosquitoes to domestic cats in a heartworm enzootic region. *Journal of Feline Medicine and Surgery* 9 (4): 309–312.

Grandi, G., Quintavalla, C., Mavropoulou, A. et al. (2010). A combination of doxycycline and ivermectin is adulticidal in dogs with naturally acquired heartworm disease (*Dirofilaria immitis*). *Veterinary Parasitology* 169 (3): 347–351.

Gruntmeir, J.M., Adolph, C.B., and Thomas, J.E. (2017). Increased detection of Dirofilaria Immitis antigen in cats after heat pretreatment of samples. *Journal of Feline Medicine and Surgery* 19 (10): 1013–1016.

Heartwormsociety.org (2016). American Heartworm Society. https://www.heartwormsociety.org/images/incidence-maps/IncidenceMap2016Final.pdf (accessed 8 January 2020).

Heartwormsociety.org (2017). American Heartworm Society – Shelter Resources. https://www.heartwormsociety.org/veterinary-resources/shelter-resources (accessed 8 January 2020).

Levy, J.K., Lappin, M.R., Glaser, A.L. et al. (2011). Prevalence of infectious diseases in cats and dogs rescued following Hurricane Katrina. *Journal of the American Veterinary Medical Association* 238 (3): 311–317.

Little, S., Munzing, C., Heise, S. et al. (2014). Pre-treatment with heat facilitates detection of antigen of Dirofilaria immitis in canine samples. *Veterinary Parasitology* 203 (1): 250–252.

McCall, J.W. (1998). Dirofilariasis in the domestic ferret. *Clinical Techniques in Small Animal Practice* 13 (2). Saunders, St. Louis: 109–112. https://doi.org/10.1016/s1096-2867(98)80015-7.

McCall, J., Guerrero, J., and Roberts, R. (2001). Further evidence of clinical prophylactic, retroactive (reach back) and adulticidal activity of monthly administrations of ivermectin (Heartgard Plus™) in dogs experimentally infected with heartworms. *Recent Advances in Heartworm Disease. American Heartworm Society. Batavia*: 189–200.

McCall, J., Genchi, C., Kramer, L. et al. (2008). Heartworm disease in animals and humans. In: Advances in Parasitology (eds. D. Rollinson and S. Hay), 193–285. New York;: Academic Press.

McCall, J.W., Kramer, L., Genchi, C. et al. (2014). Effects of doxycycline on heartworm embryogenesis, transmission, circulating microfilaria, and adult worms in microfilaremic dogs. *Veterinary Parasitology* 206 (1): 5–13.

McCall, J., Hodgkins, E., Varloud, M. et al. (2016). Blocking transmission from dogs to mosquitoes and from mosquitoes to dogs, using repellents and ectoparasiticides (insecticides and macrocyclic lactone preventives) as part of a multimodal approach – shifting the paradigm in Dirofilaria immitis prevention. 15th Triennial Symposium, New Orleans.

Mckay, T., Bianco, T., Rhodes, L. et al. (2013). Prevalence of *Dirofilaria immitis* (Nematoda: Filarioidea) in mosquitoes from Northeast Arkansas, the United States. *Journal of Medical Entomology* 50 (4): 871–878.

Mobley, E. (2010). VIN Discussion Boards: Chronic HW Dz in Ferrets. http://www.vin.com/Members/Boards/DiscussionViewer.aspx?documentid=4440268andViewFirst=1 (accessed 24 April 2017).

Morchón, R., Carretón, E., González-Miguel, J. et al. (2012). Heartworm disease (*Dirofilaria immitis*) and their vectors in Europe – new distribution trends. *Frontiers in Physiology* 3 (196): 75–85.

Morrissey, J. and Kraus, M. (2012). Cardiovascular and other diseases. In:

Ferrets, Rabbits and Rodents, 3e (eds. K. Quesenberry and J. Carpenter), 71. St. Louis: Elsevier.

Nelson, C.T., McCall, J.W., Carithers, D. et al. (2020a) Current Canine Guidelines for the Prevention, Diagnosis, and Management of Heartworm (*Dirofilaria Immitis*) Infection in Dogs. American Heartworm Society. Revised 2020. Accessed January 16, 2021. https://d3ft8sckhnqim2.cloudfront.net/images/pdf/AHS_Canine_Guidelines_11_13_20.pdf

Nelson, C.T., McCall, J.W., Carithers, D. et al. (2020b) Current Feline Guidelines for the Prevention, Diagnosis, and Management of Heartworm (*Dirofilaria Immitis*) Infection in Cats. American Heartworm Society. Revised 2020. Accessed January 16, 2021. https://d3ft8sckhnqim2.cloudfront.net/images/pdf/2020_AHS_Feline_Guidelines_11_12.pdf.

Overall, K. and Dyer, D. (2005). Enrichment strategies for laboratory animals from the viewpoint of clinical veterinary behavioral medicine: emphasis on cats and dogs. *Institute for Laboratory Animal Research (ILAR) Journal* 46 (2): 202–216.

Peterson, K.M., Chappell, D.E., Lewis, B. et al. (2014). Heartworm-positive dogs recover without complications from surgical sterilization using cardiovascular sparing anesthesia protocol. *Veterinary Parasitology* 206 (1): 83–85.

Polak, K. and Smith-Blackmore, M. (2014). Animal shelters: managing heartworms in resource-scarce environments. *Veterinary Parasitology* 206 (1): 78–82.

Rawlings, C., Bowman, D., Howerth, E. et al. (2001). Response of dogs treated with ivermectin or milbemycin starting at various intervals after *Dirofilaria immitis* infection. *Veterinary Therapeutics* 2 (3): 193–207.

Supakorndej, P., Lewis, R.E., McCall, J.W. et al. (1995). Radiographic and angiographic evaluations of ferrets experimentally infected with *Dirofilaria immitis*. *Veterinary Radiology & Ultrasound* 36 (1): 23–29.

Tzipory, N., Crawford, P., and Levy, J. (2010). Prevalence of Dirofilaria immitis, Ehrlichia canis, and Borrelia burgdorferi in pet dogs, racing greyhounds, and shelter dogs in Florida. *Veterinary Parasitology* 171 (1–2): 136–139.

Velasquez, L., Blagburn, B.L., Duncan-Decoq, R. et al. (2014). Increased prevalence of Dirofilaria Immitis antigen in canine samples after heat treatment. *Veterinary Parasitology* 206 (1–2): 67–70. https://doi.org/10.1016/j.vetpar.2014.03.021.

Venco, L., Genchi, M., Genchi, C. et al. (2011). Can heartworm prevalence in dogs be used as provisional data for assessing the prevalence of the infection in cats? *Veterinary Parasitology* 176 (4): 300–303.

Venco, L., Marchesotti, F., and Manzocchi, S. (2015). Feline heartworm disease: a 'Rubik's-cube-like' diagnostic and therapeutic challenge. *Journal of Veterinary Cardiology* 17: S190–S201.

Wang, D., Bowman, D., Brown, H. et al. (2014). Factors influencing U.S. canine heartworm (*Dirofilaria immitis*) prevalence. *Parasites & Vectors* 7 (1): 264.

Zaffarano, B. (2015). Diagnosis, treatment, and prevention of heartworm disease in ferrets. *Today's Veterinary Practice* 5 (4): 80–83.

19

External Parasites

Dwight D. Bowman[1], Araceli Lucio-Forster[1], and Stephanie Janeczko[2]

[1] Cornell University College of Veterinary Medicine, Ithaca, NY, USA
[2] Shelter Medicine Services, American Society for the Prevention of Cruelty to Animals (ASPCA), New York, NY, USA

19.1 Introduction

External parasites (ectoparasites) that commonly affect cats and dogs are all arthropods. Arthropods and arthropod-vectored diseases may represent a direct threat to cat and dog populations and may also pose human health concerns. Some are directly zoonotic, while dogs and cats may serve as sentinels for others that pose a threat to humans. It is not unusual for stray and neglected animals to be presented to shelters with heavy flea and tick infestations. Common challenges in shelters that exacerbate the impact of external parasites on the population include high levels of direct and indirect animal contact resulting from high rates of animal intake, high-density housing, and rapid population turnover, as well as inadequate funding and resources to treat and manage arthropods preventively (Foley 2009).

The presence of some ectoparasitic diseases may be readily detected by the visualization of the parasite and the characteristic pattern of skin lesions, such as with fleas and flea-bite dermatitis, while others are less apparent and require additional diagnostics. Parasites may be present on the host at all times (e.g. lice and most common mites), only during some part of their lifetime (e.g. adult fleas, larval flies), or may not spend any significant time in association with their hosts, requiring only a blood meal from time to time (e.g biting flies, hematophagous bugs, and ticks). While skin lesions may also be caused by several other agents, including some helminths that are capable of skin penetration (e.g. schistosomes, hookworms and *Strongyloides* spp), and protozoans like *Leishmania*, these are not ectoparasitic infestations that require management in a shelter environment in the United States and will therefore not be considered in this chapter. (Internal parasite infections of importance in shelters in the United States are discussed in Chapter 17.)

The focus of the chapter is on those common arthropod infestations seen in cats and dogs that may be of concern in a shelter setting. Ectoparasites that may be present in the external environment, and that might be a consideration in certain locations (e.g. biting flies and mosquitos) are also briefly discussed, as some have important implications with respect to the transmission of important diseases, such as heartworms.

The arthropods with parasitic potential that can affect dogs and cats include biting flies, maggots, mosquitoes, fleas, lice, bugs, mites,

Infectious Disease Management in Animal Shelters, Second Edition.
Edited by Lila Miller, Stephanie Janeczko, and Kate F. Hurley.

and ticks. Of these, only lice and *Demodex* mites have strict host specificity and do not cause infestations in hosts of a different species. Other mites may also have undergone a great degree of host adaptation and are unlikely to be found on hosts other than their preferred host (e.g. *Sarcoptes scabiei*). However, mosquitos, biting flies, maggots, fleas, bugs, and most ticks are capable of feeding on any of the hosts of concern in this chapter (cats, dogs, and humans).

As with internal parasite infections, the transmissibility of ectoparasites among animals or between animals and humans, and the establishment of these populations in a shelter environment, is most closely linked to the biology of the parasites themselves. Thus, a discussion of some relevant ectoparasites, and biological factors that may allow for their transmission, presence, or establishment in a shelter environment, will be highlighted in this chapter.

For more information regarding other feline and canine parasites, or more detailed information on the parasites discussed here, including their biology, specifics for diagnosis and identification, and clinical manifestations of disease, the reader is directed to the many texts on veterinary and diagnostic parasitology. Vector-borne diseases are also not covered in this chapter as there are numerous other resources with in-depth and up-to-date information about the epidemiology, diagnosis, and treatment of these diseases that are of increasing importance to both shelters and the general community. The reader is directed to Chapter 24 for information on external parasites of ferrets, rabbits, guinea pigs, and rodents.

See Table 19.1 for a list of some of the vector-borne diseases of concern to shelters and Table 19.2 for a list of resources.

See Appendix 19.1 for a list of commonly encountered ectoparasites in shelter animals.

Table 19.1 List of zoonotic vector-borne diseases that are relevant for animal shelters.

Pathogen	Route of Transmission
Anaplasma (A) phagocytophilum	Ticks (*Ixodes scapularis* or *I. pacificus*)
A. platys	Suspect tick (*Rhipicephalus sanguineus*)
Ehrlichia canis, E. chaffeensis, E. ewingii	Ticks (primarily *Rhipicephalus sanguineus* for *E. canis*, *Amblyomma americanum* for *E. chaffeensis* and *E. ewingii*)
Bartonella spp. (cat scratch fever)	Fleas Bites or scratches
Borrelia burgdorferi (Lyme Disease)	Ticks (*Ixodes scapularis* or *I. pacificus*)
Francisella tularensis (tularemia)	Direct skin contact with infected animal tissues
Leishmania spp.	Sandfly
Rickettsia felis and *R. typhi* (Typhus)	Fleas
R. rickettsii (Rocky Mountain Spotted Fever)	Ticks (primarily *Dermacentor* or *Rhipicephalus* spp.)
Trypanosoma cruzi (Chagas Disease)	Triatomine insects ("Kissing bugs")
Yersinia pestis (plague)	Fleas Aerosol

Source: Wiley Blackwell

Table 19.2 List of resources for ectoparasites and vector-borne diseases.

Companion Animal Parasite Council (www.capcvet.org)
Canine and Feline Infectious Diseases and Parasitology, 2nd ed., Blackwell's Five-Minute Veterinary Consult Clinical Companion[a]
Merck Veterinary Manual, 11th edition or online (http://www.merckvetmanual.com/)[a]
Greene's Infectious Diseases of the Dog and Cat, 4th edition, Elsevier, St. Louis[a]
Georgis' Parasitology for Veterinarians, 11th edition, Elsevier, St. Louis
Centers for Disease Control Division of Vector-Borne Diseases (DVBD) https://www.cdc.gov/ncezid/dvbd/about.html
Compendium for Veterinary Products (https://bayerall.naccvp.com/chartindex/main?type=anth)

[a] This reference is current at the time of publication, but a new edition is anticipated.

19.2 Ectoparasites with all Life Stages on the Host

Ectoparasites with all life stages spent on the host (and that are discussed here) require the animal itself to be the main focus of treatment efforts. Animals determined to be infested may need to be isolated for the duration of their treatment depending on how easily the parasite can be transmitted between animals. Repeat treatments for ectoparasitic infestations are often needed, as the eggs present at the time of treatment are expected to survive and the parasites will need to be killed after they have hatched, but before they reach sexual maturity and lay eggs of their own. It should be noted that while the environment in which the animal is housed may become contaminated if these ectoparasites are dislodged from their host, it is unlikely this will be a large number of individuals; furthermore, this population will not be able to multiply without a host. The exception to this would be ticks. *Rhipicephalus sanguineus* can and has on multiple occasions found its way into shelters and caused long-term problems that may require the assistance of professional exterminators. Newly hatched larvae of the Asian Longhorn tick (*Haemaphysalis longicornis*, introduced to the United States in 2017) tend to massively attack one or two animals, requiring significant effort to treat the dogs to get the many ticks off as quickly as possible. These ticks are also likely to do the same thing with humans. Thus, overall good care with respect to decontamination of the environment, including any bedding or grooming materials used for the animal, should be taken in order to prevent reinfestation or transmission to another host, but it is also important to examine new arrivals for replete and oviparous ticks that need to be removed and destroyed.

19.2.1 Lice

The lice of cats and dogs are members of the Orders Anoplura (sucking lice) and Mallophaga (chewing lice). Lice of each of these orders can be readily differentiated by comparing the width of their head to the width of their thorax. As a simple rule, the width of the head of sucking lice is close to equal of that of the thorax, while the width of the head of a chewing louse is greater than that of the thorax. Anopluran lice are blood-suckers while chewing lice eat skin debris, hair, and sebaceous secretions. Both types of lice and their eggs (nits) are readily visible to the naked eye or with the aid of a magnifying glass.

Cats are only infested by a single louse, the mallophagan louse *Felicola subrostratus*, while dogs are hosts to three lice: the anopluran, *Linognathus setosus*, and the mallophagans, *Trichodectes canis* (Figure 19.1) and *Heterodoxus spiniger* (though this latter louse is not present

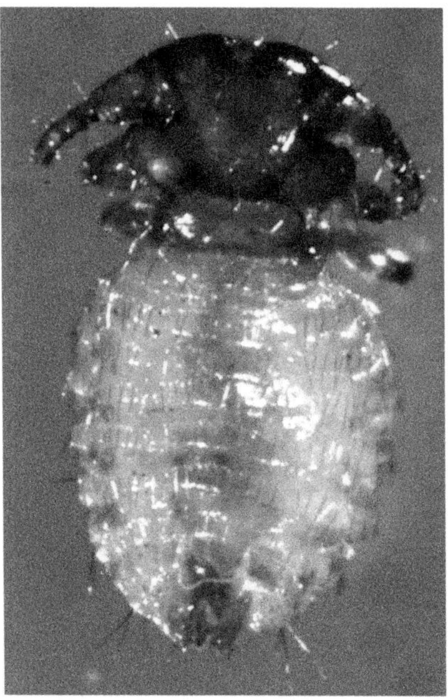

Figure 19.1 *Trichodectes canis*, the chewing louse of dogs. Note that the width of the head is greater than that of the thorax.

in the United States). Lice on cats and dogs typically do not cause a great degree of irritation unless present in large numbers. In such cases, intense pruritus, alopecia, and excoriations may be seen. Large populations of lice are most likely to occur on very young, old and/or debilitated animals, thus, low numbers of lice that may occur on many infested animals are likely to go unnoticed.

In all cases, adult lice of cats and dogs glue their eggs to the hair of their host. The nymphal stage that hatches from the egg looks like the adult stage and should be easily recognizable. After completing its simple development through a couple of molts, mature adults reproduce sexually and produce more eggs. The entire lifecycle takes about one month to complete and occurs solely on the host. Lice are unlikely to persist in the environment for more than a few days, and though transmission by fomites (especially brushes and combs) can occur, the most common mode of transmission is through direct contact, as these parasites are unable to jump or fly and require a "bridge of hair" to cross between hosts. Routine washing and drying of bedding will kill any stages that may have fallen off a host. (See Chapter 8 for more information about sanitation and fomites.)

Lice are host-species-specific, and though they may crawl onto caregivers, they do not establish infestations on humans. However, infested animals can be a source of lice for other hosts of the same species and should be isolated throughout treatment. Products with activity against fleas also work well against lice: these include sprays, shampoos, and topical products containing fipronil, imidacloprid, selamectin, or, for dogs, permethrin (Arther 2009; Bowman 2014). Nits are not susceptible to insecticides and thus a population of lice will remain on animals after treatment if nits are not mechanically removed. Upon hatching one to two weeks later, this newly emerged population of lice can reestablish an infestation on the animal and be a source of infestation for other in-contact animals. For this reason, it is also recommended that infested individuals be separated from other animals and be treated at least twice, with treatments performed one week apart. The topical application of many monthly preventive products will also be effective in controlling louse infestations.

19.2.2 Mites

Most mites that commonly infest cats and dogs spend their entire life on these hosts and are unable to persist in the environment for extended periods of time. As with lice, the transmission of these ectoparasitic infestations occurs primarily through direct contact, though fomite transmission can also occur and should be prevented. While similar types of mites may be found on cats and dogs, each of these hosts is usually infested by a different species of a given mite, as discussed below. Cross-infestations with some of these mites are possible if close contact between cats and dogs occurs, so while transmission of this sort may take place in some home environments, it is unlikely in a typical shelter setting.

Information on specific treatments of infestations is included below in association with the particular mite under discussion. However, it is worth mentioning that the new isoxazoline class of ectoparasiticides (i.e. afoxolaner, fluralaner, lotilander, and sarolaner) has been investigated for its efficacy against *Sarcoptes*, *Demodex*, *Otodectes*, and *Lynxacarus* with very promising results (Fourie et al. 2015; Becskei et al. 2016; Beugnet et al. 2016a; Beugnet et al. 2016b; Carithers et al. 2016; Chavez 2016; Han et al. 2016; Romero et al. 2016; Six et al. 2016; Taenzler et al. 2017). However, at the time of publication of this textbook, label-claims for treatment of any of these mites have not yet been acquired for the available products on the market; extra-label use would be necessary for the treatment of any of these infestations.

19.2.2.1 *Demodex* spp.

Several species of *Demodex* are found as normal fauna in hair follicles, sebaceous glands and on the skin of cats, dogs, humans, and other mammals; each is specific to its host. Species of *Demodex* found on cats include *Demodex cati*, *Demodex gatoi* (Figure 19.2), and perhaps a third species, which is (at the time of publication of this text) unnamed. Those found on dogs are *Demodex canis*, *Demodex cornei*, and *Demodex injai*. Though *Demodex* is acquired from lactating females by their young while nursing, these mites are not contagious, nor is the disease that may be present in some individuals. The exception to this statement is *D. gatoi*, which is a very superficial mite found in the stratum corneum of the skin of cats. This mite is transmissible and its mere presence on a host is thought to incite pruritus; it has been suggested the same may be true of *D. cornei* of dogs. Perhaps as a result of a hypersensitivity reaction and subsequent overgrooming, *D. gatoi* infestations may lead to patches of alopecia in cats (Beale 2012).

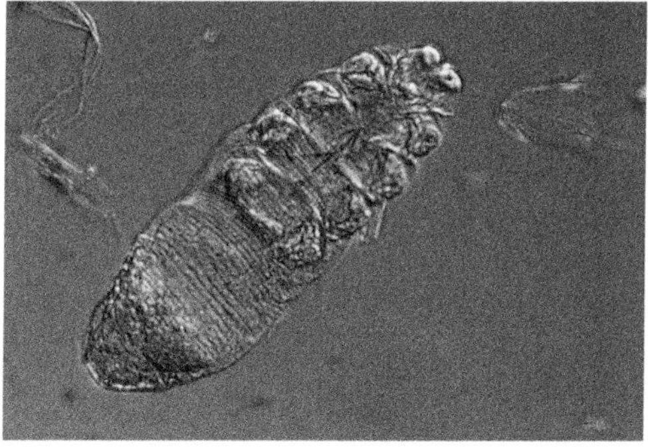

Figure 19.2 *Demodex gatoi* recovered on a skin scraping from an affected cat.

Demodicosis typically presents in three classic forms, localized, generalized, and adult-onset. Dogs are more likely to present with the disease than cats, and the species of *Demodex* most commonly involved is *D. canis*. Affected animals may or may not require treatment depending on the extent of the lesions present. Localized demodicosis, loosely defined as the presence of small numbers of isolated lesions most often found on the head, neck, and forelimbs, occurs most commonly in puppies and often resolves spontaneously within a few months. Generalized demodicosis occurs in adult and young animals and results in severe, dramatic skin disease, often with deep pyoderma and signs of systemic illness that requires treatment of mites. In most cases, generalized demodicosis is a result of immunosuppression stemming from an underlying condition, which then allows for the growth of large populations of these mites. Secondary bacterial infection may lead to scaling, crusting, exudation, and ulceration with draining tracts, which can be associated with hyperpigmentation, lymphadenopathy, lethargy, and fever. In the most severe cases, dogs may become septic as a result of bacterial translocation. The third form, adult-onset demodicosis, can be localized or generalized and requires an attempt to identify and address the underlying condition(s) predisposing the animal to the disease. Minimizing stressors should be part of the treatment protocol, as stress is believed to be a factor in the development of this disease. There is mounting evidence and good consensus that generalized demodicosis has a hereditary basis, therefore, it is recommended that animals that have a history of this condition be neutered so the overall incidence of the disease in the population may be decreased (Rosenkrantz 2016; Mueller et al. 2020).

Diagnosis of demodicosis requires the demonstration of mites on deep skin scrapes or plucked hairs from affected areas. Samples may be collected with curettes, spatulas, or scalpel blades. Some experts recommend that scalpel blades are **not** to be used because of the risks of injury to the animal as well as to the staff, and instead to utilize skin scrape spatulas that can be resterilized (Moriello et al. 2009). Primary lesions (i.e. follicular papules or pustules) should be chosen to sample from whenever possible, but material can be collected from erythematous, alopecic areas as well. After placing a drop of mineral oil on the instrument to improve adherence of the collected material, multiple scrapings should be performed in the direction of hair growth while squeezing the skin continuously or intermittently (to improve yield) until capillary bleeding occurs (Mueller et al. 2020).

Tape impressions may be more useful for the *Demodex* spp. present in the stratum corneum, *D. gatoi* and *D. cornei*. (See the section on *Cheyletiella* for a description of an acetate tape preparation.) In cats with suspected *D. gatoi*, when these methods have not revealed mites, a fecal examination may recover mites that have been ingested through grooming. Trichograms may also be useful, particularly for areas that are difficult to scrape (i.e. localized periocular lesions). A hair trichogram is a microscopic examination of a hair shaft. Hairs should be gently plucked or pulled in the direction of growth via gentle traction, making sure to obtain the hair bulb (or root). The hairs are carefully placed in a drop of mineral oil on a glass microscope slide. A glass coverslip is highly recommended to make examination of the hairs easier. Examination for *Demodex* mites should concentrate on the hair bulb and the proximal third of the hair. Mites can be seen at 10X magnification, but usually, 40X magnification is needed for confirmation (Moriello et al. 2009).

Amitraz remains the only Food and Drug Administration (FDA)-approved treatment for generalized demodicosis, but it requires an extended period of time for treatment and has the potential for severe side effects. Since the development of the macrocyclic lactone class of compounds, (e.g. ivermectin, milbemycin oxime, moxidectin, and selamectin), treatment of canine and feline demodicosis has most often relied on repeated treatment regimens with these compounds, in various formulations (Mueller et al. 2020; Paterson et al. 2014). Treatment of feline demodicosis with these compounds has been variable, and lime sulfur dips may be the treatment of choice (Beale 2012). *D. gatoi* has been successfully treated in some cats with 10% imidacloprid and 2.5% moxidectin (Short and Gram 2016). Some situations may require intervention with the topical use of amitraz or lime sulfur dips, or the long-term use of weekly oral ivermectin (Saari et al. 2009).

Updates on the management of demodicosis were recently published and include consideration of the use of isoxazolines for the treatment of demodicosis in dogs (Koch 2017); no studies have been performed to evaluate the efficacy or safety of such use in cats. Numerous studies, trials, and clinical reports support the use of isoxazolines for the treatment of demodicosis (Zhou et al. 2020), and anecdotally, many shelters have reported success with using isoxazolines for treatment, often obtaining clearance of the parasite with a single dose. Due to the ease of administration and comparatively short treatment time, safety, and overall affordability, isoxazolines are likely to be the treatment of choice for animals with generalized demodicosis in most shelters. Animals should be evaluated monthly and treatment continued for one to two months after the last negative skin scraping. Detailed clinical consensus guidelines for the diagnosis and treatment of demodicosis in dogs and cats have been issued by the World Association for Veterinary Dermatology (Mueller et al. 2020).

19.2.2.2 *Otodectes cynotis*

Otodectes cynotis is the ear mite of cats, dogs, and ferrets. It infests the external ear canal and may be found on the surrounding skin as well. These mites are more commonly seen in cats than dogs. Eggs, larvae, nymphs, and adults are all found on the host, with no stages of the lifecycle being capable of survival in the environment for prolonged periods of time. However, mites can be mechanically transferred from one animal to another by fomites as well as through direct contact. Infested animals may be asymptomatic or suffer from severe aural pruritus leading to head shaking, ear scratching and ear drooping. Ear-mite infestations can also lead to secondary infections, purulent otitis externa/media and may be involved in the development of chronic otitis media in adult cats. Severe ear-mite infestations can occur over the entire body, resulting in a pruritic, papular skin disease that can mimic many other parasitic and nonparasitic diseases. Self- trauma can lead to the formation of an aural hematoma of the pinna, especially in cats (Moriello et al. 2009).

A presumptive diagnosis is by the visualization of the dark brown, coffee-ground appearance of ear-mite debris, blood and cerumen in the ear canal, and confirmed by finding mites by direct examination with an otoscope or ear-swab cytology. Ear-swab cytology involves rolling the debris from the ear in a drop of mineral oil on a glass microscope slide and examining it for the presence of the mite.

Infested animals can serve as a source of ear-mite infestation for others and should be housed separately until treatment is completed; however, in the shelter environment, it is not uncommon to have a group of animals, such as a litter of kittens, in which multiple animals are infested. In these cases, the entire litter should be treated rather than attempting to separate and socially isolate the affected animals in individual housing. Topically applied milbemycin oxime, moxidectin/imidacloprid, ivermectin, and selamectin, as well as orally administered afoxolaner, fluralaner, and sarolaner are either labeled for this parasite or have been shown to be effective (Barr and Bowman 2012; Lynn and Duquette 2020). Additionally, cleaning of the ear canal is recommended, and the removed material should be immediately and carefully disposed of. Eggs are expected to be resistant to treatment and thus repeat treatment is warranted. It may take one month to clear an infestation; adopters should be advised if follow-up care is needed, and precautions to take if other animals, particularly cats, are in the household.

19.2.2.3 *Cheyletiella* spp.

Cheyletiella blakei and *Cheyletiella yasguri* are the "walking dandruff" mites of cats and dogs, respectively. These hair clasping mites are relatively fast-moving, superficial, non-borrowing, and have little host-specificity. This parasite is highly contagious and capable of establishing cross-infestations between hosts. Though they cannot persist on humans, contact with infested animals may result in temporary infestations and skin lesions.

Infestations in cats and dogs may be inapparent or may be exacerbated by a hypersensitivity reaction (Deplazes et al. 2016). Common presentations may include eczema with pruritus and the production of varying degrees of dandruff, apparent on the dorsum of the animal. Cats may present with miliary dermatitis. Scaling is the most important clinical sign and is most severe in animals with chronic infestations or those that are debilitated (Barr and Bowman 2012). These signs are a result of mite bites and a reaction to mite antigens. Cats may be capable of removing a portion of the population through grooming, and it is possible to recover eggs and mites on fecal examination.

As these mites are superficial and attach their eggs to the hairs of the host, recovery and examination of mites and eggs in skin debris and hairs, with the aid of a flea comb or acetate tape impression, is diagnostic. An acetate tape impression is obtained by pressing the sticky side of a clear piece of acetate tape against the suspect area and placing it on a glass microscope slide over a drop of mineral oil. Another drop of mineral oil is placed on top of the tape and then a coverslip is added to enhance visualization of mites. The slide is then examined under increasing magnification (Moriello et al. 2009). Eggs should be differentiated from lice nits, which are also attached to hair but will have an operculum (cap) on the pole of the egg not attached to the hair.

Cheyletiella is known to be one of the hardiest mites of cats and dogs, able to survive in the environment for up to 10 days. Fomite transmission is also possible, so care should be taken to avoid this. This mite is susceptible to common flea-control agents and macrocyclic lactones (Barr and Bowman 2012), though no products are labeled for this use. All in-contact animals should be treated, the environment disinfected (with insecticidal products), and bedding and grooming materials should be washed and thoroughly dried.

19.2.2.4 *Sarcoptes scabiei* var. *canis*

The only species of the genus *Sarcoptes* is *S. scabiei*. Different, specialized, host-adapted variants are present on different hosts, such as dogs, pigs, cattle, humans, and other mammals. Cross-infestation of animal species (and humans) to which the variant of *Sarcoptes* mite is not adapted results in mild, transient, and usually self-limiting infestations with reduced severity of disease manifestation. Notably, cats do not have a host-adapted species of *Sarcoptes*; however, temporary infestations of cats are possible if cats have been in regular, close contact with infested dogs or humans.

S. scabiei var. *canis* (Figure 19.3) is the mite responsible for sarcoptic mange (also known as scabies), a highly contagious skin condition that is diagnosed fairly frequently in dogs in the United States. These mites remain on their host at all times and, as a result, they are primarily transmitted through direct contact of an infested dog with others, or relatively immediate fomite transmission (e.g. via bedding, clothing, or clipper blades). Mites tunnel in the epidermis, where female mites lay eggs that adhere to the inside of the tunnel. Some proportion of the mites will also wander onto the surface of the skin to mate or search for new locations to penetrate the skin and resume their development (Arther 2009); it is these mites that are the most likely to be transmitted between animals.

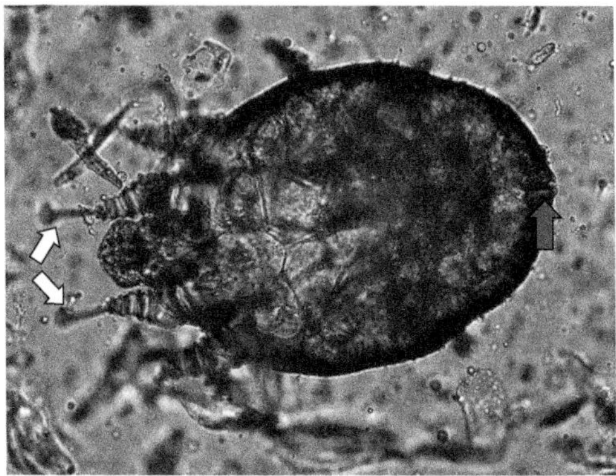

Figure 19.3 Large female *Sarcoptes scabiei* var. *canis* with adult male superimposed on top. The characteristic pretarsi can just be seen protruding on the anterior of the mites (white arrows), and the anus of the female is also visible on the posterior edge of her body (red arrow).

Sarcoptic mite infestations may be inapparent, especially upon initial colonization of the animal, but often elicit a hypersensitivity reaction in the host that leads to intense pruritus and alopecia, as well as marked changes in the skin, including thickening and lichenification. These signs are further compounded by self-trauma as a result of the host's scratching, and by the acquisition of secondary bacterial infections. Commonly affected areas include the pinnae, elbows, head, and back of the neck. The mites often become distributed to other areas of the body, including the hocks and ventral abdomen.

The diagnosis of an infestation can be difficult and may rely on presumptive treatment of symptomatic animals and evaluation of response to treatment. A positive pinnal-pedal reflex may be suggestive of the disease; this is demonstrated when the affected ear is rubbed and the dog responds by scratching with the ipsilateral hindlimb. Examination of skin scrapings is the routine diagnostic method used, though an antibody enzyme-linked immunoassay (ELISA) test for *Sarcoptes* is also available from IDEXX Laboratories. Multiple skin scrapings may be necessary before mites are demonstrated, if at all, as the test is fairly insensitive. Mites are small, round, and have long, unsegmented pretarsi attached to the end of their anterior sets of legs.

Infested animals should be isolated for the duration of treatment and any in-contact animals should also be treated. Though the disease in humans is usually mild and self-limiting, scabies is still considered to be zoonotic; therefore, as a best practice, staff and volunteers interacting with the dogs during the first three to five days of treatment should wear gloves and gowns or clothing that covers their arms and legs. (People who develop skin lesions after handling a dog with scabies should seek care from a physician or dermatologist if the lesions persist.) Leashes and collars, grooming equipment, etc., should be dedicated to individual animals and/or thoroughly cleaned and disinfected after each use. Clipping of hair is not recommended except in the most severe or refractory cases; treatment with antiseborrheic products should facilitate the resolution of clinical signs when used in conjunction with miticidal treatments. Several therapies for the treatment or control of *Sarcoptes* in dogs are available in a variety of formulations, including topical (e.g. dips, sprays and spot-ons) and internal products. If dips are to be used, the face and ears of the animal should not be neglected. Products with efficacy against *Sarcoptes* include the macrocyclic lactones (ivermectin, moxidectin, selamectin, milbemycin oxime), amitraz, lime sulfur, and fipronil (Barr and Bowman 2012). As mentioned earlier, the off-label use of an isoxazoline has also been shown to be efficacious against this mite. Routine use of these products should prevent an infestation with *Sarcoptes*. The use of premise sprays that are effective for killing fleas and ticks may sometimes be needed as an extra precaution for killing mites that may be in the environment even for just a short period of time.

19.2.2.5 *Notoedres cati*

Notoedres cati is a *Sarcoptes*-like mite that is found on cats. It is sometimes referred to as "feline scabies" because it causes an intensely pruritic disease on cats that is similar to *S. scabiei* on dogs. Like *S. scabiei*, it may cause pruritus on humans without establishing self-sustaining human infestations. The disease in cats manifests as keratitis, often around the ears, face, and extremities, but it can become generalized. In severe cases with heavy mite infestations, the presentation can be dramatic, with severe dermal thickening and lichenification, particularly around the ear tips and face. *N. cati* can be rapidly spread between cats by direct contact.

Macrocyclic lactones are typically used for the treatment of notoedric mange. In a shelter setting, if infestations are present in several animals, it may be more cost-effective to treat infested and in-contact animals with a subcutaneous injection of ivermectin (0.1–0.3 mg/kg) as was done for 500 cats during an outbreak among the feline population on one of the Florida Keys (Foley 1991a). Treatment can also be performed with one or two applications of topical formulations of selamectin or 10% imidacloprid with 2.5% moxidectin, which may be preferable due to the ease and speed of administration, particularly if animals are fearful, anxious, or stressed by handling. It may be expected, based on results with other mites, that the isoxazoline class may also be effective against this mite. Additionally, in Europe, a spot-on formulation containing fipronil, (S)-methoprene, eprinomectin, and praziquantel has been shown to be effective for the treatment of this mite (Knaus et al. 2014). Mite clearance is expected to require repeat treatments to target hatched populations that may have survived the initial treatment.

19.2.2.6 *Lynxacarus radovskyi*

Lynxacarus radovskyi is a superficial hair-clasping fur mite of cats. It is found around the world and has a lifecycle more like that of *Cheyletiella* than *Notoedres* in that it lives on the surface of the cat and glues its eggs to hairs.

Infested cats present with multiple nonspecific signs that include a dull, dry, rust-colored haircoat and hairballs associated with excess grooming. There may be alopecia of the inguinal and tail-head area, and hair-mowing, hair-pulling, and self-traumatic dermatitis. Definitive diagnosis is by finding the mites on skin scrapings or acetate tape preparations, but it may be difficult to find them; treatment is often based upon suspicion of an infestation.

Treatment options include the use of pyrethrins (spray, powder, shampoo, or dip) or 2.5% lime sulfur dips (Foley 1991b). Recently, topical administration of 10% imidacloprid with 2.5% moxidectin and oral fluralaner have both been shown to be effective treatments for individual cases (Han et al. 2016).

19.3 Ectoparasites with Environmental and Host Stages

Fleas and myiasis-inducing flies inhabit the host (as adults or larvae, respectively) and also have developmental stages that are present in the environment, posing additional considerations for the management and prevention of infestations. This section will review flea biology and highlight some of the considerations in controlling infestations or infections in a shelter environment. A brief mention of myiasis is also included for completeness, and to reinforce the mode of transmission and infection with these parasites. However, it should be understood that while myiasis infections are important on an individual animal basis, they pose no risk of transmission to other animals or humans and cannot establish a breeding population within the shelter environment.

19.3.1 Fleas

Fleas are members of the Order Siphonaptera, a name reflective of their ability to suck blood in a manner similar to anopluran lice and mosquitoes, and their inability to fly due to their lack of wings. These insects are laterally compressed, have long jumping legs to reach their host, and thick, comb-like structures and hairs that aid in maintaining them on their host. Fleas have particular importance due to (i) their ability to take blood from the host, especially important in young, old, or already-debilitated animals, in whom a large enough infestation may result in flea bite anemia and/or death; (ii) their propensity to cause hypersensitivity reactions in certain hosts, leading to severe pruritus with only a few bites; and (iii) their role in the transmission of other pathogens. The cat flea, *Ctenocephalides felis* (Figure 19.4) is an intermediate host of *Dipylidium caninum*, the tapeworm of cats, dogs, and sometimes humans, and may also transmit *Acanthocheilonema* (*Dipetalonema*) *reconditum*, the subcutaneous filariid of dogs. Fleas may also transmit *Rickettsia typhi*, *Rickettsia felis*, *Bartonella henselae*, hemoplasmas, and *Francisella tularensis*. Other species of fleas play an important role in the transmission of *Yersinia pestis* (plague) as well as several other pathogens.

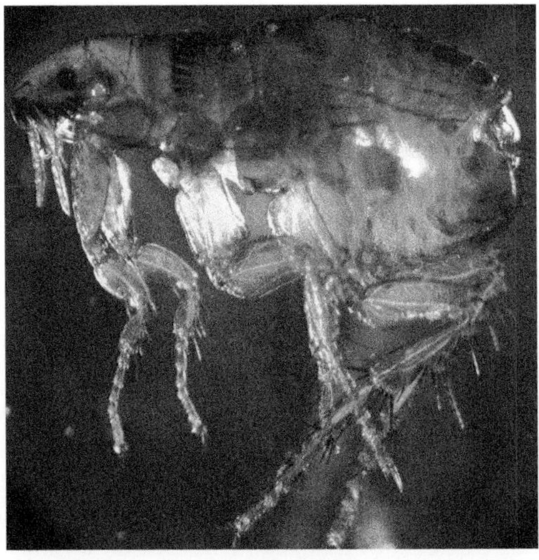

Figure 19.4 *Ctenocephalides felis* adult flea recovered from a student's apartment in Ithaca, NY.

The cat flea, *C. felis* is the most common flea of cats and dogs alike, though other flea species may occasionally be encountered (Blagburn and Dryden 2009). Only the adult flea is generally present on the animal but, in rare instances, larvae have been recovered from animals with matted hair coats with trapped eggs. Environmental populations can quickly be established if infested animals are left untreated and eggs produced by females are deposited into suitable environments.

Fleas develop in the environment through complete or complex metamorphosis. Eggs laid by adults on the host roll off the animal in areas where they rest. They hatch as caterpillar-like, legless larvae. After three larval stages, these creatures spin silken pupal cases around themselves in areas that are unlikely to be disturbed. Pupae are the hardiest stage of the lifecycle and can persist in certain environments for months awaiting the introduction of a host. Host cues such as heat, carbon dioxide and vibration (movement) stimulate the adult to eclose from its pupal case. The newly emerged adult then jumps onto the host and feeds almost immediately. Thus, animals acquire fleas from environments where infested animals have been housed and where eggs have fallen, and larvae and pupae have developed, even if an infested animal has not been present in the environment for an extended period of time. Though it is not impossible for adult fleas to jump off a host and onto another, this is not the most common method of transmission.

Control of animal infestations must include adulticidal treatments to remove the feeding and breeding populations from the animals, as well as addressing populations in the environment. Insect growth regulators can prevent the development of environmental stages and can preclude the establishment of the lifecycle in areas where animals are housed. Mechanical removal of environmental stages through washing and vacuuming of contaminated materials and areas (with proper disposal of vacuum bags) will also aid in this regard. It must be remembered that wild animals can be reservoirs for flea infestations and the lifecycle can easily become established outdoors in temperate climates. Eggs falling off infested animals as they rest outdoors in yards with shaded areas and adequate humidity levels can "seed" that environment with larvae and eventually pupae from which animals can re-acquire infestations. It should also be noted that though flea infestations are most common during warm weather, they can be encountered year-round, even in climates with cold winters.

For optimal control in a shelter or any environment where new animals are going to be introduced, it is prudent to always thoroughly examine animals for evidence of fleas at the time of intake and, at minimum, treat animals that are infested. Tapeworms may be suggestive of a flea problem since they may result from flea ingestion. It may be helpful to use a flea comb to find evidence of fleas, flea eggs or flea excreta (dark specks on the skin also known as flea dirt). In some cases, especially in allergic animals, fleas may not be seen because of the animal's fastidious grooming (or overgrooming). Signs of a flea allergy include alopecia over the lumbosacral and hind legs in dogs and cats (often referred to as "hot spots"), while cats may also suffer from miliary dermatitis and areas of exudation and crusts on the back, face and abdomen. If the flea allergy causes a secondary bacterial infection, appropriate antimicrobial treatment should be provided.

In areas where fleas are more common, such as warm, humid environments, it may be beneficial and worth the initial cost to treat all cats and dogs at the time of intake, as a single female flea is likely to be missed. The use of a combination product effective against both adults and developing larvae would be optimal to prevent environmental contamination in the event that some eggs or female fleas are not killed by the initial treatment. If an animal is suffering from an obvious flea infestation at admission, the animal should be treated with nitenpyram to immediately kill adult fleas in addition to a product effective against developing larvae. Routine flea prevention may be warranted if shelter animals have access to the outdoors, are walked outside regularly, or have contact with animals that have such exposure. Numerous products are available for control and prevention of flea infestations, many of which also have efficacy in the control of other ecto- and endoparasites. Resources that summarize new and other currently available products and their indications can be helpful in evaluating and selecting which one(s) will be most appropriate for use in a particular population and animal shelter; one example of such listings can be found on CAPC's website (https://capcvet.org/parasite-product-applications/).

It is important to make every effort to ensure the shelter does not adopt out animals with fleas; they should be treated promptly at intake and reexamined at the point of adoption for any signs of an ongoing problem. Besides being a nuisance, fleas may transmit disease, cause an allergic reaction in both humans and animals, and may quickly infest the adopter's home.

19.3.2 Larval Flies (Myiasis)

The infection of vertebrate hosts by larval flies is termed myiasis. Primary myiasis is the result of an obligatory need of the fly for larval development in living tissue, while secondary myiasis occurs as an opportunistic infection by flies that generally lay eggs on carrion or decaying organic matter. As the term indicates, the only stages infecting the host in these cases are larval fly (maggot) stages. In the cases discussed here, maggot infections are a result of the direct placement of eggs by adult flies on wounds on the host, with the notable exception of *Cuterebra*, as discussed below. Though myiasis can occur in any animal under the right circumstances, these infections are not contagious. The prevention of infection is achieved by preventing access of flies to open wounds or injured or debilitated animals. This may require a combination of fly-control methods including keeping cats and dogs housed indoors in screened-in areas, ensuring animals are kept clean and dry, and treating and covering any wounds. For *Cuterebra*, prevention is achieved through the control of an animal's access to areas where adult bot flies have laid their eggs (rodent or rabbit runs and burrows), i.e. the prevention of hunting behaviors. Thus, in most shelter situations, the acquisition of cuterebriasis is unlikely. The reader is also directed to Chapter 17 for additional information on *Cuterebra*.

19.3.2.1 Primary Myiasis-Inducing Flies in Cats and Dogs

Within the group of flies that can lead to primary myiasis in cats and dogs is the bot fly, *Cuterebra* (discussed in Chapter 17), and the still uncommon, but very important calliphorid fly, *Cochliomyia hominovorax* also known as the New World or American Screwworm. *C. hominovorax* was eradicated from North America through the release of sterile males to control and eventually eliminate the population. However, reintroductions are possible and remain a source of concern. The 2016/2017 outbreak in the Florida Keys, which primarily affected deer but also included small numbers of companion animals, was successfully contained but underscores the need for continued vigilance and prompt and aggressive intervention concerning this fly (Skoda et al. 2018; Hennessey et al. 2019). It is also important to note this is a reportable disease and relevant authorities must be notified of suspected cases.

The calliphorid fly requires living flesh for the development of its immature stages. Typically, infections occur at wound sites, though mucous membranes have also been reportedly colonized by these flies. The fly is attracted to these areas and will lay several hundred eggs from which maggots hatch and then invade the tissue. These maggots cause a great degree of tissue damage through their voracious appetites and mechanical tissue destruction. The maggots' destruction of living, healthy tissue is the distinguishing factor between this type of myiasis and the much more common secondary myiasis where maggots feed on diseased tissue. The tissue necrosis that results from *C. hominovorax* maggot activity can attract more primary, as well as secondary, myiasis-inducing flies. Severe debilitation or even death may occur with untreated infections. Treatment would be the same as for other more commonly seen maggot infections, described below.

19.3.2.2 Secondary Myiasis-Inducing Flies in Cats and Dogs

Secondary (or facultative) myiasis is caused by the invasion of devitalized tissue by the maggots of opportunistic flies. These types of infections most commonly occur in animals with soiled, matted hair-coats, skin or ear infections, or open wounds that are attractive to flies that would typically lay their eggs in decaying flesh or other organic matter. These flies can be any one of several calliphorid (bottle or blow), sarcophagid (flesh) or even muscid (filth) flies (Figure 19.5). The rate of development for immature forms of these flies is temperature-dependent and varies by species, and infections can develop remarkably quickly on a debilitated or sleeping animal in the right environmental conditions, such as a warm summer day.

Cases of arthropod-infested, abandoned or abused animals are sometimes brought to veterinarians with the requirement for a full forensic evaluation as part of the investigation of a cruelty complaint. In these situations, the use of forensic entomology is an important pathology tool since the presence of the various arthropod life stages for a variety of insects, especially of blowflies, can be used to determine the appropriate amount of time that has passed since colonization. In deceased animals, this is most commonly utilized to infer the approximate time since death (postmortem interval or PMI), and in living animals with myiasis, this can indicate the duration of the neglect or timing of an injury (Merck 2012; McGarry et al. 2018). Veterinarians who deal with the evaluation and documentation of cruelty cases are advised to be familiar with how to preserve this important evidence. There are several articles and veterinary necropsy and forensic textbooks that deal with this subject in depth.

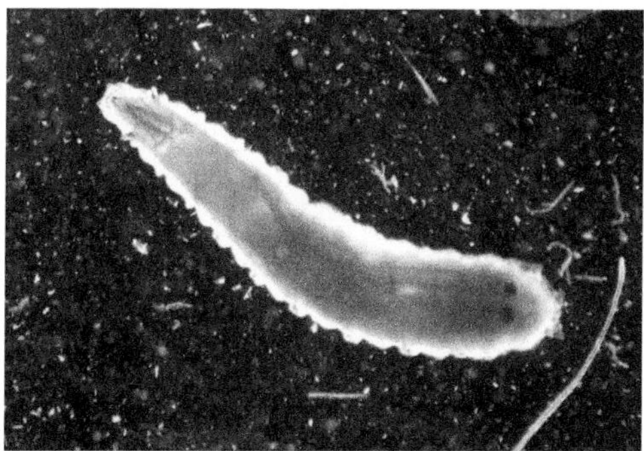

Figure 19.5 Third instar calliphorid maggot recovered from an infected wound in the peri-anal folds of the skin of a dog.

Once the eggs hatch into maggots, they begin to feed upon the diseased flesh of the animal. Careful treatment of the wound(s) and/or other underlying conditions predisposing the animal to secondary myiasis is necessary, along with concomitant treatment with nitenpyram or topical 10% imidacloprid/2.5% moxidectin, pain medications, and antibiotics (if indicated).

19.4 Temporary Ectoparasites Associated with Hosts Only While Feeding

These ectoparasites (biting flies, mosquitos, bugs, ticks) are blood-feeders that inflict pain and discomfort through their feeding action and may transmit disease. Control of these ectoparasites relies on integrated pest-management strategies, which include the use of repellants/insecticides on the hosts, minimizing exposure, and environmental alterations. Steps should be taken to limit access of these arthropods to animals (e.g. use of screens for windows, porches, or outdoor enclosures) as well as to eliminate or reduce hazardous environmental conditions in and around animal shelters (e.g. removal of standing water, garbage, decomposing organic matter, and long grass). Products are available for use in dogs to repel and kill mosquitoes and biting flies, but at the time of publication, no products were licensed for such use in cats.

19.4.1 Biting Flies and Mosquitoes

Shelters with unscreened outdoor runs or pens will provide biting flies and mosquitoes with access to animals that may have difficulty escaping from the discomfort caused by these pests. Stable flies and deer flies are mainly important as pestiferous biters that cause pain with the bites they inflict. Blackflies can also inflict markedly painful bites and when in high numbers, can greatly disturb animals. Additionally, blackflies have been incriminated as vectors of *Onchocerca lupi* infection in dogs. Mosquitoes serve as the vector of *D. immitis* (heartworm) as well as numerous other pathogens of concern for dogs, cats, and humans. Finally, in some parts of the country, sandflies can transmit *Leishmania* spp., and biting midges can be the source of allergic dermatitis if enough bites are received.

19.4.2 Bugs

Kissing bugs (triatomines) are flying insects that could gain access to shelters and kennels. These parasites feed on sleeping hosts at night, in a manner reminiscent of bedbugs. In addition to their blood-feeding, however, their greater importance lies in that some of these bugs have the capability of transmitting *Trypanosoma cruzi* to people and animals alike. (The reader is referred to Chapter 17 for additional information on *T. cruzi* infections, also known as Chagas Disease.) Transmission to humans is generally through the contamination of bite wounds or mucous membranes with the feces of the bug (in which the trypanosomes are shed). In dogs and cats, a more likely mode of transmission would be the ingestion of the bug itself.

Triatomid bugs capable of transmitting *T. cruzi* have been reported in 28 states, with the highest prevalence reported in southern states. Blood meal typing from such bugs has shown that they routinely feed on cats and dogs; a finding supported by the high seropositivity of *T. cruzi* in southern domestic dogs (Kjos et al. 2013), including shelter animals (Tenney et al. 2014). These bugs are frequently reported from outdoor dog-sleeping areas in Texas (Curtis-Robles et al. 2015), and dogs have been suggested to serve a reservoir role for the parasite in peri-domestic environments (Kjos et al. 2013). Therefore, in some areas of the country, it may be necessary to implement strategies to keep these insects out of the shelter environment by using screens on windows and fixing cracks in walls and floors. Housing animals in outdoor environments at night is discouraged.

Bed bugs (*Cimex lectularius*) are mentioned briefly here only because they are an emerging or re-emerging concern in many areas of the United States, and questions sometimes arise as to their association with cats and dogs. Though animals are not likely to have any bed bugs on them at the time of admission, these bugs can be introduced into a shelter via used furniture, bags, or other items where bugs from homes or other buildings that were infested could hide. Following this introduction, the bed bugs could feed on both shelter personnel and animals if they are in close proximity to either. Thus, bed-bug infestations could occur in a shelter much as in any other building where people spend time, but they are unrelated to the animals housed there. As is the case with the tick *R. sanguineus* (discussed below), bed-bug infestations will likely require the services of a certified pest-control officer to oversee their removal from a premise.

19.4.3 Ticks

Ticks are efficient blood-sucking parasites that gain access to and attach firmly to a wide variety of hosts as they pass by them in grass or shrubs.

They feed slowly and often go unnoticed while feeding. They are arachnids like scorpions, spiders, and mites, with four pairs of legs as adults and no antennae. They only crawl; they cannot fly or jump but can crawl several feet toward a host. In general, they feed on the host for three to five days before they drop off. Female ticks lay their eggs usually after feeding. The greatest risk of being bitten by a tick exists in the spring, summer, and fall, but adult ticks may be out searching for a host any time winter temperatures are above freezing.

There are two types of ticks, argasid or "soft ticks" and ixodid or "hard ticks." *Otobius megnini* is a soft tick that commonly infests the ears of many wild and domestic animals, and occasionally humans. *Rhipicephalus, Ixodes, Dermacentor*, and *Amblyomma* are the most common ixodid ticks. In addition to causing blood-loss anemia (usually as a result of heavy infestations in young, old or debilitated animals), pain and discomfort, ticks can also cause tick paralysis or transmit several systemic infections, including Rocky Mountain Spotted Fever (RSMF), *Babesia*, canine ehrlichiosis, canine granulocytotropic anaplasmosis, *Cytauxzoon felis*, and other diseases. The black-legged ticks, *Ixodes scapularis* and *Ixodes pacificus,* are responsible for transmitting the bacterium *Borrelia burgdorferi* that causes Lyme Disease in dogs, humans, and potentially cats. It is important to note that the tick transmits these diseases, and pets are not an immediate source of infection for people. A description of tick-borne diseases and how to identify the ticks can be found at https://www.cdc.gov/ticks/tickbornediseases/tickID.html.

Most ticks can be removed from animals at the time of shelter entry by the administration of one of the many excellent acaricides that are currently on the market today. If there are no funds for such products, the ticks can be manually removed by an experienced staff member; it is important to examine the animal's entire body, paying close attention to the ears and between the toes. Ticks should be removed by grasping them as close to the skin's surface as possible with fine-tipped forceps (never bare hands), pulling gently in the direction of hair growth, making certain to remove the entire tick; if the mouthparts of the tick are not removed, it can cause an inflammatory reaction. It is important to be sure the tick is dead before it is disposed of. Some animals may be heavily infested and very small ticks may be missed, so the recommendation is still to treat with a topical (e.g. whole body dips and sprays) or isoxazoline product and carefully inspect the animal afterward. Prompt removal of ticks may be key to preventing the transmission of some systemic diseases such as Lyme Disease because of the amount of time feeding that is necessary before the pathogens pass across the tick's salivary glands.

Fortunately, even if the fully engorged female of most ticks were to drop off the dog in the shelter, most species of ticks (e.g. *Ixodes, Dermacentor*, and *Amblyomma*) would be unlikely to persist in the shelter environment due to their need to feed on smaller hosts, e.g. rodents, birds, or reptiles, as larvae. The one important exception is *R. sanguineus* (the brown dog tick) because it is fully adapted so that all stages readily feed on dogs. This tick has long been the bane of shelters, boarding kennels, and domiciles. It originated in the arid areas of North Africa and other Mediterranean climes and has the ability to undergo all its development within the dry environs of human habitations. This, and the fact that all its life stages readily feed on dogs, has allowed it to be transported around the world. This tick thrives in the tropics, but it is now virtually everywhere one finds dogs and human beings, and it has recently been found doing quite well even in Alaska (Durden et al. 2016). In the case of *R. sanguineus*, the infestation of a shelter that is not recognized early can spread quickly and widely and will likely require professional pest control to treat the premises. Thus, it is important that inspections occur that routinely look for signs of this tick (and bedbugs) along cracks, behind cages, and in other sites where these parasites can hide in the daytime.

19.5 Conclusion

It is important for shelters to consider the various ectoparasites that may be encountered due both to the geographic region as well as the types of animals that enter the shelter. In addition to causing discomfort and pain to the animals, some ectoparasites are also capable of causing serious disease in both animals and humans from the transmission of vector-borne pathogens. In addition to providing animals with appropriate treatment, every animal shelter needs to develop a plan for treating and preventing environmental infestation of parasites of concern. As with other parasites, in order to develop a plan appropriate for the specific facility and population, the shelter will need to consider the risks and costs of not preventing and treating against the resources required to provide necessary treatments or other interventions. Finally, adopters should be provided with straightforward and easy to understand information about any ectoparasite diagnosis, treatment and follow-up care instructions to ensure the health and welfare of humans and other animals in the home as well as the new pet. In providing this information, it is especially important to make sure adopters understand that vector-borne disease is spread by the vector and not the pet.

19.A Ectoparasites Potentially Affecting Shelter Animals

Parasite	Common Name/ Condition	Species Affected	Zoonotic Potential	Major Clinical Sign	Distribution of lesions
Otobius megnini	Spinous ear tick, soft ticks	Warm-blooded animals	Yes	Irritation, blood loss	Primarily ear canals
Rhipicephalus *Dermacentor* *Amblyomma* *Ixodes* *Haemaphysalis*	Hard ticks	Warm-blooded animals	Yes. Many species transmit blood-borne parasites or other infectious diseases	Irritation, blood loss	Any body part
Lynxacarus radovsky	Cat fur mite	Cat	Not reported	Pruritus	Generalized
Otodectes cynotis	Ear mite	Cat and dog	Rare, but possible	Obvious pruritic otitis externa, hypersensitivity reaction	Ears and whole body in severe cases
Cheyletiella	"Walking dandruff" mite	Cats, dogs, rabbits, other small mammals	Yes	None to severe scaling with variable pruritus	Primarily dorsal distribution
Demodex canis	Demodectic mange, follicular mange, red mange	Dogs	No	Highly variable, commonly causes hair loss, pruritus, scaling, deep pyoderma	Local to generalized
Demodex cati	Feline demodicosis	Cats	No	Highly variable	Local or generalized

Parasite	Common Name/ Condition	Species Affected	Zoonotic Potential	Major Clinical Sign	Distribution of lesions
Demodex gatoi	Feline demodicosis	Cat	No	Most commonly moderate to intense pruritus, evidence of contagion	Usually generalized lesions, pattern of contagion often present
Sarcoptes scabiei var *canis*	Scabies	Dogs	Yes	Intense pruritus	Ventral distribution, ears and elbows, will rapidly become generalized, highly contagious
Notoedres cati	"Feline scabies"	Cats	Yes	Intense pruritus and scaling	Often starts on the head, highly contagious
Trichodectes canis *Linognathus setosus* *Felicola subrostratus*	Lice	Lice are species-specific	No	Pruritus, inflammation, sucking lice can cause anemia	Generalized
Ctenocephalides spp. *Echidnophaga* spp.	Fleas, stick-tight fleas	Warm-blooded animals	Yes	Pruritus, inflammation, anemia	Highly variable
Flies	Fly bite/ strike dermatitis	Warm-blooded animals	N/A	Pruritus, hemorrhagic crusts	Ears, face
Myiasis	Maggots	Warm-blooded animals	N/A	Secondary invaders to open wounds	Any open wound is susceptible
Cuterebra	Bot	Dogs, cats, rabbits	N/A	Maturing maggots in skin with cutaneous nodule, breathing pore commonly seen	Any skin location possible, dorsal back and face common; respiratory, ocular, or neurologic signs

Courtesy: Wiley Blackwell

References

Arther, G.A. (2009). Mites and lice: biology and control. *Veterinary Clinics of North America-Small Animal Practice* 39: 1159–1171.

Barr, S.C. and Bowman, D.D. (2012). *Canine and Feline Infectious Diseases and Parasitology, Blackwell's Five-Minute Veterinary Consult Clinical Companion*, 2e. Chichester, West Sussex: Wiley Blackwell.

Beale, K. (2012). Feline demodicosis: a consideration in the itchy or overgrooming cat. *Journal of Feline Medicine and Surgery* 14: 209–213.

Becskei, C., de Bock, F., Illambas, J. et al. (2016). Efficacy and safety of a novel oral isoxazoline, sarolaner (Simparica™) for the treatment of sarcoptic mange in dogs. *Veterinary Parasitology* 222: 56–61.

Beugnet, F., de Vos, C., Liebenberg, J. et al. (2016b). Efficacy of afoxolaner in a clinical field study in dogs naturally infested with *Sarcoptes scabiei*. *Parasite* 23: 26.

Beugnet, F., Halos, L., Larsen, D. et al. (2016a). Efficacy of oral afoxolaner for the treatment of canine generalised demodicosis. *Parasite* 23: 14.

Blagburn, B.L. and Dryden, M.W. (2009). Biology, treatment, and control of flea and tick infestations. *Veterinary Clinics of North America, Small Animal Practice* 39: 1173–1200.

Bowman, D.D. (2020). *Georgis' Parasitology for Veterinarians*. 11th edition. St. Louis: Elsevier.

Carithers, D., Crawford, J., de Vos, C. et al. (2016). Assessment of afoxolaner efficacy against *Otodectes cynotis* infestations of dogs. *Parasites and Vectors* 9: 636.

Chavez, F. (2016). Case report of afoxolaner treatment for canine demodicosis in four dogs naturally infected with *Demodex canis*. *International Journal of Applied Research in Veterinary Medicine* 14: 123–127.

Curtis-Robles, R., Wozniak, E.J., Auckland, L.D. et al. (2015). Combining public health education and disease ecology research: using citizen science to assess Chagas disease entomological risk in Texas. *PLoS Neglected Tropical Diseases* 9 (12).

Deplazes, P., Eckert, J., Mathis, A. et al. (2016). *Parasitology in Veterinary Medicine*. The Netherlands: Wageningen Academic Publishers.

Durden, L.A., Beckmen, K.B., and Gerlach, R.F. (2016). New records of ticks (Acari: Ixodidae) from dogs, cats, humans, and some wild vertebrates in Alaska: invasion potential. *Journal of Medical Entomology* 53: 1391–1395.

Foley, J. (2009). Vector borne diseases. In: *Infectious Disease Management in Animal Shelters* (eds. L. Miller and K. Hurley), 331. Ames: Wiley Blackwell.

Foley, R.H. (1991a). A notoedric mange epizootic in an island's cat population. *Feline Practice* 19: 8–10.

Foley, R.H. (1991b). An epizootic of a rare fur mite in an Island's cat population. *Feline Practice* 19: 17–19.

Fourie, J.J., Liebenberg, J.E., Horak, I.G. et al. (2015). Efficacy of orally administered fluralaner (Bravecto™) or topically applied imidacloprid/moxidectin (advocate®) against generalized demodicosis in dogs. *Parasites & Vectors* 8: 187.

Han, H.S., Noli, C., and Cena, T. (2016). Efficacy and duration of action of oral fluralaner and spot-on moxidectin/imidacloprid in cats infested with *Lynxacarus radovskyi*. *Veterinary Dermatology* 27: 474–e127.

Hennessey, M.J., Hsi, D.J., Davis, J.S. et al. (2019). Use of a multiagency approach to eradicate New World screwworm flies from Big Pine Key, Florida, following an outbreak of screwworm infestation (September 2016–March 2017). *Journal of the American Veterinary Medical Association* 255 (8): 908–914.

Kjos, S.A., Marcet, P.L., and Yabsley, M.J. (2013). Identification of bloodmeal sources and *Trypanosoma cruzi* infection in triatomine bugs (Hemiptera: Reduviidae) from residential settings in Texas, the United States. *Journal of Medical Entomology* 50: 1126–1139.

Knaus, M., Capári, B., and Visser, M. (2014). Therapeutic efficacy of Broadline® against notoedric mange in cats. *Parasitology Research* 113: 4303–4306.

Koch, S.N. (2017). Updates on the management of canine demodicosis. *Today's Veterinary Practice* 4: 77–85.

Lynn, R.C. and Duquette, R.A. (2020). Antiparasitic Drugs. In: *Georgis' Parasitology for Veterinarians*, 11e (ed. D.D. Bowman), 286–348. St. Louis, MO: Elsevier Saunders.

McGarry, J.M., Ratsep, E., Ressel, L. et al. (2018). Introducing forensic entomology in cases of suspected animal neglect. *Veterinary Record* 182 (5): 139.

Merck, M. (2012). Forensic entomology. In: *Veterinary Forensics: Animal Cruelty Investigations* (ed. M. Merck), 273. Ames: Wiley Blackwell.

Moriello, K., Newbury, S., and Diesel, A. (2009). Ectoparasites. In: *Infectious Disease Management in Animal Shelters* (eds. L. Miller and K. Hurley), 278. Ames: Wiley Blackwell.

Mueller, R.S., Rosenkrantz, W., Bensignor, E. et al. (2020). Diagnosis and treatment of demodicosis in dogs and cats: clinical consensus guidelines of the World Association for Veterinary Dermatology. *Veterinary Dermatology* 31 (1): 4–e2.

Paterson, T.E., Halliwell, R.E., Fields, P.J. et al. (2014). Canine generalized demodicosis treated with varying doses of a 2.5% moxidectin+10% imidacloprid spot-on and oral ivermectin: Parasiticidal effects and long-term treatment outcomes. *Veterinary Parasitology* 205: 687–696.

Romero, C., Heredia, R., Pineda, J. et al. (2016). Efficacy of fluralaner in 17 dogs with sarcoptic mange. *Veterinary Dermatology* 27: 353–e88.

Rosenkrantz, W. (2016). Update on canine demodicosis. NAVC Conference Small Animal and Exotics, Orlando.

Saari, S.A.M., Juuti, K.H., Palojarvi, J.H. et al. (2009). *Demodex gatoi*-associated contagious pruritic dermatosis in cats – a report from six households in Finland. *Acta Veterinaria Scandinavica* 51: 40.

Short, J. and Gram, D. (2016). Successful treatment of *Demodex gatoi* with 10% imidacloprid/1% moxidectin. *Journal of the American Animal Hospital Association* 52: 68–72.

Six, R.H., Becskei, C., Mazaleski, M.M. et al. (2016). Efficacy of sarolaner, a novel oral isoxazoline, against two common mite infestations in dogs: *Demodex* spp. and *Otodectes cynotis*. *Veterinary Parasitology* 222: 62–66.

Skoda, S.R., Phillips, P.L., Welch, J.B. et al. (2018). Screwworm (Diptera: Calliphoridae) in the United States: response to and elimination of the 2016–2017 outbreak in Florida. *Journal of Medical Entomology* 55 (4): 777–786.

Taenzler, J., de Vos, C., Roepke, R.K.A. et al. (2017). Efficacy of fluralaner against *Otodectes cynotis* infestations in dogs and cats. *Parasites & Vectors* 10: 30.

Tenney, T.D., Curtis-Robles, R., Snowden, K.F. et al. (2014). Shelter dogs as sentinels for *Trypanosoma cruzi* transmission across Texas, USA. *Emerging Infectious Diseases* 20: 1323–1326.

Zhou, X., Hohman, A., and Hsu, W.H. (2020). Review of extralabel use of isoxazolines for treatment of demodicosis in dogs and cats. *Journal of the American Veterinary Medical Association* 256 (12): 1342–1346.

20

Dermatophytosis

Sandra Newbury

Shelter Medicine Program, Department of Medical Sciences, University of Wisconsin-Madison School of Veterinary Medicine, Madison, WI, USA

20.1 Introduction

Dermatophytosis, commonly referred to as ringworm, is a fungal disease that causes a superficial skin infection in many species, including humans. It has long been considered to be one of the most complex infectious disease problems facing shelters. Whereas the disease itself is not life-threatening, in the absence of effective diagnostic, management and treatment strategies, the impact of dermatophytosis itself on a shelter can truly be devastating because of fear or panic often based on misperceptions about this disease. At the time of writing of the first edition of this text, it had been widely accepted that the disease was too difficult for most shelters to diagnose and treat, and that successful environmental decontamination of the long-lived, resistant spores was virtually impossible to achieve. More recently, however, there have been tremendous advances in understanding and increasing lifesaving capacity in the face of this complex and confusing disease. Simple treatment options, relatively short expected times to achieve a cure, rapid identification and diagnostics, risk reduction for humans, and effective environmental management have all been well studied and described.

However, a great deal of fear still surrounds ringworm in shelter settings, and understandably so; the fungus is extremely durable in the environment, resistant to many disinfectants commonly used in shelters and can be highly contagious to cats and other animals, including humans. If given enough time, a cat in good health in a stress-free environment may self-cure from this disease; however, unrecognized and untreated ringworm in a shelter setting can lead to widespread infection throughout the facility. Treatment becomes increasingly difficult and more resource intensive when less effective treatments prolong recovery times.

In the author's experience, the most common life-threatening dermatophytosis management issue seen in shelters is confusion about diagnostics, second only to the desire to find treatments of short duration that do not involve the use of topical lime sulfur, which has a noxious odor.

Fortunately, successful screening and treatment programs have been established at multiple facilities, including a model program established by the author and her colleagues at the Dane County Humane Society (DCHS) in Madison, WI in 2003 and other programs modeled after this one. These programs, along with

Infectious Disease Management in Animal Shelters, Second Edition.
Edited by Lila Miller, Stephanie Janeczko, and Kate F. Hurley.

extensive consultation work with numerous shelters and facilities housing multiple animals, have demonstrated that dermatophytosis can be treated and managed successfully without panic or resorting to widespread depopulation (Carlotti et al. 2010; Newbury and Moriello 2014; Newbury, Verburgge and Moriello 2005; Newbury, Verbrugge and Steffen 2005; Newbury et al. 2007, 2015.)

Because outbreaks of dermatophytosis in shelter cats have been reported so much more frequently as a problem severe enough to debilitate an entire organization than in dogs, this chapter will emphasize management of feline dermatophytosis in a shelter setting, though information on the treatment of dogs and other animals in shelters is also included.

20.2 Etiology

20.2.1 Agent Description

The dermatophytes consist of a group of fungi of the genera *Microsporum*, *Trichophyton*, and *Epidermophyton*. These organisms have adapted to digest keratinous debris. Pathogens in these genera infect the stratum corneum, hair shafts, and claw. The species are divided into three classes, anthropophilic, zoophilic, and geophilic. The anthropophilic species have evolved on humans and rarely affect animals. The zoophilic species are adapted to animal hosts but may spread to in-contact humans. The soil-adapted geophilic species are less often a cause of human disease, but sometimes affect animals.

Though there are more than 30 species of dermatophytes that affect dogs, cats, and birds, the most commonly isolated pathogens from cats and dogs are *Microsporum canis* (*M. canis*), *Microsporum gypseum*, and *Trichophyton spp. M. canis* is the most important pathogen of cats; approximately 90% or more cases of feline dermatophytosis are caused by *M canis*. Cats can also be infected with alternate species such as *Microsporum persicolor* or *Trichophyton spp.*, but these infections are uncommon. *M. gypseum* is isolated more frequently from dogs, but they may also be infected with *M. canis,* or rarely *Trichophyton mentagrophytes. Trichophyton* infections that are clinically significant are rare, but are more common in dogs than in cats, though the latter may also be affected. *Trichophyton spp.* infections are also more common in rodents and hedgehogs. This chapter will focus primarily on the identification and control of *M. canis* as its primary management goals because it is the pathogen of greatest significance in shelters.

20.2.2 Key Factors Affecting Susceptibility to Infections

In many regions, there is a strong seasonality associated with dermatophyte infection. Infections in animals tend to be more common in warm, humid geographic regions of the world. In more temperate climates, infections may be more common in warm months than in winter. In regions with colder winters, infection in dogs is uncommon. Increased incidence of infection in shelters may also coincide with breeding season, i.e. "kitten season." For example, in the northern Midwest of the United States, October and May tend to have the largest influx of infected cats and kittens (Newbury, Verbrugge and Moriello 2005; Verbrugge et al. 2006). Kittens are more susceptible to infection, and often present to shelters in poor body condition, stressed, and infected with internal and external parasites. Shelters in the warm, humid southern regions of the United States and northern shelters that receive transports from more southern regions report problems with dermatophytosis in dogs more frequently than northern shelters. Infections are rarely reported as problematic in shelter dogs originating from the Northeast and northern Midwest.

There are many factors that influence infection but, in general, age is the most important factor. Juvenile animals (under one year of age) are most commonly affected by this disease. Young animals are also relatively likely to suffer from severe, generalized infections (i.e. skin lesions covering much of the body) while infections in adult animals are more commonly limited or focal infections/lesions. Infection tends to be most common in cats who have been living in close proximity to other cats and outgoing, friendly cats, probably because of the increased chance for exposure through contact. Long-haired cats, such as Persians and Himalayans, may be more susceptible because they are less efficient at grooming themselves and thus mechanically removing the spores.

Overcrowding of cats in shelters should be considered a major risk factor, whether singly or group-housed or free-roaming. Animals that come from environments where many animals are present, such as barns or hoarding situations, are also at higher risk of infection (Polak et al. 2014). No correlation with intake status, such as stray or owner surrendered, has been found (Verbrugge et al. 2006).

Dermatophytosis more commonly affects cats than dogs. Dogs housed outside in dirt runs or that run free, hunting dogs, and dogs housed in over-crowded environments are at increased risk of infection (Cafarchia et al. 2004). Yorkshire terriers are one well-known dog breed that is predisposed to infection; the reason is unknown and may relate to the hair length or that dogs that require frequent grooming are at higher risk for contagious skin diseases (Cafarchia et al. 2004; Cerundolo 2004).

Dermatophytosis may also be encountered in other species sometimes housed in shelters, including rabbits, ferrets, mice, rats, guinea pigs, hedgehogs, etc. Clinical signs will be similar, as the pathogenesis of the disease is the same. Treatment protocols acceptable for kittens are generally safe for use in these other species; however, the reader is cautioned to always check for species susceptibility and potential toxicity to systemic antifungals before using them in species other than cats and dogs.

20.3 Pathogenesis

Exposure occurs from contact with another infected animal, a fomite or a contaminated environment. Simply being exposed to spores does not necessarily result in an infection. For an infection to become established, spores must reach the skin surface and defeat host protective mechanisms. Natural skin flora, sebum, grooming, and the skin immune system are the first lines of defense.

Dermatophyte spores require some type of microtrauma or trauma to gain access to the skin and cause an infection. An often-overlooked source of "microtrauma" is maceration of the skin due to high humidity. External parasitism is another common source of microtrauma to the skin that can predispose animals to infection. Infection is usually the result of exposure to infected spores coupled with one or more predisposing factors, including but not limited to, youth or old age, debilitating disease, compromised immunologic status, poor body condition; matted hair coat, and/or predisposing environmental factors associated with poor husbandry. These factors are often found in combination. In settings where animals are not stressed, ill, or in poor body condition, an infective spore that reaches the hair coat may simply fall off, be groomed off or simply be mechanically carried and never trigger an infection. In shelter animals, where stress, parasitism, and concurrent illness may be impediments to normal grooming behavior, as well as having a negative impact on the immune system, exposure may more readily lead to infection.

20.4 Disease Course

20.4.1 Incubation Period

In general, the incubation period from exposure until the development of clinically obvious lesions is approximately two to four weeks. In experimentally induced infections, infected hairs have been noted in less than a week (DeBoer and

Moriello 1994). Lesions may be detected earliest by highly trained observers. The development of clinical lesions is preceded by infection of the hair follicle. The relatively long incubation period compared to many other infectious diseases must be considered when attempting to map an outbreak or determine the potential origin of infections (in-shelter spread vs. community source). Due to the long incubation period and variable clinical signs, simply quarantining potentially exposed animals to observe them for the appearance of clinical lesions is not recommended. (Please see the section on risk evaluation and response in Section 20.8.)

20.4.2 Immunity After Recovery

Studies on the immune response of cats have shown that cats develop both a humoral and cell-mediated immune response to infection, but recovery is associated with a strong cell-mediated response, not the humoral response. This contrasts with recovery from many other infections (DeBoer and Moriello 1993; Sparkes et al. 1996). Lack of a cell-mediated response is associated with prolonged infection. Immunity is also relative. Most recovered infected animals are immune from re-infection, but when challenged with large numbers of spores, infection is possible. Recovered animals should be protected from exposure in order to prevent re-infection. The duration of immunity after recovery from infection is unknown.

20.4.3 Carrier State

The author has not seen any cases in a shelter setting of unaffected "carrier state" animals, nor animals with persistent infections in the face of appropriate treatment. Studies on the fungal flora of cats have shown that *M. canis* is **NOT** part of the normal fungal flora of cats (Moriello and DeBoer 1991a, b). A positive fungal culture from a cat indicates one of three situations: a cat with obvious clinical lesions, a cat with subtle lesions, or a cat that is mechanically carrying spores on its hair coat. All three situations require some type of "action" as these spores can be transmitted to other animals and humans. The concept of "asymptomatic carriers" with respect to dermatophyte infections is unlike that of other diseases encountered in shelters where "latent" infections can be activated. The author strongly discourages the use of the term "carrier" or "asymptomatic carrier."

Differentiation between animals that culture positive for dermatophytes because they are truly infected or because they simply have spores resting like dust on their hair coat is essential because they present very different challenges and risks. "Dust mops" (cats mechanically carrying spores on their hair coat) may become infected if the spores are not removed but, in many cases, most healthy cats will remove those spores themselves by grooming.

It is unclear what risk these "dust mop" cats pose to other animals or the shelter environment. Though the hair coat of animals often carry spores representative of those found in their environment, dermatophytes are not considered part of the normal flora of dogs or cats. When large quantities of spores are carried on the hair coat, at least some risk exists that infection may develop, or spores may be shed into the environment. When the number of spores carried is low, the risk diminishes. Quantitative fungal culture can help distinguish between these two scenarios; please see the section on risk evaluation in Section 20.8.

20.5 Transmission

Naturally infective hairs and spores are easily shed into the environment from infected animals. Infective spores are small, approximately the size of dust particles, and can easily collect on, or be transferred to, the hair coats of other animals who are either housed in or passing through a contaminated area. Infective spores can be transmitted to a susceptible host by direct contact, via contaminated fomites (such as environmental surfaces, bedding, blankets, toys, brushes, lab coats, or human hands) or even by external parasites such as fleas.

In some cases, such as when handling cats, it is possible for staff to mechanically transmit dermatophytes when moving sequentially from one cat to the next medicating, feeding, socializing or providing other nursing care. These activities can also cause microtrauma to the skin that increases the likelihood that infection will become established.

Airborne transmission is a commonly reported concern of shelters and other facilities housing multiple animals. Many questions have arisen about the likelihood of environmental contamination resulting from the travel of spores through heating and cooling ducts. Though airborne transmission of dermatophyte spores is possible via infective spores "floating" across distances, in most cases, when husbandry and disinfection practices are adequate, airborne transmission is of minimal significance. In the author's work in an off-site annex facility at a shelter with a heating and cooling unit similar to that of a home, airborne transmission of spores did not occur. In this facility, infected cats were confined to cages; caretakers swept floors daily and used detergent to mop floors once or twice weekly. On multiple occasions, when the facility was completely filled with infected cats, fungal culture plates were left open and exposed to the air throughout the facility. In addition, fungal culture plates were placed directly (culture-medium side down) over heating vents to see if spores were being spread through forced air heating vents. All plates were consistently negative even when infective spores could be isolated from areas where contamination was expected (e.g. cages of actively infected cats). However, fungal cultures of the furnace filter were always positive. These results indicate that infected hairs and spores were drawn into the air-vents and trapped in the furnace filter and not being blown throughout the facility. This example also suggests that, in most shelter situations, dermatophyte transmission can be effectively controlled without providing separate air circulation, *provided adequate treatment and appropriate sanitation are concurrently provided to minimize infectious dose and environmental contamination*. However, airborne transmission was reported in a cattery where the owner used fans to cool cats and circulate air in the isolation room (Moriello and Newbury 2009). The potential for airborne transmission should be minimized whenever possible, but large investments of resources for separate air circulation or duct cleaning are probably not warranted unless a problem has been demonstrated.

Dermatophyte transmission in shelters can be reduced by paying rigorous attention to sanitation methods that promote effective fomite and environmental control. Mechanical cleaning and disinfection at regular intervals substantially lower the likelihood of environmental contamination that could lead to disease transmission. Environmental contamination is greatest in foster homes and shelters, in areas where hair has been allowed to accumulate or in homes where there are large numbers of infected kittens (Mancianti et al. 2003).

Spores will persist in the environment, remaining potentially infectious for weeks to months, unless the area is thoroughly cleaned, including specific steps to mechanically remove infective material, and disinfected. (See section 20.9.4.1 on decontamination.)

Increased infectious dose and frequency of exposure increase the likelihood of transmission. Transmission of dermatophytes is particularly problematic in situations such as shelters and rescue homes when animals are housed together, whether in cages or cage-free environments. Though high turnover shelters, with their constant influx of new, potentially infectious cats, may present a higher risk of introduction and/or greater exposure to a critical mass of infective material, any time an infectious animal is admitted to a group setting, especially when the infection goes unrecognized, infection may be transmitted to others in the population.

20.6 Clinical Presentation and Differential Diagnoses

Dermatophytosis is one of the most pleomorphic skin diseases encountered in veterinary dermatology. Classic lesions of dermatophytosis are usually described as circular areas of alopecia with inflammation and scaling. Those "classic" round, hairless lesions gave rise to the initial theory that a worm running in a ring within the skin was causing the lesions, giving rise to the name "ringworm." Many cases of dermatophytosis will present with those classic clinical signs, but many others will not. In addition to the classic presentation, dermatophytosis has a wide variety of presentations.

Clinical signs in dogs and cats include, but are not limited to, any combination of the following: hair loss (alopecia) that varies from focal to generalized in severity, erythema, easily broken hairs, excessive shedding, minimal to marked pruritus, follicular plugging, hyperpigmentation of the skin, otitis externa, ear-margin inflammation, pododermatitis, papules, pustules, "feline symmetrical alopecia," mild to severe scaling and crusting, and presentations severe enough to mimic immune-mediated skin diseases. See Figures 20.1–20.6.

Lesions can be any shape or size. The degree of inflammation, crusting, and hair loss vary widely. Lesions most often involve some degree of inflammation with or without hair loss. Skin lesions may mimic or be hidden by many other non-contagious, non-infectious skin diseases.

In many cases, subtle lesions may be overlooked without a careful, complete examination of the entire body. In other cases, lesions that have the "classic" appearance may not be due to dermatophytosis at all. While cats with a "classic" appearance of dermatophytosis are often actually infected with dermatophytes, skin lesions in adult dogs that look like "classic" ringworm lesions are much more likely to be caused by a bacterial pyoderma or demodicosis rather than dermatophytosis. Skin lesions in puppies are more likely a result of dermatophytosis than in adult dogs but may also be caused by bacterial pyoderma or Demodex. Because dermatophytosis may present in so many forms, diagnosis cannot be based solely on the presence of "classic" skin lesions, though examination of lesions is an integral part of identification, diagnosis and outbreak response (See Section 20.7).

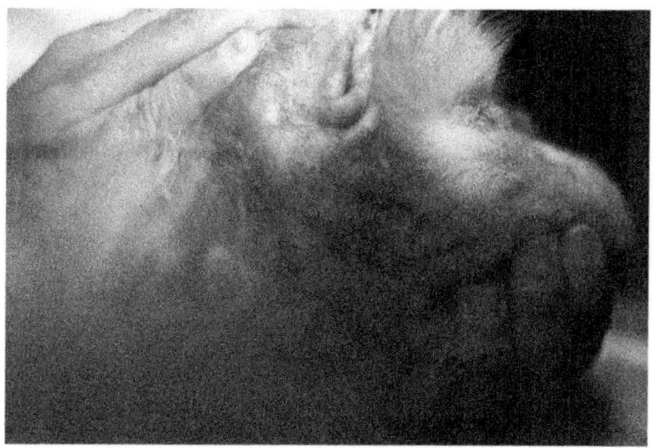

Figure 20.1 Puppy with an area of hair loss caudal to the ear. This was caused by *M. gypseum*, but other differential diagnoses included demodicosis and bacterial infection.

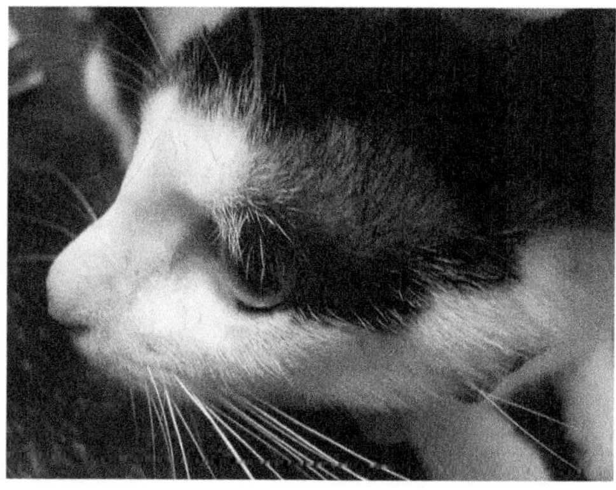

Figure 20.2 Hair loss in the pre-auricular area of a cat. It was initially assumed to be "normal" until the cat was examined with a Wood's lamp and glowing hairs were found.

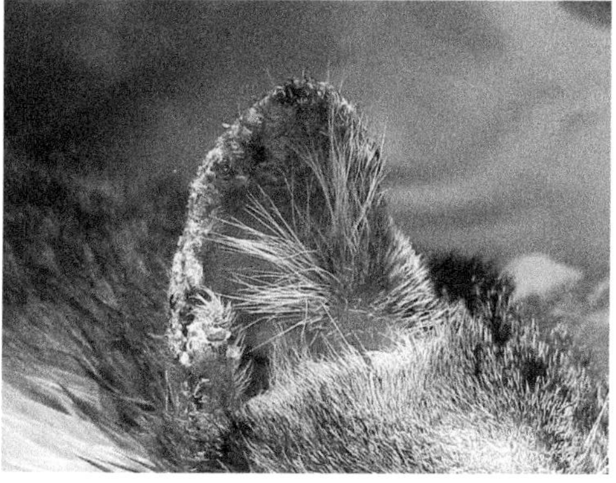

Figure 20.3 Ear margin crusting due to dermatophytosis. This was caused by a Trichophyton spp. infection. Ear margin infections are common presentations of Trichophyton spp. infections in the author's experience.

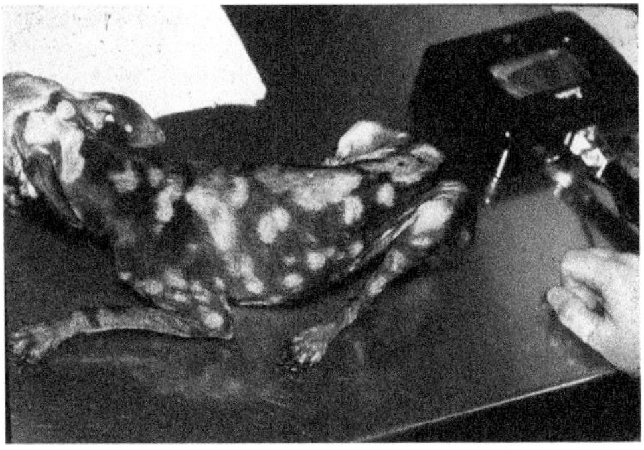

Figure 20.4 Multifocal areas of hair loss on the trunk of a dog caused by a dermatophyte infection. Note that the lesions extend to the head. The most common cause of circular areas of hair loss in an adult dog is bacterial pyoderma, however, it is rare for bacterial pyoderma to involve the face. *Source:* Courtesy of Dr. Gail Kunkle.

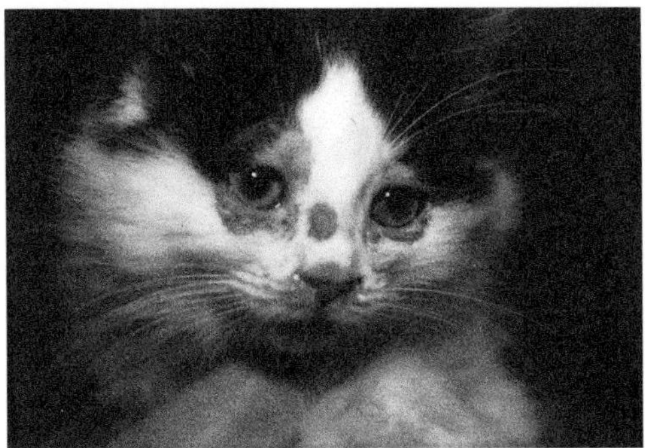

Figure 20.5 Kitten with common "classical" lesions of dermatophytosis in the periocular and muzzle region. The site of this infection is difficult to treat because it is close to the eyes.

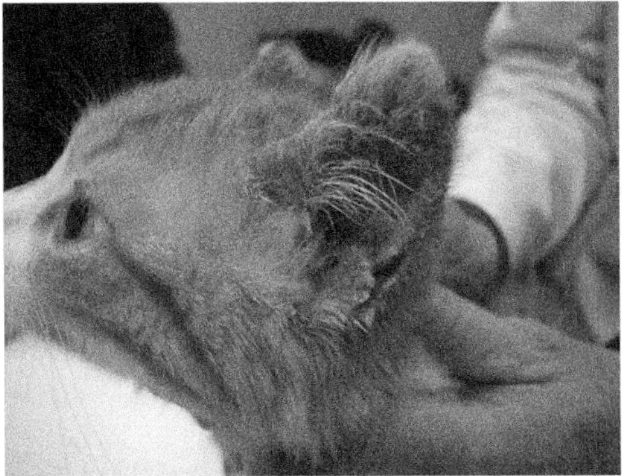

Figure 20.6 *Microsporum canis* infection on the ear of a kitten. The initial clinical signs were ear pruritus. Not only did the ear pinna glow but also the hairs inside the bell of the ear. It is important in these cases to be sure to treat the inside of the ear. Also, note that suspect cats should be handled with gloves!

20.7 Diagnosis

Diagnosis of dermatophytosis in animals in shelters can be quite challenging, but a good visual exam and use of a Wood's lamp can help to simplify the process. Decisions about which animals can go to foster care or adoption are eased when good screening practices are in place. Because of the potential for humans and other animals to become infected, early identification and prompt responses are essential to control disease spread. A detailed description of the recommended systematic screening process, including specifics of how each diagnostic tool can be effectively used in animal shelters and welfare organizations, is provided below.

20.7.1 Basic Diagnostic Tools

A meticulous dermatologic examination is the foundation for the appropriate use of all other diagnostics. The diagnostic tools described below should be used as part of an overall screening process that includes a thorough physical examination of the entire skin and hair coat by a veterinary professional or designated staff who have been carefully trained to detect clinically suspicious lesions. Every reasonable effort should be made to obtain a history of the source of the animal, previous housing situation, and prior health problems. Information about potential for exposure can be very helpful to identify higher risk animals.

After obtaining the history and performing a physical examination, the most common and practical diagnostic tools include the use of a Woods' lamp, direct microscopic examination of suspect hairs, and fungal culture as indicated. Skin biopsies are rarely used, though biopsy of unusual skin lesions may surprisingly reveal dermatophytosis as the cause, especially when dermatophytosis has not been previously ruled out. Information regarding the use of these tools has been incorporated in the systematic screening process steps described below.

20.7.2 Diagnostic Protocols for Preventive Management and Control: Systematic Screening Protocol

The recommended systematic screening protocol described here consists of coordinated and consistent use of the five basic diagnostic tools:

1) History
2) Visual (physical) examination
3) Wood's lamp examination
4) Direct examination of fluorescing hairs
5) Fungal culture.

A thorough understanding of all five components of this process is required to develop an effective protocol for dermatophyte screening, prevention, and treatment in a shelter. In some cases, specific staff may be trained to focus on particular steps of the protocol (e.g. reading fungal culture plates). The use of these five basic diagnostic tools simplifies early recognition and helps guide housing and treatment decisions. This systematic screening protocol can be used at admission, any important control point, or when responding to an outbreak. (The use of diagnostic tools to monitor treatment is discussed in Section 20.9.)

Screening is crucial at the time of admission to the shelter to prevent disease transmission. Screening at admission provides an opportunity to identify infected, potentially contagious animals, take preventative action, and start treatment quickly when resources allow. Screening for dermatophytosis using this systematic process adds only a few minutes to admission procedures if the designated area is properly equipped for the screening examination and intake staff have been properly trained. At a minimum, the examination steps of the screening process should be repeated at critical infectious disease control points (such as moving animals into public areas, group housing, or foster or adoptive homes) in order to identify any lesions or infections that may have been missed or developed since intake. This systematic screening process is also essential as part of an outbreak response plan. Other diagnostics work best in conjunction with information gathered during the screening process to help guide treatment and management decisions.

20.7.2.1 Step One: History

All relevant historical information for each individual animal and group of animals examined should be reviewed at or prior to admission. Animals from the same household with other infected animals should be treated as highly suspect (i.e. high-risk). Littermates or cage mates of confirmed infected animals should be treated as infected because of the close exposure and direct contact even though not all members of a litter will show clinical signs.

20.7.2.2 Step Two: Visual (Physical) Examination

Animals should be examined for skin lesions under a bright light. The examiner should always wear disposable exam gloves when handling the animal. A strong, directed examination light greatly helps identify subtle lesions. If this is not available, a strong-beamed flashlight should be utilized. Sometimes more lesions are found using only the light from a flashlight rather than with overhead lights because the beam is concentrated on one area. Particular attention to the following areas is needed because these are common sites where lesions are overlooked: muzzle, lips, periocular area, ear margins, the skin inside the cone of the ear, digits and nail-bed area, abdomen, medial aspects of limbs, and the tail. Staff must be trained to differentiate scars or other quiet, non-inflammatory skin lesions from possible dermatophyte lesions. All inflammatory lesions should be noted, even if another obvious cause has been identified. As an example, ear mites may cause inflammation in the ear canal and inner pinnae of cats. The infestation or the associated self-trauma may seem like an obvious cause of inflammation or hair loss in and around the ears. However, the ear-mite infestation does not rule out concurrent dermatophytosis. In the author's experience, an ear-mite infestation can actually increase the likelihood of dermatophytosis because the associated microtrauma facilitates the development of infection. Fleas have been found to be culture positive and may be another way spores can spread in a shelter. Also, even if there is an obvious cause of an animal's pruritus (e.g. louse infestation), it is important to remember that cats, especially kittens, may have more than one disease present. In addition, this careful visual examination of animals is a valuable way to identify other medical problems.

20.7.2.3 Step Three: Wood's Lamp Examination

The next step is to examine animals with a Wood's lamp for fluorescing hairs. A Wood's lamp is an ultraviolet light with a wavelength of 365 nm. Wood's lamps are screening tools to identify infected hairs for microscopic examination. The only veterinary pathogen of importance that can produce apple-green fluorescence is *M. canis*. A positive examination is strongly indicative of infection and allows one to select hairs for microscopic examination. A negative examination does not rule out dermatophytosis, but, in an animal with no lesions, it suggests infection is not present. A negative Wood's examination in an animal with lesions suggests the animal is much less likely to be infected.

A plug-in Wood's lamp should be used; battery powered UV lamps rarely give sufficient illumination of appropriate wavelength to be diagnostic. Smaller hand-held models make examination easier than bulky wands or lamps with built-in magnification. If additional magnification is needed, a hand-held magnifying glass works nicely.

Lamps can be used without taking time to warm up, but it often takes several minutes for the examiner's eyes to adapt to the light; otherwise glowing hairs can be missed. The room should be dark and the lamp held close to the hair coat and skin; the entire body should be examined slowly and carefully to avoid missing any affected areas. Attention should be focused on the examination of common sites of infection and the frequently overlooked lesion sites described previously when using the Wood's lamp.

Fluorescence associated with dermatophytosis is seen at the base of the hairs, near the hair follicle, and not just on the tips of the hairs. Infected hairs fluoresce because the fungus in the hair follicle deposits a metabolite on the hair shaft as it grows. In many cases, it will look as though the whole hair shaft is glowing. The metabolite coating on the hair does not make the hairs stick together. In some cases, infected hairs will be broken and only the stubble will glow at the base, very close to the skin.

Fluorescence from infected hairs will most commonly have a bright apple-green appearance (See Figure 20.7). During a study conducted by the author in which cats were examined daily, very early fluorescence was blue-white, eventually turning apple green. Other colors are most often artifact. Sebum on the skin that may or may not be associated with inflammation will glow a fainter, dull yellow color that is not indicative of dermatophyte infection. Doxycycline or terramycin give a yellow glow when smeared or crusted on the fur

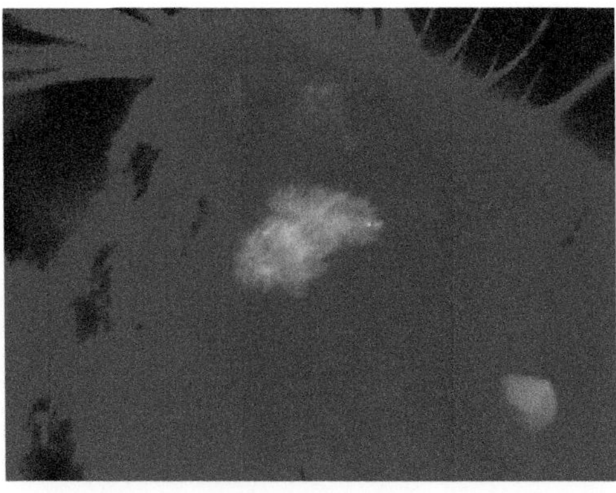

Figure 20.7 "Classic" fluorescence of hairs with a Wood's lamp.

and should not be confused with infection. It is not possible to brush off the fluorescing substance if it is caused by a dermatophyte infection. If there is any uncertainty, gently pluck hairs and examine the roots for fluorescence.

If thick crusting is present, it is important to gently remove the crusts and look for infected hairs because crusting may obscure them. In many cases, broken hairs underlying the crusts will be Wood's positive while the crusting is not.

It has been commonly cited that approximately 50% of cases of dermatophytosis caused by *M. canis* will fluoresce with a Wood's lamp. Only *M. canis* produces the metabolite that creates the fluorescent glow and not every strain of *M. canis* will produce the metabolite. However, in the author's experience examining hundreds of infected cats at animal shelters, careful examination with the Wood's lamp revealed glowing hairs on the vast majority of the cats with lesions. In many cases, cats who appear to be non-lesional on a visual examination will have fluorescing hairs that suggest pre-clinical infection or help to identify subtle lesions that were missed on initial examination.

20.7.2.4 Step Four: Direct Examination of Fluorescing Hairs

Direct microscopic examination of fluorescing hairs is a quick and simple method of obtaining an immediate diagnosis of *M. canis* dermatophytosis when a Wood's lamp examination is positive. Interpretation of the microscopic examination takes some training and practice but is not difficult to master. When initial training is conducted to evaluate direct examinations, each procedure should be confirmed by a fungal culture until an acceptable accuracy rate has been achieved. When performed properly, Wood's lamp and direct examinations of hairs are very cost effective and may save the cost and time of performing a fungal culture. There is one area of caution: If any legal circumstances surround the case, a fungal culture should always be performed even if the Wood's lamp and direct examination of hairs confirm the diagnosis.

Fungal cultures are the "gold standard" for diagnosis of dermatophytosis. In addition, if legal issues are present, it is prudent to take both gross photographs of the animal and photographs of any microscopic examinations. This is easily performed by aiming a digital camera through the microscope lens. A Wood's lamp, microscope, and a curved-tip hemostat are the only required equipment. Supplies needed are glass microscope slides, microscope coverslips and mineral oil as a suspension solution. Clearing agents such as potassium hydroxide (KOH) can be used instead of mineral oil. Clearing agents cause the background material to swell, rendering hairs and spores more refractile. Caution should be used with the KOH solution because it can be caustic to the animals' skin and microscope lenses. Mineral oil is a good, readily available, benign alternative for use in shelter settings.

Procedure:

1) A drop of mineral oil (or KOH) should be placed on a microscope slide that should be set aside where it will not be easily knocked to the floor but is still close to the examination area.
2) A few glowing hairs should be plucked following the direction of growth to ensure getting the hair root for examination. This process requires at least one assistant to hold the animal and the Wood's lamp while the other person identifies and carefully plucks the glowing hairs. The Wood's lamp can be used to carefully examine the hairs in the hemostat before they are placed in the suspension solution on the slide.
3) The hairs should be placed on the drop of mineral oil or KOH on the microscope slide and the coverslip placed on the slide. Again, the Wood's lamp can be used to confirm glowing hairs are present on the slide (See Figure 20.8).
4) The slide should be placed on the microscope stage and examined with 4× magnification with the microscope light off and the room lights dim. The Wood's lamp

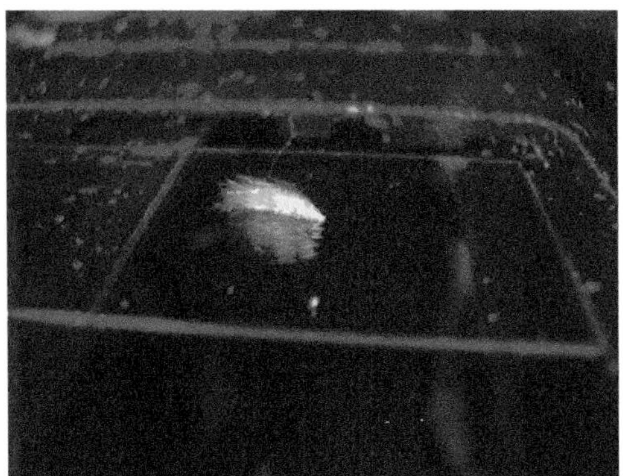

Figure 20.8 Glowing hairs on a glass slide.

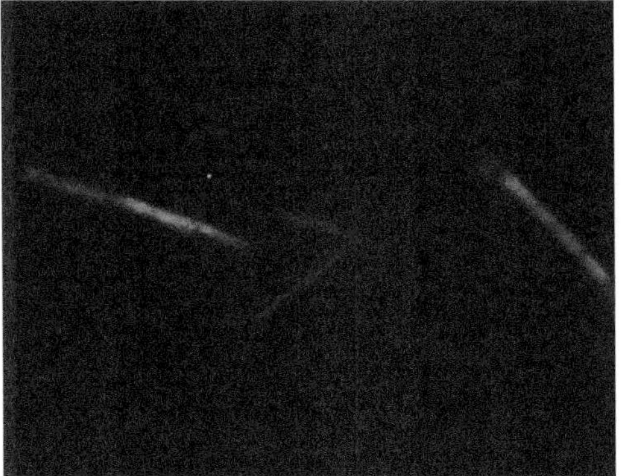

Figure 20.9 The Wood's lamp can be used to locate hairs on a glass microscope slide to facilitate examination.

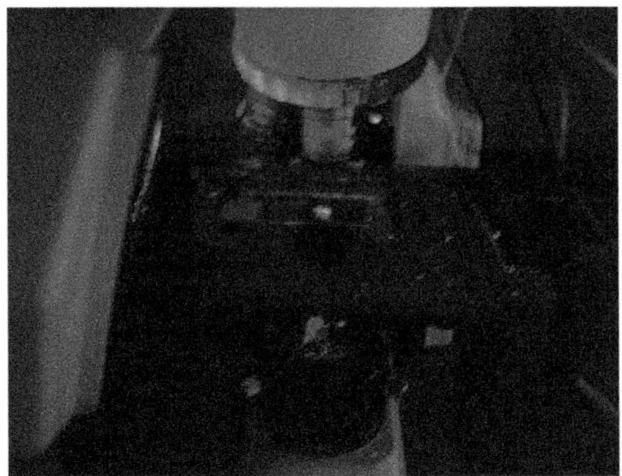

Figure 20.10 Note the glowing hairs on the glass slide on the microscope stage. This allows the specimen to be positioned beneath the lens.

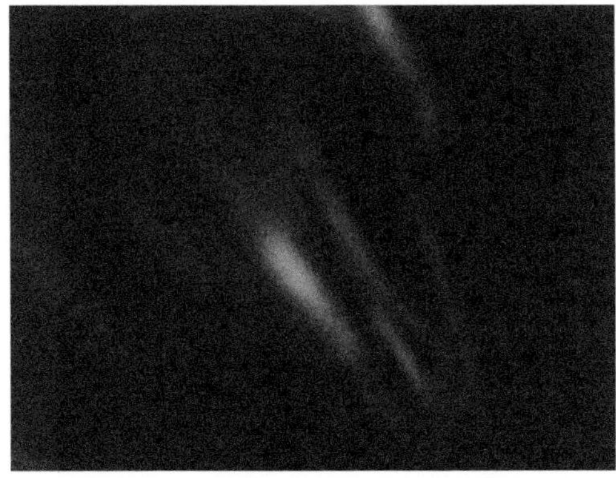

Figure 20.11 Glowing hairs seen through the microscope lens. In this situation, the Wood's lamp is being held to the slide of the stage. Once the hairs are located, the Wood's lamp is not needed and the slide can be examined normally.

should be held next to the microscope stage and directed toward the slide. This process highlights glowing hairs so they can be placed within view through the eyepiece and lens (See Figures 20.9 and 20.10). Once the fluorescing hair can be seen through the eyepiece, the Wood's lamp is no longer needed and both the microscope and room lights can be turned on (See Figure 20.11).

5) Infected hairs are wider, irregular and appear more filamentous than normal hairs at low power (See Figure 20.12). At higher magnification, cuffs of refractile spores and hyphae can be seen. A 10× lens is usually sufficient to confirm infected hairs, but a 40× magnification lens may be needed to confirm the presence of ectothrix spores. Oil immersion is not needed. Again, the examiner is looking for stacks or rows of small beads on either side of the hair shaft and/or hair shafts that appear swollen, broken, filled in or frayed in appearance compared to normal hair shaft structure (See Figure 20.13).

Please note: After completing these first four steps, an initial risk assessment and response should be made. Please see section 20.8 for risk evaluation and response information.

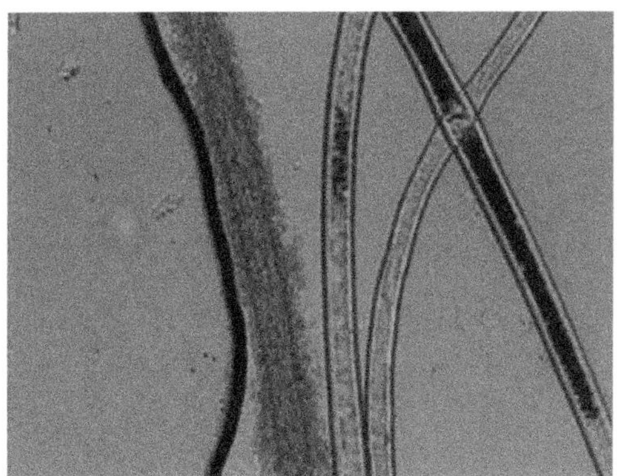

Figure 20.12 Normal and affected hairs are present. Note that the infected hairs are lighter in color, wider, and more filamentous in appearance (10×).

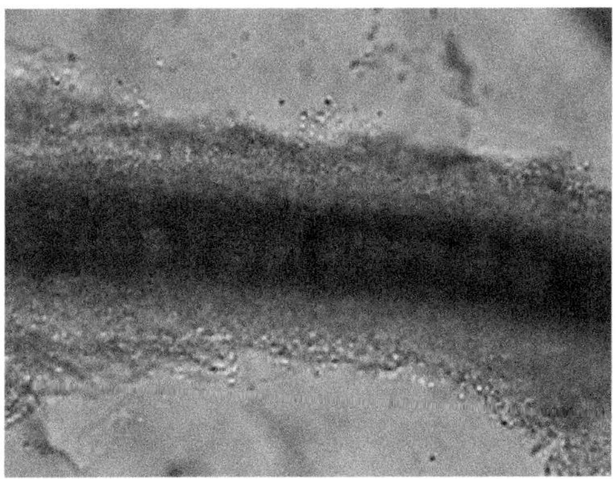

Figure 20.13 Cuffs of ectothrix spores seen around an infected hair (40×).

20.7.2.5 Step Five: Fungal Cultures

When the first edition of this textbook was published, performing a fungal culture of all animals entering the shelter, regardless of whether lesions were present, was believed to be the best or most prudent option for detecting the disease. A fungal culture is considered the gold standard for the diagnosis of dermatophytosis in individual animals and was therefore the most cautious approach for shelters; it offered a safety net to pick up any infectious animals that may have been missed by visual and Wood's lamp exams.

However, this practice is too highly resource intensive and complex to implement in most shelters. While comprehensive fungal culture screening of all cats at intake did effectively control dermatophytosis in a shelter (Newbury, Verbrugge and Steffen 2005), the same shelter, as well as many others, adapted to culturing only Wood's positive cats and those with suspicious inflammatory lesions while maintaining similar levels of control over the infection.

Careful intake evaluation using the first four diagnostic tools described previously (history, visual physical examination, Wood's lamp and a direct examination of fluorescing hairs) will identify the vast majority of suspect and infectious cats, greatly reducing the infectious risk from dermatophytosis. Selective fungal culture screening supports this process by confirming or ruling out infections in positive or suspect animals and is most needed to diagnose infection for animals with suspicious lesions that do not fluoresce. If the screening process is effective, most often culture results from non-fluorescing lesions will be negative because the vast majority of infected cats will have fluorescing lesions. In short, fungal cultures are best utilized for definitive diagnosis of dermatophytosis in animals who have fluorescing lesions or for ruling out dermatophytosis in animals with inflammatory lesions that do not fluoresce. Culturing is most often performed as a safety precaution; it contributes to risk reduction by helping to rule out infection and helping cats move faster through the shelter.

Screening for all animals is most important for shelters that commonly:

- house animals in group or community settings
- house animals in rooms that are difficult to disinfect
- send animals to private temporary homes for foster care.

Visual and Wood's exam screening should be a standard part of the protocol for moving cats into group-housing rooms or foster homes. The highest priority for fungal culture should be given to cats who have some type of inflammatory skin condition or hair coat abnormality. Tables 20.1–20.5 summarize "practice tips" from the author on setting up an in-house system and reading cultures.

Table 20.1 Practice tips for collecting samples and data.

- Package culture material into "culture kits" that have a toothbrush inside a plastic bag with a preprinted label attached.
- Use pre-printed labels that contain all of the information the organization wants documented for culture. Commercial sheets of labels are sold that contain instructions on how to format the page. Below is a sample label used by the author. Note that it asks for three key pieces of information: Wood's lamp status, presence or absence of lesions, and whether or not lesions are suspected of being caused by dermatophytosis.

ID #________________ Date: __________

Sex: M F N Hair length: S M L

Age: Kitten Juvenile (6-12 months) Adult

Wood's Positive? Y N Any Lesions? Y N

Do you suspect lesions from ringworm? Y N

- Set up an Excel sheet for recording data and making treatment plans (Tables 16.2 and 16.3)
  - This allows for the sorting of data to look for trends.
  - Excel allows for rapid searching of culture results from a particular animal via booking number
  - Macros can be made that make it easy for lay staff to enter data in a consistent manner. For example, a macro can be set up to change the status of a culture from "pending" to final once a pathogen has been identified or a week 3 culture has been entered. It can also be set up to report culture results as negative when the final outcome is no growth or contaminant growth.

Table 20.2 Sample excel sheet for recording data.

CAT ID	RESULTS	FINAL	DC	DI	LESIONS	wk 1	wk2	Day 10	wk3	P-score	Age	Sex	Hair	Source	Other comments

CAT ID: Identification number or name

RESULTS: List as "Negative" if the final culture results are no growth or contaminants. List the pathogen if Positive.

FINAL: This indicates whether or not the culture is finalized. Cultures are held for 21 days but can be finalized sooner if a pathogen is isolated or if the plate is overgrown.

DC: Date cultured

DI: Date inoculated

Lesions: List as Y or N. This is the data reported by the intake staff.

Wk 1, W2, Day 10, Wk 3: Cultures are examined daily for evidence of growth, but it is only practical to "officially" read cultures once a week. However, if a daily scan of the plates reveals a suspect colony that should be examined sooner it is appropriate to read out the culture on that day. Day 10 is a very useful data point as explained in the text.

P Score: This is P1 (1–4 cfu/plate), P2 (5–9 cfu/plate) and P3 (>10 cfu/plate). This semi-quantitative reporting system coupled with the pathogen identification is very useful in decision making.

Ng: no growth

C: Contaminant

HC: Heavy overgrowth of contaminants

S: Suspect

Table 20.3 Sample of an "ACTION PLAN" for culture positive animals.

Develop an ACTION PLAN sheet for dealing with Positive Culture results. Below is an example of one used by the author. This action plan lists the cat's ID number, location, pathogen, P Score, who will examine the animal and clinical findings, and a decision as to whether or not to move the cat to the treatment annex or treat as a "dip and go." These Action Plan sheets can be kept in an Excel file as a record of the "response" for each animal.

7/1/05	DCHS	Culture Results				Action Plan for Evaluating NEW POSITIVES				
New Positives										
Cat ID #	Name	Loc	Organism	P-Score	KM or SN	Exam? (Y/N)	Wood's (Y/N)	Lesions? (Y/N)	To Annex? (Y/N)	Needs In house Cult Dip/Go/

Table 20.4 Organizing large numbers of culture plates.

Use plastic containers to store fungal culture plates (Figure 20.14).

Use one container for Week 1, Week 2, and Week 3 plates. As plates are read each week, they are moved from one container to the next.

Each fungal culture plate should be placed in a plastic sandwich bag. This will minimize the chance of cross-contamination and minimize problems with media mites. An inexpensive digital fish tank thermometer can be used in the area where the cultures are kept to monitor the temperature (Figure 20.15).

Media mites should be suspected if the media rapidly turns red and "tracks" are seen on the plate. If this happens, this is a "laboratory emergency." The entire laboratory area should be thoroughly cleaned and the area sprayed with a pyrethrin flea spray immediately. Media mites are a common environmental mite found associated with foodstuffs (Figure 20.16).

An inexpensive incubator can be made by using a small thermal cooler and inserting a fish tank heater into the drain hole. The "correct" temperature can be monitored with the thermometer.

Key Points for the Identification of Pathogens

- Cytological identification is mandatory to identify a pathogen.
- Pathogens are never heavily pigmented either gross or microscopically.
- Pathogens ALWAYS are pale and when grown on DTM, a red color change in the medium occurs as they are growing.

For help with microscopic identification see: www.drfungus.orgor "Applied Cytology: Microscopic Examination of Fungal Cultures" at www.clinicansbrief.com, April 2008

20.7.2.6 Sample Collection and Preparation Technique

A new toothbrush must be used for sampling each animal. New toothbrushes in their original packaging are mycologically sterile. Individually wrapped toothbrushes can be purchased in bulk from various sources at a low cost. For cats, the toothbrush should be brushed vigorously over the cat's entire body until hairs are visible in the bristles of the brush. If lesions are identified, the area with the lesions should be brushed last in order to avoid spreading spores throughout the hair coat. For dogs, only areas with lesions should be sampled unless

Table 20.5 Quick guide to reading fungal culture plates.

Equipment: Clear or frosted acetate tape, new methylene blue stain or lactophenol cotton blue stain, glass microscope slides, microscope coverslips, forceps, clear nail polish

Making Slide Mounts

- The most common stain used is lactophenol cotton blue stain because it kills the organism, however, new methylene blue stain works equally well but it does not kill the spores.
- Put a drop of stain on a glass microscope slide
- It is easiest to work with clear acetate tape, but frosted tape can also be used
  - Using clear tape, touch the target colony and then place it STICKY SIDE DOWN directly over the drop of stain on the glass slide.
  - With frosted tape, touch the target colony and then place the tape STICKY SIDE UP over the drop of stain on the glass side.
  - Place a second drop of stain over the sample and coverslip.
  - Wipe off any excess stain the seeps through the edges of the "sandwich mount"
  - Wipe off any stain that touches the microscope lens IMMEDIATELY or it will damage the lens.
- If necessary, the slides of the slide can be sealed with clear nail polish making a permanent mount.

Rapid Method Sort Culture Plates (Figure 20.17**)**

- LOOK FOR THE RED AND WHITE! (Figure 20.18)
  - Possible pathogens will be pale with a red color change developing in them as they grow
  - Circle these for sampling
- IGNORE THE FOLLOWING
  - Grossly pigmented colonies regardless of whether or not a red color change in the medium occurs
  - Pale colonies WITHOUT a red color change in the medium as they grow
- SPECIAL THINGS TO NOTE
  - Toothbrush samples from cats with severe infections can sometimes grow very rapidly and the entire plate will rapidly turn red. However, the colonies all look the same (Figure 20.19).
  - Yeast or bacterial contamination will turn the plate red very quickly
- GROSSLY OVER-GROWN PLATES
  - Once the entire surface of the plate turns red, the usefulness of the color indicator is gone and all suspect colonies need to be examined. *Microsporum canis* colony (arrow). Glistening colonies are yeast or bacteria (box))
  - Once the plate is overgrown it is often difficult or impossible to find a pathogen. Reculture the animal.

Microscopic Examination of Slides

- Scan slide at 4x and 10x to find areas where there are both hyphae and spores.
- Ignore microscopic colonies that are pigmented (Figure 20.20). Pathogens are hyaline (pale) and septate hyphae.
- Microsporum genus is "boat-shaped."
  - *Microsporum gypseum* rapidly produces a large number of macroconidia compared to *M. canis* (Figure 20.21). These are thin-walled and the edges are smooth.
  - *Microsporum canis* colonies are tapered at the ends, close examination reveals the surface is rough and there is a "knob" at one end (Figure 20.22a and b).
  - Odd variations of the shape of *M. canis* can be seen, especially in cultures from shelter animals (Figure 20.23)
  - Young *M. canis* cultures can show few macroconidia or odd features. One macroconidia has the typical shape with thick walls but no subdivisions. The other shows a developing macroconidia "fingerlike" projection (Figure 20.24).
- Trichophyton spp.
  - These colonies are often slow to grow
  - Microscopically there are large numbers of round microconidia and rare macroconidia
  - Large numbers of microconidia, rare large macroconidia and spiral hyphae are the key characteristics (Figure 20.25)

For more help on microscopic identification of fungal cultures, see http://www.doctorfungus.com

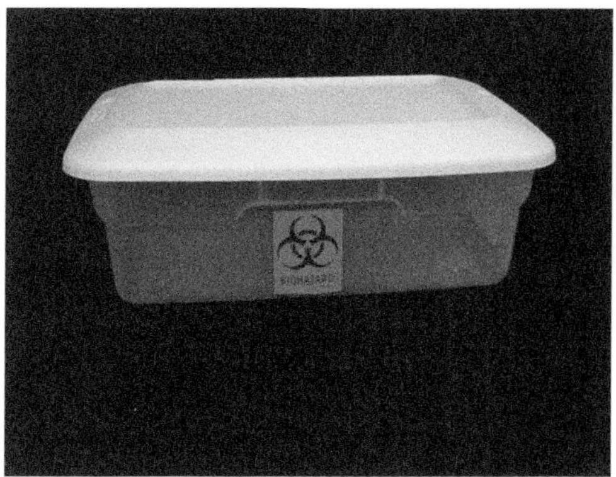

Figure 20.14 Box for cultures, legend embedded in the table.

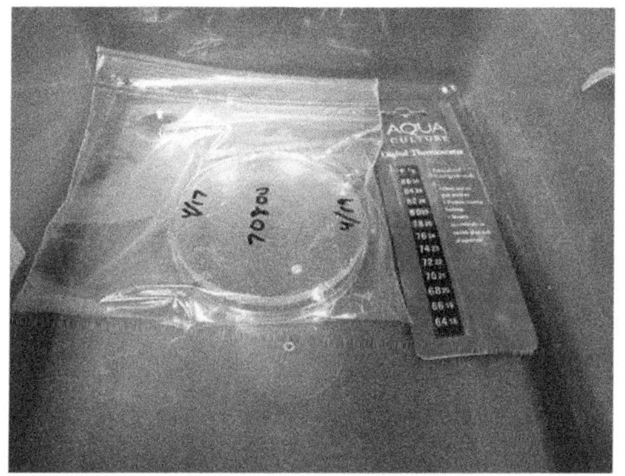

Figure 20.15 Culture in the bag with a thermometer, legend embedded in the table.

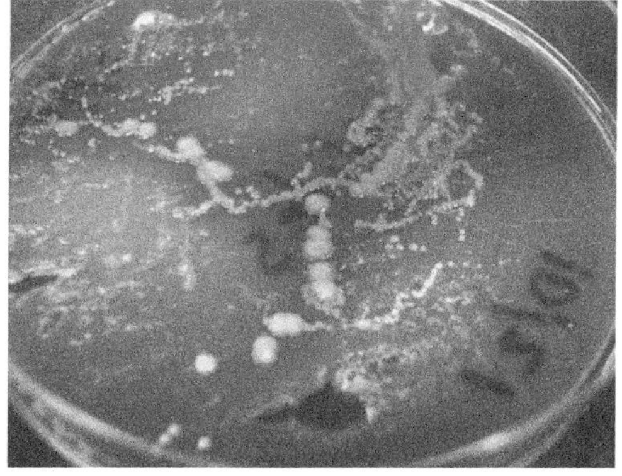

Figure 20.16 Plate showing media mite growth, legend embedded in the table.

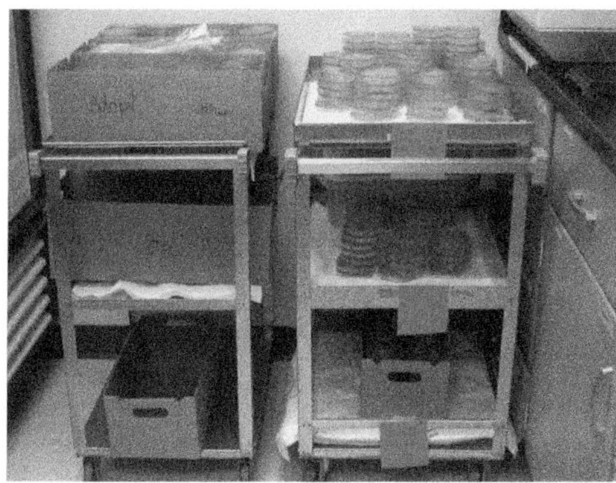

Figure 20.17 This is an actual photograph of a large number of cultures prior to being sorted for reading. Using the Quick Sort Tips in Table 20.1, these plates were examined, sorted, data recorded, and target colonies were examined in less than one hour.

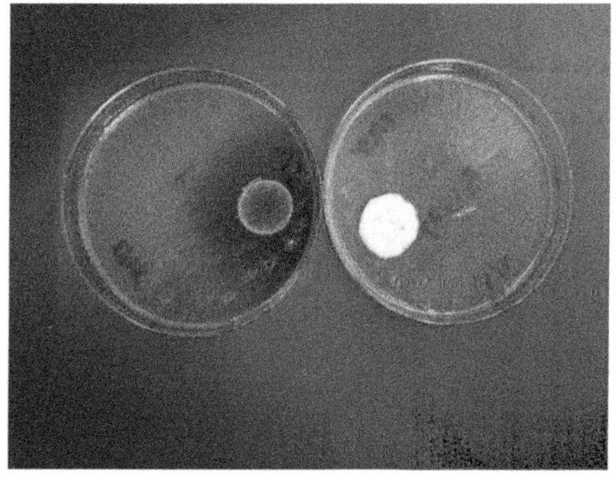

Figure 20.18 This picture demonstrates how useful the "look for the red and white" system is in sorting plates. One plate shows a red color change around the darkly pigmented colony. This is not a pathogen regardless of the "red color change" because the colony is grossly pigmented. The other plate shows a white colony. This is not a suspect pathogen because it does not have a red color change in the surrounding medium.

there are no lesions and the dog is only being sampled because there has been a known or suspected exposure. Fungal cultures from a dog's entire hair coat are commonly overgrown rapidly by contaminant organisms; these cultures should be carefully observed and dogs should be cultured again if needed.

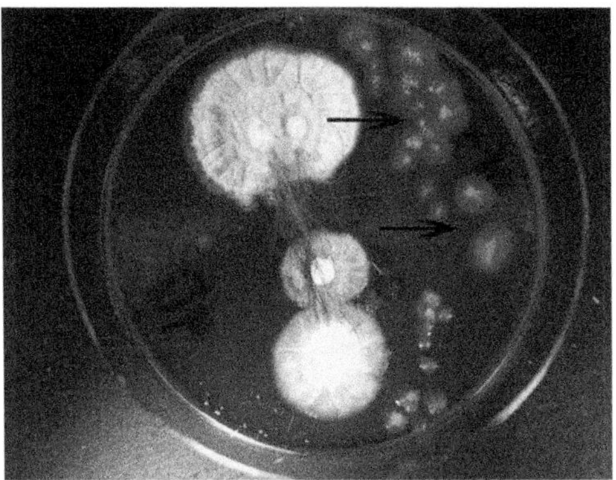

Figure 20.19 This picture shows a fungal culture plate where the entire surface is red. Close inspection of the picture shows four different grossly appearing pale colonies. Only the small white colonies (arrow) are pathogens but all four colonies need microscopic examination to determine this.

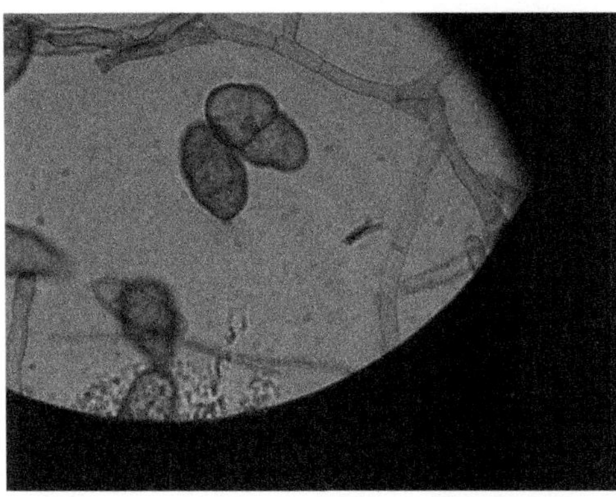

Figure 20.20 Microscopic examination of a suspect colony. Note the dark pigmentation of the spores; this is a contaminant and not a pathogen (100×).

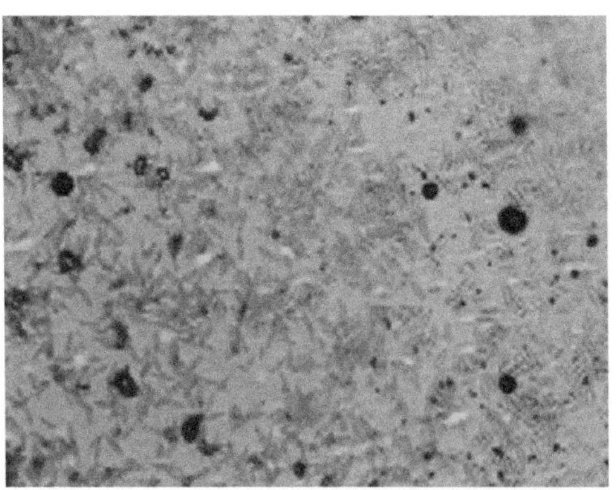

Figure 20.21 Microscopic view of tape preparation of M. gypseum. Note the large numbers of macroconidia.

(a)

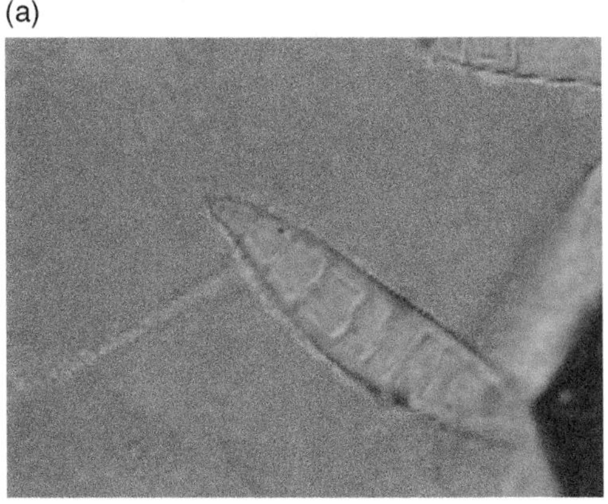

(b)

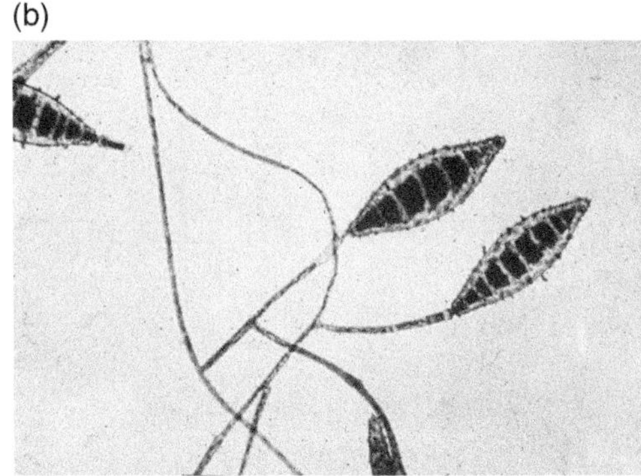

Figure 20.22 (a and b) Microscopic examination of macroconidia of M. canis. Note the thick walls, rough surface and "knob" at the end. The number of subdivisions is less reliable.

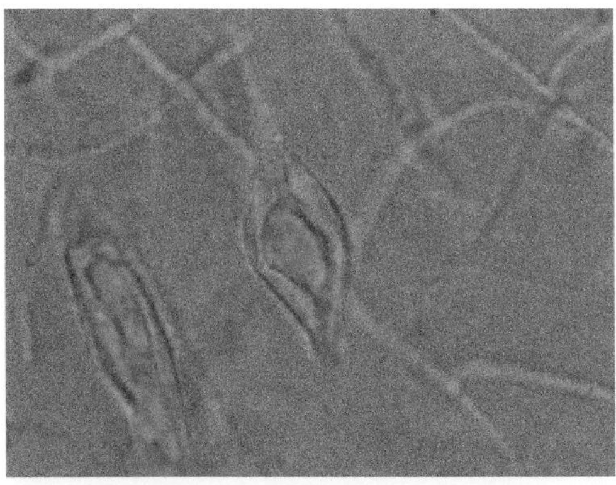

Figure 20.23 M. canis distortum. Note the distorted form of M. canis. This strain is isolated more commonly from shelter cats than from pet cats.

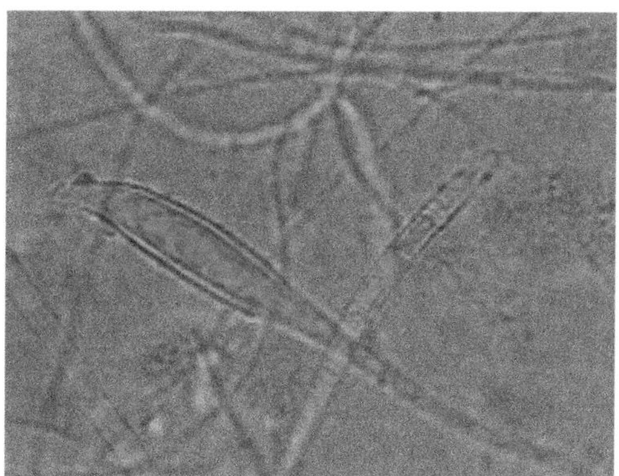

Figure 20.24 Microscopic view of a young culture of M. canis showing common features of developing macroconidia. The first is the development of a boat-shaped spore with thick walls and no subdivisions. The second is the development of thick, figure- like projections that will eventually develop into mature macroconidia.

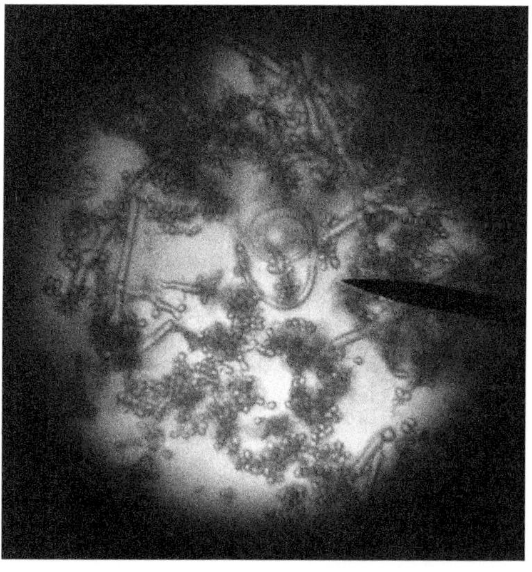

Figure 20.25 Microscopic view of a Trichophyton spp. Note the large numbers of macroconidia and spiral hyphae.

Next, the fungal culture plate should be inoculated by gently stabbing the toothbrush bristles onto the surface of a fungal culture plate. The entire plate should be covered, and a consistent system used each time to help support the pathogen scoring system described below. It is important to start in the center of the plate, working outward, and covering the entire

(a)

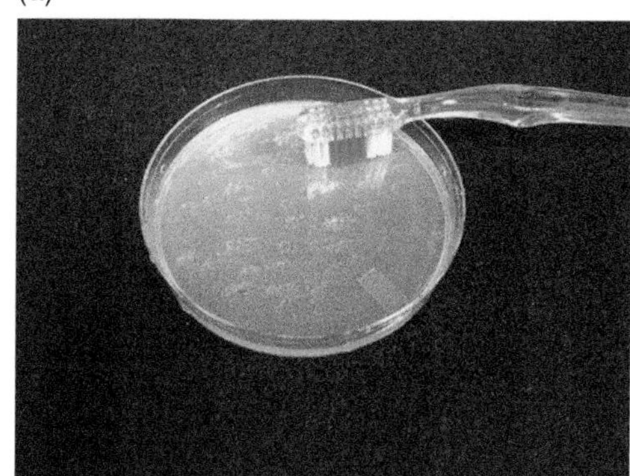

(b)

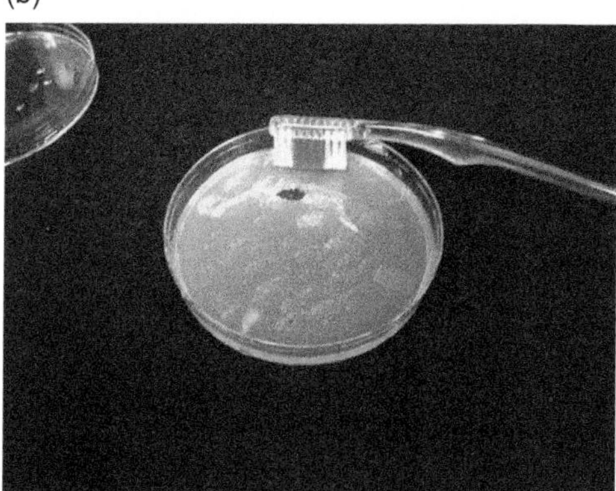

Figure 20.26 (a) Toothbrush cultures being inoculated on a plate. (b) Toothbrush culture pressed too hard into the medium, pulling the medium away from the plate.

surface of the plate, ensuring that the bristles are embedded in the plate so that the spores are transferred, but not so hard as to lift the medium off the plate (See Figure 20.26a and b).

If inoculation just after collection is not possible or practical, toothbrushes may be placed into plastic sandwich type bags and then double bagged into a sealable Ziplock™ type bag. If cultures are inoculated at a later time, this should be done in a clean area that is easily disinfected. Careful identification of toothbrush samples cannot be emphasized enough; labels with blank spaces for ID numbers and dates can be pre-printed to facilitate the process. If a sample is highly suspect, this should also be noted on the bag. When inoculating numerous samples, high-suspect samples should be inoculated last to prevent cross-contamination. Gloves should always be worn when handling samples and used toothbrushes should be discarded into trash that is sealed.

Culture plates can be difficult to mark. Plates are often wet if they have been refrigerated; the plates should be wiped dry before writing on them. If using Petri dishes, identification and dates should be marked on the bottom of the plate and not the cover to ensure that there are no mix-ups in the laboratory. Culture plates should always be marked with the animal's identification information (unique animal ID number as well as the name), the date sampled, and the date inoculated.

In a series of laboratory tests performed by the author to determine if one type of fungal culture plate was superior to another with respect to time to sporulation, Dermatophyte Test Medium (DTM) from six commercial companies was tested, including flat trays, jars, and "micromedium plates" (In-Tray) (See Figure 20.27). Some media were advertised as "rapid sporulation." Multiple replicates of each DTM brand were tested on several strains of *M. canis*, *M. gypseum*, and *Trichophyton spp.* In addition, the effects of light exposure and temperature on time to growth were tested (Verbrugge et al. 2007). With the exception of one fungal culture medium that did not perform as well as the others, there was no advantage of one brand over another with respect to time to growth. The smaller the surface area of the plate, the more difficult it was to identify growth and pathogens; once the surface turned red the usefulness of the color indicator was lost. In addition, the smaller surface area medium plates often dried up before the pathogen grew. Light had no effect on the time to growth. The most important factor affecting growth was temperature. Cultures sporulated best when grown between 27–30° C (80–86° F). Based on these findings, cultures should be performed using DTM plates that have a large flat surface area that is easily inoculated. The use of jars should be avoided because it is difficult to inoculate the surface and sample colonies. Furthermore, bacterial and yeast often swarm over the surface.

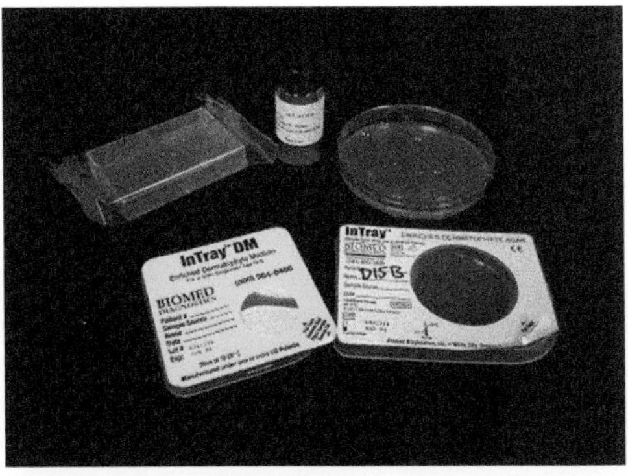

Figure 20.27 Various commercial fungal culture mediums. Small volume and small size plates are not recommended.

20.7.2.7 Animal Holding Time for Culture Results

Fungal cultures take time to incubate and grow before pathogens can be identified or the fungal culture can be deemed negative. When legal or required holding periods are similar to the time needed for culture incubation and identification, or when animals are expected to stay for long periods of time, waiting for the results of fungal cultures has little impact on the length of stay (LOS) or level of crowding. However, in many cases, holding cultured cats will lead to an increase in holding time. This could have negative consequences for individual and population health. A balance must be found between the risks of exposure to other illnesses, stress, and the contribution to shelter crowding caused by holding animals for extended periods of time as compared to the risk of potentially moving an infectious animal through the system. There is no success in ruling out dermatophytosis in an animal who has developed clinical signs of respiratory disease while waiting for culture results. In many cases, if adequate examination screening is provided as described in sections 20.7.2.1–20.7.2.3, the risks from holding animals while waiting for culture results are greater than the risk of missing a dermatophyte infection, unless there is a reason for increased suspicion. When using a comprehensive screening protocol, only truly suspect cats need to be held in isolation while awaiting culture results. If a cat is truly suspect or high-risk, treatment should be started to both minimize treatment time and decrease the risk of environmental contamination. Animals without suspect lesions should be moved to adoption.

Performing fungal cultures in-house or in a lab that will provide regular progress reports on cultures instead of only reporting results once cultures are finalized will shorten the waiting time dramatically. The author recommends performing fungal cultures in-house as this is a skill that is not difficult to learn. In-house management of fungal cultures also significantly reduces costs associated with a screening program and permits daily monitoring of cultures. Additionally, community practitioners may want to consider developing in-house culture systems as a service to clients including shelters and rescue groups. When data was retrospectively examined, over 95% of positive fungal cultures were identified between days 10 to 14 (Stuntebeck et al. 2017). Suspect growth was almost always noted in these cultures by day 7 post-inoculation. In animals with severe infections, cultures were often finalized within seven days. Cultures that are not suspect by day 7 or positive by day 10 are unlikely to be *M. canis*. Though not fool-proof, in most cases, when cultures are kept warm and evaluated in-house, decisions can be made by day 10 of fungal culture growth. Some of the Trichophyton species grow more slowly; however, these are of lesser clinical significance in shelters. See Table 20.4.

20.7.2.8 Fungal Culture Processing, Pathogen Identification and Reporting Culture Results

Typically, cultures are reported as "culture positive" with a pathogen being identified, or "culture negative." In the author's experience, this is an inadequate amount of information for designing and implementing an effective management program that minimizes infectious risk while maximizing life-saving opportunities for infected or suspect cats. The number of colony forming units (CFU) on the plate is very important for decision making when interpreting culture results, just as it is when interpreting results from bacterial cultures. The author recommends a semi-quantitative system of reporting fungal culture results that was developed for treatment studies on cats with dermatophytosis based on CFU (Deboer and Moriello 1995; Deboer et al. 2003; Moriello and DeBoer 1995; Moriello et al. 2004a).

The following is a summary of how the CFU scoring system is used to report fungal culture results, interpret the results in light of physical findings (lesions or not) and make treatment decisions. To make the language of CFU more "user-friendly" for staff, the author refers to this as a Pathogen Score or P score. To use this system, DTM culture Petri dish plates or similar large flat bottom plates should be used. The following describes an in-house system for inoculating, incubating, and reading fungal culture plates.

1) As discussed in section 20.7.2.6, plates must be properly identified in a systematic manner. Plates should be labeled with the animal's ID/Name, date of sample collection (DC) and date of inoculation (DI). Other information such as age, sex, hair length, and source can be entered on the ID label and entered into a spreadsheet for identification of trends for infection in a particular organization or community.
2) Recording both the DC and the DI is important when plates are not immediately inoculated at the time of sampling. If the time between DC and DI is long and the culture is positive in a cat that was not suspect, it may explain an unexpected outbreak in a previously unaffected facility.

3) Samples are inoculated onto DTM, preferably on a Petri dish style plate.
4) The key to early and fast identification of suspects and prompt diagnosis of pathogens is daily examination of fungal culture plates. Contrary to popular belief, this is NOT a time-consuming activity. One hundred or more plates can be quickly evaluated in less than 7–10 minutes. Any small white colonies with a red ring of color around them as they are growing should be considered suspect. Often the colonies may be too young for definitive identification, but once a plate is identified as "suspect," it should be observed more closely. A system of communication to quickly report positives is essential to allow for rapid intervention.
5) Plates should be held for 21 days and "officially" read on day 7, day 10, day 14, and day 21. Day 10 is an especially useful time point since most positive cultures show suspect growth by this date.
6) The identification of suspect colonies is not difficult. When using DTM plates, the colonies to look for are white or buff-colored colonies with a red ring around them as they are growing. *The red color change is not diagnostic for a dermatophyte*, but it "flags" colonies that need to be microscopically identified and are suspect. Pigmented colonies are not pathogens and can be ignored. Pale or white colonies with no red ring of color can also be ignored.
7) If a suspect colony is identified and it is too small or too soon to sample, it should be circled with a marker so it can be observed.
8) If plates become rapidly overgrown with contaminants in the first 7–10 days, they are useless for screening and the animal should be re-cultured because rapid overgrowth of the plate may result in a false negative or un-interpretable fungal culture. This occurs most commonly in kittens and stray cats. These cats should be re-cultured as soon as over-growth is noted, especially if a suspect lesion was noted. In addition, once the entire surface of the plate turns red, the usefulness of the red color change is lost.
9) A shorthand system for recording culture results allows data to be easily entered into a spreadsheet. In addition, a shorthand system is easy for lay staff to understand.
   a) "NG" is for no growth; it is not uncommon for cats to have no growth on their fungal culture plate due to their fastidious grooming skills.
   b) "C" is for contaminant growth.
   c) "HC" is for heavy growth of contaminants and signals the staff to re-culture the cat. This may not be cost-effective in every shelter but minimally, cats with skin lesions or kittens with HC should be re-cultured.
   d) "S" is for suspect growth; many culture positive plates will have S growth in the first week. Identified pathogens should be listed by name. If a pathogen (e.g. *M. canis*) is identified, the number of CFU should be counted and recorded. The significance of the latter will be discussed in detail below.
10) Plates should be held for 21 days unless a pathogen is identified sooner, the plate turns completely red, or the plate is overgrown. When cultures are held in a warm room or incubator (approximately 80–86° or 27–30°C), most *M. canis* positive cats will be identified within 7–14 days of culture (Stuntebeck et al. 2017). Plates are held for 21 days because *Trichophyton spp.* dermatophytes take longer to grow. From a practical perspective, if cats are culture negative for *M. canis* after 10–14 days, they can be considered "culture negative." Holding cultures, not animals, for the full 21 days is still recommended since that is considered a standard culture incubation time by reference laboratories, and individuals infected by less common and less contagious species may still benefit from identification and treatment. See Table 20.5.

20.7.2.9 The Pathogen Scoring System: Using Colony-Forming Units to Aid in Management and Treatment Decisions

The determination of the number of CFU is an important aid to guide treatment. Simply reporting a fungal culture as positive or negative may not be very helpful as a component of a management plan because no distinction can be made between fomite carriers or "dust mops" and truly infected cats. Incorporating the number of CFU found on the plate via a Pathogen Score ("P-score") helps further guide diagnosis and treatment decisions.

If a culture has been properly obtained and inoculated, the number of CFU per plate generally corresponds to the severity of infection for cultured animals or degree of contamination when evaluating cultures of the environment. The system is very simple:

- P1 score = 1–4 CFU/plate,
- P2 score = 5–9 CFU/plate
- P3 score = 10 or more CFU/plate

(See Figure 20.28a–c).

Shelter staff can readily learn the significance of a P1, P2 or P3 cat even if they are not involved or trained in the laboratory aspect of fungal cultures. This information, along with the presence or absence of lesions at the time of culture, can help speed the identification of culture positive cats and differentiate fomite carriers from those who are truly infected. When the laboratory alerts the shelter that a positive animal has been identified, the P-score would ideally be included. The animal should be immediately re-examined for lesions. Most commercial laboratories do not currently report CFUs or P-scores; they only report one finalized result after three weeks, making in-house culture evaluation even more important for shelters.

(a)

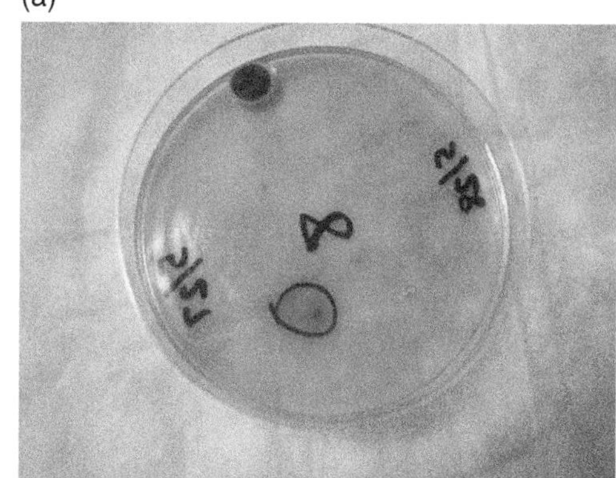

(b)

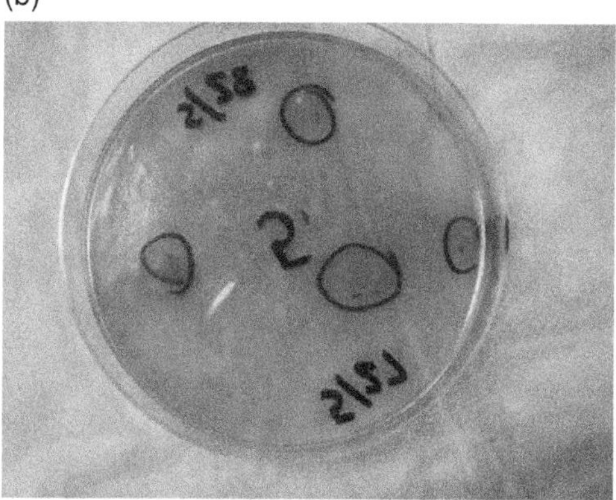

(c)

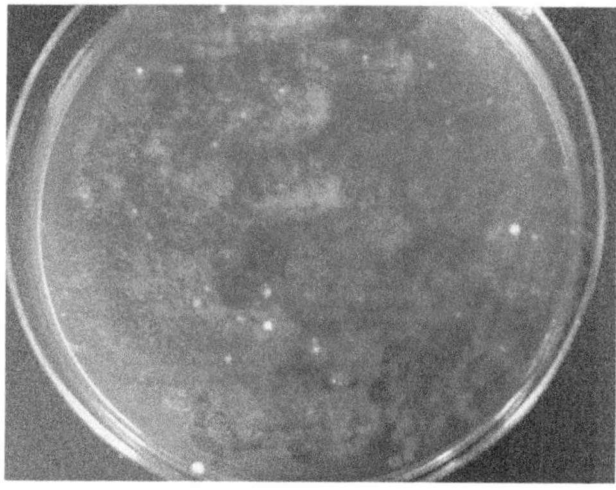

Figure 20.28 (a–c) This series of pictures is representative of a P1, P2, and P3 fungal culture scored plate. Note that many of the colonies are circled. These colonies were identified as "suspect" colonies during daily examinations; circled colonies alert staff to pay special attention to the colonies.

20.7.2.9.1 *P-1 Cats* P-1 cats fall into two categories. The first is cats that are fomite carriers. These cats are lesion free and Wood's lamp negative when carefully re-examined. On re-culture one to two weeks following an initial screening culture, non-lesional P1 and P2 cats are generally negative without any intervening treatment. These cats likely groom the spores from their coats. It also seems possible that the initial sampling process of brushing vigorously with a toothbrush may have removed the majority of the spores. These cats should be re-cultured as a safeguard and treated with one topical application of lime sulfur. These animals are referred to by the author as "Dip and Go" cats.

The second category of P-1 cats is those that were incubating infections at the time of admission. Lesions in these cats may have been very subtle and overlooked on initial examination. At the time of re-examination, lesions can still be very subtle. The face, hairs in the bell of the ear, ear margin, chin, lips, and the ear canal should be closely inspected. Wood's lamp examinations may or may not be positive depending upon the strain of *M. canis*; *Trichophyton* infections do not fluoresce. Animals whose lesions are identified after re-examination due to positive culture results should be treated as truly infected.

20.7.2.9.2 *P-2 Cats* P-2 cats most commonly fall into the "infected group" but may be fomite carriers. The major difference with these cats is that if lesions are found, they tend to be more noticeable and often shelter staff report these lesions almost simultaneously with the reporting of the fungal culture. When re-examining a cat with a "positive P-2" culture, the index of suspicion for a missed lesion should be higher than for a P-1. As with P-1 cats, those cats that are lesion-free on a very careful second examination may be dipped once in lime sulfur and placed for adoption as usual, while those with lesions must be treated as truly infected.

20.7.2.9.3 *P-3 Cats* P-3 cats should be immediately removed from the general population regardless of whether or not lesions are identified. In general, when thorough intake examinations have been performed, these cats have already been identified as suspect. Lesions are often found in -difficult-to-find locations on the re-examination of P-3 cats who were initially reported as non-lesional. P-3 cats are considered a risk to the population and should not be housed in the general population. A small number of cats with P3 cultures may have been "dust mops." These cats usually had a history of coming from a contaminated environment and often did not groom well or had a thick or long coat. When treatment data was examined, these cats were generally found to be become culture negative very rapidly, often after the first week of treatment.

20.7.2.9.4 *Use of the P-Scoring System* The P-scoring system is also very useful when monitoring treatment. Animals under treatment should be cultured once weekly with P-scores reported. As animals are cured, the P-score becomes lower. (Please see Section 20.9)

The P score system and CFU counts are also helpful when reporting the results of environmental cultures. Environmental cultures help to identify contaminated areas so that cleaning may be targeted and focused. Reporting an area as culture positive, with some indication of the level of contamination, is very helpful to staff charged with the task of cleaning and disinfecting the area. The P-score system has resulted in "buy-in" and improved compliance by shelter staff and volunteers. (Please see 20.9.4.1 on disinfection.)

20.7.3 PCR Testing

Real-time polymerase chain reaction testing (PCR) testing for dermatophytosis is available and has the potential advantage of a rapid turn-around time compared to fungal culture (results may be available within one to three days from a commercial laboratory). As with PCR tests in general, the test has high sensitivity, meaning that false negatives are unlikely. For this reason, PCR testing can be helpful to rule out dermatophyte infection in exposed cats, and the costs associated with diagnostic testing may be lower than the costs, risks, and welfare concerns associated with holding cats for prolonged periods awaiting culture results (Jacobson et al. 2018a).

However, PCR testing also has drawbacks for dermatophytosis management in shelters. Because of the exquisite sensitivity of this test, it is less reliable for identifying cats that are not, in fact, infected (lower specificity). False-positive results or those resulting from sample contamination could trigger a prolonged LOS and needless treatment in cats that were not truly infected. Additionally, PCR results do not distinguish between viable and non-viable organisms and do not provide the clinical guidance associated with the quantitative CFU scoring system described above for diagnosis or monitoring of treatment efficacy. Quantitative PCR (qPCR) is available and has shown value in distinguishing clinically important infection from the incidental presence of a pathogen, for instance in distinguishing likely vaccine virus versus true infection for canine distemper or parvovirus. However, this method provided limited value in distinguishing between culture-positive and culture-negative cats in a field study of shelter cats, nor was it useful for monitoring treatment (Jacobson et al. 2018b).

Ultimately, in many cases, careful history, visual exam, Woods lamp and direct exam as described above will be sufficient to adequately rule in or out cats requiring fungal culture and further evaluation. However, there may be situations, such as a hoarding case or transfer of a group of cats from a ringworm endemic shelter, where the entire group is considered potentially high-risk. In such cases, PCR may be a helpful adjunct to quickly identify and move low-risk cats through the shelter system. All PCR-positive animals should be confirmed with a culture, which can be initiated at the same time PCR samples are submitted. This will expedite confirming additional negative cases.

20.8 Initial Risk Evaluation and Response

As part of a systematic screening process, an initial risk evaluation and response must be made for animals as they are examined and screened. Information to consider for this initial response is collected during the first four steps of the screening process described previously. The initial response should be made at intake, or after an initial evaluation if screening is happening at a time other than intake (e.g. during an outbreak). The initial response plan should be developed *prior to incubation or confirmation of fungal culture results*. Positive, suspect and high-risk animals should be clearly identified to staff, volunteers, and the public.

A prompt, definitive response should be implemented for the management of animals with a positive diagnosis. An initial response plan for animals with Wood's positive lesions (high-risk animals) should include, at the very least, separation or isolation from the general population as described below. Additionally, animals with characteristic inflammatory lesions should be considered suspect until further results from other diagnostics are available. Isolation is ideal, but where it is not possible to isolate, adequate separation practices must be put in place for suspect animals. (Please see Section 20.8.1 for more detailed information.) Wood's positive animals must be clearly identified, including designation as a potential zoonotic health risk for staff, volunteers and public. Identification should include signage on their cages, notations in their medical record and on the cage card, and ID tags affixed to them in case they are moved around the shelter. Animals with suspicious lesions that are not Wood's lamp positive likely pose less risk, but should still be identified as possibly contagious, if suspicion is high enough to warrant holding them back for culture results. If suspicion is high and treatment would be initiated if a positive result were confirmed, starting treatment while awaiting results will help shorten the LOS while also reducing the risk of transmission.

20.8.1 Isolation and Separation

Wood's lamp positive, culture positive, and suspect animals (including PCR positive) should be isolated from the general population as soon as possible. Ideally, isolation includes a physically separate housing ward, including separate cleaning and care staff designated to work in that area only, and separate equipment. Newer facilities with designated isolation areas may be designed with separate air circulation. This can be extremely costly, and the investment is likely not warranted for dermatophytosis. Instead, strict adherence to minimizing fomite transmission and environmental contamination will likely bring a higher reward. (Please see Section 20.5) Because of the potential for zoonosis, animal attendants assigned to work in isolation areas should be required to wear protective clothing, including gowns, disposable gloves, shoe covers, and caps. All materials located in the isolation ward should be dedicated to that ward and must not be moved to other areas for use. In shelters where assigning separate staffing for an isolation area can be a problem, staff who work in multiple areas should work in isolation wards only after working in other areas if at all possible. At a minimum, staff must always completely change all garments before moving to other areas. Staff who work in isolation areas should also ideally not work with vulnerable, sick or high-risk animals, especially juveniles. All shelter staff should change clothes before going home at the end of the day. The risk of carrying infected spores home is minimal if staff members adhere to these guidelines.

Within the isolation area, "clean" and "dirty" areas should be defined. These need not be physically separate rooms or wards, but clear visual and practical separation should be maintained (e.g. by colored tape or painted lines). Areas in the immediate vicinity of the housing units should be defined as "dirty" (See Figure 20.29). In-contact bedding, litter and food should be carefully bagged within the "dirty" area in an effort to control environmental contamination with spores. Infected animals should remain within the "dirty" area.

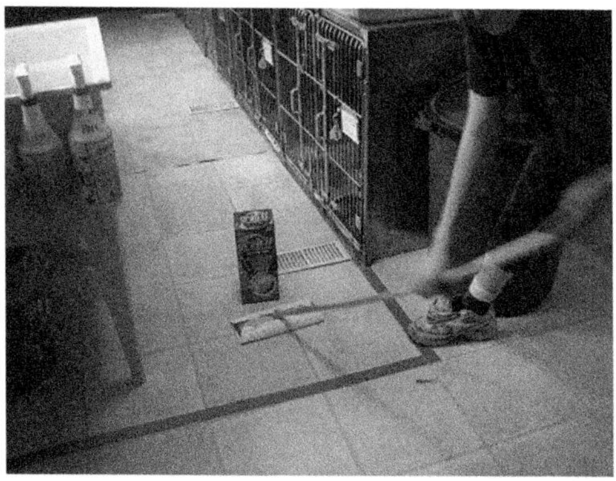

Figure 20.29 In this facility, red tape is used on the floor to designate a "dirty" area.

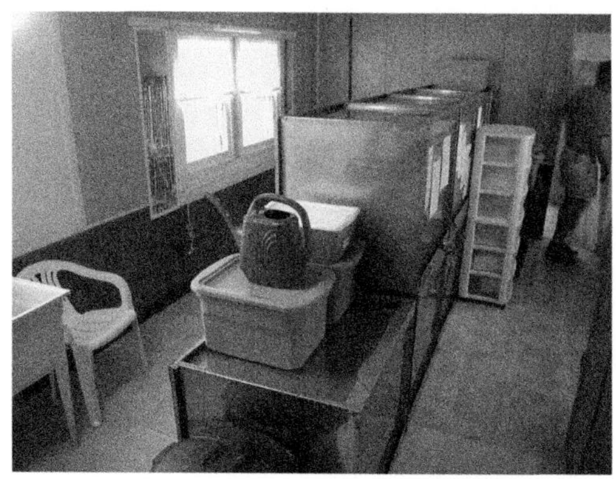

Figure 20.30 In order to control environmental contamination, a conscious effort has been made in this facility to minimize clutter and keep food, bedding, and other materials in closed containers.

Protective garments worn within the dirty area should remain in that area except when bagged and removed to be taken directly for laundering. A clean area should be designated to provide a safe area for supply storage, food preparation, or other activities (See Figure 20.30). When creating an isolation area for the treatment of cats with dermatophytosis, a separate contained section within the isolation area for cats with both dermatophytosis and upper respiratory infections may be beneficial.

When physical isolation is not possible, *temporary* separation of suspect or positive animals in a defined section may be sufficient to help control disease spread. In order for temporary separation to be effective, it must be clearly indicated that there is a possibility that the animals housed within may be infectious to humans and other animals; specific precautionary care procedures must be in place and staff must be carefully trained and comply well with control procedures. A "dirty" area or zone should be defined surrounding these housing units (See Figure 20.29). Housing suspect or high-risk animals near to or intermingled with other animals or in areas where other animals are commonly housed risks exposing the group as a whole, as well as in-contact humans. It may also contaminate the environment with infective spores that are difficult to eliminate. Treating suspect animals with topical lime sulfur reduces the infectious risk by reducing the number of spores being shed into the environment during this waiting period. It should be emphasized that fungal culture-positive animals should be housed in this area only temporarily while awaiting a definitive plan. Suspect animals should be held in this type of separation area only long enough to confirm the results of diagnostic testing. In general, incomplete physical separation for the duration of treatment should not be considered a sufficient precaution against disease transmission. Isolation is strongly recommended. (Please see 20.9.4 on treatment and housing.)

20.9 Treatment

Dermatophytosis is a treatable and curable disease. When animals have long-standing or unresolving infections, treatment choices and medications, as well as environmental contamination should be evaluated. In many cases, the animal continues to culture positive because there are spores remaining in the housing environment. The author has not encountered any cases in a shelter setting where cats with long-standing or "incurable" infections could not be cured once appropriate treatment was instituted, underlying diseases concurrently treated and resolved, and appropriate environmental treatment instituted.

Because dermatophytosis can self-cure in a healthy cat in a home environment given enough time, anecdotal reports of treatment with various substances abound. However, in the high-stakes environment of a shelter where time to cure is of the essence, a treatment protocol proven effective specifically in a shelter environment should be used. The treatment most extensively documented as effective in shelters is itraconazole orally, given once daily for 21 days, in combination with twice-weekly topical lime sulfur treatments (Newbury et al. 2007). This protocol is recommended for the treatment of dermatophytosis in shelter cats and dogs. After completion of the itraconazole, topical treatment should be continued until the animal has reached a mycological cure. Terbinafine can be substituted for itraconazole in this treatment protocol, as it achieves similar results (Moriello et al. 2013) (See section 20.9.2.).

20.9.1 Topical Treatment

Miconazole, enilconazole and lime sulfur are the most consistently antifungal agents against *M. canis* when tested *in vitro* (Moriello and Verbrugge 2007; Moriello et al. 2004b). Enilconazole is an effective topical treatment, but it is not available in the United States and is labeled for use in dogs and horses only. Miconazole alone, or in combination with chlorhexidine, has been shown to be equally as sporicidal when compared to lime sulfur *in vitro* (Moriello and Verbrugge 2007); *in vivo*, however, though it did help to hasten a cure it was not as effective as lime sulfur (Newbury et al. 2011). Several other topical products that have been used to treat dermatophytosis include povidone iodine, Captan, chlorhexidine shampoos and sodium hypochlorite (bleach) (Deboer and Moriello 1995; Moriello et al. 2004b; White-Weithers and Medleau 1995). These products are ineffective or otherwise problematic and should not be used. Local topical therapy with various ointments and creams alone is also not recommended.

20.9.1.1 Lime Sulfur

Lime sulfur is an effective topical treatment (both *in vivo* and *in vitro*) to both eliminate infection and reduce shedding of spores that lead to environmental contamination (Moriello and Verbrugge 2007; Moriello et al. 2004b; Newbury et al. 2007). When diluted and applied properly, lime sulfur has been shown consistently to be inexpensive, available, safe and effective; and, therefore, is the best choice to use as a component of a shelter treatment protocol.

Commercial lime sulfur products are equivalent to one another in efficacy, including commercial products with masking agents for the odor (Diesel et al. 2011). Though lime sulfur tends to be malodorous and may stain certain fabrics, the odor disappears fairly quickly and should not be a deterrent to its use. Because animal shelters should prioritize treatments that minimize animal care days and the potential for contagion or environmental contamination, the application of topical lime sulfur any time an animal shelter is going to treat animals for dermatophytosis is strongly recommended.

20.9.1.1.1 Application of Lime Sulfur Dip

Lime sulfur should be used at a dilution of 8 oz (236 ml) to the gallon (3.78 l) of warm water (the higher dilution of the two given most commonly on the commercially available products). When mixing the product, it is important to put 8 oz (236 ml) of the concentrated lime sulfur in the mixing container FIRST and then add the warm water. Though the term "dip" is commonly used, it is not necessary to immerse the animal in the solution. Instead, the solution should be applied topically to the animals' coat. A simple, inexpensive and portable "dip" sink can be made using a laundry sink that is set up to drain into a bucket (See Figure 20.31).

The cat should not be bathed or pre-wet prior to treatment. The properly diluted lime sulfur solution is easily applied with a gallon or half-gallon garden rose sprayer (See Figure 20.32). The nozzle of the sprayer should be held very close to the cat's skin so the spray flows over them like a gentle shower. Often, the solution will bead up and roll off the hair coat initially. The solution should coat the entire hair, reaching the base of the hairs. The cat must be soaked to the skin in order for the treatment to be effective. Cloths should be used to gently sponge the dip on around the face and inside the ears, on the nose, etc. These

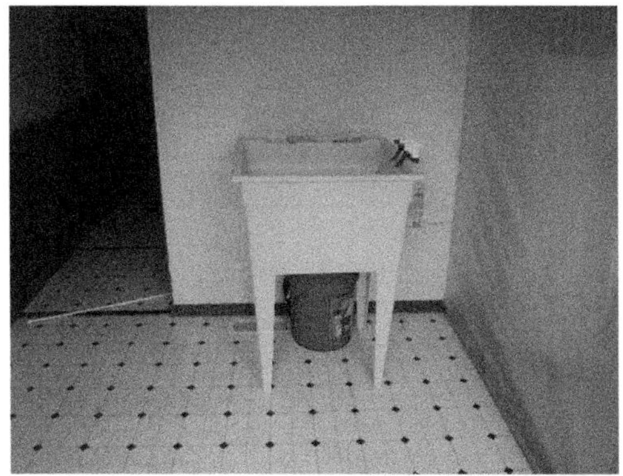

Figure 20.31 This is a portable treatment station. It is comprised of a plastic utility sink with a bucket beneath to collect dip. This station is portable, allowing cats to be treated in areas with improved ventilation so that the odor of lime sulfur in a facility is minimized.

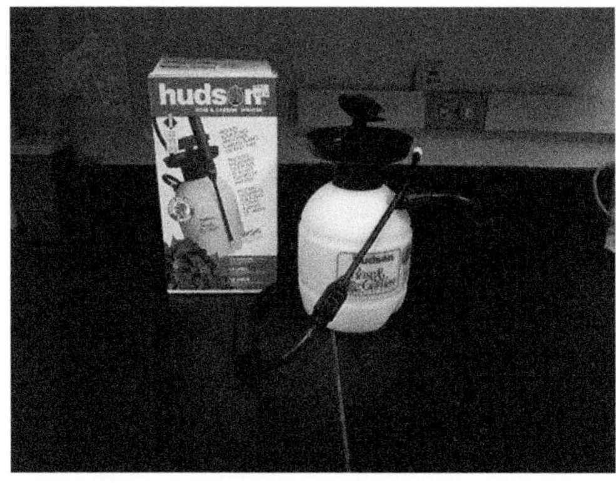

Figure 20.32 Portable rose garden sprayer used to apply topical treatment solutions.

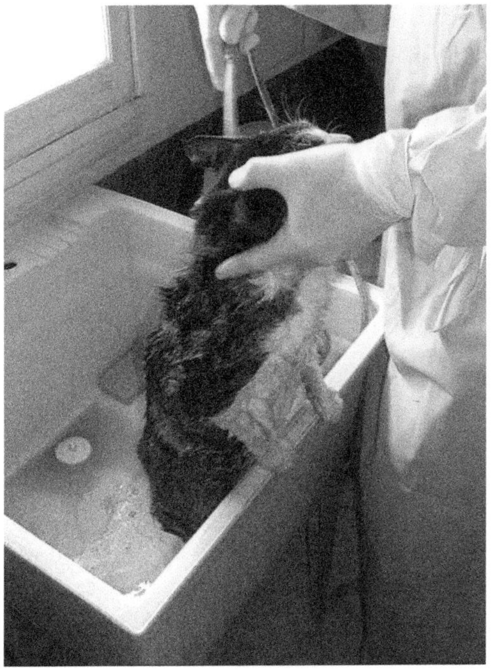

Figure 20.33 Application of lime sulfur to a cat using a garden sprayer. Note that the nozzle is held very close to the cat's skin, in effect "showering" the cat rather than spraying.

areas are most important as the lesions found there tend to be the most difficult to resolve. Surprisingly, cats appear to tolerate this application method much better than being soaked in towels or drenched with watering cans (See Figure 20.33). It is also a very cost-effective method of application. Though fractious cats can be sprayed through a wire carrier, an attempt should still be made to keep the spray close to the cat's skin since cats seem most tolerant of the treatment when the nozzle is close enough so the liquid does not spray out at them or make a hissing noise. The solution should not be rinsed off. Both rinsing and pre-wetting will cause dilution and could lead to less efficacious treatment.

Lime sulfur is safe to apply topically, even on kittens as young as four weeks of age and nursing queens; hypothermia is a concern in young kittens. When lactating queens are treated, teats should be wiped clean of the solution after dipping. Animals must be kept warm while they are wet. This is especially important for kittens, puppies or other animals that may have some difficulty with thermoregulation. Adverse side effects are uncommon. During the author's' experience treating hundreds of cats, it was not necessary to put e-collars on them after treatment. The only time oral ulcers were seen in cats treated with lime sulfur was when they had concurrent severe upper respiratory disease, and they were consistent with what would be expected in a cat with an upper respiratory infection and not from an irritant reaction.

20.9.1.1.2 Clipping the Hair Coat Prior to Topical Treatment Clipping the hair prior to topical treatment has often been recommended but the author has not found that clipping is necessary for short- or medium-haired cats. However, in a long-haired cat with a high pathogen score or a cat that appears unkempt, matted, unwilling or unable to groom, the cat's entire body should be clipped with a #7 or #10 blade (not a surgical blade). Clipping can also be helpful for cats whose coats get clumped or matted from the dipping process. Caution is advised: hair must be carefully contained in order to avoid environmental contamination that is likely to result from clipping. The environment must also be carefully and thoroughly cleaned and disinfected after clipping an infected cat.

Clipping should be done in a designated and controlled area that will not be used to house other animals, using clippers dedicated only to that purpose. Clipping should be performed cautiously to avoid causing abrasive injuries to the skin. It is recommended to alternate between two clippers, or to take breaks to allow the clippers to cool to avoid inadvertently causing thermal injuries. Deep thermal burns can result from clipping cats with overheated clippers. In some cases, these burns may not become apparent until several days after clipping when an eschar begins to form.

20.9.2 Systemic Treatment

Dermatophytosis is an intrafollicular disease. Systemic treatment is responsible for shortening the course of infection by reaching the fungus within the follicles. Itraconazole is the drug recommended for systemic treatment of dermatophytosis in shelter cats (Newbury et al. 2007). In this chapter, all treatment information is based on the combination protocol using itraconazole for systemic treatment. As part of the recommended combination topical and systemic treatment protocol, itraconazole is given orally, once daily at 5–10 mg/kg for 21 days. Terbinafine is also effective and can be used as the systemic component of combination therapy when itraconazole is not available (Moriello et al. 2013).

Though many alternative drugs and schedules for systemic treatment are available, because of either potential problems associated with the drugs or because alternative drugs or schedules have not been proven effective when times until cure are documented by fungal culture of shelter cats, they are not recommended as the treatment of first choice in this environment. The following is a summary of key points about the currently available systemic antifungal drugs.

20.9.2.1 Itraconazole

Itraconazole is currently the most commonly used drug for the treatment of dermatophytosis in both dogs and cats. Itraconazole, a triazole antifungal that accumulates and persists in hair and epidermis, can be used to treat dermatophytosis in a daily or pulse-therapy protocol, or a short-term treatment protocol when coupled with effective topical therapy.

In practice, the most common pulse-therapy protocol is a week-on/week off protocol (5–10 mg/kg) until cured; this is how the drug is licensed for use in Europe. A 14-day daily dose-loading period is required to achieve appropriate therapeutic levels before initiating pulse therapy. Pulse therapy is not ideal for animals that are ill or have limited body fat because the drug is stored in body fat. For stressed, thin, or debilitated animals, 21–28 days of daily therapy coupled with topical therapy is recommended. Since the shelter protocol that has been published used only 21 days of oral treatment, pulse therapy is not generally recommended for cats in shelter settings.

Itraconazole is available in 100 mg capsules that can be divided into smaller doses manually and repackaged in empty gelatin capsules or mixed with a small amount of food; alternatively, one can use the oral solution. Toxicity problems are rare, though occasionally animals may become inappetant. If this is persistent, the drug should be stopped, and liver enzymes should be checked.

As a note of caution, the author is aware that bulk itraconazole powder may be obtained inexpensively in foreign countries; anecdotally, this treatment often fails. There have also been many separate reports of shelters encountering unexpectedly long times to cure using compounded itraconazole; this problem resolves when a change is made to the brand name product. Itraconazole requires careful formulation in appropriate vehicles to ensure its absorption; use of any material other than official, approved products is not recommended, as it may result in treatment failure.

20.9.2.2 Terbinafine

The use of oral terbinafine (Lamisil®, Novartis) is another acceptable treatment option. Though the drug appears to offer no advantages over itraconazole, it is almost equally effective (Moriello et al. 2013). Though its occurrence is rare, when cats with *M. canis* infections have been documented to be resistant to azole drugs, they can sometimes be treated successfully with terbinafine. Various doses have been used (10–40 mg/kg, once daily, orally, but cats treated at the higher end of the dosage range cure significantly faster. It is recommended that liver enzymes be monitored; this drug may elevate alanine aminotransferase (ALT) in cats though no clinical toxicity is necessarily seen. The drug has been shown to have residual activity in the skin similar to that of itraconazole and may be useful for pulse therapy (Foust et al. 2007).

20.9.2.3 Fluconazole

Fluconazole has received some attention as an alternative to itraconazole. Fluconazole has not been used as extensively as itraconazole, and there is limited information about its use in shelter cats. Treatment of two groups of cats with fluconazole has been reported: one group at 5 mg/kg and another at 10 mg/kg (Moriello and Newbury 2009). Cats treated at 10 mg/kg were cured faster than the ones at the lower dose. If used, 10 mg/kg orally once daily is recommended until studies determine that lower doses can be used effectively.

20.9.2.4 Griseofulvin

Griseofulvin is not recommended for use in shelter cats because it has a narrow margin of safety and may require a longer time to cure dermatophytosis. In one study, griseofulvin therapy alone required a mean of 70 days of treatment to cure experimentally infected cats, compared to 56 days of treatment with itraconazole (Moriello and DeBoer 1995). It is highly teratogenic and must not be used in pregnant animals. It can cause bone-marrow suppression in cats; this side effect is severe, unpredictable and not dependent upon the dose, breed, or length of therapy. To be used safely, white blood cell (WBC) counts are recommended pre-therapy and biweekly thereafter, which makes the drug cost-ineffective. Cats should be tested for feline leukemia virus (FeLV) and feline immunodeficiency virus (FIV) infection before use because there may be an association between infection and these adverse reactions. Though the author does not recommend griseofulvin use in cats, it may be less expensive per dose than itraconazole when treating large dogs. Over the full course of treatment though, considering all costs and times to cure, itraconazole may still be the more cost-effective treatment. The dose is dependent upon the formulation (microsize vs. ultra-microsize). Absorption is enhanced with a fatty meal. Vomiting, diarrhea, and inappetence are common adverse effects. This drug is increasingly difficult to obtain.

20.9.2.5 Ketoconazole

The true clinical efficacy of ketoconazole in dermatophytosis is unknown; there are limited anecdotal reports on its efficacy. Some strains of *M. canis* are resistant to ketoconazole. The drug is not well tolerated and has a narrow therapeutic margin in cats and consequently is not recommended for use in this species. The use of ketoconazole as a systemic antifungal is best reserved for infections in dogs, particularly Trichophyton. Ketoconazole has become inexpensive over the past few years, but other than this, it has no advantage over other drugs in routine cases of dermatophytosis.

20.9.2.6 Lufenuron

A published case in 2000 caused speculation that lufenuron (Program®, Novartis) may be beneficial for the treatment of feline or canine dermatophytosis (Ben-Ziony and Arzi 2000). Though there have been anecdotal reports of "cures" using lufenuron, controlled studies using feline experimental infection models and natural exposure models consistently found that lufenuron did not prevent the initial establishment of dermatophytosis in cats, did not result in faster cure once the infections were established, (Deboer et al. 2003; Moriello et al. 2004a) and was not synergistic with terbinafine. Lufenuron is NOT recommended for the treatment of dermatophytosis.

20.9.3 Verification of Cure

Successful treatment of dermatophytosis must be verified through repeated fungal cultures to establish that a mycologic cure has been achieved. Resolution of some of the clinical signs, including reduction of scaling, erythema and pruritus, etc., may be seen within two weeks of treatment, with hair growth in clipped cats starting shortly thereafter. When effective and recommended treatment protocols are used, a mycologic cure may actually precede hair regrowth. However, when times to cure are longer or lesions are mild, cats may appear clinically cured before mycologic cure has been achieved; if released into the general population or adopted out prematurely, these cats may continue to spread infection. This is particularly likely if an ineffective treatment is used. Mycologic cure has been defined most frequently by three consecutive negative cultures at weekly intervals; cultures should be held for 21 days. Treatment monitoring should start after one week of treatment. In a shelter treatment trial using the recommended combination treatment protocol, it was found that no cats became positive again after two consecutive negative weekly fungal cultures (Newbury et al. 2007). Cats were held in the treatment facility and received continued topical treatment until the fungal cultures were finalized. Using two negative cultures rather than three to define mycologic cure shortened the waiting time for the release to adoption with no negative consequences; *however, this has only been demonstrated to be reliable when using the combined lime sulfur and systemic itraconazole treatment described above.* Using any other treatment still requires three negative cultures to be reasonably certain of cure.

As treatment progresses, P-score values are expected to drop rapidly. Fluorescence of hairs on Wood's examination becomes increasingly faint. In fact, monitoring animals under treatment with a Wood's lamp examination can be an effective means of verifying that topical treatment is being correctly applied. Most commonly, in the author's experience, when a topical solution is not applied carefully enough to the face, probably because of caution around the eyes and nose for the animal's sake, brightly fluorescing, minimally treated hairs located in these areas contribute to prolonged times to cure. Showing these hairs to treatment staff who were applying topical treatment resulted in more attention being paid to these areas, which dramatically changed the amount of fluorescence seen on re-examination.

In the treatment trial discussed above, the mean number of days of treatment required for cure was 18.4 ± 9.5 SEM (standard error of the mean) (range 10–49 days). Cats with more severe infections required longer therapy. This time to cure data does not include an additional 21 days required to finalize the fungal cultures in order to demonstrate a mycologic cure. In general, an average treatment and housing time of at least one month should be estimated when considering an animal for treatment. The time it takes to cure and release an animal back into the population for adoption may be an especially important consideration for kittens. In some cases, kittens that undergo treatment may be young adults by the time mycologic cure has been verified. Culturing animals weekly during treatment helps reduce total treatment time by limiting the time wasted between when a cat has actually reached mycologic cure, but no culture has been taken.

20.9.4 Housing of Animals Undergoing Treatment

If infected or suspect animals are permitted to roam freely throughout any part of the facility, the risk of environmental contamination will rise, times to cure may be extended, and the zoonotic risk increases. Animals should be treated for dermatophytosis in an isolation area, as described above, in small family groups, bonded pairs or housed individually. Housing animals individually or separating them into small groups of two or three kittens helps prevent cross-infection and potential cross-contamination with spores that could confound the fungal culture process; it also allows better monitoring of general health and behavior. Animals should be released for adoption only when all co-housed animals have reached mycologic cure, so housing fewer animals per housing unit may also prevent delays in release.

Since animals are likely to be housed and treated for at least one month without an opportunity to roam freely, housing size and quality should be adequate for an extended stay. Behavioral and environmental enrichment should be provided, including toys and regular positive interactions with humans. Staff or volunteers must be trained to follow isolation protocols for enrichment as well as treatment. Bedding may be provided for animals undergoing treatment but should be changed each time the animal is treated topically, identified as contaminated, and kept contained when transported dirty to the laundry area. In the treatment trial referenced above, all cats had bedding in their cages. Bedding was removed and laundered each day in the shelter's standard washing machine and heated dryer. Though separate laundry facilities were not used, bedding was washed and dried separately from all other shelter laundry.

20.9.4.1 Environmental Decontamination: Cleaning, Disinfection, and Preventative Planning

Environments can become contaminated with naturally infective hairs and spores, which are resistant to many disinfectants commonly used in shelters. Mechanical cleaning and removal of spores must always be the cornerstone of decontamination. However, several effective disinfectant products are available as an adjunct to removal. Sodium hypochlorite (bleach) is effective at dilutions of 1:10 or 1:32, however, the lower dilution with a longer contact time (at least 10 minutes) is preferred in a shelter environment where animals and people are present. Accelerated hydrogen peroxide is also effective at a dilution of 1:10, as is 2% (but not 1%) potassium peroxymonosulfate (Moriello 2015; Moriello and Hondzo 2014). Enilconazole (Clinafarm™) is effective at a dilution of 1:100 and is available as a spray or a fogger and is most commonly used in poultry farms; it is usually found in agriculture supply stores. Calcium hypochlorite, 1% potassium peroxymonosulphate (Trifectant™) and the quaternary ammonium products are ineffective, as is chlorhexidine (Moriello 2015; Moriello et al. 2004b). Heat (50 °C or 122 °F) will inactivate Trichophyton spores better than repeated chilling and freezing. The same is likely true for *M. canis*, as it has been reported that toothbrush cultures from severely infected cats left in a car on a sunny day were all unexpectedly negative. Numerous studies have looked at the effect of UV light on various aspects of the growth of dermatophytes, however, data from these studies cannot be translated to practical application because the studies used the mycelial (culture plate) state and not naturally infective material.

The key to minimizing contamination and effectively decontaminating the environment is a combination of daily mechanical removal of infective material thorough sweeping or "Swiffering" of the floor and mechanical scrubbing with a good detergent (See Figure 20.34). (Swiffers™ are a line of cleaning products developed by Proctor and Gamble that include disposable cleaning cloths.) Disinfection of the environment should be performed ONLY after a thorough cleaning; its purpose is to kill any remaining spores that were not mechanically removed. The use of chemical disinfectants is recommended as an adjunct sanitation procedure because even though chemicals have been shown to inactivate spores *in vitro*, achieving sufficient contact time is difficult or impossible on many surfaces. Spores may linger in hard to penetrate cracks and crevices. In the author's expe-

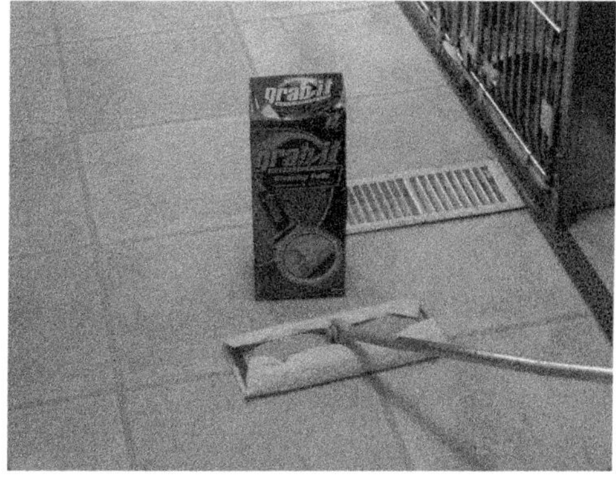

Figure 20.34 Commercial Swiffer clothes are excellent ways to mechanically remove spores from surfaces. These clothes readily collect spores, dirt and dust. The only negative is that they are expensive to use and should be on an organization "want list."

rience, meticulously cleaning an area three times in a row, followed each time by disinfection with properly prepared and applied bleach, often results in negative environmental cultures as long as there are no items in the room that could not be effectively cleaned.

In general, it is very difficult to effectively decontaminate areas containing soft, carpeted or upholstered furniture and other unwashable items. Lime- sulfur solution has been used in combination with direct sunlight to disinfect cat trees from community rooms or other indoor housing units (cat trees were placed outside because light filtered through windows will not be effective). Cat trees were cultured until two negative cultures were obtained. Steam cleaning and vacuuming may be helpful in those cases, but difficult or questionable items should be carefully evaluated for contamination after cleaning since they may remain a source of exposure and infection for humans and animals. Discarding these contaminated items is often safer and more cost-effective.

Environmental cultures of rooms and furniture are an extremely helpful tool to target cleaning efforts and verify successful decontamination. Environmental cultures can be particularly helpful to verify that difficult-to-clean areas such as group rooms or foster homes have been sufficiently decontaminated and are safe enough to admit new animals. They may also be helpful prior to investing in expensive procedures such as cleaning of ductwork; cultures may reveal that such procedures are unnecessary. Cultures can be obtained by using clean Swiffers to sample the environment, identify contamination and verify decontamination (Heinrich, Newbury and Verbrugge 2005).

In a clean area known to be free of contamination, a sheet of Swiffer should be cut into four sections and placed in a re-sealable plastic bag (See Figure 20.35). Several locations from each potentially contaminated area or room should be sampled, being sure to include locations frequented by infected animals or where hair or dust is likely to accumulate. Swiffer sheets should be wiped over an area until visibly soiled (See Figure 20.36). Items that may be particularly difficult to disinfect should also be sampled. Swiffer sections can then be used to inoculate fungal culture media by pressing firmly them onto the fungal culture plate. Fabric-covered furniture is often easier to culture using a toothbrush. The P-score system described previously can be used to evaluate relative levels of contamination in each area.

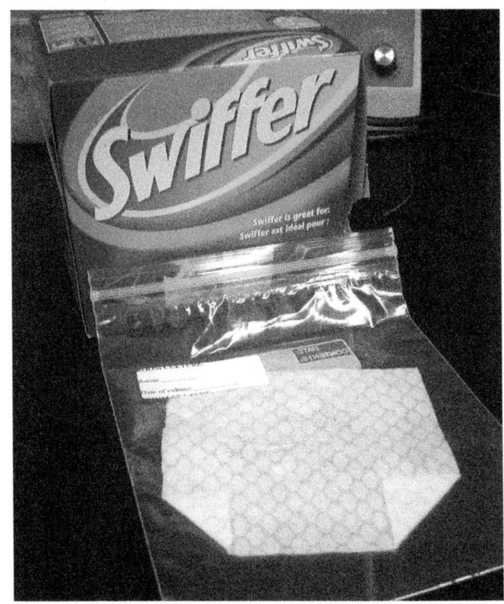

Figure 20.35 "Swiffer kit" for environmental sampling.

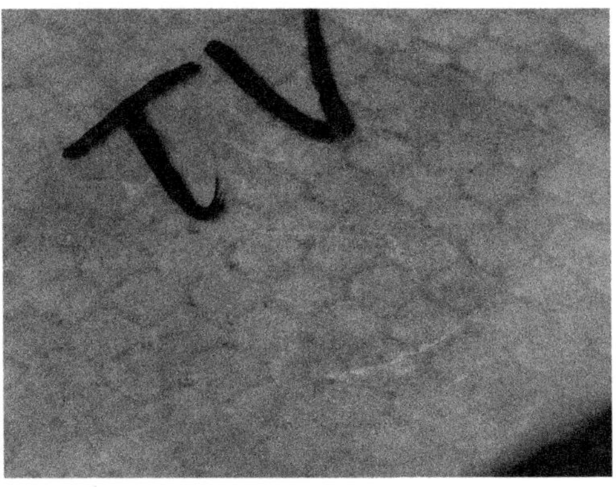

Figure 20.36 The Swiffer should be wiped over the target area until visibly soiled. The soiled side is then pressed onto the surface of a fungal culture plate to inoculate the sample.

Rooms should be designed to minimize and prevent disease transmission. They should use plastic or vinyl furniture that can be easily washed or hosed down if needed, combined with soft, removable, washable bedding and disposable items such as cardboard or a simple log to be used as a scratching post. Walls, floors, cages, and kennels should be smooth, in good repair and easily sanitized. Cracked walls and baseboards create many opportunities for spores to collect and evade efforts at disinfection. Preventative management should include performing visual/physical examinations; Wood's lamp/direct examination screening; and/or fungal cultures on higher risk animals before admitting them to difficult to clean areas such as community rooms or foster homes. It should also include regular monitoring of animals in those areas for the possible late development of lesions and regular, thorough cleaning and removal of hair from the environment. Because stress and lack of normal grooming are important risk factors for dermatophyte infection, low stress housing that facilitates normal behavioral expression is also helpful. There are no controlled studies on whether or not exposure to the outside is beneficial or not, but it is commonly observed in bovine practices that calves with dermatophytosis that are allowed to go outside in the sunshine recover faster than calves housed indoors. Management and housing issues, and their impact on the treatment of dermatophytosis, are an area of shelter medicine in need of further investigation.

20.10 Outbreak Management and Response

Successful management of dermatophytosis must be a continual preventative process, using the systematic screening protocol and environmental prevention practices described previously in this chapter. When outbreaks do occur, the same systematic screening protocol guides diagnosis, separation, and treatment decisions as well as environmental cleanup.

The first step is often answering the question, "Is this an outbreak?" It is difficult to define what number of cases or which particular situations may constitute an outbreak. Whenever in-shelter transmission is occurring, some type of intervention and organized response is necessary to assess the number of animals affected and disrupt further transmission. Outbreaks are far more common in shelter cats than shelter dogs, and in shelters or other facilities that house cats, but can affect either or both species as well as in-contact humans.

A systematic process is recommended using the basic tools described earlier for screening. When an outbreak is suspected, all potentially exposed animals should be screened and cultured. Because the response to a true dermatophytosis outbreak will be resource intensive and time consuming, the very first step should always be verifying the diagnosis via fungal culture. If there is any doubt about the accuracy of in-house fungal culture or the ability to perform and read cultures correctly, samples should be sent to a commercial laboratory for verification. In order to manage dermatophytosis outbreaks efficiently, every effort must be made to allocate appropriate resources promptly. Evaluating or responding to an outbreak or potential outbreak without a comprehensive screening of all at-risk animals will make resolution unlikely and may result in unnecessary treatment or removal from the population. In some cases, inadequate training, delayed, insufficient or inaccurate diagnostics may lead to unnecessary euthanasia. Outbreak response is time consuming, emotionally draining, and costly for any organization. Attempting to respond, without using all the tools available, will virtually ensure the need for another response in a short period.

It is equally important to recognize that outbreak responses must be accompanied by diligent prevention practices. Otherwise, the cycle may begin again almost immediately after the previous outbreak is resolved when another infected, yet unrecognized, animal enters the facility.

The following steps should be taken when responding to an outbreak or suspected outbreak of dermatophytosis:

1) Clearly identify all known cases and remove, isolate or separate infected animals from the general population.
2) Assess the potential for exposure for each animal or group of animals by mapping the location and movement of known cases in and out of each shelter area as well as the movements and routines of staff and volunteers. In some cases, exposure may have been confined to a particular area or ward. In other cases, when the number of known cases is relatively high, all cats in the shelter must be considered potentially exposed.
3) Systematically screen all at-risk animals as described previously in this chapter using the five basic diagnostic tools.
4) Discontinue the movement of exposed animals while awaiting culture results. If movement is absolutely necessary, carefully document and track locations.
5) Plan an initial response for each animal based on the results of the first four steps of the systematic screening protocol.
6) Establish a "clean break" between unexposed animals who are just entering the shelter and those who may have been exposed. Create separate housing areas for the exposed and unexposed groups. If possible, have separate staff provide care for each area and do not handle animals in the "clean" area after handling animals in the exposed group. At a minimum, ensure separate protective garments, gloves and equipment are used when handling exposed and unexposed cats.
7) Perform environmental cleanup as described previously.
8) Assess culture results as they become available, using culture results to guide treatment and other animal movement decisions as described previously.

20.11 Considerations for Adoption

Dermatophytosis is a zoonotic disease. Not everyone who is exposed to dermatophytes will become infected and develop clinical lesions. Though ringworm is most likely to affect the immune-compromised, elderly, infants and very young children, the disease can occur in immune-competent adults as well. If animals are made available for adoption or sent to foster while undergoing treatment, information should be provided about the disease, the treatment the animal has received, and what continued treatment is recommended. Potential risks to adopters, foster parents or their pets should be carefully explained, including information that their home environment could become contaminated with this durable pathogen and serve as a source of infection for other animals and people. In addition, adopters or foster parents should receive detailed guidance on how to manage risks, including complying with all treatments as prescribed and keeping the pet isolated to an easily cleaned area until resolution has been confirmed. With this information, foster parents and adopters can be empowered to decide what risks they are willing to accept for animals who are infected or under treatment. Animals who have been treated and achieved a confirmed mycologic cure pose no greater risk to adopters than any other shelter animal. In fact, since they have been so thoroughly monitored, the risk they pose to adopters is likely even lower.

20.12 Conclusion

Dermatophytosis is a treatable, curable disease that, when managed properly, has no associated long-term sequelae. In fact, left untreated, many cases will clear up on their own eventually in healthy, stress-free cats. Yet, because of the potential for widespread contagion and zoonosis, the infection may be life-threatening for both the individual shelter animal carrying the infection and the general shelter population, as well as damaging to the entire organization. The preventative management practices described in this chapter have demonstrated it is possible to effectively control dermatophytosis in a shelter setting. Defined diagnostic procedures and treatment protocols leading to relatively shorter times to mycologic cure have helped to minimize risk and allow more shelters to undertake this process, while planning and training make it possible to avoid situations that put large numbers of animals, shelter workers and the public at risk.

References

Ben-Ziony, Y. and Arzi, B. (2000). Use of lufenuron for treating fungal infections of dogs and cats: 297 cases (1997–1999). *Journal of the American Veterinary Medical Association* 217: 1510–1513.

Cafarchia, C., Romito, D., Sasanelli, M. et al. (2004). Epidemiology of canine and feline dermatophytosis in southern Italy. *Mycoses* 47: 508–513.

Carlotti, D.N., Guinot, P., Meissonnier, E. et al. (2010). Eradication of feline dermatophytosis in a shelter: a field study. *Veterinary Dermatology* 21 (3): 259–266.

Cerundolo, C. (2004). Generalized Microsporum canis dermatophytosis in six Yorkshire terrier dogs. *Veterinary Dermatology* 15: 181–187.

DeBoer, D.J. and Moriello, K.A. (1993). Humoral and cellular immune responses to Microsporum canis in naturally occurring feline dermatophytosis. *Journal of Medical and Veterinary Mycology* 31: 121–132.

DeBoer, D.J. and Moriello, K.A. (1994). Development of an experimental model of Microsporum canis infection in cats. *Veterinary Microbiology* 42: 289–295.

DeBoer, D.J. and Moriello, K.A. (1995). Inability of two topical treatments to influence the course of experimentally induced dermatophytosis in cats. *Journal of the American Veterinary Medical Association* 207: 52–57.

DeBoer, D.J., Moriello, K.A., Blum, J.L. et al. (2003). Effects of lufenuron treatment in cats on the establishment and course of Microsporum canis infection following exposure to infected cats. *Journal of the American Veterinary Medical Association* 222: 1216–1220.

Diesel, A., Verbrugge, M., and Moriello, K.A. (2011). Efficacy of eight commercial formulations of lime sulphur on in vitro growth inhibition of Microsporum canis. *Veterinary Dermatology* 22 (2): 197–201.

Foust, A.L., Marsella, R., Akucewich, L.H. et al. (2007). Evaluation of persistence of terbinafine in the hair of normal cats after 14 days of therapy. *Veterinary Dermatology* 18: 246–251.

Heinrich, K., Newbury, S., and Verbrugge, M. (2005). Detection of environmental contamination with Microsporum canis arthrospores in exposed homes and efficacy of the triple cleaning decontamination technique. (Abstract). *Veterinary Dermatology* 16: 192.

Jacobson, L.S., McIntyre, L., and Mykusz, J. (2018a). Comparison of real-time PCR with fungal culture for the diagnosis of Microsporum canis dermatophytosis in shelter cats: a field study. *Journal of Feline Medicine and Surgery* 20 (2): 103–107.

Jacobson, L.S., McIntyre, L., and Mykusz, J. (2018b). Assessment of real-time PCR cycle threshold values in Microsporum canis culture-positive and culture-negative cats in an animal shelter: a field study. *Journal of Feline Medicine and Surgery* 20 (2): 108–113.

Mancianti, F., Nardoni, S., Corazza, M. et al. (2003). Environmental detection of Microsporum canis arthrospores in households of infected cats and dogs. *Journal of Feline Medicine and Surgery* 5: 323–328.

Moriello, K.A. (2015). Kennel disinfectants for Microsporum canis and Trichophyton sp. *Veterinary Medicine International*: 853937. https://doi.org/10.1155/2015/853937.

Moriello, K.A. and DeBoer, D.J. (1991a). Fungal flora of pet cats. *American Journal of Veterinary Research* 52: 602–606.

Moriello, K.A. and DeBoer, D.J. (1991b). Fungal flora of the hair coat of cats with and without dermatophytosis. *Journal of Medical and Veterinary Mycology* 29: 285–292.

Moriello, K.A. and DeBoer, D.J. (1995). Efficacy of griseofulvin and itraconazole in the treatment of experimentally induced dermatophytosis in cats. *Journal of the American Veterinary Medical Association* 207: 439–444.

Moriello, K.A. and Hondzo, H. (2014). Efficacy of disinfectants containing accelerated hydrogen peroxide against conidial arthrospores and isolated infective spores of Microsporum canis and Trichophyton sp. *Veterinary Dermatology* 25 (3): 191–e148.

Moriello, K.A. and Newbury, S. (2009). Dermatophytosis. In: *Infectious Disease Management in Animal Shelters* (eds. L. Miller and K.F. Hurley), 243–274. Ames: Wiley Blackwell.

Moriello, K.A. and Verbrugge, M. (2007). Use of isolated infected spores to determine the sporicidal efficacy of two commercial antifungal rinses against Microsporum canis. *Veterinary Dermatology* 18: 55–58.

Moriello, K.A., DeBoer, D.J., Volk, L.M. et al. (2004a). Development of an in vitro isolated infected spore testing model for disinfectant testing of Microsporum canis isolates. *Veterinary Dermatology* 15: 175–180.

Moriello, K.A., DeBoer, D.J., Schenker, R. et al. (2004b). Efficacy of pre-treatment with lufenuron for the prevention of Microsporum canis infection in a feline direct topical challenge model. *Veterinary Dermatology* 15: 357–362.

Moriello, K.A., Coyner, K., Trimmer, A. et al. (2013). Treatment of shelter cats with oral terbinafine and concurrent lime sulphur rinses. *Veterinary Dermatology* 24 (6): 618–620, e149-150.

Newbury, S. and Moriello, K.A. (2014). Feline dermatophytosis: steps for investigation of a suspected shelter outbreak. *Journal of Feline Medicine and Surgery* 20 (5): 407–418.

Newbury, S., Verbrugge, M., and Moriello, K.A. (2005). Management of naturally occurring dermatophytosis in an open shelter: part 1: development of a cost-effective screening and monitoring program. (Abstract). *Veterinary Dermatology* 16: 192.

Newbury, S., Verbrugge, M., and Steffen, T. (2005). Management of naturally occurring dermatophytosis in an open shelter: part 2: treatment of cats in an offsite facility. (Abstract). *Veterinary Dermatology* 16: 193.

Newbury, S., Moriello, K., Verbrugge, M. et al. (2007). Use of lime sulphur and itraconazole to treat shelter cats naturally infected with Microsporum canis in an annex facility: an open field trial. *Veterinary Dermatology* 18 (5): 324–331.

Newbury, S., Moriello, K.A., Kwochka, K.W. et al. (2011). Use of itraconazole and either lime sulphur or Malaseb Concentrate Rinse (R) to treat shelter cats naturally infected with Microsporum canis: an open field trial. *Veterinary Dermatology* 22 (1): 75–79.

Newbury, S., Moriello, K.A., Coyner, K. et al. (2015). Management of endemic Microsporum canis dermatophytosis in an open admission shelter: a field study. *Journal of Feline Medicine and Surgery* 17 (4): 342–347.

Polak, K.C., Levy, J.K., Crawford, P.C. et al. (2014). Infectious diseases in large-scale cat hoarding investigations. *The Veterinary Journal* 201 (2): 189–195.

Sparkes, A.H., Gruffydd-Jones, T.J., and Stokes, C.R. (1996). Acquired immunity in experimental feline Microsporum canis infection. *Research in Veterinary Science* 61: 165–168.

Stuntebeck, R., Moriello, K.A., and Verbrugge, M. (2017). Evaluation of incubation time for Microsporum canis dermatophyte cultures.

Journal of Feline Medicine and Surgery 20 (10): 997–1000. https://doi.org/10.1177/1098612X17729286.

Verbrugge, M., Moriello, K.A., and Newbury, S. (2006). Correlation of skin lesions and dermatophyte culture status in cats at the time of admission to a shelter. (Abstract). *Veterinary Dermatology* 17: 213.

Verbrugge, M., Kesting, R., and Moriello, K.A. (2007). Effects of light exposure and temperature on time to growth of dermatophytes using commercial fungal culture media. (Abstract). *Veterinary Dermatology* 19: 110.

White-Weithers, N. and Medleau, L. (1995). Evaluation of topical therapies for the treatment of dermatophyte infected hairs from dogs and cats. *Journal of the American Animal Hospital Association* 31: 250–253.

21

Zoonosis

Brian A. DiGangi and Lila Miller

American Society for the Prevention of Cruelty to Animals (ASPCA), New York, NY, USA

21.1 Introduction

A zoonotic disease is strictly defined as an infectious disease that is naturally transmitted from living animals to humans. There are over 1,400 pathogens (viruses, bacteria, fungi, protozoa and helminths) known to infect man (Microbiology 2011); 60% of them are considered zoonotic. These numbers are subject to change as scientists estimate that 75% of newly emerging diseases in humans are of animal origin (NCEZID 2018). There are many reasons why emerging and reemerging diseases are an increasing public health concern. Intensive agriculture systems, increasing globalization, climate change, habitat destruction, increased tourism, etc. can all facilitate infections in crossing species barriers and traveling into new ecologic environments (Cutler et al. 2010).

Anthroponosis (also known as reverse zoonosis) refers to infections that can be transmitted from humans to animals; examples include Methicillin-resistant *Staphylococcus aureus* (MRSA) and *Streptococcus*. Anthroponotic diseases are generally of less concern in shelters; however, disease prevention practices and associated animal management issues have similar impacts on shelter operations as zoonotic diseases.

Shelter personnel should be aware that zoonotic (and anthroponotic) pathogen transmission may occur in a variety of ways other than direct contact with an infected animal. It is also important to note that infected animals may appear healthy, yet still be able to transmit an infection to a susceptible host. The most common methods of pathogen transmission include:

- Direct contact with the saliva, blood, urine, mucus, feces, skin (hair) or other body fluids of an infected animal through bites, scratches, petting, contamination of wounds, etc.
- Indirect contact with fomites (e.g. clothing, equipment, animal bedding, etc.) or other objects contaminated with the pathogen, such as soil
- Inhalation or ingestion of infected body tissues, aerosols, secretions, or excretions
- Vector-borne through contact with an infected arthropod such as a tick, flea, or mosquito.

Some zoonotic diseases may be transmitted through multiple means, or the mode of transmission may be obscure. For example, tularemia (caused by *Francisella tularensis* and also known as rabbit fever) is transmitted to humans through contact with body or tissue fluids, hair, skin or tissue of an infected animal,

Infectious Disease Management in Animal Shelters, Second Edition.
Edited by Lila Miller, Stephanie Janeczko, and Kate F. Hurley.

consumption of contaminated meat, tick bites, bites or scratches from infected cats or through inhalation of the pathogen. In addition, mowing lawns was identified as a potential risk factor for acquiring tularemia in disease-endemic areas where rabbits may be killed by mowers or hedge trimmers (Agger et al. 2005).

The impact of a zoonotic disease on shelter populations (both human and animal) can be mitigated by maintaining an awareness of the mechanisms of pathogen transmission and adjusting shelter operations to minimize opportunities for infection to occur. Careful attention to the environmental characteristics of the shelter, animal-handling procedures, means of personal protection, and adherence to basic hygienic practices can support a safe working environment that is better positioned to serve the animals and people within the shelter's community.

21.2 General Guidelines for Zoonotic Disease Prevention

21.2.1 The Shelter Environment

The shelter environment presents a disease-management challenge because animals of unknown medical backgrounds and unknown exposure histories must coexist in a congregate living environment. Often, asymptomatic animals are carriers of infection, and the congregate environment facilitates animal-to-animal and animal-to-human pathogen transmission.

It is unrealistic to expect shelters to ensure that all animals in their care are free of every potential zoonotic condition, but they must take reasonable precautions to avoid releasing infected animals into the community. Depending on the source of information, estimates are that anywhere from 30 to 40 zoonotic diseases affect companion animals (Greene and Levy 2006). According to the Centers for Disease Control (CDC), it is estimated that more than 6 out of every 10 known infectious diseases in humans can be spread from animals, and 3 out of every 4 new or emerging infectious diseases in humans come from animals (CDC 2017). Though there is at least one report of a higher percentage of zoonotic enteric pathogens in shelter cats compared to client-owned cats (Hill et al. 2000), another study found no difference in the prevalence of zoonotic enteric pathogens in cats less than one year of age (Spain et al. 2001). Furthermore, another report found that the shelter management model was an important factor in the type of feline enteric pathogens found (Andersen et al. 2018). Regardless of the prevalence and risk factors for zoonoses in a given shelter population, which is largely unknown outside of the research setting, similar disease mitigation efforts can be applied to maximize the benefits of pet ownership and reduce the risks of contracting a zoonotic disease. Most human infections with zoonoses come from livestock, including pigs, chickens, cattle, goats and sheep; only a relatively small percentage of zoonotic infections in humans can be traced to direct contact with pets (Greene and Levy 2006).

It should not come as a surprise that shelters (and veterinary practice environments) can present a high risk of exposure to various infectious pathogens that can transmit disease from animals to humans. Many of the stray animals that enter shelters are debilitated, immunocompromised, and have vague or unknown histories of disease-exposure risk. Many zoonotic diseases present no overt clinical signs in animals; it is therefore imperative that shelter personnel be vigilant about the potential for exposure to zoonotic diseases. Infection control measures should be implemented in all animal-care facilities to minimize the risk of pathogen transmission. A variety of resources designed for private veterinary practices, including model infection control plans and infection control audit checklists are accessible and easily adaptable to the animal shelter setting. See Box 21.1.

Box 21.1 Infection Control Resources

American Animal Hospital Association
2018 AAHA Infection Control, Prevention, and Biosecurity Guidelines
https://www.aaha.org/globalassets/02-guidelines/infection-control/icpb_guidelines.pdf
Centers for Disease Control and Prevention
National Center for Emerging and Zoonotic Infectious Diseases (NCEZID)
https://www.cdc.gov/ncezid
National Association of State and Public Health Veterinarians (NASPHV)
Compendium of Veterinary Standard Precautions for Zoonotic Disease Prevention in Veterinary Personnel, 2015
http://www.nasphv.org/Documents/VeterinaryStandardPrecautions.pdf
Model Infection Control Plan for Veterinary Practices
http://www.nasphv.org/documents CompendiaVet.html

The shelter environment should be set up to enable easy access to basic disease prevention tools and personnel should be trained in their proper use. This may mean that duplicate sets of equipment and supplies may need to be purchased to avoid personnel traveling through the facility to obtain the needed items. In some facilities or at public events, the installation of portable handwashing stations should be considered to make proper hand hygiene accessible. The adaptations needed will necessarily vary by each individual shelter scenario, though some basic recommendations for zoonotic disease prevention include:

- Practicing proper hand hygiene between examinations of individual animals or groups; before eating, drinking, or smoking; after cleaning animal cages and whenever hands are visibly soiled
- Using protective gloves, sleeves, gowns, face and hair covers, and/or shoe covers (also referred to as personal protective equipment or PPE), as dictated by individual disease risk and especially when handling animals with obvious clinical signs of infectious disease (e.g. sneezing, coughing, ocular or nasal discharge, diarrhea, fever)
- Using facial protection to protect eyes, nose, and mouth when handling animals, performing procedures (e.g. dentals), or cleaning and disinfecting the facility
- Using appropriate protective garments when cleaning, such as boots, coveralls, smocks, and eye protection (i.e. goggles, glasses)
- Wearing designated protective outerwear while in the shelter and removing it upon leaving
- Ensuring that disposable or single-use items (e.g. syringes, examination gloves) are discarded after each use.

Environmental sanitation is another critical component of zoonotic disease mitigation and is discussed in detail in Chapter 8. Spills, blood, urine, feces, etc. should be cleaned up promptly and surfaces disinfected with a disinfectant that will inactivate pathogens of concern. Infected tissues should be handled as biohazardous waste and disposed of properly. Laundry should be sorted and machine washed using hot water, detergent, and bleach, and machine dried.

Rodent and vector control are important components of any comprehensive disease control program. Care must be taken to ensure that the control methods are the most humane option available for the target species and minimize risks to shelter animals and personnel. A multi-faceted approach is likely to be most effective. Environmental factors to address include securing potential food sources, particularly overnight; eliminating potential rodent nesting areas from around the facility (e.g. piles of yard waste, wood, etc.); sealing and/or packing any obvious cracks or holes with steel wool, and draining free-standing water to eliminate mosquito breeding grounds. Ultrasonic deterrents may decrease the population for a few days, but target species are likely to return if their food source remains accessible (Mason and Littin 2003).

When lethal means of rodent control are deemed necessary, properly used snap traps may be the most humane method that is feasible in a shelter environment (Mason and Littin 2003). If a decision is made to use a rodenticide, consideration should be given to the type and formulation of rodenticide; the means of handling partially poisoned animals; provisions for disposal of dead animals; and for non-target species, the toxicity of the rodenticide, the likelihood of relay toxicosis, and the potential for treatment following accidental ingestion. The Universities Federation for Animal Welfare is a good source for information regarding the humane control of unwanted rat and mouse populations (www.ufaw.org.uk/rodent-welfare/rodent-welfare).

21.2.2 Personal Protective Equipment and Hand Hygiene

PPE is equipment worn to minimize exposure to serious workplace injuries and illnesses. The specific type of PPE indicated in any given situation will depend on the type of pathogens known or suspected to be present, the routes of transmission of those pathogens, and the likelihood and degree of contact with potentially infective material. Shelters must train all personnel who use PPE to know when and what kind is necessary, how to put it on ("don"), adjust, wear, and take it off ("doff") correctly, the limitations of the equipment and its proper care, maintenance, useful life, and disposal. PPE must be of good quality, in adequate supply, and readily accessible. The type of PPE required for entering each area of the shelter should be readily visible and accessible. Instructional display posters and training videos for shelter personnel are available online through the Centers for Disease Control and Prevention (CDC) (https://www.cdc.gov/hai/pdfs/ppe/ppe-sequence.pdf) and the American Society for the Prevention of Cruelty to Animals (ASPCA) (https://www.aspcapro.org/resource/personal-protective-equipment-posters-and-how-video).

Gloves are an important—and perhaps the most commonly used—piece of PPE as well as a key component of proper hand hygiene for the prevention of pathogen transmission and, as such, warrant special mention. Gloves do not replace the need for handwashing, but act as an additional barrier to pathogen spread. Single-use, disposable gloves should be utilized whenever possible; gloves designed for such use cannot be washed, re-sterilized or otherwise re-purposed for use without loss of integrity and compromise to their function as a physical barrier to biological material. Medical or surgical grade gloves, which are composed of vinyl, latex, or nitrile should be used to ensure adequacy and consistency in puncture, abrasion, and chemical resistance (Predolich 2015). Gloves designed for use in food preparation are not subject to formal regulations or inspections of quality insurance, may not provide an equivalent level of protection and may promote the transfer of sweat and bacteria (Eagle Protect 2017; Steuven n.d.).

Hand hygiene is a key element in preventing the transmission of infections; in fact, it is the single most effective disease prevention method to use in a shelter. However, it must be performed correctly and at the appropriate times to be effective. In addition to the proper use of gloves, hand hygiene includes handwashing with soap and water and the use of alcohol-based hand rubs. Artificial nails and hand jewelry should not be worn when handling animals.

Hands should be washed with plain soap, or a soap that contains antiseptic, and water in these instances:

- When hands are visibly soiled
- Before eating
- After using the restroom
- After caring for animals with clinical signs of or known diagnoses of infectious disease, and especially after caring for animals colonized or infected with spore-forming bacteria, (e.g. *Bacillus anthracis*, *Clostridium difficile*).

If hands are not visibly soiled, an alcohol-based rub, e.g. 70–95% ethyl alcohol (ethanol) or isopropyl alcohol (isopropanol), may be used (temporarily) to decontaminate hands when soap and water are unavailable. Because hand rubs are well tolerated and can be made readily accessible in areas where sinks are not available, they are gaining acceptance for use in many clinical settings. However, alcohol-based rubs do not provide any cleaning or detergent activity and are not a substitute for handwashing. When applied properly for 20–30 seconds of contact time with visibly clean hands, hand rubs are highly effective against bacteria, many fungi, and enveloped viruses; they are not effective against bacterial spores, protozoal parasites, and some nonenveloped viruses such as parvovirus. The correct use of hand rubs should include the following steps:

1) Ensure hands are visibly clean.
2) Place alcohol-based hand rub in palms.
3) Apply to all surfaces of hands.
4) Rub hands together for 20–30 seconds, until dry.

Care should be taken to apply enough sanitizer to ensure that 20–30 seconds of contact time can be achieved.

Though not a substitute, compliance with the use of alcohol-based hand rubs may be higher than for handwashing; as such, both alcohol hand sanitizers and handwashing stations should be available to shelter staff and visitors. The use of moisturizers after handwashing can enhance the integrity of the skin and reduce skin breakdown and should also be considered when stocking hand-hygiene stations. See Box 21.2 for hand hygiene (with soap and water or an alcohol-based product) guidelines to minimize pathogen transmission and Box 21.3 for guidelines for proper handwashing.

21.2.3 Animal Handling and Other General Precautions

Animals should be examined on intake to identify those with signs of infectious disease or other illness so they may be isolated from the general population as soon as possible and handled appropriately. During animal handling, careful attention should be paid to assessing and responding to body language, and principles of low-stress animal handling should be applied to minimize opportunities for bite injuries. According to the National Association of State Public Health Veterinarians' (NASPHV) Model Infection Control Plan, animals that

Box 21.2 Hand Hygiene to Minimize Pathogen Transmission

ALWAYS WASH HANDS BEFORE:
- Direct contact with patients
- Donning gloves when inserting a central intravascular catheter
- Inserting indwelling urinary catheters, peripheral vascular catheters, or other invasive devices that do not require a surgical procedure

ALWAYS WASH HANDS AFTER:
- Direct contact with the patient's intact skin
- Contact with mucous membranes, body fluids or excretions (vomit, feces), nonintact skin, and wound dressings
- Contact with inanimate objects in the immediate vicinity of the animal or contaminated by the animal
- Emptying/cleaning litter boxes and cleaning cages or runs
- Handling known or suspected tick- or flea-infested animals
- Handling laboratory specimens
- Removing gloves

Box 21.3 Guidelines for Proper Handwashing

1) Turn on the faucet and use warm or cold water. Hot water will dry out skin and increase the risk of infections.
2) Remove rings before wetting hands.
3) Apply 1–2 oz of liquid soap. Bar soap should not be used as this increases the risk of cross-transmission of microorganisms.
4) Rub hands together to make a lather, making sure to wash the palms, the back of hands, between the fingers, and under the nails.
5) Scrub vigorously for 20–30 seconds.
6) Rinse with water.
7) Dry hands with a single-use or disposable towel.
8) Turn the faucet off using the towel, before disposing of the towel in a wastebasket.

have neurologic signs, diarrhea, respiratory signs, fever, infected wounds, chronic infections, or known exposure to an infectious agent should be placed directly into a designated exam or isolation room (NASPHV 2015). Appropriate vaccinations (see Chapter 9) and prophylactic deworming (see Chapter 17), especially for zoonotic internal parasites such as roundworms and hookworms, should be administered to all animals on intake, regardless of their source or condition on arrival. A sink with running water, soap and paper towels should be readily accessible in areas where intake examinations are conducted so that personnel may wash their hands frequently.

Food for human consumption should be stored in a refrigerator separate from animal products, vaccines, etc. The consumption of food and beverages should be prohibited in animal housing and holding areas. Fungal and other cultures and test materials should be stored separately; gloves should be worn when they are handled, and hands should be washed after gloves are removed.

Vaccines and biologics should be stored, handled and administered according to the manufacturer's instructions. Immunocompromised individuals should avoid handling and administering intranasal (IN) vaccines. Sharps containers should be readily available wherever needles are used. The practice of recapping or cutting needles before disposal is strongly discouraged to avoid needle sticks or aerosolization of certain pathogens. Shelters that perform surgeries, necropsies, or handle diagnostic specimens are advised to follow the same, if not higher, safety precautions than would be followed in a veterinary practice because there may be a greater degree of uncertainty about disease in stray animals. Nonessential personnel should not be permitted in the room, and protective garments should be worn during surgical procedures and necropsies. Hands should always be washed at the end of any procedure and before handling other equipment, rubbing one's eyes, handling contact lenses, or consuming food.

Shelters should have a written infection control plan that contains information pertinent to the protection of employee health. This section may best be written by a physician in consultation with a shelter veterinarian. Shelter veterinarians are generally more knowledgeable about the zoonotic disease risks faced by shelter personnel. Those who routinely handle animals should receive rabies preexposure and tetanus vaccinations, and there should also be a risk assessment to determine if other preventive vaccinations and procedures may be warranted. The plan should be available to all personnel and updated regularly. Training regarding zoonotic diseases, the transmission of disease, and sanitation should be provided on a routine basis. The NASPHV Model Infection Control Plan provides an excellent template for a plan that can be edited and adapted for each individual shelter's needs.

21.3 Zoonotic Diseases

A discussion of specific zoonotic diseases is beyond the scope of this textbook; the objective of this chapter is to list canine and feline diseases of most concern to shelters arranged by the most common mode of transmission and to provide principles of disease prevention and control. The reader is reminded that many diseases have multiple modes of transmission; they should refer to other veterinary and public health resources mentioned in this chapter for up-to-date information about specific zoonotic diseases, and to other chapters in this textbook for information about the management of targeted diseases, such as rabies (Chapter 22) and dermatophytosis (Chapter 20). Veterinary textbooks, such as Greene's Infectious Diseases of the Dog and Cat (Saunders/Elsevier, St. Louis), are an excellent resource for detailed disease information. Table 21.1 lists the diseases discussed below along with their implications for animal adoption.

Whenever an animal that has been diagnosed and is currently undergoing treatment for a zoonotic disease is adopted from a shelter, the veterinarian should provide complete details of the disease and a written medical record that includes treatment provided and any control measures that must be taken to prevent disease spread. The veterinarian should take special care to provide detailed information and answer any questions individuals may have regarding ownership of an animal with a potentially zoonotic condition; adopters should also be advised to consult with their physician before finalizing the adoption because of the potential increased risk. (Shelter personnel and veterinarians should exercise good judgment to avoid invading the privacy or violating the rights of immunocompromised persons when discussing health concerns associated with the adoption of shelter animals.) An excellent resource for adopters is provided by the CDC at http://www.cdc.gov/healthypets.

21.3.1 Infections Transmitted through Bites or Exposure to Saliva

Bite-inflicted wounds are one of the most common sources of zoonoses (Greene and Levy 2006). This may be particularly true in shelters where many of the animals may be highly stressed, are sick, in pain, or are strays with an unknown behavior history. Wounds may become infected with bacteria from either the flora on the victim's skin or the "normal flora" of the biter; animals should never be permitted to lick open wounds they have inflicted.

The animal inflicting the bite is often clinically normal. Risk factors for dog bites include the dog's age, breed, size, reproductive status, and medical condition. One reference indicates most cat bites are inflicted by unowned female cats on female adults (Greene and Goldstein 2006). Shelters should ensure that personnel are trained in proper animal handling that minimizes stress; how to recognize the behavior signs that indicate fear and possible aggression; how and when to use safety and restraint equipment, including tranquilizers or sedation for frightened or fractious animals; and when to leave the animal alone if performing non-essential tasks that can be postponed to another time when the animal is calmer. Shelter personnel may be reluctant to report dog and cat bites, especially if they feel the bite is minor, justified, or may hurt the animal's chances for adoption. However, they must be encouraged to do so because of the risk of pathogen transmission and increased liability for the shelter if an adopted animal bites someone and knowledge of a bite history was deliberately withheld.

Dog bites are more common than cat bites; however, cat bites are more likely to become infected because they tend to produce deep puncture wounds contaminated with highly pathogenic bacterial species. A study of cat bites to the hand found that their sharp teeth inject hard-to-treat bacteria deeply into joint and tendon sheaths where they have relative protection from blood and the immune system (Babovic et al. 2014). Dog bite wounds also reflect the dog's oral flora; they are frequently infected in descending order with *Staphylococcus aureus*, *Streptococcal* species, or *Pasteurella* species. Cat bites are more likely to

Table 21.1 List of common zoonotic pathogens (Please review detailed information in the text about adoption considerations, especially when adopting to high-risk individuals.)

Pathogen	Description	Common Routes of Transmission	Implications for Adoption[a]
Bartonella henselae, B. clarridgeiae (Cat scratch fever in humans)	Gram-negative, intracellular proteobacterium Transmitted among cats, mainly by the cat flea, *Ctenocephalides felis*	Scratch or bite from a cat with exposure to fleas or flea feces	Apply flea control Antibiotic therapy recommended prior to adoption to a high-risk person Additional cautions may be warranted for adoptions of kittens <1 year of age
Bordetella bronchiseptica (Infectious tracheobronchitis, Kennel cough, Canine Infectious Respiratory Disease)	Gram-negative bacillus Affects many species, including humans **(rare)**	Exposure to aerosol from an infected animal	Adopt after initiating treatment Advise on the indications for follow-up with a veterinarian See Chapters 10 and 13 respectively on Canine and Feline Infectious Respiratory Disease (CIRD and FIRD)
Brucella canis (Brucellosis)	Gram-negative coccobacillary organism	Contact with vaginal secretions, aborted fetuses, placenta, or lochia	Case management and eligibility for adoption may be subject to local regulations Consider adoption only after neutering and instituting long-term antibiotic therapy Lifetime laboratory testing recommended
Campylobacter jejuni, C. coli, C. helveticus, C. upsaliensis, and *C. lari*	Gram-negative bacillus	Exposure to infected animals, raw or undercooked meats, unpasteurized milk or milk products, or contaminated food and water	Adopt after completing treatment Verification of negative status recommended before adopting to high-risk individuals
Capnocytophaga canimorsus and *C. cynodegmi*	Gram-negative fusiform bacteria Commonly isolated from the oral cavity of humans and animals	Dog bites	Normal flora, no treatment or special precautions needed
Coxiella burnetti[a] (Coxiellosis or Q Fever)	Obligate, intracellular, gram-negative bacteria *May also be tick-borne (Amblyomma americanum, Dermacentor andersoni)*	Inhalation of dust contaminated by infected animal feces, urine, milk, and parturient discharges Consumption of contaminated or unpasteurized dairy products	Potential bioterrorism agent Affected animals should be isolated immediately Cases should be reported to the Department of Health Treatment or adoption **NOT** recommended

(*Continued*)

Table 21.1 (Continued)

Pathogen	Description	Common Routes of Transmission	Implications for Adoption[a]
Cryptosporidium parvum, felis, canis	Coccidian protozoan Infects many animals and humans	Ingestion of fecal-contaminated water	Adopt after completing treatment Verification of negative status recommended before adopting to high-risk individuals
Francisella tularensis[a] (Tularemia)	Gram negative bacillus	Bite wound from vector species (i.e. wild rodent or lagomorph) Bites or scratches from infected cats Insect bites (ticks)	Potential bioterrorism agent Cases should be reported to the Department of Health Treatment or adoption **NOT** recommended
Giardia duodenalis (also known as *intestinalis, lamblia*)	Flagellated protozoan Several strains (assemblages) in many species	Ingestion of fecal-contaminated water Direct hand contact with an infected person	Adopt after initiating treatment Advise on the indications for follow-up with a veterinarian Risk of humans acquiring *Giardia* infection from dogs or cats is small as the exact type of *Giardia* that infects humans is usually not the same type that infects dogs and cats Report human cases to the Department of Health
Hookworms *Ancylostoma caninum* (dogs) *Ancylostoma braziliense* (dogs and cats) *Uncinaria stenocephala* (dogs and cats) (Cutaneous larval migrans [CLM] or creeping eruption in humans)	Parasitic nematode	Direct contact with fecal-contaminated soil	Adopt after initiating treatment Advise of need for follow-up with a veterinarian if treatment is not completed before adoption

Leptospira spp.	Gram-negative spirochete	Direct or indirect contact with urine Inhalation of aerosolized urine Contact with contaminated water, soil or food Cuts and abrasions on the skin	Adopt after completing treatment
Malassezia pachydermatis	A yeast that colonizes the skin of dogs and cats	Direct contact	Adopt after initiating treatment Advise on the indications for follow-up with a veterinarian
Microsporum canis, Trichophyton mentagrophytes (Dermatophytosis or Ringworm)	Fungal infection	Direct contact with broken hairs and associated spores on the animal and in the environment Microtrauma to skin required for infection	Initiate systemic and topical treatment Consider adoption after two negative weekly fungal cultures Advise of need for follow-up with veterinarian if treatment is not completed before adoption See Chapter 20 on Dermatophytosis
Pasteurella multocida, P. stomatis and *P. dagmatis*	Gram-negative bacillus An inhabitant of the oropharyngeal and nasal cavity of cats, dogs, and other animals	Cat (most commonly) or dog bites	Normal flora, no treatment or special precautions needed
Rabies (*Lyssavirus* in the Rhabdoviridae family)	Virus maintained in wildlife	Bite from a mammal, especially wildlife	Dogs and cats exposed to confirmed or suspected rabid animals are subject to quarantine periods and reporting as outlined by local regulations Do not adopt See Chapter 22 on Rabies
Roundworms *Toxocara canis* (dogs) *Toxocara cati* (cats) *Baylisascaris procyonis* (raccoons) (Visceral Larval Migrans (VLM), Ocular Larval Migrans (OLM), and Neural Larval Migrans)	Parasitic nematodes	Ingestion of fecal-contaminated soil	Adopt after initiating treatment Prior to adopting to families with young children, verification of negative status or counseling on the need for follow-up with a veterinarian if treatment is not completed is recommended

(*Continued*)

Table 21.1 (Continued)

Pathogen	Description	Common Routes of Transmission	Implications for Adoption[a]
Sarcoptes scabiei var. canis (Sarcoptic mange, Acariasis)	Highly contagious mite found on the skin surface of dogs	Direct contact	Adopt after initiating treatment Advise of need for follow-up with a veterinarian
Threadworms *Strongyloides stercoralis*	Parasitic nematode	Direct contact with fecal-contaminated soil	Adopt after initiating treatment Advise of need for follow-up with a veterinarian
Toxoplasma gondii	Obligate coccidian parasite Infects all mammals, including humans The cat is the definitive host	Consumption of raw or undercooked meat Exposure to cats fed raw meat diets	Adopt after initiating treatment Advise on the indications for follow-up with a veterinarian See text for precautions regarding pregnant women
Salmonella enterica	Gram-negative bacillus	Contaminated food, water, fomites Ingestion of contaminated products of animal origin Direct and indirect contact with reptiles, backyard poultry	Adopt after completing treatment Report human cases to the Department of Health

[a] Caution should be exercised whenever adopting animals that have been diagnosed with zoonotic diseases to high-risk persons, such as those who are immunocompromised, elderly, <5 years of age, or have chronic disease. See the text for more detailed information about adoption considerations.

become infected with *Pasteurella* species (Zurlo 2005). *Pasteurella multocida* subsp. *septica* has a greater prevalence in cats, and *P. canis biotype 1* is found only in dog bites.

Bite wounds, in general, typically include lacerations, avulsions, punctures, and scratches. Persons who wait more than 8 hours to seek treatment after a bite will usually have an infected wound. Typical signs of infection include pain at the site of the injury, a purulent discharge, gray color, and a foul odor. Approximately 2–30% of all bite wounds for which medical care is sought will become infected and may result in hospitalization of the patient. Puncture wounds are more likely than avulsions to become infected and result in abscess formation. Wounds near bones and joints may cause septic arthritis, tenosynovitis, or osteomyelitis. Osteomyelitis should be considered whenever there is joint pain or limited range of motion.

21.3.1.1 Bite Wound Management

All bite wounds and scratches should be washed immediately with soap, preferably an antiseptic agent with virucidal activity such as povidone-iodine, and water. First aid should consist of immediate irrigation with copious amounts of normal saline. Puncture wounds should be irrigated under pressure using a 20-ml syringe and an 18-gauge needle. The wound should be covered with a bandage and evaluated immediately by a physician. If the hand is injured it should be elevated; it is strongly suggested that physicians administer aggressive antibiotic treatment to puncture wounds near joints, especially on the hands. Failure to adequately treat hand-bite wounds can lead to deep infection, structural damage and permanent loss of function, with the possibility of sepsis in high-risk patients (Jha et al. 2014). One should always collect a history about the bite that will help in determining the circumstances surrounding the bite. Appendix 21.A is an example of a comprehensive animal bite investigation form. Animal bites are reportable to the local health department in many jurisdictions, so it is advisable to check on their regulations.

21.3.2 Infections Transmitted through Scratches, Close Physical, or Mucosal Contact

Scratch wounds (which may contain oral pathogens from grooming), close physical contact with the skin of an infected animal or the animal's contaminated environment, and contact with an animal's mucosal surfaces (such as through licking or kissing) can all serve as routes for pathogen transmission to humans. Prevention is largely through careful animal handling to avoid scratches, good sanitation to minimize environmental contamination, and regularly practicing good hand hygiene (wearing gloves and frequent handwashing).

21.3.3 Infections Transmitted Via the Fecal–Oral Route

Some diseases that can be spread to humans by the fecal-oral route, such as Toxoplasmosis, Salmonellosis, Campylobacteriosis, etc. have been highly publicized. For example, a case of multidrug-resistant *Campylobacter jejuni* affected 30 people that had contact with infected puppies or associated pet stores across 13 states (CDC 2019a). Over 1,000 people across 49 states were infected with *Salmonella* that was traced back to contact with backyard poultry; this outbreak resulted in two human deaths (CDC 2019b).

Toxoplasmosis has received a great deal of publicity as a zoonotic disease because of its ability to cause fetal injury when pregnant women are infected; it also causes central nervous system disease in patients with acquired immunodeficiency syndrome (AIDS). Though cats are the definitive host of *Toxoplasma gondii* and the only species that shed infective oocysts, the overall risk of infection from cats is very low; the disease is more likely to be acquired through ingestion of contaminated soil by children in rural areas, ingestion of undercooked meat, handling or inhaling contaminated dust, or drinking contaminated water than by direct contact with a cat (Greene and Levy 2006). Rather than avoid cat ownership, pregnant women should be advised to adopt cats that are healthy and at least 1 year old because these cats are less likely to be infected with *Toxoplasma gondii*. If possible, someone else in the household should change the litter pan during the pregnancy period; the litter pan should be changed daily, and the litter should be disposed of properly. If the pregnant woman must change the litter pan herself, she should wear gloves, remove the fecal waste daily, and wash her hands with soap and hot water afterward.

21.3.3.1 Prevention Measures

Exposure to diseases spread by feces can be reduced by wearing utility or disposable gloves, and by removing gloves and handwashing immediately after finishing a task that involves contact with animal feces. When reusable utility gloves are used, these must be cleaned and disinfected after each use. To reduce fecal splashes to the oral cavity, care should be taken to physically remove all visible fecal material from environmental surfaces before using hoses, and workers should wear a mask when hosing or cleaning cages or runs. Eating should not be allowed in animal treatment, housing, or holding areas. All surfaces contaminated with feces should be thoroughly cleaned first and then disinfected using a disinfectant with demonstrated efficacy against the pathogen of concern. Note that the infective stages of many parasites are not susceptible to common disinfectants. Particularly in these cases, physical cleaning with a detergent and thorough rinsing and drying of the exposed environmental surfaces are critical steps in the sanitation process to remove infective particles from the environment. Food dishes should be cleaned and disinfected or autoclaved between uses. Cages should be cleaned and disinfected between use by different animals.

Adopters and the public should be advised that washing hands after handling feces and before eating and preventing children from ingesting fecal material (including soil contaminated with feces) is key to preventing the fecal-oral spread of disease. As an additional precaution, pets should not be permitted to hunt and consume their prey or eat raw or undercooked meat.

21.3.4 Infections Transmitted Via Contact with Urine or Genital Secretions

In order to minimize the risk of pathogen spread through contact with contaminated urine, personnel should ensure that cages and runs are cleaned and disinfected on a regular schedule to remove urine contamination. Dogs should be walked outdoors and allowed to eliminate in a designated area if appropriate given the pathogen of concern and level of risk anticipated. Appropriate facial protection (i.e. a mask with a face shield or goggles), rubber boots, and gloves should be considered when cleaning and disinfecting enclosures and runs contaminated with urine or genital secretions. Particular care should be taken to cover all cuts and abrasions on the hands with a bandage before donning gloves, and hands should be washed with soap and water after removing gloves.

Infection with *Brucella canis* has been of increasing concern to animal shelters and public health authorities in recent years and warrants special attention. Detection of antibodies against *B. canis* has been reported in at least two populations of shelter dogs (Hubbard et al. 2018; Whitten et al. 2019). Particular attention should be paid to assessing risk in dogs from active breeding operations where dogs are housed in close contact and are subject to frequent movement for breeding or sale (Hensel 2018); many puppy mill operations and hoarding cases encountered by animal shelters share such risk factors. The United States Department of Agriculture (USDA) does not consider brucellosis to be a curable disease in dogs and recommends against re-homing of confirmed brucellosis positive dogs (USDA 2015); however, the risk of zoonosis from a neutered dog is thought to be extremely low (Greene and Levy 2006). For this reason, if re-homing is pursued, it is recommended that dogs undergo surgical sterilization and long-term antibiotic therapy including lifetime laboratory testing to evaluate infective potential (USDA 2015). There must be full disclosure and counseling provided about brucellosis to anyone who chooses to adopt an animal infected with this disease; animals should not be adopted out to the immunocompromised or members of the high-risk categories. Canine brucellosis is a reportable disease in most states and, in some areas, local laws or directives may prohibit the adoption of affected dogs.

21.3.5 Infections Transmitted through Airborne Exposure

Diseases that are acquired through exposure to airborne pathogens often have multiple modes of transmission. Animals may or may not have clinical signs of infection, yet transmission to humans can still cause severe disease. Personnel interacting with animals that have been diagnosed with airborne pathogens of concern should avoid close facial contact with such animals and consider wearing protective equipment sufficient to prevent inhalation of aerosolized pathogens (e.g. fitted face masks, face shield and/or goggles) when such contact is required.

21.3.6 Vector-Borne Pathogens

Dogs and cats, like humans, are not the reservoir for most vector-borne diseases; they are accidental hosts. They serve as a mechanism of transmitting the infected vectors (i.e. ticks or fleas) to humans. Shelters should maintain an effective vector-control program to treat affected animals and ensure that tick or flea infestations are not a problem within the shelter; treatment plans for vector-borne diseases in individual animals should also address the vector itself. When handling tick-infested animals, personnel should wear gloves, be sure that exposed skin surfaces (i.e. arms, legs) are covered, and wash their hands after glove removal.

Ticks should be removed promptly because many diseases are transmitted only after the tick has been attached to the animal for a few days. Ticks should also be removed systematically to ensure that the removal process does not create or exacerbate problems for the animal or create a vector-borne pathogen risk to the humans involved. Several topical and systemic acaricides are labeled for such use in dogs or cats (note that products must be used only for the species identified on the label); however manual removal may be desirable or necessary in some cases. A purpose-made tick removal device or fine hemostatic or thumb forceps may be employed for this purpose; ticks should not be removed directly by hand. Ticks should be grasped as close to the skin as possible and extracted using slow, steady pressure. Avoid crushing, twisting, or jerking the tick out of the skin so as not to increase the animals' exposure to pathogens within the tick or cause the mouthparts to break off in the skin, which can lead to granuloma formation (CAPC 2020). Ticks should be killed by submersion in isopropyl alcohol and disposed of in an appropriate biomedical waste container; they should not be crushed or flushed down a sewage system. The use of appropriate sedation and analgesia should be considered if manual removal of multiple ticks is necessary. Hand hygiene (handwashing is preferable) must be performed after glove removal. Table 21.2 lists common zoonotic vector-borne pathogens.

21.3.7 Anthroponoses

Anthroponoses are diseases that are spread from humans to animals. They are considered less common than zoonotic diseases. Most anthroponoses are unlikely to be of concern to shelters, but veterinarians should be particularly aware of diseases such as MRSA that are a growing concern in human hospitals and for animals involved in pet therapy programs. Measures that can be taken by shelters to prevent the spread of MRSA include judicious use of antibiotics to avoid creating resistance, handwashing, and strict attention to sanitation. Table 21.3 lists common anthroponotic pathogens.

21.4 Adoption Considerations

Whenever making medical decisions about adoption potential, in addition to complying with state regulations regarding the manage-

Table 21.2 Common zoonotic vector-borne pathogens.

Pathogen	Domestic species	Vector	Description
Anaplasma phagocytophilum (Anaplasmosis)	Dogs	*Dermacentor, Amblyomma, Ixodes, Rhipicephalus, Haemaphysalis,* and *Otobius* tick spp. (depends on region)	Gram-negative, obligate, intracellular bacterium
Borrelia burgdorferi (Lyme disease)	Dogs	*Ixodes* tick spp.	Bacterial spirochete
Ehrlichia chafeenisis, E. ewingii (Ehrlichiosis)	Dogs	*Dermacentor, Amblyomma, Ixodes, Rhipicephalus, Haemaphysalis,* and *Otobius* tick spp. (depends on region)	Gram-negative, obligate, intracellular bacterium
Rickettsia rickettsii (Rocky Mountain spotted fever)	Dogs	*Dermacentor, Amblyomma,* and *Rhipicephalus* tick spp.	Gram-negative, intracellular, coccobacillus
Rickettsia felis, R. typhi (Typhus)	Cats	*Ctenocephalides* fleas	Gram-negative, obligate, intracellular bacterium
Yersinia pestis[a] (Plague)	Dogs, Cats, Rodents	Fleas	Gram-negative bacillus Transmitted via flea bites, contact with contaminated fluid or tissue (including ingestion of infected rodents), aerosol

[a] *Y. pestis* is a potential bioterrorism agent. Cases of plague in a domestic animal or human should be reported to the Department of Health. Treatment in the shelter is **NOT** recommended, nor should animals with this disease be adopted from a shelter.

Table 21.3 Common anthroponotic pathogens.

Pathogen	Description	Common Routes of Transmission
Clostridium difficile	Gram-positive bacillus	Direct contact or environmental
Group A *Streptococcus* and *Streptococcus pneumoniae*	Gram-positive cocci	Direct or close contact to dogs and cats
Methicillin-resistant *Staphylococcus aureus* (MRSA)	Gram-positive cocci Identified in dogs	Readily spread via direct contact or fomites
Mycobacterium tuberculosis (Tuberculosis)	Pathogenic bacteria Identified in dogs	Aerosolized droplets and close contact

ment of the disease, veterinarians must also consider the shelter's ability to treat the disease successfully and verify the cure. This may be difficult for some zoonotic diseases (e.g. brucellosis). The handling of some animals may require input from the Department of Health or be subject to local regulations. Regardless of the resources consulted, outside of legal restrictions, the ultimate responsibility for determining medical suitability for adoption and the need to provide adopter counseling regarding medical issues should rest with the veterinarian. Good written medical records and adopter counseling are essential to protect the health of the adopter and the adopted animal and help limit the shelter's liability if a zoonotic disease should occur.

Shelters should be mindful that the populations most at risk for contracting zoonotic diseases include veterinarians and animal care workers, the immunocompromised, elderly, infants, and children under the age of five. It is important to take appropriate precautions to ensure their safety when handling and adopting animals. A risk analysis should be performed to minimize the possibility of spreading infection to staff, volunteers, and the public, and adopters should be educated about precautions to prevent pathogen transmission from animals. The decision to release an animal from the shelter when that animal is known to have been infected with a zoonotic disease should be based on: (i) the risk of transmission from the animal to the caregiver and other members of the household; (ii) the risk of disease actually developing in the owner and other members of the household; and (iii) the risk of fatality in humans. For example, one would not release a dog or cat for adoption that had been potentially exposed to rabies via a bite from a wild animal. However, a puppy who has completed treatment for giardiasis might be released to immunosuppressed owners as long as they are made aware of the presumed risks (i.e. there is scant direct evidence that transmission of *Giardia* from dogs to humans occurs so the risk is considered very small) and advised of preventive measures needed to protect themselves.

Shelter veterinarians are often asked for advice about human health when a zoonotic disease is encountered because veterinarians are frequently at the forefront of such knowledge, including the symptoms found in both humans and animals. Veterinarians are cautioned to use their best judgment, and to refrain from offering an opinion that could be interpreted as practicing human medicine. Questions about human health should always be referred to a physician.

21.4.1 Adopting to High-Risk People

Immunocompromised individuals are at higher risk for contracting a zoonotic disease, but there is no reason to avoid adopting clinically healthy animals to high-risk individuals if they are informed of the risk and precautions to take to protect themselves. Though the public often associates immunocompromise solely with human immunodeficiency virus (HIV) infection and AIDS, other groups of individuals should be considered at high-risk. These include, but are not limited to, people who have chronic renal failure, diabetes mellitus, cancer, severe or extensive burns, or liver cirrhosis; are malnourished or on long-term steroid therapy, chemotherapy, or have undergone organ transplantation; pregnant women; newborns; children under 5 years of age; the elderly; and people who have been recently hospitalized, especially if they have (or had) indwelling catheters, tubes, or synthetic implants. In general, high-risk individuals should consider avoiding adopting pets that:

- Are younger than 6 months of age
- Have active cases of diarrhea
- Have fleas or ticks
- Have long, unclipped nails
- Are overly aggressive in behavior or play.

Other precautions that high-risk individuals should be advised to take to avoid contracting a zoonotic disease include frequent handwashing during the day, especially after handling their pet or their pet's excretions, and before eating, smoking, brushing or flossing teeth, or handling contact lenses. They should avoid letting pets lick them on the mouth or wounds, and wear gloves whenever administering oral medications. They should avoid feeding pets raw food, unprocessed meat, or unpasteurized dairy products and should be conscious of pet food recalls such as the one that linked multidrug-resistant *Salmonella* to pig ear pet treats (CDC 2019c). High-risk pet owners should dispose of cat and dog excrement promptly, keep cats indoors and dogs on a leash when outside to avoid hunting and eating their prey and to make sure the pet's environment is clean. It is very important that they take their pets to the veterinarian for regular examinations, including fecal analysis and routine deworming, to ensure the pet is clinically healthy and parasite free (Greene and Levy 2006). Screening for diseases that cause immunosuppression in animals, such as FeLV and FIV in cats, should be considered. Though FeLV and FIV are not zoonotic, they may render the animals more susceptible to other diseases.

21.5 Consulting with the Department of Health

All shelters should establish a working relationship with their state public health veterinarian or state veterinarian. This relationship will facilitate the two-way flow of information and provide the shelter personnel with the professional support they will need before and during events of public health concern, including outbreaks of zoonotic diseases, disasters, or emergencies. State public health veterinarians are local and state veterinarians who are employed by the state health department and consult with physicians, emergency rooms, legislators, local officials, schools, health departments and the general public on preventing exposures to and controlling zoonosis (NASPHV n.d.). A list of state public health veterinarians is available online at http://www.nasphv.org/Documents/StatePublicHealthVeterinariansByState.pdf. State animal health officials are employed primarily by the state agriculture department and mostly target livestock diseases (some of which can be zoonotic). Their activities may concentrate on benefits and protection to livestock and the livestock industry, but they conduct disease surveillance and other activities to improve animal health by preventing, controlling and eliminating animal disease (USDA 2020) A list of state animal health officials is available online at http://www.aphis.usda.gov/animal_health/vet_accreditation/downloads/state-animal-health-officials.pdf.

The National Notifiable Disease Surveillance System (NNDSS) helps monitor, control and prevent serious diseases. Some infectious diseases are nationally notifiable; diagnosis or suspicions of these diseases must be reported to the local health/agriculture agency which, in turn, notifies the national health/veterinary agency (CDC) of a disease. Some factors that determine whether a disease is notifiable include the nature of the infectious agent, the danger to the public and the likelihood that it will develop into an epidemic. In some urgent cases, the veterinarian may contact the CDC directly and bypass the state agency. Other diseases must be reported, a process that requires practitioners to inform the local health or veterinary agency of a suspected or confirmed case of a disease. Some diseases are reportable only at the state or local level; that is, each state or local health department decides what conditions, in addition to the nationally notifiable conditions, they require veterinarians to report. Shelters should contact their local or state health departments to obtain a list of reportable and notifiable diseases. The list of notifiable diseases is updated periodically as new and emerging pathogens are identified; diseases may also be removed from the list. The current list may be found on the NNDSS website (https://wwwn.cdc.gov/nndss/conditions).

21.6 Conclusion

Many families consider pets to be members of the family, and the emotional and physical benefits of pet ownership have been demonstrated repeatedly. While shelters must be vigilant about the prevention of zoonosis, the risk of contracting a zoonotic disease is low for the immune-competent population when basic practices in personal hygiene and preventive pet care are practiced. High-risk individuals can also enjoy pet ownership if a few precautions are taken regarding careful pet selection, regular health checks, and routine preventive care.

A broad, responsible, and balanced approach to handling diseases in shelters that have the potential to be zoonotic is warranted. Managing the shelter environment, using PPE effectively, practicing safe animal handling and maintaining shelter operations should all be conducted with the most likely pathogens to be encountered and their means of transmission in mind. Not only will this approach ensure due diligence in protecting and promoting public health, but it will ensure that shelter personnel and animal populations are set up for a healthy and successful shelter experience.

21.A Sample Animal Bite Investigation Form

Shelter name: ____________________ Shelter phone number: ____________________

Shelter address: ____

Veterinarian in Charge of Shelter: ____

Employee last name: ____________________ Employee first name: ____________________

1. Date of Injury: ___/___/_____ (mm/dd/yyyy)   2. Time of Injury: ___ am/pm (circle one)
3. Location where the injury occurred? (Check one box only)
   - ☐ Examination Room
   - ☐ Procedure Room *(X - ray, EKG,* etc.*)*
   - ☐ Kennel
   - ☐ Euthanasia Room
   - ☐ Outside Patient Care Area *(hallway, unloading bay,* etc.*)*
   - ☐ Other, describe: ____________________
4. What is employee's job category? (Check one box only)
   - ☐ Veterinarian
   - ☐ Veterinary Technician
   - ☐ Kennel Personnel
   - ☐ Other: (describe): ____________________
5. How was employee employed at the time of the injury? ☐ Full time ☐ Part-time
6. Was this the employee's regular shift? ☐ Yes ☐ No
7. Was the employee working overtime? ☐ Yes ☐ No
8. What species of animal caused the injury? ☐ Cat ☐ Dog ☐ Other (describe) ____
9. Animal ID #_____
10. Was the animal that caused the injury previously owned? ☐ Yes ☐ No ☐ Don't know
11. Was the animal vaccinated against rabies? ☐ Yes ☐ No ☐ Don't know
12. If yes; date of rabies vaccination___/___/_____ (mm/dd/yyyy)
13. Describe the signs and symptoms the animal had or has

    ____

    ____

    ____

    ____

    ____
14. Is the animal available for observation? ☐ Yes ☐ No
15. Date animal was placed under observation ___/___/_____ (mm/dd/yyyy) ☐ NA
16. Disposition of animal (Check one)
    - ☐ Died   Date ___/___/___ (mm/dd/yyyy)
    - ☐ Euthanized   Date ___/___/___ (mm/dd/yyyy)
    - ☐ Released from observation   Date ___/___/___ (mm/dd/yyyy)
    - ☐ Other (describe) _____date ___/___/_____ (mm/dd/yyyy)
17. Was the animal tested for rabies? (Check one) ☐ Yes ☐ No ☐ Don't know
18. If yes; date of test _____/_____/_____ (mm/dd/yyyy)

19. Type of specimen sent (Check all) ◻ Brain stem ◻ Cerebellum ◻ Cerebrum ◻ Entire head ◻ Other (specify) ___________

20. If yes; name of laboratory: ____

21. Circle on the diagram below the location(s) of the injury(ies):

22. For each injury site identified in the figure above, indicate the type of wound obtained (A = avulsion; L = laceration; P = puncture; S = scratch)

Injury site #	Wound type (Letter)	Injury site #	Wound type (Letter)
________	________	________	________
________	________	________	________
________	________	________	________

23. Describe the circumstances leading to this bite injury: ______________________________
____
____
____
____

24. Did the employee complete a tetanus vaccination series? ◻ Yes ◻ No ◻ Don't know

25. When was the last tetanus vaccine given? ___/___/___ (mm/dd/yyyy) ◻ Don't know

26. Did the employee complete a rabies vaccination series? ◻ Yes ◻ No ◻ Don't know

27. When was the employee's last rabies vaccine given? ___/___/___ (mm/dd/yyyy) ◻ Don't know

28. When was the employee's last rabies vaccination titer taken? ___/___/___(mm/dd/yyyy) ◻ Don't know

29. Was the employee's rabies RFIT titer ≥ 1: 5? □ Yes □ No □ Don't know
30. Was the employee referred to a physician/ER for follow-up? □ Yes □ No
31. Physician/ER name ______
    Address____________
    Physician's/ER's phone number______
32. Reported to □ State DOH □ Local DOH (Check one) on ___/___/___ (mm/dd/yyyy)
32. Follow up recommendations and other information ____
    ____
    ____
    ____
    ____

Source: Wiley Blackwell

References

Agger, W.A., Goethert, H.K., and Telford, S.R. III (2005). Tularemia, lawn mowers, and rabbits' nests. *Journal of Clinical Microbiology* 43: 4304–4305.

Andersen, L.A., Levy, J.K., McManus, C.M. et al. (2018). Prevalence of enteropathogens in cats with and without diarrhea in four different management models for unowned cats in the Southeast United States. *Veterinary Journal* 236: 49–55.

Babovic, N., Cayci, C., and Carlsen, B.T. (2014). Cat bite infections of the hand: assessment of morbidity and predictors of severe infection. *Journal of Hand Surgery* 39 (2): 286–290.

Centers for Disease Control (2019a). Outbreak of Multidrug-resistant *Campylobacter* Infections Linked to Contact with Pet Store Puppies. https://www.cdc.gov/campylobacter/outbreaks/puppies-12-19/index.html (accessed 22 April 2020).

Centers for Disease Control (2019b). Outbreaks of *Salmonella* Infections Linked to Backyard Poultry. https://www.cdc.gov/salmonella/backyardpoultry-05-19/index.html (accessed 22 April 2020).

Centers for Disease Control (2019c). Outbreak of Multidrug-Resistant *Salmonella* Infections Linked to Contact with Pig Ear Pet Treats. https://www.cdc.gov/salmonella/pet-treats-07-19/index.html (accessed 22 April 2020).

Centers for Disease Control (2017). Zoonotic Diseases. https://www.cdc.gov/onehealth/basics/zoonotic-diseases.html (accessed 30 April 2020).

Centers for Disease Control and Prevention (2018). Zoonotic Diseases. https://www.cdc.gov/onehealth/basics/zoonotic-diseases.html (accessed 20 June 2018).

Companion Animal Parasite Council (2020). Ticks. https://capcvet.org/guidelines/ticks (accessed 22 April 2020).

Cutler, S.J., Fooks, A.R., and van der Poel, W.H. (2010). Public health threat of new, reemerging, and neglected zoonoses in the industrialized world. *Emerging Infectious Diseases* 16 (1): 1–7. https://doi.org/10.3201/eid1601.081467. (Accessed May 13, 2020).

Eagle Protect (2017). Why Medical Grade Disposable Gloves are Essential for Food Safety. http://blog.eagleprotect.com/why-medical-grade-disposable-gloves-are-essential-for-food-safety (accessed 22 April 2020).

Greene, C.E. and Goldstein, E. (2006). Bite wound infections. In: *Infectious Diseases of the Dog and Cat*, 3e (ed. C.E. Greene), 495–510. St. Louis: Elsevier Inc.

Greene, C.E. and Levy, J.K. (2006). Immunocompromised people and shared human and animal infections. Zoonoses, sapronoses, and anthroponoses. In: *Infectious Diseases of the Dog and Cat*, 3e (ed. C.E. Greene), 1051–1068. St. Louis: Elsevier.

Hensel, M.E., Negron, M., and Arenas-Gamboa, A.M. (2018). Brucellosis in dogs and public health risk. *Emerging Infectious Diseases* 24 (8): 1401.

Hill, S., Cheney, J., and Taton-Allen, G. (2000). Prevalence of enteric pathogens in cats. *Journal of the American Veterinary Medical Association* 216: 687–692.

Hubbard, K., Wang, M., and Smith, D.R. (2018). Seroprevalence of brucellosis in Mississippi shelter dogs. *Preventive Veterinary Medicine* 159: 82–86.

Jha, S., Khan, W.S., and Siddiqui, N.A. (2014). Mammalian bite injuries to the hand and their management. *Open Orthopedics Journal* 27 (8): 194–198.

Mason, G. and Littin, K.E. (2003). The humaneness of rodent pest control. *Animal Welfare* 12: 1–38.

Microbiology, N.R. (2011). Microbiology by numbers. *Nature Reviews Microbiology* 9: 628.

National Association of State Public Health Veterinarians (n.d.). About State Public Health Veterinarians. http://www.nasphv.org/aboutPHVs.html (accessed 30 April 2020).

National Association of State Public Health Veterinarians (2015). Model Infection Control Plan for Veterinary Practices. http://www.nasphv.org/Documents/ModelInfectionControlPlan.docx (accessed 23 April 2020).

Predolich, M. (2015). What's the Difference Between Industrial and Medical Grade Gloves. https://www.yourglovesource.com/blogs/glove-knowledgebase/49932161-whats-the-difference-between-industrial-and-medical-grade-gloves (accessed 22 April 2020).

Spain, C.V., Scarlett, J.M., Wade, S.E. et al. (2001). Prevalence of enteric zoonotic agents in cats less than 1 year old in Central New York State. *Journal of Veterinary Internal Medicine* 15: 33–38.

Steuven, H. (n.d.). Not All Gloves are Equal and it Matters in Food Safety. https://www.dininggrades.com/blog/not-all-gloves-are-equal-and-it-matters-in-food-safety (accessed 11 April 2020).

United States Department of Agriculture (2015). Best Practices for *Brucella canis* Prevention and Control in Dog Breeding Facilities. https://www.aphis.usda.gov/animal_welfare/downloads/brucella_canis_prevention.pdf (accessed 23 April 2020).

United States Department of Agriculture (2020). Animal Health Program Overview. https://www.aphis.usda.gov/aphis/ourfocus/animalhealth/program-overview (accessed 30 April 2020).

Whitten, T.V., Brayshaw, G., Patnayak, D. et al. (2019). Seroprevalence of *Brucella canis* antibodies in dogs entering a Minnesota humane society, Minnesota, 2016-2017. *Preventive Veterinary Medicine* 168: 90–94.

Zurlo, J.J. (2005). Pasteurella species. In: *Principles and Practice of Infectious Diseases*, 6e (eds. G.L. Mandell, J.E. Bennett and R. Dolin), 2687–2691. Philadelphia: Elsevier Inc.

22

Rabies

G. Robert Weedon[1,2] and Catherine M. Brown[3]

[1] TLC PetSnip, Inc., Lakeland, FL, USA
[2] College of Veterinary Medicine, University of Illinois, Urbana, IL, USA
[3] Massachusetts Department of Public Health, Jamaica Plain, MA, USA

22.1 Overview of Rabies

Rabies is a perfect example for the One Health initiative, recognizing that human health, animal health, and ecosystem health are inextricably linked. It is a highly fatal zoonotic disease that affects the central nervous system (CNS) of mammals. The disease has been around for centuries; it was first described in the twenty-third century BCE (Baer 2007). The Centers for Disease Control and Prevention (CDC) estimates that 40,000–50,000 people in the United States receive treatment annually in the form of post-exposure prophylaxis (PEP) after contact with a potentially rabid animal (CDC 2015); the US public health cost associated with rabies is estimated to be as high as $500 million annually. The World Health Organization (WHO) estimates that more than 15 million people worldwide receive PEP. The CDC and WHO also estimate that worldwide, 59,000 people die annually from the disease.

Rabies, and rabies-like diseases, are caused by neurotropic viruses that are members of the genus Lyssavirus in the family Rhabdoviridae. These agents are enveloped, bullet-shaped ribonucleic acid (RNA) viruses that usually measure 75 × 180 nm (Greene 2012). Antigenic and molecular genetic techniques have demonstrated that several viruses within this genus cause diseases clinically similar to rabies. The only one of these viruses found in the United States is classical rabies virus and the information in this chapter refers solely to that pathogen. Rabies virus is often regarded or referred to as a single viral entity with multiple mammalian hosts (Cleaveland et al. 2001; Dobson and Foufopoulos 2001); however, it may be better described as a metapopulation in which genotypically and phenotypically distinguishable rabies virus variants are adapted to and maintained by a single or a few mammalian species (Childs and Real 2007). The reservoirs for rabies are the mammalian host species that circulate different rabies virus variants, with variable rates of spillover into humans, depending on the virus variant and the natural history of the host species. Rabies can be found worldwide, though several countries are free of any rabies virus variant maintained in terrestrial animals. This information is used by the CDC for the purpose of waiving canine vaccination importation requirements. However, rabies virus variants in bats may still occur in these countries, and the list of countries is subject to change.

Infectious Disease Management in Animal Shelters, Second Edition.
Edited by Lila Miller, Stephanie Janeczko, and Kate F. Hurley.

It is critically important that sheltering and veterinary professionals are knowledgeable about rabies. Though the disease is relatively rare in domestic animal shelters in the United States, the frequency with which animal shelters deal with rabies is higher than in most other settings. This is because shelters handle stray animals that are often unvaccinated, may be immunosuppressed, have a greater risk of exposure to potentially rabid animals, and have been admitted to shelters without background information or a history to indicate whether or not such exposure may have occurred. In addition, some shelters may be involved in international animal rescue programs which, while important for animal welfare concerns, pose a constant risk for the introduction of rabies into the United States depending on the country of origin. Furthermore, changes in behavior that typically signal concerns about rabies are more difficult to discern in stray and relinquished animals whose normal behavior is unknown and which may be altered in unpredictable ways due to the stress experienced in an unfamiliar shelter environment.

22.1.1 Rabies Epidemiology

More than 27,000 cases of animal rabies are reported annually in the world (Greene 2012), but the actual number of cases is estimated to be many times greater for several reasons. First, wildlife that die from the disease are usually unobserved. Second, rabies surveillance relies on a passive public health system that only captures data on cases that involve human and sometimes domestic animal exposures. Third, access to public health services and animal rabies diagnostics is limited in many parts of the world and suspect animals may not be reported or tested. Though all mammals are susceptible to rabies, dogs are the main source of infection in people worldwide (Greene 2012). In the United States, the overall incidence of rabies in domestic animals has decreased since the 1950s (see Figure 22.1). This decrease has largely been driven by a decreasing incidence in dogs due to the institution of mandatory municipal and state vaccination requirements and stray animal control programs. In fact, though dogs may still contract the disease from

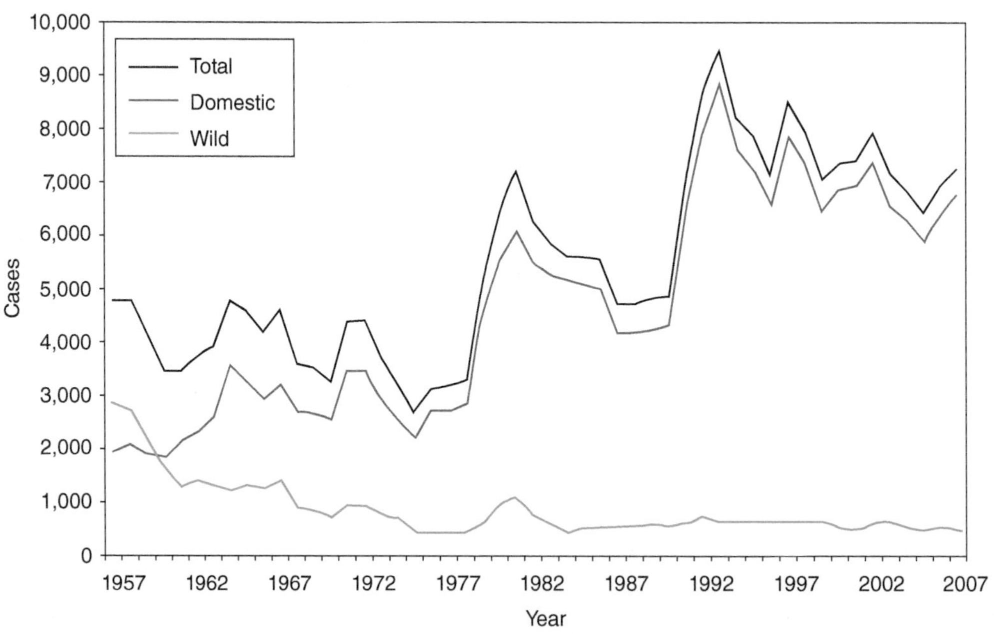

Figure 22.1 Cases of animal rabies in the United States 1957–2007. (*Source:* Blanton (2008) © 2007 American Veterinary Medical Association).

other wild animals, circulation of the canine rabies virus variant has been eliminated in the United States. However, the incidence of rabies in wildlife has skyrocketed during the same time, which is thought to be due, in part, to human encroachment on wildlife habitats (see Figure 22.2). The abrupt increase in wildlife rabies cases in the mid-1970s coincided with the translocation of rabid raccoons from southern Florida to West Virginia, and the subsequent geographic expansion of the raccoon rabies virus variant throughout most of the east coast (Nettles et al. 1979). Despite the dramatic reduction in the incidence of domestic animal rabies cases in the United States, it remains a significant concern due to the severe consequences to human and animal health following exposure and the ongoing potential for exposure arising from contact with wildlife and free-roaming animal populations. An additional source of concern, particularly for animal shelters, is the illegal importation of dogs from rabies endemic countries since appropriate screening and vaccination protocols may not always be followed.

22.1.2 Prevalence and Distribution in the United States

The prevalence and distribution of rabies in the United States and Puerto Rico are driven largely by existing terrestrial wildlife host species and their associated rabies virus variants. While some variation in the geographic distribution of the California skunk and Arizona fox virus variants has occurred, the distributions of the raccoon variant on the east coast, the north-central and south-central skunk variants, the arctic fox variant in Alaska and the mongoose variant in Puerto Rico have remained fairly consistent for several decades (Krebs et al. 1999; Ma et al. 2020) (See Figure 22.2). Spillover of the raccoon virus variant into other wildlife species as well as dogs and cats are reported more frequently than spillover of any other virus variant in the

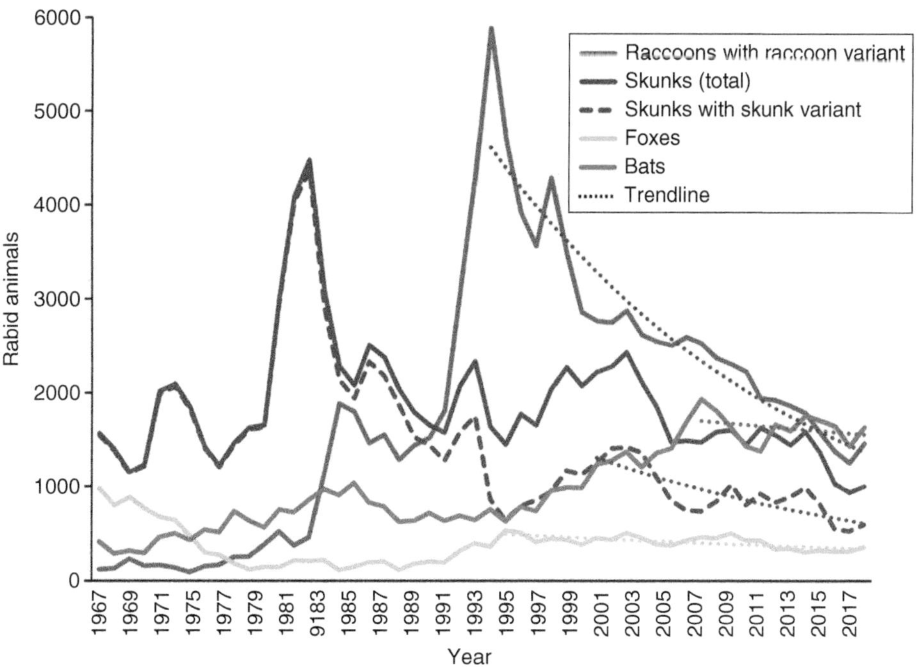

Figure 22.2 Cases of rabies among wildlife in the United States, by year and species, for 1966 through 2017. (*Source:* Graph courtesy of CDC/ Ma et al. *2020*).

United States as identified by confirmed cases of animal rabies (Figure 22.3). This is less likely to represent a specific characteristic of the raccoon virus variant and is probably due to the density of human, domestic dog and cat and urban/suburban wildlife populations in the mid-Atlantic and northeast areas of the country, as well as the relatively social nature of raccoons working in concert to create more opportunities for exposure to other species. Rabies in bats has been documented in every state except Hawaii, and spillover to dogs, cats and wild mammals occurs across the United States. Exposure to bats remains the most common source of rabies transmission to people in the United States. See Figure 22.4a–f for a map of the reported cases of rabies in the United States in several species of wild and domestic animals during 2018.

Animal rabies is a reportable[1] disease in all 50 US states and Puerto Rico. It is also nationally notifiable[2]. Shelters and jurisdictions should know the protocol for how and when to report suspect animal rabies cases to local and state public health departments. The CDC maintains a list of local and state contacts for consultation and notification of rabies cases (https://www.cdc.gov/rabies/resources/contacts.html). The CDC also summarizes and publishes data annually in the Journal of the

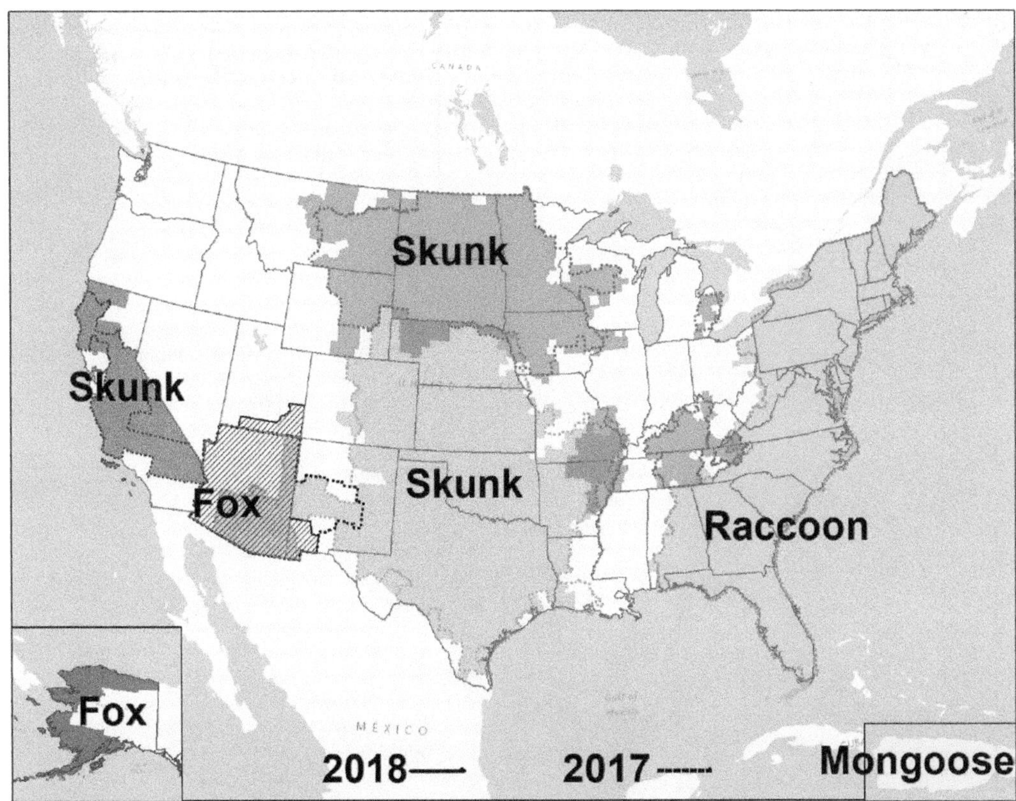

Figure 22.3 Distribution of major rabies virus variants in mesocarnivores in the United States (*Source:* Map courtesy of CDC; Ma et al. 2020).

[1]Reporting, which is mandated, is the act of a veterinarian or laboratory informing the local health/agriculture agency of a suspected or confirmed case of a disease.

[2]Notification is the process of the local health/agriculture agency voluntarily informing the national health/veterinary agency of a disease.

American Veterinary Medical Association (JAVMA), which provides a useful way to stay current on any changes in the epidemiology of rabies. In 2018, the most recent year for which national data was available at the time of submission of this manuscript, 50 states and Puerto Rico reported 4,951 rabid animals and three human cases of rabies to the CDC, representing an 11.2% increase from the 4,454 rabid animals reported in 2017. Of the 4,951 animal cases of rabies, almost 92% (4589) were in a wildlife species, which is a consistent finding. Cats accounted for 67% of rabid domestic animals (Ma et al. 2020); they have been the most commonly identified rabid domestic animal species since 1990. Though data show that more post-exposure prophylaxis regimens are administered for dog bites than cat bites and confirmed cases of rabies in cats are relatively rare (241 rabid cats in 2018, 4.9% of all rabid animals and 1.1% of all cats tested) (Ma et al. 2020), shelters should be aware that cats are more likely than dogs to be carrying rabies virus (Moran et al. 2000) and are the most common domestic animal source of human exposures to the rabies virus in the United States. Rabies in exotic companion mammals, including small rodents (i.e. hamsters, guinea pigs, gerbils, rats, and mice), and lagomorphs can occur but is considered very rare.

22.2 Rabies Pathophysiology

22.2.1 Transmission, Incubation Period and Disease Course

The transmission of rabies virus begins when saliva from an infected host is introduced into

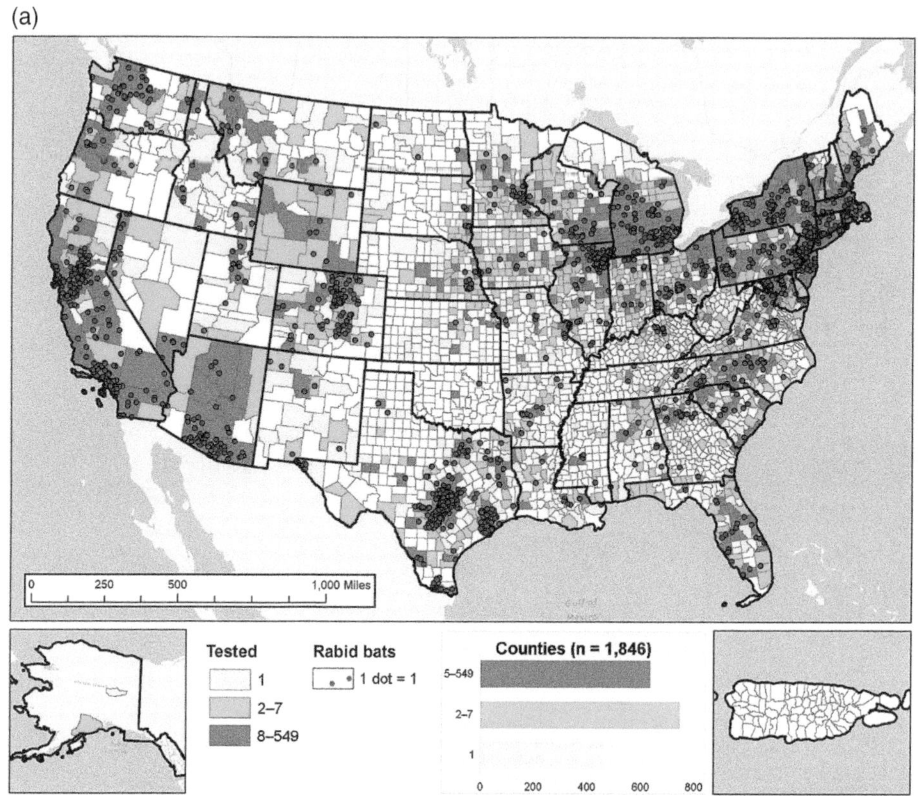

Figure 22.4 (a–f) Reported cases of rabies in several species of wild and domestic animals during 2018 (*Source:* Map courtesy of CDC; Ma et al. 2020).

(b)

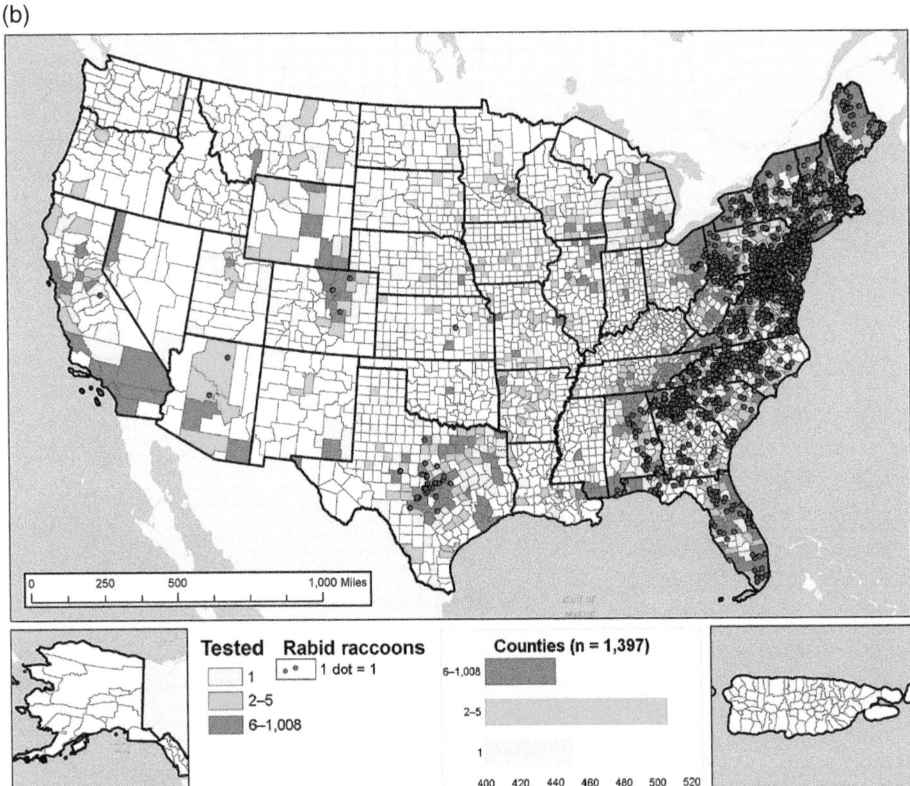

(c)

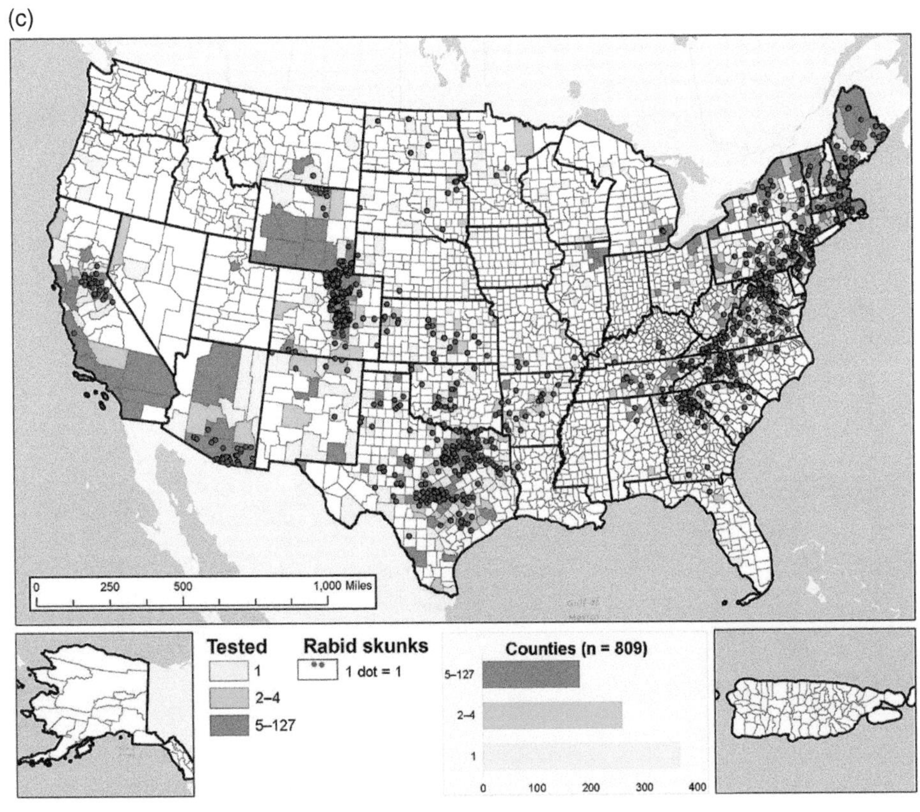

Figure 22.4 (Continued)

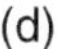

(d)

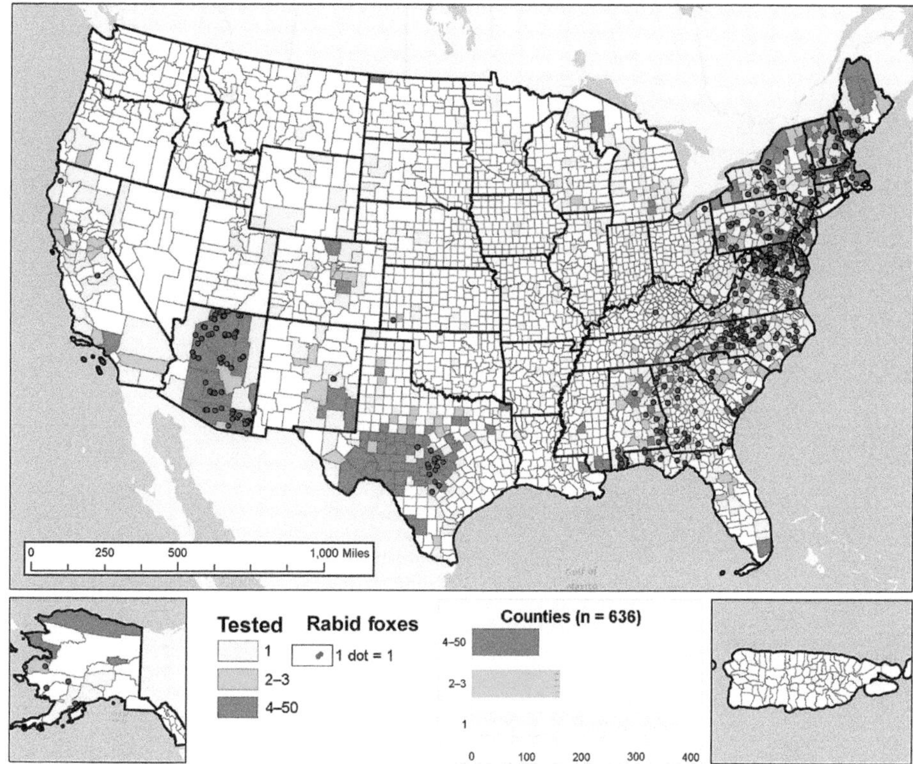

(e)

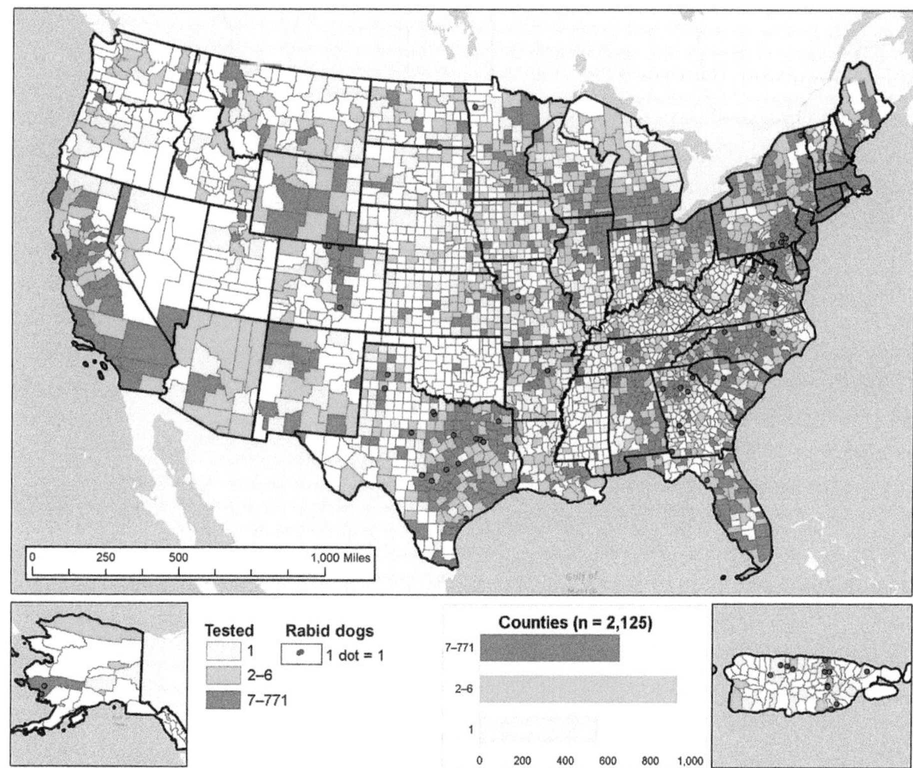

Figure 22.4 (Continued)

(f)

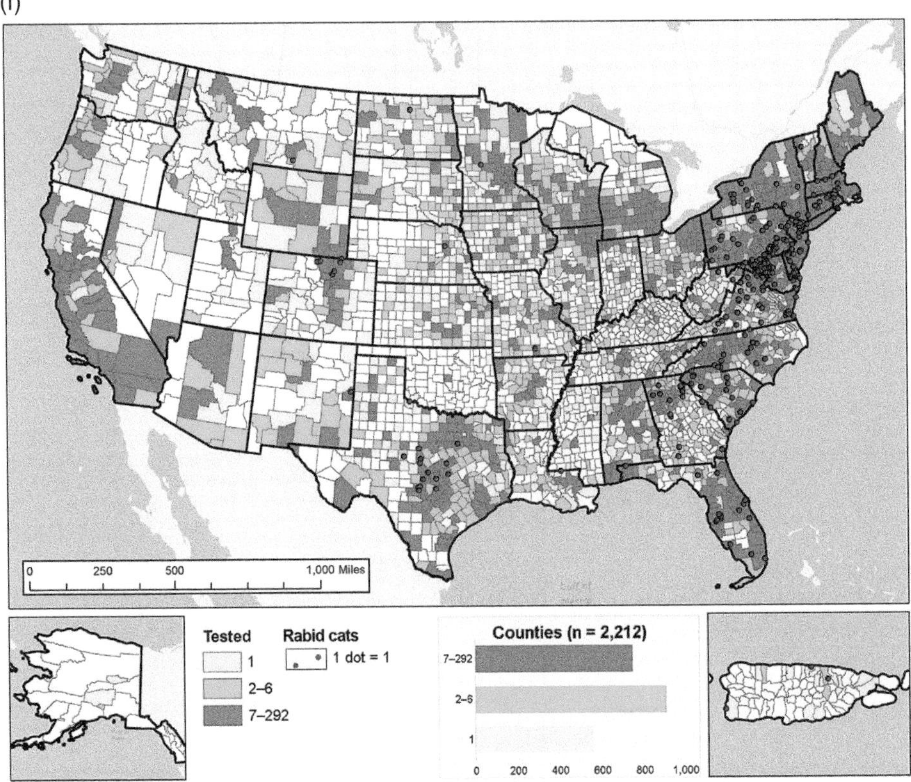

Figure 22.4 (Continued)

an uninfected animal. Bites are the most common way that virus is transmitted (CDC 2016a); less common non-bite routes of exposure include the introduction of infective saliva, or other potentially infectious material such as cerebrospinal fluid (CSF) or neural tissue, into a fresh open wound or mucous membrane (Manning et al. 2008). Aerosol transmission has occurred extremely rarely and only in specific circumstances (e.g. aerosol exposure to rabies virus being used for vaccine preparation and inhalation of aerosolized bat saliva in a cave). Transmission through corneal and solid organ transplantation has also been documented. Oral exposure (ingestion) may result in infection, but with relatively low efficiency (Hanlon et al. 2007). Unlike many other pathogens of concern in shelters, fomites are not considered a route of transmission for rabies and the virus is easily inactivated by most disinfectants.

It is often pointed out that there have been cases of bat rabies virus variants in humans in which the exposure scenario has never been determined (Greene 2012). This is because by the time the diagnosis is made, opportunities to question the patient about possible exposures are no longer available. In all cases, the most likely explanation is that the patient received an unnoticed bite from a bat. Bat bites are very small and these exposures may go undetected. National recommendations include consideration of PEP for persons who awake to find a bat in the room; have direct contact with a bat and are unable to rule out that a bite or scratch has occurred; or for children or mentally incapacitated persons who are found in the room with a bat and are unable to report if they had direct contact with the bat, unless the bat is available for testing and tests negative. If a bat is observed under any of these circumstances and cannot be submitted for testing, it is important to consult with the local health department to determine if an exposure has occurred and PEP is recommended.

The incubation period for rabies is highly variable in all species. In domestic animals, it is generally 3–12 weeks, but can range from several days to months, rarely exceeding six months (Beran 1994). In humans, incubation periods of several days to years have been reported, however, the typical incubation period is one to three months (Iowa State University 2012). Once introduced into a susceptible animal, the virus may replicate in muscle tissue at the site of inoculation before invading local nerves. It is then transported through peripheral nerves to the CNS. Centrifugal spread from the brain to organs throughout the body, including the salivary glands, results in an infected animal capable of transmitting the virus (Jackson and Fu 2013). Disease progression is rapid, and animals may show clinical signs for only a short time before death.

It is important to note that exposure to the rabies virus does not mean that infection and ultimately disease will occur. Not all rabid animals will transmit the virus to animals or people that they bite. Viral shedding is estimated to occur in 50–90% of infected animals, and the amount of virus in the saliva varies from a trace to high titers. Variability in clinical signs and incubation periods may be related to the specific site(s) of the primary CNS lesion(s) or the viral variant, and the dose and route of infection (Hanlon et al. 2007). The disease may also be influenced by host factors such as the age and immune status of the patient.

22.2.2 Clinical Signs

Rabies causes an encephalitis that results in varying neurologic signs. The clinical signs and progression of rabies have been classically divided into two major types: the psychotropic, or "furious" form, and the paralytic, or "dumb" form. This classification and progression of infection are artificial because rabies can be quite variable in its presentation, and atypical signs are commonly seen. Not all animals progress through all the clinical stages (Greene 2012). It is important to note that in the shelter setting, particularly with the dumb form, it may be difficult to distinguish infected animals from animals that have altered behavior and may be withdrawn due to the stress of the shelter environment.

There are no known definitive or species-specific clinical signs of rabies (Hanlon et al. 2007) and rabies should be considered as a differential diagnosis even if "classic" clinical signs are not present. It is also critical to note that viral shedding in saliva can begin before the onset of clinical signs, increasing the opportunity for human exposure to the virus. While the absence of dramatic neurologic abnormalities cannot be used to absolutely rule out the possibility of rabies infection (Greene 2012), in domestic animals, clinical signs will develop within the short period of time that observation of the animal is required (e.g. 10 days) following possible exposure of a person or another domestic animal by the animal.

Clinical signs of rabies are variable but include inappetence or increased appetite, dysphagia, cranial nerve deficits, abnormal behavior, ataxia, paralysis, altered vocalization, dilation of the pupils and seizures; they can also include common signs of infectious disease, i.e. vomiting, diarrhea, fever, etc. It is particularly important for shelters holding animals for rabies observation to be aware of the range of non-neurologic as well as neurologic clinical signs that rabid animals may exhibit. Progression to death is rapid. There are currently no known effective rabies antiviral drugs (NASPHV 2016).

During the prodromal or early phase in dogs, which usually lasts two to three days, apprehension, nervousness, anxiety, solitude, variable fever, or licking, chewing or scratching at the site of the bite may be noted (Greene 2012). The dumb or paralytic form of the disease, which may be more common in dogs, usually develops within two to four days after the first clinical signs are observed. Dogs may exhibit a dropped jaw and begin to salivate or froth excessively, which is thought to be a result of the inability to swallow. These signs resemble choking, and this may lead to human exposure when staff react by assuming there is a foreign object in the dog's throat and open its mouth to try to remove it. Respiratory failure is often the final cause of death. The furious form of the disease is rarer in dogs, usually lasts for one to seven days and is associated with forebrain involvement. Dogs become restless and irritable and are hypersensitive to auditory and visual stimuli. They frequently become excitable, photophobic, and hyperesthetic, and may bark or snap at imaginary objects or eat unusual objects (pica). Dogs confined in cages in shelters may attack or bite the cage. They often have seizures and die as a result of the seizure or paralysis.

Cats more consistently develop the furious form of the disease, showing erratic and unusual behavior. They may appear anxious and may stare or have a blank look in their eyes. They may make vicious, striking movements and attempt to bite or scratch at moving objects (Greene 2012). However, cats may develop the paralytic or dumb form, or transition to paralytic signs, after the initial furious manifestations by day five of onset of clinical signs, or directly after the prodromal phase with few or no signs of excitement. In the author's experience, hind limb paralysis is frequently reported. Cats generally die after three to four days of illness (Greene 2012).

22.2.3 Diagnosis

There are currently no ante-mortem diagnostic tests available to reliably diagnose rabies in a case of suspected human or animal exposure due to the limited and variable distribution of the virus outside of the CNS. Definitive diagnosis requires submission of brain tissue following death or euthanasia of the animal. A diagnosis of rabies can be made if the virus is detected in any part of the brain from the suspected animal. However, in order to effectively rule out rabies, the lack of virus in neural tissue taken from both a complete cross-section of the brain stem and from at least one additional location must be confirmed. The cerebellum is preferred as the second sample, but the hippocampus may be substituted if the cerebellum is unavailable. The gold standard for the detection of rabies virus within brain tissue is the direct fluorescent antibody test (dFA), and this is currently the only recommended diagnostic method for routine rabies determination in animals involved in a human or domestic animal exposure in the United States (CDC 2016b).

The head or body of the suspect animal should be cooled, but not frozen, and shipped as soon as possible with hazardous laboratory specimen labeling on the shipping container. If a suspect animal is accidentally frozen prior to collecting the brain specimens, the tissue should be prepared and shipped frozen as freeze–thaw cycles will destroy brain tissue architecture and make the sample untestable. In the case of bats and other small mammals, the entire body may sometimes be submitted for testing (Greene 2012). Guidelines for testing can be found on the CDC website, but veterinarians should always consult with their local rabies diagnostic laboratory to ensure proper timing, preparation, storage, and preservation of samples.

Though not approved for routine testing in this country, other test methodologies are available for rabies diagnosis, including histopathology, immunohistochemistry, electron microscopy, and virus amplification techniques. Recently, a Direct Rapid Immunohistochemical Test (dRIT) has been developed. The test is simple, requires no specialized equipment or infrastructure, and can be successfully performed on samples preserved in glycerol solution for 15 months or frozen for 24 months and in variable conditions of preservation. These qualities make it ideal for testing under field conditions and in developing countries. In one study, when compared to the dFA test, the traditional standard in rabies diagnosis, the dRIT was 100% sensitive and specific (Lembo et al. 2006). The test is currently in use in the United States to enhance routine public health passive surveillance efforts but is appropriate for use only on specimens from animals not involved in a human or domestic animal exposure.

Very recently, the CDC has developed and validated a pan-lyssavirus real-time reverse transcription polymerase chain reaction (RT-PCR) assay, LN34, which shows promise for rabies diagnostics (Gigante et al. 2018). The test is highly sensitive, easy to implement and has the potential for use on deteriorated tissues which are not currently testable using standard diagnostic methods.

22.3 Rabies Prevention and Control

Multiple, jurisdiction-specific issues exist in the practice of rabies prevention and control in animals, and it is ultimately the responsibility of the shelter and the veterinarian to know the local and state regulations and abide by them. Questions about these regulations should be addressed to the local public health authority or the agency that has rabies control authority in the relevant jurisdiction. Best practice guidelines for rabies prevention and control are produced by the National Association of State Public Health Veterinarians (NASPHV) and published as the Compendium of Animal Rabies Prevention and Control. The most current version is accessible through the NASPHV website, www.nasphv.org. Though these guidelines are not legally binding, they do form the basis for many local statutes.

22.3.1 Rabies Vaccination in Animals

Vaccination is the mainstay of worldwide rabies prevention efforts. Rabies is rare in properly vaccinated animals (Frana et al. 2008; Murray et al. 2009). Multiple vaccines are licensed for use in domestic animal species. Shelters often receive animals other than dogs and cats and also operate vaccination clinics for the public; it is essential that vaccines are administered by authorized personnel to the approved species in accordance with the manufacturer's guidelines and state regulations. (State regulations should be followed if they differ from the manufacturer's recommendations.) A list of available vaccines, including inactivated and modified-live virus-vectored products, products for both intramuscular (IM) and subcutaneous (SQ) administration, products with durations of immunity for periods of one to three years, and products with various minimum ages of vaccination can be found in the Rabies Compendium (NASPHV 2016).

22.3.1.1 Legal Requirements

State and/or local laws and regulations govern what species of animals must be vaccinated as well as age requirements, including the youngest age at which vaccination will be recognized and the age by which time vaccination is required. Not all states require rabies vaccination in dogs and/or cats. In those states that do require it, the minimum age for initial vaccine administration, based on the vaccine label, in dogs and cats is three months, and four months is often the age by which the vaccination must legally be given. Regardless of the age of the animal at initial vaccination, booster vaccinations should be given in a manner consistent with the manufacturer's label and in accordance with relevant laws, including a booster vaccination administered one year following the initial vaccination. A valid rabies vaccination certificate should always be issued and signed by authorized personnel. Within twenty-eight days of initial vaccination, a peak rabies virus antibody titer is expected, and the animal can be considered immunized.

Figure 22.5 shows the states that require rabies vaccination in dogs and cats (green), dogs only (yellow), and no requirements (pink); there are no states that require

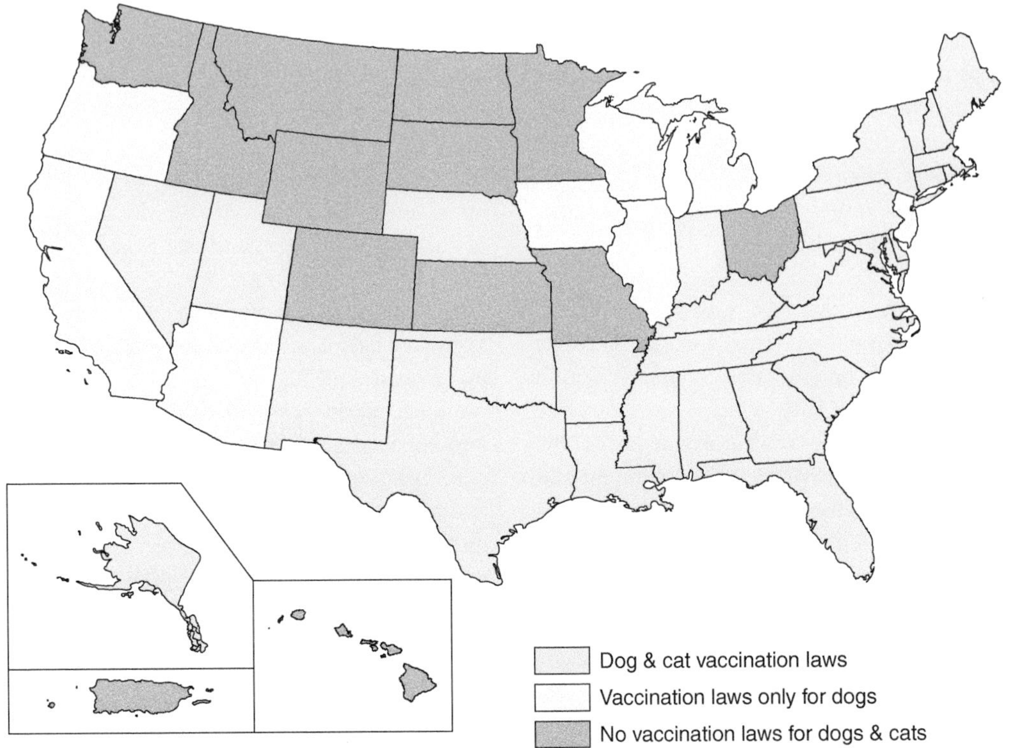

Figure 22.5 Map of vaccination laws by state in the United States and Puerto Rico *Source:* Blanton (2010) © 2007 American Veterinary Medical Association).

vaccination in cats but not dogs. Slightly more than half of the states in the United States require rabies vaccination for both dogs and cats (CDC 2010).

True medical contraindications to rabies vaccination are rare and many jurisdictions do not allow veterinarians to waive the rabies vaccination requirement. Increasingly, however, some jurisdictions have created criteria under which a vaccination exemption for medical reasons can be issued. In jurisdictions that do permit a veterinary exemption, owners should be aware that in the event of a possible rabies exposure, the animal will be subject to the unvaccinated animal protocol that may result in a lengthy quarantine/observation period or euthanasia and testing. As with all other rabies prevention and control measures, shelter staff and veterinarians are responsible for making themselves aware of local requirements.

22.3.1.2 Personnel Authorized to Administer Rabies Vaccinations

Of primary concern to shelters and veterinarians is the question of who can legally administer rabies vaccinations. The Rabies Compendium recommends that "Parenteral animal rabies vaccines should be administered only by or under the direct supervision of a licensed veterinarian on premises" (NASPHV 2016). However, the Compendium also recommends "Rabies vaccines may be administered under the supervision of a licensed veterinarian to animals held in animal shelters before release." State and local laws vary on the matter. It is interesting to note that one state, Utah, specifically mentions that, "Animal shelter employees acting under the indirect supervision of a veterinarian who is under contract with the animal shelter" are legally allowed to administer rabies vaccine

(AVMA 2016). Some jurisdictions mandate that rabies vaccine only be administered by a licensed, accredited veterinarian (e.g. Michigan for vaccinating dogs), others say a licensed veterinarian, while some allow for veterinarians to supervise non-veterinarians administering the vaccine. A small number of states allow for rabies vaccine to be administered by a licensed veterinarian or other qualified/approved individuals, though the requirements for qualification/approval are variable. Texas state law allows a licensed veterinarian to sell a rabies vaccine to a client with whom he/she has a veterinarian-client-patient relationship (VCPR) for the purpose of vaccinating their own livestock. Several states do not specify administration requirements in their laws. Table 22.1 lists the breakdown of states and their requirements compiled by the AVMA in 2016. However, because local and state laws and regulations can and do change, veterinarians and other animal care employees working in any jurisdiction should ensure that they remain current on local requirements.

A related rabies prevention and control issue is the question of who is required to sign a rabies certificate if the vaccine is administered by an individual other than a veterinarian. This is an important point as the signatory is the individual that can be held legally responsible for the administration of that vaccine. There is also jurisdiction-specific variability as to whether or not the signature can be electronic or stamped as opposed to handwritten. Again, these requirements vary by jurisdiction and it is essential that shelter personnel responsible for vaccination be aware of and adhere to local requirements.

22.3.1.3 Frequency and Timing of Revaccination

Another aspect of rabies vaccination that can be a particular source of confusion for veterinarians, as well as the public, is the duration for which an administered rabies vaccination is considered valid. The initial rabies vaccination is legally valid for one year, regardless of the type of vaccine, route of administration, or the age of the animal at the time of administration. Thus, a booster vaccination should be given one year following the initial administration according to all rabies vaccine labels (NASPHV 2016). When prior documentation of a rabies vaccination is not available, the rabies certificate issued for a rabies vaccination administered at the shelter would be for one year. Subsequent vaccinations would be legally valid for either a one-year or three year period depending on the specific product used. Ideally, all rabies vaccine should be handled,

Table 22.1 Individual State Requirements Regarding Rabies Vaccine Administration (AVMA 2016).

Licensed Veterinarians Only	Licensed Veterinarians and Other (Approved) Individuals	Licensed Veterinarians and Others Under the Supervision of a Veterinarian	Not Specified
Colorado, Connecticut, Delaware, District of Columbia, Florida, Georgia, Illinois, Indiana, Iowa, Kentucky, Louisiana, Massachusetts, Michigan, Missouri, Montana, Nebraska, New Hampshire, New Jersey, and Wyoming.	Alabama, Alaska, Arkansas, Mississippi, North Carolina, Oregon, Pennsylvania, Utah, Washington, and West Virginia.	California, Idaho, Kansas, Maine, Maryland, Minnesota, New Mexico, New York;, Oklahoma, Rhode Island, South Carolina, Tennessee, Texas, Vermont, Virginia, and Wisconsin.	Arizona, Hawaii, Nevada, North Dakota, Ohio, and South Dakota.

stored, and administered in accordance with the label on the vaccine product used, though certain jurisdictions may have legal requirements that deviate from that standard; it is incumbent on whoever is administering the vaccine to be aware of the relevant laws and regulations in their jurisdiction.

If a previously vaccinated animal is overdue for any booster rabies vaccination, including the first booster vaccination (due one year after initial vaccination), it should be given another vaccine at that time. Though local laws and regulations may apply, in general, the animal is considered currently vaccinated immediately following the administration of this vaccine and should be placed on a booster vaccination schedule consistent with the label of the vaccine used. There are no laboratory or epidemiologic data to support the annual or biennial administration of three-year vaccines after completion of the initial vaccine series (NASPHV 2016), though, in some cases, local law may require such a protocol.

22.3.1.4 Use of Rabies Virus Antibody Titers

Rabies virus antibody titers are indicative of a response to vaccine or infection. Titers do not directly correlate with protection because other immunologic factors also play a role in preventing rabies and the ability to measure and interpret those other factors is not well-developed. Some jurisdictions (including Hawaii) require evidence of vaccination and rabies virus antibodies for animal importation purposes, but evidence of circulating rabies virus antibodies should not be used as a substitute for current vaccination in managing rabies exposures or determining the need for booster vaccination (NASPHV 2016).

22.3.1.5 Vaccination of Shelter Animals

Various approaches are recommended in different sets of guidelines for vaccination of dogs and cats against rabies in the shelter setting. The American Association of Feline Practitioners (AAFP) (www.catvets.com) has classified rabies as a core vaccine in their 2020 Feline Vaccination Guidelines, and notes rabies vaccination is necessary for all cats in a shelter setting where legally mandated or in an endemic region (Figure 22.3). In jurisdictions where rabies vaccination may not be mandated, the Guidelines advise shelters to consider the benefits of vaccinating more cats against rabies. For a shelter adopting out virtually all of its cats, or where the LOS is commonly months or longer, rabies vaccine should be administered on intake. For shelters with shorter LOS or where not all cats are adopted, rabies vaccination at the time of release is acceptable. If local regulations prohibit the issuance of a rabies certificate for vaccines administered at the shelter by non-veterinary staff, cats should receive a rabies vaccination from a local veterinarian within four weeks of adoption (Stone et al. 2020).

For dogs, the American Animal Hospital Association Canine Vaccination Taskforce (www.aaha.org) recommends that all dogs be vaccinated for rabies before their release from a shelter. If a long-term stay is anticipated or for shelters where virtually all dogs will be adopted, rabies vaccine should be administered on intake with the other core vaccines (Ford et al. 2017).

According to the Association of Shelter Veterinarians *Guidelines for Standards of Care in Animal Shelters*, rabies vaccination on intake is not considered a priority in most shelters, as the risk of exposure to this disease is not high within most shelter environments. However, animals should be vaccinated against rabies when a long-term stay is anticipated, when the risk of exposure is elevated, or when mandated by law (Newbury et al. 2010).

At a minimum, animals over three months of age should be vaccinated for rabies at or shortly following release from the shelter (Newbury et al. 2010). Though rabies vaccination guidelines from national organizations such as the Association of Shelter Veterinarians (ASV), AAFP, the American Animal Hospital Association (AAHA), and NASPHV recommend vaccination before release from the shelter as an animal and public health priority to prevent disease, it is the authors' opinion that since it is critical for new adopters to establish a relationship with a veterinarian as soon as possible, obtaining a legally required rabies vaccination could be seen as a means to try to drive new adopters to see a private practice veterinarian. However, vaccinating in the shelter prior to adoption ensures that the animal receives at least one single rabies vaccine to protect itself and public health; whereas deferring vaccination leaves the animal and the public unprotected for some period of time if a rabies exposure occurs. Deliberate failure to vaccinate eligible animals against rabies prior to release may cause serious liability issues for shelters if it contravenes local laws mandating rabies vaccination of animals by a certain age or recommended shelter vaccination protocols. Since the rabies vaccine must be administered by a licensed veterinarian in most states, if the animal is not going to be vaccinated prior to adoption because it is under three months of age or a veterinarian is not available to administer the vaccination, the adopter must be strongly advised, preferably in writing, to take the pet to a local private practitioner as soon as possible to receive the vaccine.

22.3.2 Management of Potential Rabies Exposure

Shelters, particularly those with animal control functions within their community, have a tremendous impact on the response to and prevention of rabies exposures. It is critical for them to establish contact with the appropriate local and state public health officials before an exposure occurs to understand the rabies regulations and be able to implement necessary control measures as soon as possible to limit the impact of any such exposures.

According to the NASPHV, from a strict public health point of view, stray dogs, cats, and ferrets should be removed from the community, and mechanisms should be put in place to facilitate voluntary surrender of animals to prevent abandonment (NASPHV 2016). However, population management solutions need to be adapted to the local situation (Sparkes et al. 2013) and include sheltering and animal welfare considerations. Therefore, shelters should consult with the local health department to design a mutually agreeable and safe stray animal policy. The following subsections provide general guidance for the management of animals with potential rabies exposure when the biting animal is not available for observation. In cases where the animal that caused that exposure is available for a 10-day observation period, the lengthier holding periods described below are often unnecessary; such determination should be made by the local public health authority.

22.3.2.1 Rabies Exposure in Vaccinated Animals

NASPHV recommends that exposed dogs, cats, and ferrets that are current on rabies vaccination should immediately receive veterinary medical care for assessment, wound cleansing, and booster vaccination. Verification of rabies vaccination status requires the production of a valid rabies certificate, not just a rabies tag on the collar or an owner's verbal assertion. Generally, the animal should be kept under the shelter or owner's control and observed for 45 days (NASPHV 2016) for signs of illness, though local laws and regulations apply and may vary. It is particularly important to know how "owner's control" is defined in local regulations.

A recently published study indicated that the anamnestic responses of dogs and cats with an out-of-date rabies vaccination status were similar to the responses in animals with a current rabies vaccination status (Moore et al. 2015). Accordingly, the Rabies Compendium (NASPHV 2016) updated recommendations for this situation. Dogs and cats that are overdue for a booster vaccination and that have appropriate documentation of having received a USDA-licensed rabies vaccine at least once previously should immediately receive veterinary medical care for an assessment, wound cleansing, and booster vaccination. The animal should be kept under the shelter or owner's control and observed for 45 days for signs of illness or behavior changes. Any changes should be reported immediately to the appropriate authority. It is recommended to check with the local rabies control authority to determine how and if this recommendation has been implemented locally (See Table 22.2).

22.3.2.2 Rabies Exposure in Unvaccinated Animals

NASPHV also recommends that exposed dogs, cats, and ferrets without a documented prior vaccine history should be euthanized immediately (NASPHV 2016). There are currently no USDA-licensed biologics for post-exposure prophylaxis of previously unvaccinated domestic animals, and there is evidence that the use of vaccine alone will not reliably prevent the disease in these animals (Hanlon et al. 2002). Decision making about euthanasia should only be done after it is determined that an exposure has truly occurred, as scratches or contact with certain animals, especially in non-rabies endemic areas, may or may not be deemed an exposure by the local public health authority and recommendations will vary accordingly. Exposure to blood, feces, or urine from a rabid animal is not considered an exposure.

If a shelter or the owner of an exposed but unvaccinated animal is unwilling to have the animal euthanized, advice on recommendations should be obtained from the local public health authority. Current Rabies Compendium (2016) recommendations are that the animal should be placed in strict quarantine for four (dogs and cats) or six (ferrets) months. Strict quarantine in this context means confinement in an enclosure that precludes direct contact with people and other animals. Decisions about strict quarantine should not be undertaken lightly as the social isolation the animal may experience can be detrimental to its welfare. A rabies vaccine should be administered as soon as possible at the time of entry into quarantine to bring the animal up to current rabies vaccination status. It is recommended that the period from exposure to vaccination not exceed 96 hours (See Table 22.2).

22.3.2.3 Animals with Wounds of Unknown Origin

Another often-encountered situation in the shelter setting is the intake of animals with wounds of unknown origin. It can be very

Table 22.2 Summary NASPHV Recommendations for Management of Rabies Exposure.

Scenario	Vaccination Status	General response – NASPHV recommendations[a]
Healthy dog or cat bites another person or animal	May or may not have a current rabies vaccination	Hold and observe for **10 days** for physical or behavioral changes. Do not vaccinate until the observation period is over
Dog or cat exposed to a potentially rabid animal (Includes animals with wounds of unknown origin)	Current or a lapsed rabies vaccination	Administer a rabies booster vaccine and keep under the owner's control and observe for **45 days** for physical or behavioral changes.
Dog or cat exposed to a potentially rabid animal (Includes animals with wounds of unknown origin)	No prior vaccination history documented	Euthanize and test or vaccinate immediately and hold in strict quarantine **for 120 days** (4 months)

[a] This column summarizes current NASPHV recommendations. Final determination regarding the need for observation, revaccination, euthanasia, and/or testing is made by the local public health authority or the agency that has rabies control authority in the jurisdiction where the exposure occurred.

difficult for the shelter to determine if the wound qualifies as a rabies exposure without a history. The way to handle these animals may be dictated by law but otherwise, there is little guidance on this area and, in many cases, there is no clear threshold or certainty with which the cause of a wound must be determined before it is considered to be a potential rabies exposure. Conventional wisdom for owner relinquished animals suggests considering the number of previous rabies vaccinations, interval since the most recent vaccination, current health status, and local rabies epidemiology to determine the most appropriate course of action, but there is no way to apply the same considerations to strays. Decision making must involve the local rabies control authority, and for public protection, include consideration of options referenced in the most recent *Compendium of Animal Rabies Prevention and Control* for dogs and cats that have a known exposure to a rabid or presumably rabid animal (e.g. four to six month quarantine or euthanasia). Though it is time-consuming, some shelters handle these situations with the local rabies control authority on a case-by-case basis, rather than try to create a single blanket policy.

22.3.3 Rabies Prevention in Humans

Shelter staff should always exercise care when handling live animals whose potential for rabies exposure and vaccination history is unknown. All staff and volunteers with animal contact should receive training in appropriate animal handling and use of any personal protective equipment (PPE) that is available to help prevent bites (e.g. towels, gloves, muzzles, cages, etc.) during handling. Suspect rabid animals and wild animals should always be handled with extreme caution, especially if they are ill, injured, or behaving abnormally. Tranquilizers, catchpoles, squeeze cages, and other safety equipment are all important measures to use to avoid being bitten or scratched when humanely handling or euthanizing suspect animals. Staff should know which species in their area are at high risk for rabies. Due to a higher risk of exposure, persons who routinely handle companion animals or wildlife (including veterinarians, veterinary technicians and animal shelter personnel) should receive pre-exposure vaccinations against rabies as well as routine serologic (titer) monitoring and booster vaccinations (if needed based on titer), in accordance with the most current recommendations of the Advisory Committee on Immunization Practices (ACIP) (CDC 2008a; Newbury et al. 2010). Pre-exposure rabies prophylaxis is administered for several reasons. First, though pre-exposure vaccination does not eliminate the need for additional medical evaluation after a rabies exposure, it simplifies management by eliminating the need for human rabies immune globulin and decreasing the number of doses of vaccine required. Second, pre-exposure prophylaxis might offer partial immunity to persons whose post-exposure prophylaxis is delayed. Finally, pre-exposure prophylaxis might provide some protection to persons at risk for unrecognized exposures to rabies (Manning et al. 2008). According to the 2008 ACIP guidelines, vaccine titers should be checked every two years thereafter to ensure that measurable antibody persists (CDC 2008a).

Animal bite wounds and scratches that penetrate the skin should be washed immediately with soap and water for 10 minutes. Povidone iodine can be applied locally to wounds; bites can be irrigated with a 1–4% quaternary ammonium product or 20% aqueous soap solution. Deep puncture wounds can be irrigated with a sterile saline solution. Prompt treatment has been shown to be effective in reducing the chance of rabies virus infection (Greene 2012). Regardless of whether or not a bite was provoked, medical attention should be sought promptly to assess the need for additional wound care, tetanus vaccination, antibiotics, and rabies post-exposure prophylaxis. The local public health authority should be consulted to determine if an exposure has occurred and to learn what the appropriate course of action should be. Regardless of rabies vaccination status, a healthy dog, cat, or ferret that exposes a person or animal should be reported to the local authorities and confined and observed daily for 10 days from the time of the exposure; administration of rabies vaccine to the animal is not recommended during the observation period to avoid confusing signs of rabies with rare adverse vaccine reactions (NASPHV 2016).

It is important to note that human exposure to parenteral animal rabies vaccines does not constitute a risk for rabies virus infection, but human exposure to vaccinia vectored oral rabies vaccines should be reported to state health officials (NASPHV 2016).

Staff in rabies endemic areas should have the proper equipment and training to safely prepare the tissues from rabies suspect animals for submission for diagnostic testing. Individuals tasked with the preparation of specimens for rabies testing should wear appropriate PPE, i.e. heavy rubber gloves, laboratory gown and waterproof apron, boots, surgical masks, protective sleeves, and a face shield during tissue sample handling. The use of band saws or other procedures likely to result in aerosolization of brain tissue or cerebrospinal fluid (CSF) should be avoided. Fortunately, the virus is easily inactivated by most disinfectants, including sodium hypochlorite, 45–75% ethanol, iodine preparations, quaternary ammonium compounds, potassium peroxymonosulfate, accelerated hydrogen peroxide, formaldehyde, phenols, ether, and some other detergents. Standard cleaning and disinfection protocols should be sufficient for environmental decontamination. It is also inactivated by a very low or high pH (below 3 or greater than 11), and is susceptible to ultraviolet radiation, sunlight, and drying (Iowa State University 2012).

22.4 Additional Considerations for Shelters and Shelter Animals

While the incidence of rabies in animal shelters is thought to be rare, the consequences of even a single case to the public, shelter, and other animals can be significant. It is critical to remain vigilant regarding the potential for animals with an unknown history to be admitted to a shelter while incubating the disease. On more than one occasion, a confirmed case of rabies in an animal shelter has sparked a public search for visitors and volunteers who may have been exposed (CDC 2011; O'Quin 2013). In addition to the human health risks, the presence of a rabid animal in a shelter can result in otherwise healthy and adoptable animals having to be euthanized. In one case, 36 dogs had to be euthanized because employees and volunteers might not have consistently followed the shelter's policy of preventing muzzle-to-muzzle contact between dogs (CDC 2011). Finally, though the active circulation of the canine rabies virus variant associated with dog-to-dog transmission has been eliminated in the United States, importation of animals from areas where the variant still actively circulates poses a continual risk for reintroduction (Castrodale et al. 2008; CDC 2008b).

Shelters with a contract to perform animal control duties are often responsible for holding rabies suspect animals, both stray and owned, for 10 days to observe them for signs of rabies if they are responsible for biting a human or another animal. These animals should be housed humanely in isolation in double-sided compartments to minimize staff handling and provided with exercise and behavioral and environmental enrichment during their stay. Feeding, cleaning, and husbandry tasks should be limited to one or two experienced staff members who, in the absence of a veterinarian, have been trained to observe for any changes in physical or behavioral health that should be reported to the veterinarian and public health authorities. Severely ill or injured animals who cannot be humanely held for the 10-day observation period should be euthanized with permission from, and as directed by, the local health department or relevant authority, and tested if deemed appropriate. Shelters that elect to hold animals for 45 days or a four to six-month quarantine need to balance individual animal and population considerations (i.e. their ability to provide humane physical and behavioral care in the shelter during that time).

22.4.1 Rabies Considerations in Animal Translocation

As a result of aggressive spay/neuter messaging and programs, there are areas of the United States where shelters have difficulty finding adoptable puppies, whereas there are other regions of the country where more puppies are relinquished to shelters than can be adopted. As a result, programs have been developed to rescue apparently healthy dogs and cats from euthanasia by transporting them out-of-state to shelters where they will have a better chance of finding a home. For interstate transport, current rabies vaccination is an import requirement for dogs in all states in the United States, and all interstate movement requires a valid USDA health certificate for each animal. The majority of states also require rabies vaccination for cats (Newbury et al. 2010). Stray puppies from rabies endemic areas whose vaccination history is unknown should be at least 12 weeks of age in order to receive a rabies vaccination prior to shipping (ASPCA 2016). Changes to import requirements were introduced by CDC in 2017 and require owners of dogs without proof of sufficient rabies vaccination to apply at least 10 business days prior to travel to obtain an entry permit to import dogs from countries where rabies is endemic in dogs (CDC 2017).

22.4.2 Rabies Vaccination in Community (Feral and Free-Roaming) Cats

Rabies vaccination is an important aspect of the management of feral and free-roaming cats. Having a population of animals with immunity to rabies creates a barrier to help prevent the spread of rabies to pets and people from wildlife vectors. Rabies vaccination is also an important feature of the public and animal health aspects of Trap-Neuter-Vaccinate-Return (TNVR) programs, and should be considered a mandatory component of those programs

Ideally, feral and free-roaming cats should be managed in accordance with the guidelines established by the AAFP (Fischer et al. 2007; Scherk et al. 2013). This includes capturing animals to administer initial vaccines, especially rabies, and recapturing them to administer booster vaccinations. Because the ideal may not always be achievable, research regarding the response to a single vaccination has been conducted. In one study, nearly all cats developed high antibody titers against rabies after a single dose of inactivated rabies vaccine (Fischer et al. 2007). Licensing studies have demonstrated a three to four-year duration of immunity following a single rabies vaccine administered to laboratory kittens. This suggests that, while the first rabies vaccine may only be labeled as valid for a single year, it is likely that most vaccinated cats will be protected longer (Scherk et al. 2013). The effectiveness of vaccinating cats at the time of surgery for practicality and to minimize handling has also come into question. There is evidence in dogs and cats that vaccination against various viruses at the time of neutering appears to induce excellent immune responses as determined by the assessment of serum antiviral antibody titers measured approximately 10 weeks later (Fischer et al. 2007).

For practical purposes, one of the authors (GRW) routinely uses three-year licensed rabies vaccines in community (feral and free-roaming) cat programs. According to the Code of Federal Regulations 9, Animals and Animal Products, in order to license a three-year rabies vaccine, that product must protect 22/25 (88%) or 26/30 (86.7%) of immunologically naïve animals who receive one dose of vaccine and are then challenged three years later (CFR9 2000). As such, there is reason to be confident that the administration of such a product will protect cats for an extended period of time. However, because of the legal mandate regarding rabies vaccination and subsequent boosters, there may be little leeway in some jurisdictions regarding the need to booster feral and free-roaming cats in a timely fashion to comply with the law. Legal requirements aside, there are likely individual animal and herd immunity benefits to revaccination and recapturing animals periodically to allow for other veterinary care to be provided.

22.4.3 Shelters as a Source of Public Education

When an animal is adopted from a shelter, the shelter staff has a tremendous opportunity to educate adopters about the important public health aspect of rabies prevention and vaccination for their new pet. Though vaccination may only be required for certain species, livestock species may benefit from rabies vaccination in rabies endemic areas. Owner education should include stressing a prompt visit to a veterinarian to update the rabies vaccination status (if necessary), as well as to provide the opportunity for the adopters to learn about the importance of preventative healthcare, including other necessary vaccines, and prevention and control of internal and external parasites. All of this may be invaluable for first-time pet owners and will contribute to the health and wellbeing of the recently-adopted animal for its lifetime.

22.5 Conclusion and Sources of Additional Information

Rabies continues to be of great concern globally because it is a zoonotic disease that can infect all mammals and is invariably fatal. The United States is fortunate because it has reliable access to post-exposure prophylaxis biologics to prevent disease following exposure in humans and to safe and effective vaccine products to prevent disease in domestic animals. This relative success in preventing human deaths from rabies and dramatically reducing the number of rabies cases in domestic animals can lead to some complacency about the disease; the authors are familiar with numerous cases where the veterinarians and/or shelter staff had not even considered rabies infection as a differential diagnosis.

Animal shelters are often on the front lines of dealing with the disease because they handle, shelter, and transport thousands of animals with unknown exposure and vaccination histories and may hold exposed and rabies suspect animals for rabies observation. They are also instrumental in prevention efforts as many shelters vaccinate pets for rabies before they are released for adoption, offer free and discounted rabies vaccination clinics for pets or vaccinate feral and free-roaming cats in TNVR programs. Shelters must understand the disease; be familiar with applicable laws and regulations; establish open lines of communication with state and local regulatory agencies, the local rabies laboratory and state or local public health contacts; educate the public; and take steps to inform and protect staff and volunteers to be prepared to handle an exposure situation before it occurs.

As has been referenced throughout this chapter, the *Compendium of Animal Rabies Prevention and Control* is an invaluable source of information for veterinarians and shelter personnel (http://www.nasphv.org/Documents/NASPHVRabiesCompendium.pdf). Another resource is the CDC rabies page (https://www.cdc.gov/rabies). This page includes a link to State and Local Public Health Contacts (https://www.cdc.gov/rabies/resources/contacts.html), which lists contact information for all 50 states, including daytime and after-hours phone numbers for consultation. A list of designated and acting state public health veterinarians can be found on the NASPHV web site (http://www.nasphv.org/Documents/StatePublicHealthVeterinariansByState.pdf). Specific information about pre- and post-exposure prophylaxis administration and protocols for serologic monitoring of animal care workers at frequent and infrequent risk of exposure is also available on the CDC site (https://www.cdc.gov/rabies/resources/acip_recommendations.html). The Rabies Awareness Initiative is developing a national, online resource to address "must-know" issues about companion animal rabies; state-specific information is presented. This information is currently available at www.rabiesaware.org, but is being transitioned to and permanently housed on the NASPHV site (http://www.nasphv.org/rabiesaware).

Though not specific to rabies, the Compendium of Veterinary Standard Precautions for Zoonotic

Disease Prevention in Veterinary Personnel (NASPHV 2015) provides extensive information on infection control practices to help protect staff and volunteers who have direct animal contact.

Finally, Figure 22.6 shows algorithms for handling animals exposed to rabies and for animals that may have exposed humans to rabies. These algorithms are not

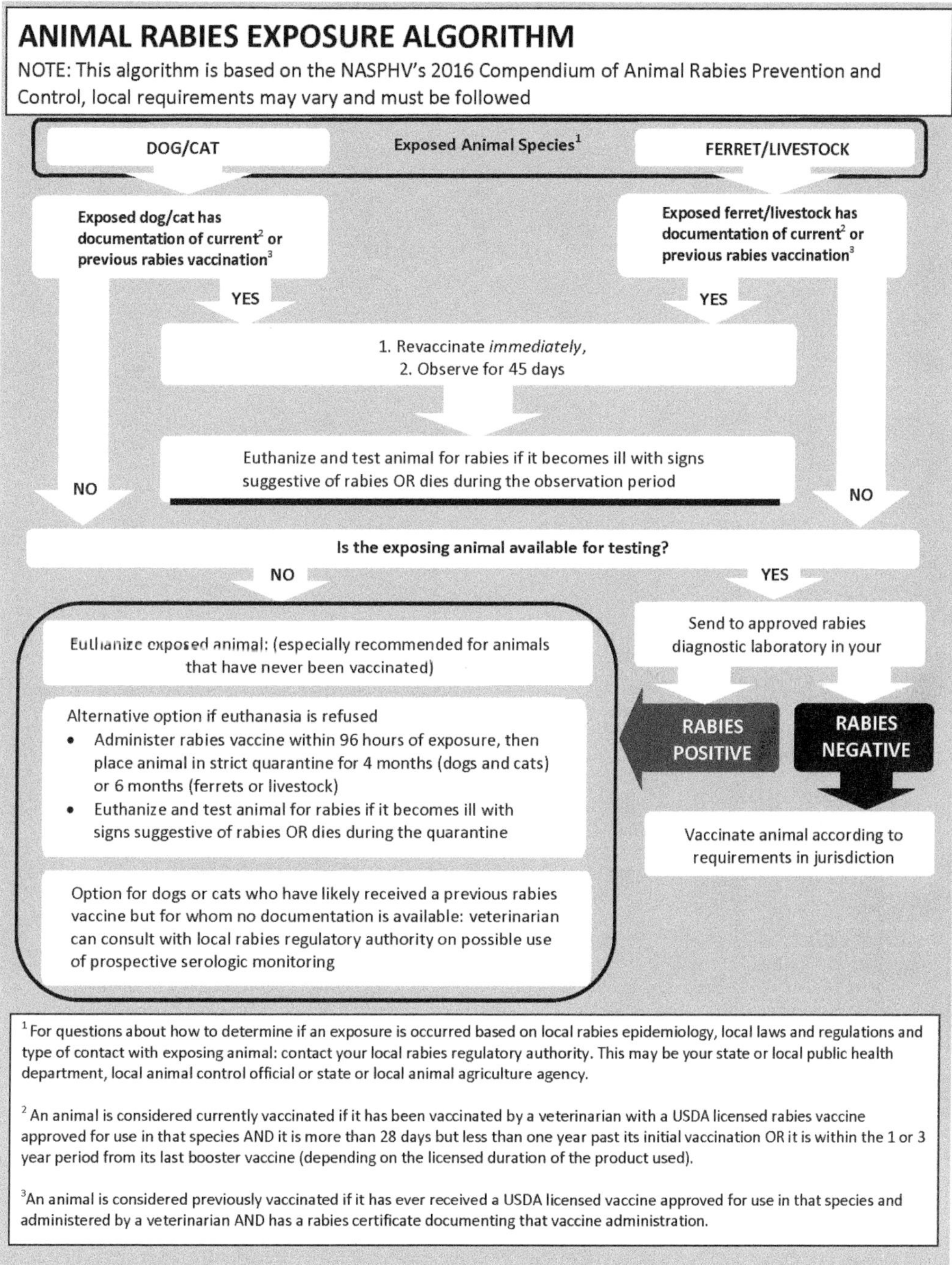

Figure 22.6 Template algorithms for handling animals and humans exposed to rabies. Jurisdictional requirements may vary and take precedence. (*Source:* Michigan Rabies Assessment, Michigan Department of Health and Human Services. © 2020 State of Michigan).

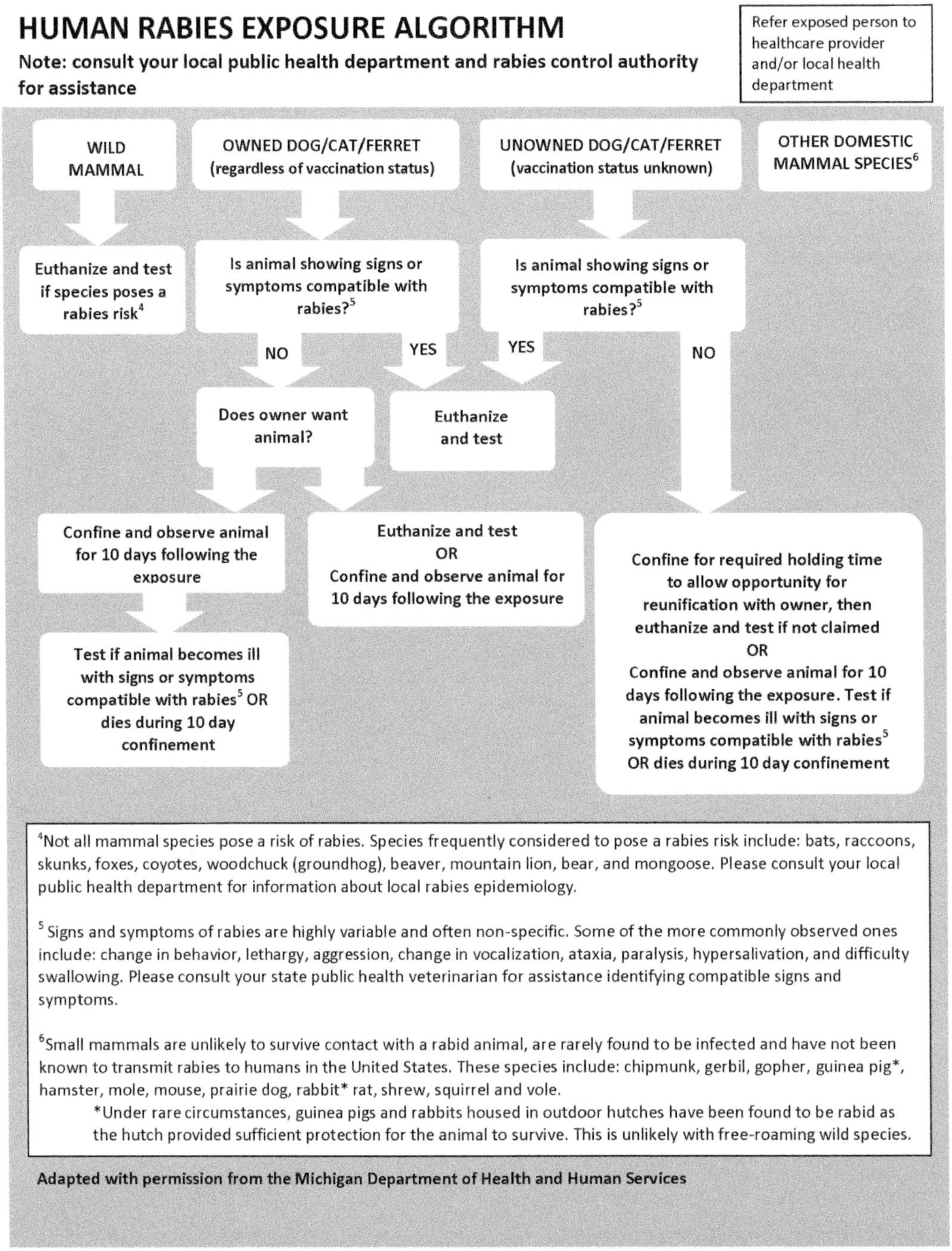

Figure 22.6 (Continued)

jurisdiction-specific and should only be used as a general guide for readers. Jurisdictional requirements may vary and must always be followed. Most, if not all, jurisdictions have similar documents with information that applies to that location.

References

American Society for the Prevention of Cruelty to Animals (2016). Position Statement on Animal Transport for Adoption. https://www.aspca.org/about-us/aspca-policy-and-position-statements/animal-transport-adoption (accessed 23 September 2018).

American Veterinary Medical Association (2016). Administration of Rabies Vaccination State Laws. https://www.avma.org/Advocacy/StateAndLocal/Pages/rabies-vaccination.aspx (accessed 23 September 2018).

Baer, G.M. (2007). The history of rabies. In: *Rabies*, 2e (eds. A.C. Jackson and W.H. Wunner), 1–22. San Diego: Academic Press.

Beran, G.W. (1994). Rabies and infections by rabies-related viruses. In: *Handbook of Zoonoses, Section B: Viral*, 2e (ed. G.W. Beran), 307–357. Boca Raton: CRC Press.

Blanton, J.D., Palmer, D., and Rupprecht, C.E. (2008). Rabies surveillance in the United States during 2007. *Journal of the American Veterinary Medical Association* 233 (6): 884–897.

Blanton, J.D., Palmer, D., and Rupprecht, C.E. (2010). Rabies surveillance in the United States during 2009. *Journal of the American Veterinary Medical Association* 237 (6): 646–657.

Castrodale, L., Walker, V., Baldwin, J. et al. (2008). Rabies in a puppy imported from India to the USA, March 2007. *Zoonoses Public Health* 55: 427–430.

Centers for Disease Control and Prevention (2017). Bringing an Unimmunized Dog into the United States. https://www.cdc.gov/importation/bringing-an-animal-into-the-united-states/dogs.html. (accessed 23 September 2018).

Centers for Disease Control and Prevention (2008a). Recommendations of the Advisory Committee on Immunization Practices (ACIP). https://www.cdc.gov/mmwr/preview/mmwrhtml/rr57e717a1.htm (accessed 25 October 2020).

Centers for Disease Control and Prevention (CDC) (2008b). Rabies in a dog imported from Iraq–New Jersey, June 2008. *Morbidity and Mortality Weekly Report* 57: 1076–1078.

Centers for Disease Control and Prevention (2010). Rabies Vaccination Laws, by State. http://www.cdc.gov/rabies/resources/publications/2009-surveillance/vaccination-laws.html (accessed 23 September 2018).

Centers for Disease Control and Prevention (CDC) (2011). Public Health Response to a Rabid Dog in an Animal Shelter — North Dakota and Minnesota, 2010. *Morbidity and Mortality Weekly Report* 59 (51 & 52): 1678–1680.

Centers for Disease Control and Prevention (2015). Cost of rabies prevention. https://www.cdc.gov/rabies/location/usa/cost.html (accessed 23 September 2018).

Centers for Disease Control and Prevention (2016a). How is rabies transmitted? http://www.cdc.gov/rabies/transmission/index.html (accessed 23 September 2018).

Centers for Disease Control and Prevention (2016b). Protocol for Postmortem Diagnosis of Rabies in Animals by Direct Fluorescent Antibody Testing. https://www.cdc.gov/rabies/pdf/rabiesdfaspv2.pdf (accessed 23 September 2018).

Childs, J.E. and Real, L.A. (2007). Epidemiology. In: *Rabies*, 2e (eds. A.C. Jackson and W.H. Wunner), 123–199. San Diego: Academic Press.

Cleaveland, S., Laurenson, M.K., and Taylor, L.H. (2001). Diseases of humans and their domestic mammals: pathogen characteristics, host range and the risk of emergence. *Philosophical Transactions of the Royal Society of London B Biological Sciences* 356: 991–999.

Code of Federal Regulations, 9 (2000). Animals and Animal Products. § 113.209 Rabies Vaccine, Killed Virus. Office of the Federal Register National Archives and Records Administration, Washington, DC.

Dobson, A. and Foufopoulos, J. (2001). Emerging infectious pathogens of wildlife. *Philosophical Transactions of the Royal Society of London B Biological Sciences* 356: 1001–1012.

Fischer, S.M., Quest, C.M., Dubovi, E.J. et al. (2007). Response of feral cats to vaccination at the time of neutering. *Journal of the American Veterinary Medical Association* 230: 52–58.

Ford, R.B., Larson, L.J., McClure, K.D. et al. (2017). 2017 AAHA Canine Vaccination Guidelines. *Journal of the American Animal Hospital Association* 53: 243–251.

Frana, T.S., Clough, N.E., Gatewood, D.M. et al. (2008). Post marketing surveillance of rabies vaccines for dogs to evaluate safety and efficacy. *Journal of the American Animal Hospital Association* 232: 1000–1002.

Gigante, C.M., Dettinger, L., Powell, J.W. et al. (2018). Multi-site evaluation of the LN34 pan-lyssavirus real-time RT-PCR assay for post-mortem rabies diagnostics. *PLoS One* 13 (5): e0197074.

Greene, C.E. (2012). Rabies and other *Lyssavirus* infections. In: *Infectious Diseases of the Dog and Cat*, 4e (ed. C.E. Greene), 179–197. St. Louis: Elsevier/Saunders.

Hanlon, C.A., Niezgoda, M., and Rupprecht, C.E. (2002). Postexposure prophylaxis for prevention of rabies in dogs. *American Journal of Veterinary Research* 63: 1096–1100.

Hanlon, C.A., Niezgoda, M., and Rupprecht, C.E. (2007). Rabies in terrestrial animals. In: *Rabies*, 2e (eds. A.C. Jackson and W.H. Wunner), 201–258. San Diego: Academic Press.

Iowa State University Center for Food Security and Public Health (2012). Rabies and Rabies-Related Lyssaviruses. http://www.cfsph.iastate.edu/Factsheets/pdfs/rabies.pdf (accessed 5 May 2017).

Jackson, A.C. and Fu, Z.F. (2013). Pathogenesis. In: *Rabies: Scientific Basis of the Disease and its Management*, 3e (ed. A.C. Jackson), 299–349. San Diego: Elsevier, Inc.

Krebs, J.W., Smith, J.S., Rupprecht, C.E. et al. (1999). Rabies surveillance in the United States during 1998. *Journal of the American Veterinary Medical Association* 215 (12): 1786–1798.

Lembo, T., Niezgoda, M., Velasco-Villa, A. et al. (2006). Evaluation of a direct, rapid immunohistochemical test for rabies diagnosis. *Emerging Infectious Diseases* 12 (2): 310–313.

Ma, X., Monroe, B.P., Cleaton, J.M. et al. (2020). Rabies surveillance in the United States during 2018. *Journal of the American Veterinary Medical Association* 256 (2): 195–208.

Manning, S.E., Rupprecht, C.E., Fishbein, D. et al. (2008). Human rabies prevention – United States recommendations of the advisory committee on immunization practices. *Morbidity and Mortality Weekly Report Recommendations and Reports 2008* 57 (RR-3): 1–28.

Moore, M.C., Davis, R.D., Kang, Q. et al. (2015). Comparison of anamnestic responses to rabies vaccination in dogs and cats with current and out-of-date vaccination status. *Journal of the American Veterinary Medical Association* 246: 205–211.

Moran, G.J. et al. (2000). Appropriateness of rabies postexposure prophylaxis treatment for animal exposures. *Journal of the American Medical Association* 284: 1001–1007.

Murray, K.O., Holmes, K.C., and Hanlon, C.A. (2009). Rabies in vaccinated dogs and cats in the United States, 1997–2001. *Journal of the American Veterinary Medical Association* 235: 691–695.

National Association of State Public Health Veterinarians (NASPHV) (2015). Compendium of veterinary standard precautions for zoonotic disease prevention in veterinary personnel. *Journal of the American Veterinary Medical Association* 247 (11): 1252–1271.

National Association of State Public Health Veterinarians (NASPHV) (2016). Compendium of animal rabies prevention and control. *JAVMA* 248 (5): 505–517.

Nettles, V.F., Shaddock, J.H., Sikes, R.K. et al. (1979). Rabies in translocated raccoons. *American Journal of Public Health* 69: 601–602.

Newbury, S., Blinn, M.K., Bushby, P.A. et al. (2010). Guidelines for Standards of Care in Animal Shelters. The Association of Shelter Veterinarians. https://www.sheltervet.org/assets/docs/shelter-standards-oct2011-wforward.pdf (accessed 2 June 2020).

O'Quin, J. (2013). Outbreak Management. In: *Shelter Medicine for Veterinarians and Staff*, 2e (eds. L. Miller and S. Zawistowski), 349–367. Ames: Wiley Blackwell.

Scherk, M.A. et al. (2013). 2013 American Association of Feline Practitioners (AAFP) feline vaccination advisory panel report. *Journal of Feline Medicine and Surgery* 15: 785–808.

Sparkes, A., Bessant, C., Ellis, S.L.H. et al. (2013). ISFM Guidelines on Population Management and Welfare of Unowned Domestic Cats (Felis catus). *Journal of Feline Medicine and Surgery* 15: 811–817.

Stone, A.E., Brummet, G.O., Carozza, E.M. et al. (2020). 2020 AAHA/AAFP Feline Vaccination Guidelines. *Journal of Feline Medicine and Surgery* 22: 813–830.

23

Feline Leukemia and Feline Immunodeficiency Viruses

Julie K. Levy

Maddie's Shelter Medicine Program, College of Veterinary Medicine, University of Florida, Gainesville, FL, USA

23.1 Introduction

The prevalence of feline leukemia virus (FeLV) and feline immunodeficiency virus (FIV) in shelters mirrors the rates found regionally in pet cats (Burling et al. 2017). In the United States, thousands of infected cats are likely to pass through shelters each year. Shelters should have policies in place for testing, preventing and responding to positive test results. Identification and segregation of infected cats is the most effective method for preventing new infections with FeLV and FIV. Though characteristics such as sex, age, lifestyle, and health status can be used to assess the likely risk of FeLV and FIV infections, cats in all categories are at risk.

23.1.1 Epidemiology and Course of the Disease

23.1.1.1 Etiologic Agent and Susceptible Species

FeLV (oncornavirus) and FIV (lentivirus) are both in the family *Retroviridae*. The primary host species for FeLV and FIV is the domestic cat. With the exception of endemic infection in the European wildcat and epizootics in the Florida panther, FeLV is uncommonly reported in free-ranging nondomestic felids (Chiu et al. 2019; Leutenegger et al. 1999).

Domestic cat FIV is also uncommonly transmitted to nondomestic felids, but at least seven felid species and the spotted hyena harbor their own FIV strains that are genetically distinct from domestic cat FIV. The transmission of these viruses between species is infrequent. The prevalence of FIV infection is higher in some species than in domestic cats and may exceed 80% in some wild populations. It is generally observed that the nondomestic felid lentiviruses are less pathogenic in their natural hosts than FIV is in the domestic cat, but virus-associated immune alterations have been documented (Troyer et al. 2005).

23.1.1.2 Zoonotic Potential

FeLV and FIV are not zoonotic. Both viruses can replicate in human cell lines, and FIV infection has been experimentally induced in nonhuman primates, but there is no evidence that either virus is capable of infecting humans (Butera et al. 2000; Johnston et al. 2001; Terry et al. 2017).

23.1.1.3 Prevalence

FeLV and FIV are found worldwide, with increased risk of infection among male cats and cats experiencing illness, roaming outdoors, having inter-cat aggressive encounters, or originating from cat hoarding conditions

Infectious Disease Management in Animal Shelters, Second Edition.
Edited by Lila Miller, Stephanie Janeczko, and Kate F. Hurley.

(Gleich et al. 2009; Goldkamp et al. 2008; Polak et al. 2014). In a global study of 2.9 million test results from 68 countries (Buch et al. 2017), results were grouped into the following regions:

- North America (FeLV 3.9%; FIV 5.0%)
- Caribbean (FeLV 9.2%; FIV 12.6%)
- Latin America (FeLV 12.6%; FIV 7.4%)
- Northern Europe (FeLV 7.5%; FIV 7.5%)
- Southern Europe (FeLV 12.4%; FIV 12.4%)
- Middle East-Africa (FeLV 14.2%; FIV 14.2%)
- Asia-Pacific (FeLV 6.1%; FIV 13.0%).

In the United States, seroprevalences of FeLV and FIV are less than 2% in healthy cats, and 5–40% in high-risk cats and cats that are tested during illness (Burling et al. 2017). Indoor lifestyle and sterilization are associated with reduced infection risks. This protection is likely due to the reduced risk of encountering and fighting with infected cats.

In a study of more than 62 000 cats tested in the United States. and Canada, 3.1% were seropositive for FeLV antigen, and 3.6% were seropositive for FIV antibody (Burling et al. 2017). For both viruses, seroprevalence was higher among cats tested at veterinary clinics (FeLV 3.4%; FIV 4.0%) than among cats tested at animal shelters (FeLV 2.6%; FIV 2.6%), and higher in pet cats allowed outdoors (FeLV 3.9%; FIV 5.0%) than in pet cats kept indoors (FeLV 2.0%; FIV 1.7%). For cats tested at animal shelters, FeLV and FIV were higher in stray (FeLV 3.3%; FIV 3.7%) and feral cats (FeLV 5.6%; FIV 11.6%) than in owner-relinquished cats (FeLV 2.1%; FIV 1.8%). Specific disease conditions commonly associated with infection include cutaneous wounds and abscesses (FeLV 5.5%; FIV 12.5%), oral diseases (FeLV 4.7%; FIV 9.7%), and respiratory diseases (FeLV 8.0%; FIV 6.4%).

23.1.1.4 Morbidity, Mortality, and Prognosis

FeLV and FIV cause chronic infections with a generally low transmission rate, so outbreaks are not expected. Though infected cats may experience a prolonged period of clinical latency, a variety of disease conditions are associated with retroviral infections, including anemia, lymphoma, chronic inflammatory conditions, and susceptibility to opportunistic infections (Burling et al. 2017; Hosie et al. 2009; Lutz et al. 2009; O'Connor et al. 1991).

Multiple studies indicate that on average, cats with FeLV infection have a reduced lifespan. In contrast, studies reporting survival times in cats with FIV are more variable, with some reporting normal lifespans and some indicating a reduction (Gleich et al. 2009; Ravi et al. 2010). Long-term monitoring of a 26-cat household with endemic FeLV and FIV revealed that all FeLV-infected cats died within 5 years of the 10-year observation period, but FIV infection did not affect survival (Addie et al. 2000). A large study compared the survival of more than 1000 FIV-infected cats to more than 8000 age- and sex-matched uninfected control cats (Levy et al. 2006). The cats represented a mix of healthy cats presented for well-care visits and those presented for evaluation of health problems. Of cats that were not euthanized around the time of diagnosis, the median survival rate of the FIV-infected cats was 4.9 years after diagnosis compared to 6.0 years for control cats. A similar comparison was made between more than 800 FeLV-infected cats and more than 7000 controls. The median survival of FeLV-infected cats was 2.4 years after diagnosis compared to 6.3 years for controls.

With proper care, many retrovirus-infected cats may live from several years to a normal lifespan, with a good quality of life. Thus, a decision for treatment or euthanasia should never be based solely on the presence of a retrovirus infection.

23.1.1.5 Mode of Transmission

Viremic cats act as a source of FeLV infection since the virus is shed in saliva, nasal secretions, feces, milk, and urine (Willett and Hosie 2013). Cats typically acquire FeLV via the oronasal route by nursing, mutual grooming, or sharing dishes, but also through bites. Most infections are likely acquired as kittens born to infected queens, either due to in utero infection, or more commonly, through nursing and grooming. Though age-related resistance to infection is reported in experimental infections, the epidemiology of natural infections indicates that cats of all ages are susceptible (Burling et al. 2017). In the early days following the discovery of FeLV, multi-cat households with infected cats were studied to determine the mechanisms of transmission. In one study of 70 such households, 26% of cats were already infected at the time of screening. Infection was completely eliminated in most of the 45 households that removed the infected cats. In contrast, an additional 12% of cats became infected in the households that did not remove infected cats, suggesting that cats residing with infected cats are at risk for acquiring infection (Hardy et al. 1976). Similar studies regarding the co-mingling of FeLV-infected and uninfected cats in animal shelters have not been reported.

The primary mode of FIV transmission is through bite wounds. Transmission of FIV from infected queens to their kittens has been reported in laboratory-reared cats, but appears to be an uncommon event in nature. Sexual transmission does not appear to be a threat, in contrast to other lentiviruses. A recent report demonstrated a lack of transmission between FIV-infected and uninfected comingled cats in a shelter, suggesting that FIV-infected cats can cohabitate with compatible FIV-negative cats with little risk (Litster 2014). As a result, it is increasingly common for shelters to forgo firm restrictions against adopting an FIV-infected cat into a household with FIV-negative cats. In addition, some shelters have stopped segregating FIV-infected cats from uninfected cats in group housing as long as there is no fighting. See Figure 23.1

Both viruses are efficiently transmitted via cross-contamination during invasive procedures or by blood transfusions (Wardrop and Birkenheuer 2016).

23.1.1.6 Incubation Period and Persistence of Infection

Much of what is known about the pathogenesis of retroviral infections in cats is gathered from experimental infections in relatively small numbers of laboratory cats. These findings may or may not represent all the potential outcomes of natural infections. Few naturally infected cats have been monitored throughout their lifetimes, which contributes to uncertainty regarding their long-term prognosis.

Acute infection with either virus is rarely associated with any observable clinical signs and is likely to go unnoticed by shelter staff and cat owners. Using commonly available diagnostic tests, the outcome of exposure to either virus is likely to be evident within 16 weeks. FIV causes a life-long infection with continuous excretion of infectious virus (Hosie et al. 2009).

Most cats infected with FeLV will carry the virus for life, though it may be suppressed in an undetectable regressive form (Beall et al. 2017; Lutz et al. 2009). The pathogenesis of FeLV infection is complex, and several outcomes are possible. In many cases, it is not possible to assign cats to a simple categorical classification scheme of positive or negative. The status of cats can change over time depending on each cat's immune response and its subsequent shift along the spectrum of regressive-progressive infection (Figure 23.2).

1) Abortive FeLV infection

   Abortive infection occurs when a robust immune response completely eliminates the virus shortly after infection and before it can disseminate in the cat's body. Soluble antigen, immunofluorescence assay (IFA), and polymerase chain reaction (PCR) tests are negative (20–30% of cats).

2) Regressive FeLV infection

   Regressive infection occurs when an early transient viremia is suppressed by a partial immune response, but not before provirus (viral DNA) has permanently settled into organs and/or bone marrow. Cats with regressive infection are not believed to shed large amounts of virus and are at low risk to develop FeLV-associated diseases. Immune suppression leading to reactivation of viral replication in regressively infected cats, sometimes years after the initial exposure is possible, at which time they become infectious

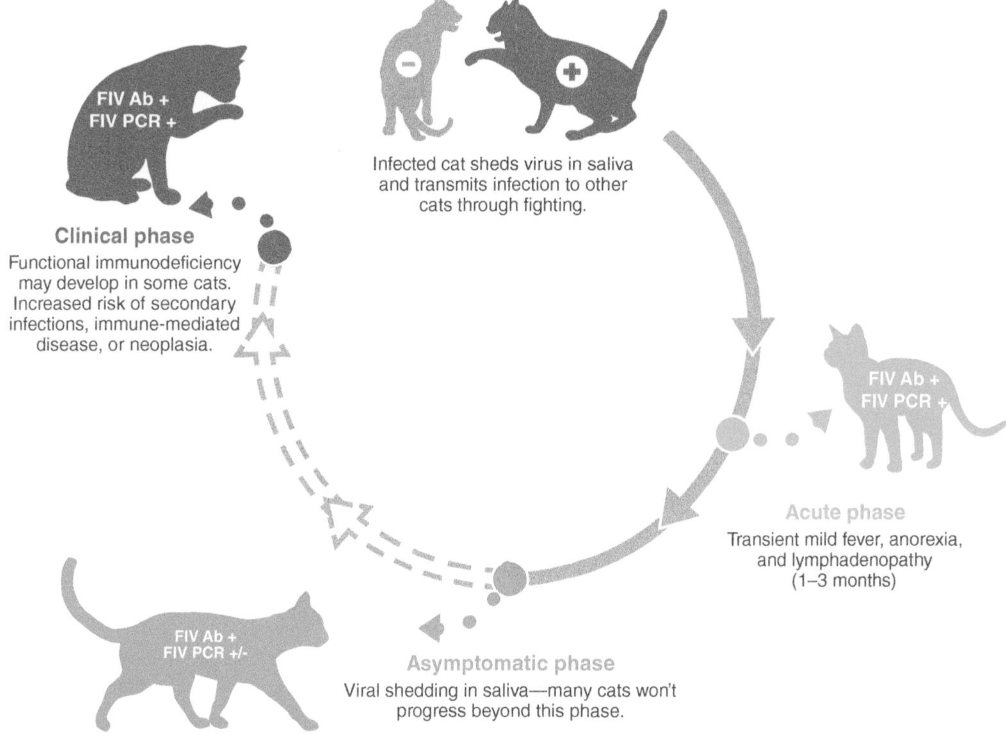

Figure 23.1 The most common mode of FIV transmission is from bite wounds. A brief acute phase of infection may be associated with mild nonspecific signs or go unnoticed. The asymptomatic phase commonly lasts for the rest of a cat's life. After several years, some cats enter a clinical phase in which they develop signs such as stomatitis, chronic inflammatory conditions, or lymphoma. Cats remain infected for life.

to other cats and may develop FeLV-related diseases. In regressive infections, low amounts of circulating antigen and viral DNA may or may not be detected in the blood via antigen and PCR tests, whereas IFA tests are negative. Regressive infections may escape detection in routine screening protocols. (30–40% of infected cats).

3) Progressive FeLV infection

Progressive infection occurs when the immune response fails to contain viremia and virus replication subsequently spreads from the local lymphoid tissues to multiple organ systems. Infection of glandular and mucosal tissues results in shedding of virus in bodily secretions. Cats are continuously infectious to other cats and are at risk of developing FeLV-related disease conditions. Soluble antigen, IFA, and PCR tests are generally positive (30–40% of infected cats).

23.1.1.7 Shedding

Viral shedding in saliva begins within a few weeks post-infection for both viruses (Hosie et al. 2009; Lutz et al. 2009). The virus is subsequently shed in high concentrations in saliva and milk throughout viremic infections, with lesser amounts found in other body secretions. Interestingly, the infectivity of FIV in milk is counteracted by the concurrent shedding of FIV antibodies, which protect most nursing neonates from infection (Pu et al. 1995). This protection does not occur with FeLV, for which nursing is considered to be a major mode of transmission.

23.1.1.8 Clinical Signs

There are no pathognomonic clinical signs for retroviral infections in cats, and many infected cats will live for a significant period of time without any signs of disease attributable to infection. Although FeLV can contribute to

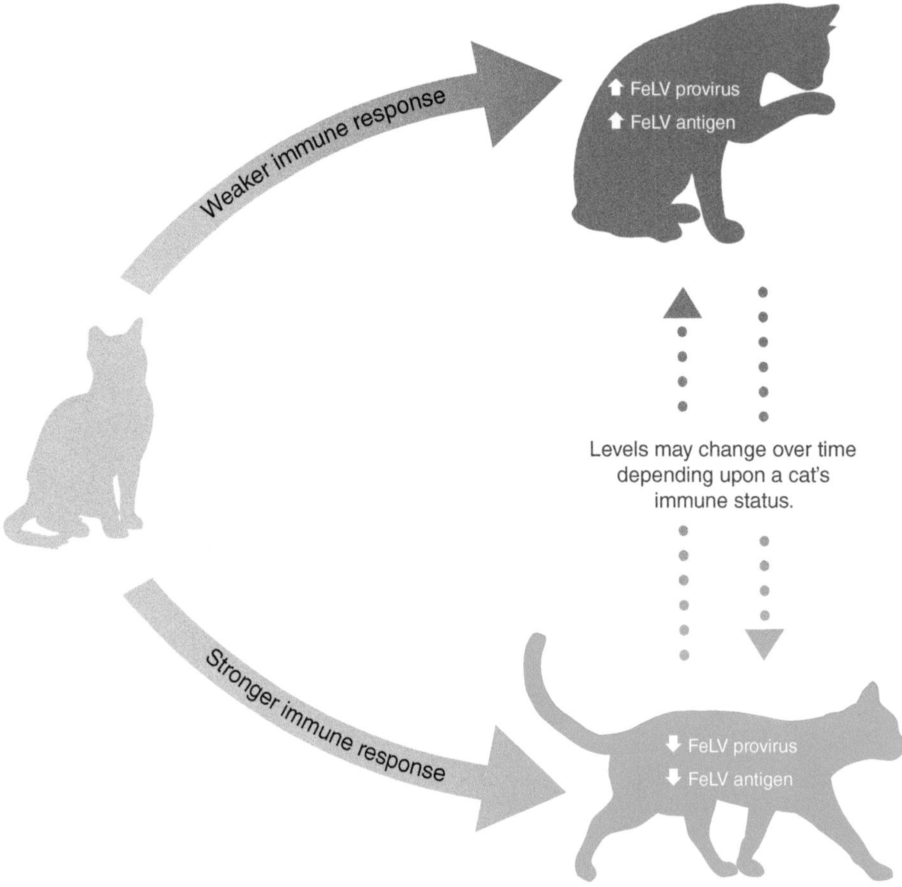

Figure 23.2 Following FeLV infection, a strong immune response suppresses viral replication and dissemination. This is characteristic of regressive infection. Viral shedding and the development of FeLV-associated disease are uncommon. Regressive infection is believed to occur in 30–40% of infected cats. A weak immune response allows for the dissemination of FeLV throughout the body, shedding of infectious virus, and clinical disease. This is characteristic of progressive infection. Progressive infection occurs in 30–40% of infected cats. The immune response to FeLV can vary over time in response to various stressors, resulting in shifting of patterns between regressive and progressive infections. This explains why cats may change from testing negative to positive and back over time in the absence of new exposures.

fading kitten syndrome in neonatal cats, most clinical signs are associated with the effects of chronic retroviral infections leading to anemia, chronic inflammatory conditions, neoplasia, and opportunistic secondary infections. Nonspecific clinical signs that can raise suspicion for retroviral infection include pale mucous membranes, enlarged lymph nodes, oral inflammation, persistent upper respiratory infection, and failure to respond as expected to treatment for other conditions.

23.1.2 Diagnosis

23.1.2.1 Diagnostic Tests

Many of the advanced diagnostic tools used by researchers to define retroviral status in cats, such as viral culture, antibody titers, and quantitation of antigens and nucleic acids, are not routinely available. As a result, shelters must rely on a more limited suite of diagnostic tests, including viral antigen detection (FeLV), antibody detection (FIV), or PCR (FeLV and FIV), to determine the most likely infection status of cats.

1) Combination FeLV/FIV point-of-care (POC) screening tests

   Combination FeLV/FIV POC screening tests are rapid assays that detect soluble FeLV p27 antigen (protein) and FIV antibodies in whole blood, serum, and plasma. In these tests, whole blood is more sensitive for p27 detection than plasma or serum, likely due to the adherence of viral proteins to the surfaces of blood cells and platelets. Plasma has a low amount of cellular material, whereas serum is the most cell-free blood component, and therefore the least sensitive. Combination tests also detect antibodies against FIV that appear following infection or vaccination. These POC tests are the most commonly used method for routine screening in shelters.

2) Microwell plate enzyme-linked immunosorbent assays (ELISAs)

   Microwell plate ELISAs detect FeLV p27 or FIV antibodies in multiple samples tested at the same time. These are used most commonly in reference laboratories for high-volume testing. They can also be used in shelters but are more technically challenging to perform than the individual POC tests and are best reserved for batch testing of multiple samples.

3) IFA tests for FeLV

   IFA tests for FeLV detect p27 within the cytoplasm of circulating white blood cells and platelets. IFA is typically negative in regressive infection and positive in progressive infection, provided sufficient time has elapsed since infection to allow infection of the bone marrow. IFA is performed in reference laboratories on fresh blood smears.

4) PCR tests for FeLV and FIV

   PCR tests for FeLV and FIV detect provirus (viral DNA) and/or viral RNA. PCR tests for FeLV are typically positive in progressive infection but are sometimes negative in regressive infection. Low proviral copy number in FeLV quantitative PCR is a reliable marker for regressive infection associated with prolonged survival, whereas high proviral copy number is found in progressive infection and increased risk for morbidity and early mortality. PCR is positive in FIV infection in most cases, but some field strains can escape detection due to variability in viral genetic sequences. PCR is usually performed in a reference laboratory.

5) Western blot tests

   Western blot tests detect FIV antibodies induced by infection or vaccination. This test does not add significant value to the diagnosis of FIV in shelters and has been largely replaced by PCR when follow-up on a positive screening test is desired.

Negative screening test results in healthy cats are generally reliable due to the low prevalence of infection in most populations. Since the consequences of a positive test may affect management and outcome options, a second level of testing using PCR can be utilized to further investigate the infection status of cats as needed. This is especially important in low-risk and asymptomatic patients in which the risk of a false-positive result is higher (Hosie et al. 2009; Lutz et al. 2009). Advances in diagnostic molecular biology now make PCR the most practical confirmatory test for both FeLV and FIV.

Discordant test results occur when the results of two different tests disagree. This occurs most commonly when screening tests are positive, but follow-up IFA or PCR tests are negative. This situation makes it difficult to define the true infection status of a cat since it is not often possible to determine which of the conflicting results is correct (Gomes-Keller et al. 2006). The status of the cat with discordant results may eventually become clear by repeat testing over time until the test results agree, but some cats remain persistently discordant. Cats with discordant test results are best considered as potential sources of infection for other cats and managed accordingly.

23.1.2.2 Testing in Shelters

In principle, retroviral testing and management guidelines developed for owned pet cats apply to shelter cats as well. However, shelter managers must also take into consideration the allocation of available resources, the diagnostic value of testing cats at a single point in time, the value of test results in critical decision making, and the protection of other cats in the facility and the homes of adopters.

Shelter cat intake continues to outstrip the capacity of many shelters to provide optimal care and to assure positive outcomes, especially during kitten season. The sheltering industry is in a state of flux as rising community demand to save healthy and treatable animals challenges traditional animal control paradigms. A trend also exists for shelters to provide more positive alternatives to keep animals in the home or community when admission to a shelter is not the best choice. These increased expectations require shelter managers to continuously re-evaluate their protocols and resource allocations to achieve the best overall results.

At a minimum, protection of the health and welfare of cats in shelters requires vaccination on intake against acute life-threatening infections, parasite treatment, treatment of illness or injury (including appropriate analgesia), wholesome nutrition, species-appropriate housing, enrichment, and behavioral care (http://www.sheltervet.org/assets/docs/shelter-standards-oct2011-wforward.pdf). Decisions regarding additional care, including retroviral management, should be made based on the best allocation of resources to support the shelter's goals and the most current evidence-based medicine.

Though the results of a single screening test for FeLV and FIV are accurate in many cases, there are exceptions, and results can change over time. Thus, it must be accepted that it is not always possible to prove an individual cat's infection status with certainty, especially if there are discordant results. Each shelter must assess the value of routine screening tests, second level testing, and investigation of discordant results within the context of the shelter's resources and goals.

Costs of testing can be minimized by enrolling in vendor shelter discount programs or using reference laboratories for multiple samples submitted at a time. However, some tests and laboratories are more accurate than others, so cost should not be the only consideration when selecting tests for use in shelters (Levy et al. 2017). Shelter medical records should identify each cat individually and accurately reflect the actual testing procedures, sample types, and test brands used.

Shelters electing to screen cats for retroviral infection have several options. One example is provided in Figure 23.3. In this protocol, Level 1 testing uses a small volume (<0.5 ml) of anticoagulated whole blood a POC rapid assay. This sample is selected because it is relatively easy to collect and does not require any processing before testing. Whole blood is also the most sensitive sample for FeLV detection. In contrast, some shelters prefer to use serum for FeLV detection, or to follow-up a positive whole blood test with a serum test, specifically because the lower sensitivity of serum may reduce the detection of cats with less clinically significant regressive infections.

Some shelters may perform only the Level 1 "one and done" screening protocol since it will correctly identify the status of most cats at the point of time of testing. Cats with negative screening tests can be presumed to be free of FeLV and FIV infection altogether or to have undetectable regressive FeLV infection. Positive screening test results can be furth investigated with optional Level 2 diagnostics if resources exist. Increased costs, delays, and difficulty in interpreting discordant results are reasons that some shelters do not pursue Level 2 testing. Attempting to resolve the status of cats with persistent discordant results by repeated testing can lead down a path of diminishing returns.

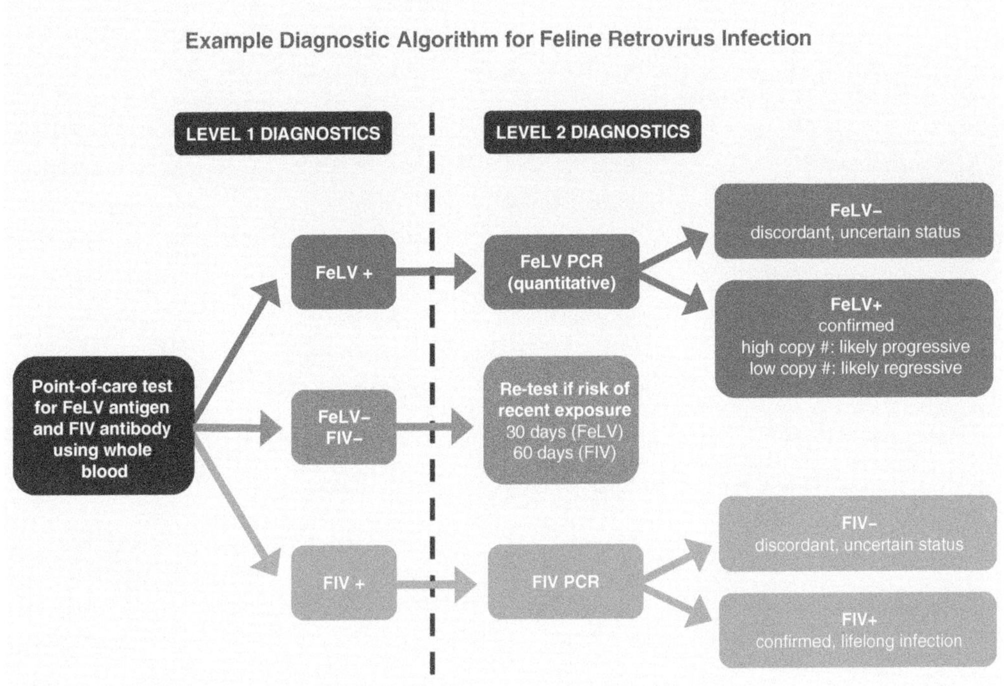

Figure 23.3 Sample FeLV and FIV screening protocol beginning with point-of-care screening of whole blood with a rapid assay in the shelter for Level 1 diagnostics, which will correctly identify the infection status of most cats. Optionally, Level 2 diagnostics (PCR) may be used to further investigate the infection status in cats as needed. Quantitative FeLV PCR is used to detect infection and to measure proviral burden, which can distinguish progressive infection from regressive infection. Recent exposure, atypical responses, occult infections, and variability among different test brands complicate the interpretation and reliability of tests performed at a single point in time. The true status of cats with discordant results can be difficult to determine with certainty.

Shelter testing protocols can be tailored to meet the needs of specific subgroups of cats, including (See Table 23.1):

Adoptable cats: If cats are not tested in the shelter, they should be housed singly and a recommendation for post-adoption testing be clearly explained to the adopter and documented in the medical record provided to the adopter. Arrangements should be made by the adopter to have the new pet tested by the pet's veterinarian as soon as possible. The new pet should be kept separate from other cats until the test result is known. Though more than 95% of sheltered cats are free of infection, post-adoption testing is likely to result in some new pet owners confronting difficult decisions about what to do with a newly adopted cat that is subsequently diagnosed with a retrovirus infection. If one cat in a litter or group reported to be infected, the adopters of other cats with exposure to the infected cat should be contacted and informed.

Blood Donors: Blood transfusions are occasionally performed in animal shelters, and often a resident cat is selected as a donor during emergencies. Both FeLV and FIV are efficiently transmitted via blood transfusions. All donors should be screened for FeLV antigen and FIV antibodies and excluded if either is positive. FeLV can be transmitted via blood

Table 23.1 FeLV and FIV testing and vaccination recommendations for cats in animal shelters.

	FeLV/FIV Testing	FeLV vaccination	FIV vaccination
Healthy individually housed cats	Optional	Not recommended	Not recommended
Group-housed cats	Recommended[a]	Recommended	Not recommended
Foster cats	Recommended	Optional	Not recommended
Resident cats in foster homes	Recommended	Recommended	Not recommended
Long-term sanctuary cats	Recommended	Recommended	Not recommended
Adopted cats	Recommended[b]	Optional[b]	Not recommended
Trap-neuter-return cats	Not recommended	Not recommended	Not recommended
Blood donor cats	Essential	Recommended	Not recommended

[a] Testing for both FeLV and FIV is most comprehensive, but due to lower transmission risk, testing for FIV in group housing may be optional when cats are compatible and stress is low.
[b] May be performed in the shelter before adoption or by the pet's new veterinarian after adoption.

transfusions from cats with undetected regressive FeLV infection, even when antigen screening tests are negative (Nesina et al. 2015). Optimally, donors should also be tested for FeLV by PCR to rule out regressive infection (Pennisi et al. 2015; Wardrop and Birkenheuer 2016). While emergencies often preclude delaying the procedure until PCR test results are received, shelters that keep an in-house donor or who rely on volunteered pets can plan ahead for PCR testing. Details about the blood transfusion procedure and donor used should be recorded in the recipient's record.

Foster cats: If foster cats are likely to mingle with resident cats, both should be tested free of FeLV.

Group-housed cats: Cats should have negative test results for FeLV prior to being introduced to group housing.

Group testing: The presence of infection can vary within individual litters, community cat colonies, and households. Therefore, it is not appropriate to reduce costs by testing one cat as a proxy for the others. Practices such as testing a queen and not her kittens or testing only a few members of a litter, colony, or household are both unreliable and a poor use of resources. In addition, test procedures must be performed as indicated by the manufacturer to maintain accuracy. Pooling multiple samples for use in a single test reduces test sensitivity and should not be performed.

High-risk cats: Demographic factors associated with FeLV and FIV infection include increasing age, male sex, inter-cat aggression, illness, and high-risk environments, such as animal hoarding. When testing only a subset of cats is possible, shelters should prioritize testing of the highest risk cats. Additionally, cats removed from high-risk environments should be retested at least two months after removal to detect the outcome of recent exposure.

Individually housed cats: Testing is optional for healthy cats housed in single-cat enclosures.

Kittens: The most common reason for false-positive FIV results is the passive transfer of maternal FIV antibodies from infected queens to their kittens via colostrum. Though infection of kittens is uncommon, a positive antibody test indicates the queen was infected (or vaccinated) and the kittens were exposed. Kittens with positive FIV antibody tests should be retested up to five months of age, by which time, maternal antibodies will no longer be present. Kittens in which FIV antibodies persist past six months can be considered infected.

Neonates: Unweaned motherless kittens are frequently tested at intake for FeLV, especially if they will be fostered by a surrogate queen or co-mingled with unrelated kittens. However, it is not unusual for incubating FeLV infections to be unapparent on the initial test. In addition, approximately 50% of neonates that initially test positive for FeLV antigen in whole blood turn negative by the time adoption age is reached. The reason for this is unknown but could theoretically be caused by the transfer of FeLV antigens without infectious virus from an infected queen to her newborn or to an unusual form of neonatal regressive infection. For these reasons, neonates should be retested at adoption age since they appear to be especially prone to changes in FeLV testing results early in life.

Sanctuaries: Long-term confinement in densely populated environments amplifies the risk of introduction and spread of infections even if all cats are screened when they are first added to the group. Cats can be incubating undetected infections or regressive infections and can revert to transmissible progressive infections following the initial screening. It is ideal to repeat testing following a two-month quarantine before integrating cats into the general population, to retest cats at regular intervals, such as annually, and to vaccinate against FeLV. Cats diagnosed with FeLV should be segregated from uninfected cats.

Trap-Neuter-Return (TNR) programs: Though the American Association of Feline Practitioners (AAFP) broadly recommends testing all cats for retroviral infection, an exception exists for free-roaming stray and feral community cats in TNR programs. An overarching objective of TNR is to spay, neuter, and vaccinate a sufficient number of free-roaming cats in order to eventually reduce their population, mitigate nuisance, and improve feline welfare. The success of TNR programs hinges on deploying adequate financial and personnel resources to sterilize cats faster than they can reproduce. The prevalence of FeLV and FIV infection is within a few percentage points in outdoor owned pet cats and unowned community cats, so positive community cats do not increase the existing threat to pets if they remain in the environment (Burling et al. 2017). However, neutering reduces the two most common modes of transmission: queen to the kitten for FeLV and fighting among males for both FeLV and FIV (Goldkamp et al. 2008). Because the prevalence of disease is generally low and population control of community cats requires a commitment to neutering the largest number possible, TNR programs do not routinely test cats at the time of surgery (Wallace and Levy 2006).

23.2 Prevention and Control

23.2.1 Housing

Cats known to be infected with FeLV should be housed in individual enclosures or in groups according to their infection status to avoid in-shelter transmission (Westman et al. 2019). Evidence available to date suggests that the risk of FIV transmission among compatible shelter cats is low (Bęczkowski et al. 2015). Therefore, it is increasingly popular for shelters to include FIV-infected cats in group housing with uninfected cats or to forego FIV testing altogether.

Due to the immune-suppression experienced by some retroviral-infected cats, they should not be housed in isolation wards where they may be exposed to other infectious diseases such as upper respiratory infections, panleukopenia virus, or dermatophytosis.

Both FeLV and FIV are short-lived in the environment and are not transmissible via the air or casual handling. Therefore, no special sanitation procedures are required when infected cats are housed near uninfected cats. Signage used to promote the adoption of infected cats is most effective when it features their positive attributes and avoids alarming warnings. More detailed information about the infection is reserved for an in-person discussion.

23.2.2 Vaccination

23.2.2.1 FeLV Vaccination

Several FeLV vaccines are available and have been reported to protect a high proportion of cats against progressive infection and, presumably, subsequent FeLV-associated fatal conditions (Lutz et al. 2009). However, experimental studies suggest that vaccination does not always protect against regressive infection (Hofmann-Lehmann et al. 2006). Because protection is not induced in all vaccinates, vaccination against FeLV does not diminish the importance of testing cats to identify and to segregate infected cats. Therefore, the FeLV infection status of all cats should be determined before beginning FeLV vaccinations. Although FeLV vaccination will not affect testing results, there is no value in administering FeLV vaccines to individuals confirmed to be infected.

FeLV vaccines are considered noncore (See Chapter 9 on Vaccinations and Immunology). The AAFP recommends FeLV vaccination for cats at risk of exposure, such as cats permitted outdoors, residing in multiple-cat environments with frequent cat turnover, living with FeLV-infected cats, or residing with cats in which FeLV infection status is not known or in which the introduction of new cats is common. While these conditions are uncommon in shelters, they may be present in foster homes. Due to the difficulty in determining the true infection status of some cats, potential interaction of foster cats with resident cats, and the often-prolonged period of residence in foster homes, ideally, both resident cats and foster cats should be vaccinated against FeLV in multi-cat households. This is especially true for kittens, which are more easily infected with FeLV than adults.

Because of the low risk of transmission, vaccination against FeLV is not recommended for individually housed cats (Little et al. 2020). In facilities in which unfamiliar cats are group-housed for prolonged periods of time, testing, followed by FeLV vaccination, is recommended if resources permit. However, population management protocols should favor reduced length of stay rather than delays designed to assure cats are fully vaccinated against FeLV. FeLV vaccination is also recommended in sanctuaries because long-term group housing increases the chances of exposure to infected cats inadvertently admitted with negative intake screening tests due to recent infection or regressive status (Westman et al. 2019).

When FeLV vaccination is determined to be appropriate, a two-dose primary series is required, with the first dose administered as early as eight weeks of age followed by a second dose administered three to four weeks later. Annual booster vaccinations should be administered as long as the risk of exposure remains. FeLV vaccines should be administered as low as possible on the left hind leg, which is usually just above the hock. Since two doses are required to provide initial protection, there is little value in giving a single dose in the shelter. In most cases, discussion of FeLV vaccination should be referred to the adopter's veterinarian.

23.2.2.2 FIV Vaccination

As is the case for other lentiviruses, it has been difficult to develop a vaccine against FIV that protects against the broad range of virus subtypes that are found in the field. One vaccine has been brought to market, a whole-virus, dual-subtype (subtypes A and D), inactivated product combined with an adjuvant. The vaccine was removed from the market in the United States and Canada in 2015 but is still available in several other countries.

Vaccinated cats develop antibodies that are indistinguishable from those caused by natural infection in two commonly used POC diagnostic tests, IDEXX SNAP® and Abaxis VetScan®, but not in two others, Zoetis Witness® and Anigen Rapid™ (Crawford et al. 2016; Westman et al. 2015). Since these antibodies have been shown to persist for up to eight years after the last vaccination, positive FIV antibody test results should be interpreted in light of the assays used in regions where FIV vaccination is available. FIV vaccination does not interfere with diagnosis by PCR.

FIV vaccination is considered noncore, with use limited to cats at high risk of exposure, such as those who fight with other cats. As such, it is not recommended for use in shelters. An initial series of three doses is administered SC two to three weeks apart; annual revaccination is recommended after the initial series as long as the risk of exposure continues.

Vaccination against FIV is not recommended in shelters. Transmission of FIV among compatible co-housed cats is rare (Litster 2014), vaccine-induced immunity is not predictable (Westman et al. 2016), and vaccine-induced positive antibody test results complicate the future confirmation of the true FIV infection status of vaccinated cats.

23.2.3 Disinfection (Environmental Control)

Retroviruses are unstable outside their hosts and can be inactivated by detergents and common hospital disinfectants (Little et al. 2020). However, retroviruses in dried biological deposits can remain viable for more than a week. Simple precautions and routine sanitation procedures will prevent transmission of retroviruses in shelters. (See Chapter 8 for more information on sanitation.)

Dental and surgical instruments, needles, tattoo equipment, endotracheal tubes, anesthesia monitoring equipment, and other items potentially contaminated with body fluids should be thoroughly cleaned and sterilized between uses (Griffin et al. 2016). The re-use of suture between patients has been shown to transmit FIV and should not be performed (Druce et al. 1997). Care should be taken to avoid cross-contamination of items potentially shared among multiple patients, such as fluid administration tubing and multi-dose medication vials.

23.2.4 Treatment and Management

A great many antiviral and immune-boosting treatments have been proposed for retrovirus-infected cats; unfortunately, none have been proven effective in promoting health or prolonging survival (Hartmann 2015). At this time, the best recommendations for optimizing long-term health in infected cats are similar to those for uninfected cats: good nutrition, husbandry, and routine veterinary care. Lifestyle-based vaccination following the usual AAFP guidelines for uninfected cats should be administered, as well as routine annual physical examinations, parasite control, and disease screening as for uninfected cats (Hoyumpa et al. 2010; Little at al. 2020).

Physical health and emotional welfare require that the complex environmental needs of cats must be met (Ellis et al. 2013). There is evidence that insufficient enrichment and confinement in incompatible social groups have a negative impact on the health of cats (Stella and Croney 2016). (See Chapter 2 on Wellness for more information.)

The health of retrovirus-infected cats is especially sensitive to chronic stress, and their long-term wellbeing is best supported by placement in stable homes with few other cats. A study comparing FIV-infected cats living in homes with at most one other cat to cats living in a sanctuary housing 60 cats found striking differences over a 22-month observation period. Survival rates over a 22-month monitoring period were 94% for FIV+ cats in homes and 37% for FIV+ cats in the sanctuary (Bęczkowski et al. 2015). A study comparing FeLV infection rates in 440 household pets compared to 89 cats in two sanctuaries found that not only were sanctuary cats 18 times more likely to be infected (prevalence 46%), but they were also 42 times more likely to have the more lethal progressive form of disease (Westman et al. 2019). Since stress can exacerbate the clinical course of either virus, adoption into a home-like setting is likely to result in better long-term outcomes than would occur with long-term institutionalization.

23.2.5 Euthanasia Guidelines

With proper care, retroviral-infected cats can live many years and may die at an advanced age from causes unrelated to their infection. In addition, there is little chance of viral transmission within a shelter when simple procedures for segregating infected cats are adhered to. Both the AAFP and the Association of Shelter Veterinarian (ASV) recommend against routine euthanasia of healthy retrovirus-infected cats (Little et al. (2020) http://www.sheltervet.org/assets/docs/position-statements/managementofcatswhotestpositive.pdf). Thus, a decision for treatment or euthanasia should never be based solely on the diagnosis of a retrovirus infection.

23.2.6 Client Education and Implications for Adoption

In response to goals to save healthy and treatable cats, a growing number of shelters have expanded their adoption programs to include cats with FeLV and FIV infections. Due to evidence of longer survival, adoption into a home is preferred over confinement in sanctuaries for most cats. Shelters should develop specific marketing and education programs to assure that these cats do not linger unnecessarily in shelter confinement, receive the post-adoption care they require, and to minimize the risk of spreading the infection to other cats in their new homes.

When a cat owner already has an infected cat, the adoption of another cat carrying the same virus offers an ideal opportunity for placement of retrovirus-infected cats and for companionship for the resident cat. Because the risk of FIV transmission within a household of compatible neutered adult cats appears to be very low (Litster 2014), it may also be appropriate to allow well-informed adopters to add FIV-infected cats into their homes, even if they have resident cats that are not infected. The risk of FeLV transmission is higher, and the potential health impacts of infection more severe, so it is not recommended to place FeLV-infected cats with uninfected ones.

Little is known about the satisfaction of adopters who acquire pets with medical conditions or uncertain prognosis. However, post-adoption survey data gathered by one large FeLV adoption program is encouraging. Though less than a quarter of the adopters had previous experience with FeLV, 95% reported a positive experience, 74% said they were likely to adopt another FeLV-infected cat in the future, and only 4% of cats were returned (Lockhart et al. 2020).

23.3 Conclusion

Retroviral infections remain common and important conditions of cats throughout the world. Shelters that care for cats will almost certainly encounter these infections and should have strategic and transparent policies in place regarding testing, management, outcomes, and education.

Mass testing in shelters is not always the best approach, and testing of individually housed cats is not essential if other needs are greater. There is a current shift away from routine in-shelter testing in favor of transferring that function to the adopter and their veterinarian. Regardless of where testing is performed, it is vital to follow proper testing protocols, which include performing a separate test for each cat and not extrapolating the results for one cat to others in the group. Despite rigorous testing efforts, the true infection status is not always clear, especially for FeLV.

Placement of cats with retroviral infection should be approached with optimism, education, and support. While the lifespan of some infected cats may be unpredictable, this is also true of many other populations of shelter pets, such as the elderly and those with chronic diseases.

References

Addie, D.D., Toth, S., Reid, S. et al. (2000). Long-term impact on a closed household of pet cats of natural infection with feline coronavirus, feline leukaemia virus, and feline immunodeficiency virus. *Veterinary Record* 146: 419–424.

Beall, M., Buch, J., Cahill, R.J. et al. (2017). Staging feline leukemia virus infections using quantitative p27 ELISA and real-time PCR results. *Journal of Veterinary Internal Medicine* 31: 1314.

Bęczkowski, P.M., Litster, A., Lon, T.L. et al. (2015). Contrasting clinical outcomes in two cohorts of cats naturally infected with feline immunodeficiency virus (FIV). *Veterinary Microbiology* 176: 50–60.

Buch, J., Beall, M. et al. (2017). Worldwide clinic-based serologic survey of FIV antibody and FeLV antigen in cats. *Journal of Veterinary Internal Medicine* 31: 1315.

Burling, A.N., Levy, J.K., Scott, H.M. et al. (2017). Seroprevalences of feline leukemia virus and feline immunodeficiency virus infection in cats in the United States and Canada and risk factors for seropositivity. *Journal of the American Veterinary Medical Association* 251: 187–194.

Butera, S.T., Brown, J., Callahan, M.E. et al. (2000). Survey of veterinary conference attendees for evidence of zoonotic infection by feline retroviruses. *Journal of the American Veterinary Medical Association* 217: 475–479.

Chiu, E.S., Kraberger, S., Cunningham, M.W. et al. (2019). Multiple introductions of domestic cat feline leukemia virus in endangered Florida panthers. *Emerging Infectious Diseases* 25: 92–101.

Crawford, P.C., Levy, J.K., and Tucker, S.J. (2016). Does a DIVA test exist for differentiating FIV infection from FIV vaccination? *Journal of Veterinary Internal Medicine* 30: 1475.

Druce, J.D., Robinson, W.F., Locarnini, S.A. et al. (1997). Transmission of human and feline immunodeficiency viruses via reused suture material. *Journal of Medical Virology* 53: 13–18.

Ellis, S.L., Rodan, I., Carney, H.C. et al. (2013). AAFP and ISFM feline environmental needs guidelines. *Journal of Feline Medicine and Surgery* 15: 219–230.

Gleich, S.E., Krieger, S., and Hartmann, K. (2009). Prevalence of feline immunodeficiency virus and feline leukaemia virus among client-owned cats and risk factors for infection in Germany. *Journal of Feline Medicine and Surgery* 11: 985–992.

Goldkamp, C.E., Levy, J.K., Edinboro, C.H., and Lachtara, J.L. (2008). Seroprevalences of feline leukemia virus and feline immunodeficiency virus in cats with abscesses or bite wounds and rate of veterinarian compliance with current guidelines for retrovirus testing. *Journal of the American Veterinary Medical Association* 232: 1152–1158.

Gomes-Keller, M.A., Gonczi, E., Tandon, R. et al. (2006). Detection of feline leukemia virus RNA in saliva from naturally infected cats and correlation of PCR results with those of current diagnostic methods. *Journal of Clinical Microbiology* 44: 916–922.

Griffin, B., Bushby, P.A., McCobb, E. et al. (2016). The Association of Shelter Veterinarians' 2016 veterinary medical care guidelines for spay-neuter programs. *Journal of the American Veterinary Medical Association* 249: 165–188.

Hardy, W.D., Hess, P.W., MacEwen, E.G. et al. (1976). Biology of feline leukemia virus in the natural environment. *Cancer Research* 36: 582–588.

Hartmann, K. (2015). Efficacy of antiviral chemotherapy for retrovirus-infected cats: what does the current literature tell us? *Journal of Feline Medicine and Surgery* 17: 925–939.

Hofmann-Lehmann, R., Tandon, R., Boretti, F.S. et al. (2006). Reassessment of feline leukaemia virus (FeLV) vaccines with novel sensitive molecular assays. *Vaccine* 24: 1087–1094.

Hosie, M.J., Addie, D., Belák, S. et al. (2009). Feline immunodeficiency. ABCD guidelines on prevention and management. *Journal of Feline Medicine and Surgery* 11: 575–584.

Hoyumpa, V.A., Rodan, I., Brown, M. et al. (2010). AAFP-AAHA: feline life stage guidelines. *Journal of Feline Medicine and Surgery* 12: 43–54.

Johnston, J.B., Olson, M.E., Rud, E.W., and Power, C. (2001). Xenoinfection of nonhuman primates by feline immunodeficiency virus. *Current Biology* 11: 1109–1113.

Leutenegger, C.M., Hofmann-Lehmann, R., Riols, C. et al. (1999). Viral infections in free-living populations of the European wildcat. *Journal of Wildlife Diseases* 35: 678–686.

Levy, J.K., Lorentzen, L. (2006). Long-term outcome of cats with natural FeLV and FIV infection (abstract). Eighth International Feline Retrovirus Research Symposium, Washingon, DC.

Levy, J.K., Crawford, P.C., and Tucker, S.J. (2017). Performance of 4 point-of-care screening tests for feline leukemia virus and feline immunodeficiency virus. *Journal of Veterinary Internal Medicine* 31: 521–526.

Litster, A. (2014). Transmission of feline immunodeficiency virus (FIV) among cohabiting cats in two cat rescue shelters. *Veterinary Journal* 201: 184–188.

Little, S., Levy, J., Hartmann, K., et al. (2020). 2020 AAFP Feline Retrovirus Testing and Management Guidelines. *Journal of Feline Medicine and Surgery* 22: 5–30.

Lockhart, H.L., Levy, J.K., Amirian, E.S., et al. (2020). Outcome of cats referred to a specialized adoption program for feline leukemia virus-positive cats. *Journal of Feline Medicine and Surgery* 22: 1160–1167.

Lutz, H., Addie, D., Belák, S. et al. (2009). Feline Leukaemia: ABCD guidelines on prevention and management. *Journal of Feline Medicine and Surgery* 11: 565–574.

Nesina, S., Helfer-Hungerbuehler, A.K., Riond, B. et al. (2015). Retroviral DNA-the silent winner: blood transfusion containing latent feline leukemia provirus causes infection and disease in naive recipient cats. *Retrovirology* 12: 105.

O'Connor, T.P. Jr., Tonelli, Q.J., and Scarlett, J.M. (1991). Report of the national FeLV/FIV awareness project. *Journal of the American Veterinary Medical Association* 199: 1348–1353.

Pennisi, M.G., Hartmann, K., Addie, D.D. et al. (2015). Blood transfusion in cats: ABCD guidelines for minimizing risks of infectious iatrogenic complications. *Journal of Feline Medicine and Surgery* 17: 588–593.

Polak, K.C., Levy, J.K., Crawford, P.C. et al. (2014). Infectious diseases in large-scale cat hoarding investigations. *Veterinary Journal* 201: 189–195.

Pu, R., Okada, S., Little, E.R. et al. (1995). Protection of neonatal kittens against feline immunodeficiency virus infection with passive maternal antiviral antibodies. *AIDS* 9: 235–242.

Ravi, M., Wobeser, G.A., Taylor, S.M., and Jackson, M.L. (2010). Naturally acquired feline immunodeficiency virus (FIV) infection in cats from western Canada: prevalence, disease associations, and survival analysis. *Canadian Veterinary Journal* 51: 271–276.

Stella, J.L. and Croney, C.C. (2016). Environmental aspects of domestic cat care and management: implications for cat welfare. *Scientific World Journal* 2016: 6296315. https://doi.org/10.1155/2016/6296315.

Terry, A., Kilbey, A., Naseer, A. et al. (2017). Barriers to infection of human cells by feline leukemia virus: insights into resistance to zoonosis. *Journal of Virology* 91: e02119–e02116.

Troyer, J.L., Pecon-Slattery, J., Roelke, M.E. et al. (2005). Seroprevalence and genomic divergence of circulating strains of feline immunodeficiency virus among *Felidae* and *Hyaenidae* species. *Journal of Virology* 79 (13): 8282–8294.

Wallace, J.L. and Levy, J.K. (2006). Population characteristics of feral cats admitted to seven trap–neuter–return programs in the United States. *Journal of Feline Medicine and Surgery* 8: 279–284.

Wardrop, K.J. and Birkenheuer, A. (2016). Update on canine and feline blood donor screening for blood-borne pathogens.

Journal of Veterinary Internal Medicine 30: 15–35.

Westman, M.E., Malik, R., Hall, E. et al. (2015). Determining the feline immunodeficiency virus (FIV) status of FIV-vaccinated cats using point-of-care antibody kits. *Comparative Immunology, Microbiology and Infectious Diseases* 42: 43–52.

Westman, M.E., Malik, R., Hall, E. et al. (2016). The protective rate of the feline immunodeficiency virus vaccine: an Australian field study. *Vaccine* 34: 4752–4758.

Westman, M., Norris, J., Malik, R., et al. (2019). The diagnosis of feline leukaemia virus (FeLV) infection in owned and group-housed rescue cats in Australia. Viruses 11: 503

Willett, B.J. and Hosie, M.J. (2013). Feline leukaemia virus: half a century since its discovery. *Veterinary Journal* 195: 16–23.

24

Exotic Companion Mammals (Ferrets, Rabbits, Guinea Pigs and Rodents)

Jennifer Graham[1] *and S. Emmanuelle Knafo*[2]

[1] *Department of Clinical Sciences, Cummings School of Veterinary Medicine at Tufts University, Grafton, MA, USA*
[2] *Avian and Exotics Department, Red Bank Veterinary Hospital, Tinton, NJ, USA*

24.1 Introduction

Ferrets, rabbits, and other exotic companion mammals are often admitted to animal shelters. It is imperative for shelters to be aware of the unique anatomic features, husbandry requirements, and safe handling techniques for these species. Additionally, knowledge of common infectious disease is important to manage and maintain the welfare of these small mammals as well as prevent the spread of disease to other animals, the staff handling them and the public. This chapter will review some of the most important aspects of appropriate care for these animals in a shelter setting. Though some recommendations for treatment and drug dosages are provided in this chapter, the reader is advised to also refer to other current veterinary exotic animal reference materials and formularies for the most current treatment protocols.

24.2 Ferrets

24.2.1 Anatomy, Husbandry, Handling, and Routine Healthcare

24.2.1.1 Terminology, Anatomy, and Physiology

Derived from the Siberian or European polecat, the domestic ferret (*Mustela putorius furo*) has been domesticated for 2000–3000 years (Johnson-Delaney 2017a; Powers 2012). Also known as a "mouse-eating (*Mustela*) smelly (*putorius*) thief (*furo*)," ferrets were historically used for hunting rabbits throughout Europe (Powers 2012). Ferret ownership is illegal in some areas of the United States (California, Hawaii, New York City) and permits for ownership must be obtained in some locations (Georgia) (Johnson-Delaney 2017a). "Jill" is the term used for an intact female ferret while an intact male ferret is referred to as a "hob." An ovariectomized female ferret is a "sprite" and a castrated male ferret is a "gib." With over 30 variations recognized by the American Ferret Association, ferrets can be classified by coat color and pattern, eye color, mask type, and nose pattern (Johnson-Delaney 2017b). A long-haired ferret is known as an Angora ferret. Ferrets undergo a heavy shed in the spring and fall coinciding with seasonal change, and variations in hair length and color can be noted seasonally in some ferrets (Powers 2012).

Ferrets have a strong musky odor caused by active sebaceous glands. Intact animals have an increased odor during the breeding season along with oily fur and a yellow to orange discoloration of the undercoat. The skin on the dorsum of the neck is thickened which allows "scruffing" for restraint. Ferrets are susceptible to overheating in

Infectious Disease Management in Animal Shelters, Second Edition.
Edited by Lila Miller, Stephanie Janeczko, and Kate F. Hurley.

part because they lack sweat glands in the skin. Ferrets have well-developed anal glands that are routinely removed at large commercial breeding facilities in the United States (Powers 2012).

Ferrets have 34 adult teeth with a dental formula of 2(I 3/3; C1/1; P 3/3; M 1/2). Ferrets are prone to dental and periodontal pathology, likely related to being fed a kibble diet combined with inappropriate chewing behavior. Broken and discolored canine teeth are commonly noted on oral examination. The same principles of dental disease management in dogs and cats apply to ferrets. Ferrets have five pairs of salivary glands and salivary mucoceles have been described in ferrets (Johnson-Delaney 2017c; Powers 2012).

Ferrets lack a true gastroesophageal sphincter and can vomit. The gastrointestinal (GI) transit time of ferrets is short at three to four hours and ferrets should not be fasted more than three hours prior to surgery. Ferrets are obligate carnivores with an intestinal length to body length ratio of 5 : 1. Foreign body ingestion is common, particularly in ferrets under one year of age. Ferrets imprint on food smells within the first few months of life which can make dietary transitions later in life particularly challenging (Johnson-Delaney 2017c; Powers 2012).

The heart of the ferret is located between the sixth and eighth ribs, which requires auscultation caudal to the point of the elbow. Sinus arrhythmia can be a normal finding on examination. The lymph nodes of ferrets are surrounded by fat and increased fat around nodes in an obese ferret can be mistaken for lymphadenopathy. Moderate splenomegaly can be noted in normal ferrets (generally associated with benign extramedullary hematopoiesis) (Johnson-Delaney 2017c; Powers 2012).

Male ferrets are generally larger than females and have an os penis with a J-shaped tip which can make urinary catheterization challenging. Most ferrets presenting in a shelter situation have likely been neutered, but a prepuce located on the ventral abdomen in males makes sexing ferrets straightforward. Males have a prostate gland that can become enlarged and cause urinary tract obstruction in association with adrenal gland disease (excessive sex hormone production by the adrenal glands). The urogenital opening is a small slit in females but the vulva can become considerably enlarged during estrus or in association with adrenal gland disease. Jills are seasonally polyestrous and, if not bred, can remain in persistent estrus that can be associated with anemia due to bone marrow suppression (Johnson-Delaney 2017a; Powers 2012). Many commercially bred ferrets in the United States have a two-dot tattoo in the right ear indicating the ferret has been descented and neutered (Johnson-Delaney 2017c; Powers 2012).

24.2.1.2 Housing and Husbandry

Ferrets can be housed indoors or outdoors depending on weather conditions; ferrets do not tolerate temperatures above 90 °F (32° C) and a heated shelter should be provided if the temperature drops below freezing. Enclosures should be "ferret proofed" to ensure safety and prevent escape (Figure 24.1a). Wire multi-level caging is ideal for ferret housing, but caging used for dogs and cats can be adapted for ferrets (Figure 24.1b). Ferrets are social animals and are ideally housed with other ferrets. Ferrets are predators and the odors of ferrets can be stressful to prey species like rabbits and rodents; it is important to house ferrets away from these species. Ferrets are susceptible to canine distemper virus (CDV) and should not be housed near dogs at risk for shedding this virus (Johnson-Delaney 2017d).

Water should always be available in heavy bowls to prevent them from tipping over. Some ferrets prefer water bottles over bowls. Ferrets love hammocks and to burrow; covered baskets, blankets, and towels can provide enrichment. A corner litter tray can be provided though not all ferrets are litter trained. Toys should be provided but care should be taken to prevent ingestion. No soft rubber or foam objects should be available since these are frequently swallowed. Polyvinyl chloride (PVC) tubing, ramps, and boxes can provide environmental enrichment. Boxes filled with clean soil or uncooked long-grain rice allow for natural digging behavior (Johnson-Delaney 2017d).

Commercially available ferret-specific diets are available, though cat food can also

(a)

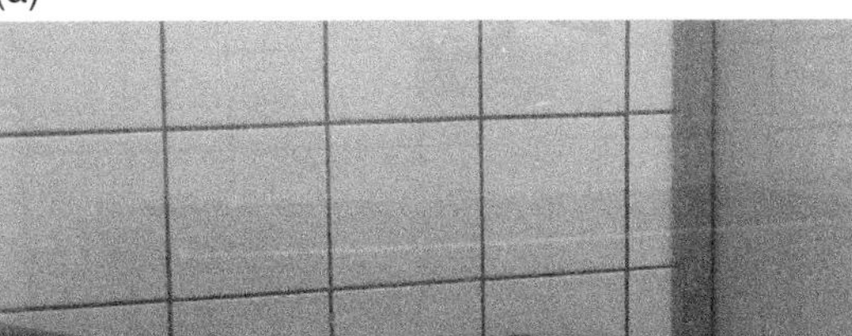

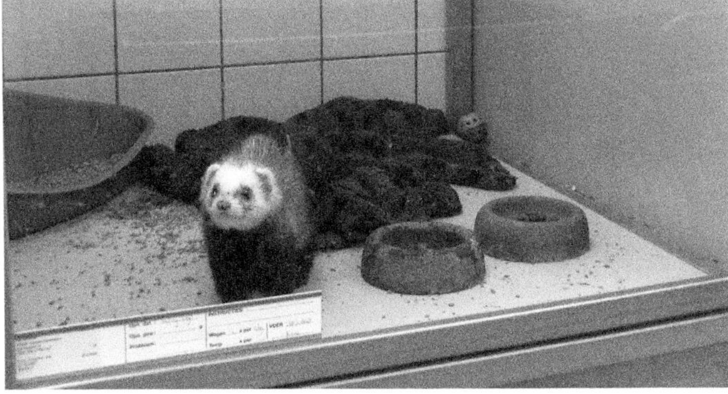

(b)

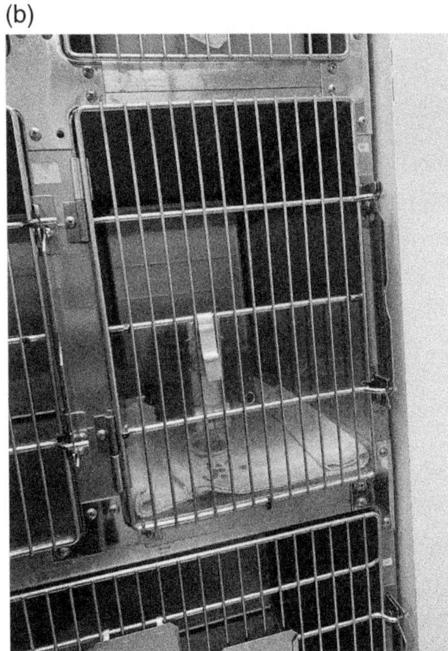

Figure 24.1 (a) Ferret cage. *Source:* Courtesy N.J. Schoemaker and Yvonne Van Zeeland. (b) Caging used for dogs and cats can be adapted for use in ferrets. In this picture, a plastic barrier has been affixed to the lower part of the cage to cover gaps between cage bars. *Source:* Courtesy Jennifer Graham.

be used. A diet composed of high-quality meat sources with 30–35% crude protein, 15–30% fat, and minimal carbohydrates and fiber is suitable for non-breeding adult ferrets. An adult ferret will eat about 43 g/kg body weight of dry food daily. Plant proteins in the diet may lead to urolithiasis (Johnson-Delaney 2017e).

24.2.1.3 Handling

Most ferrets can be handled for examination or treatment by holding by the scruff at the back of the neck (Figure 24.2). If the ferret is calm it can be examined on a table without scruffing, but most ferrets require this technique when taking a rectal temperature and administering oral or injectable medications. Ferrets can bite without

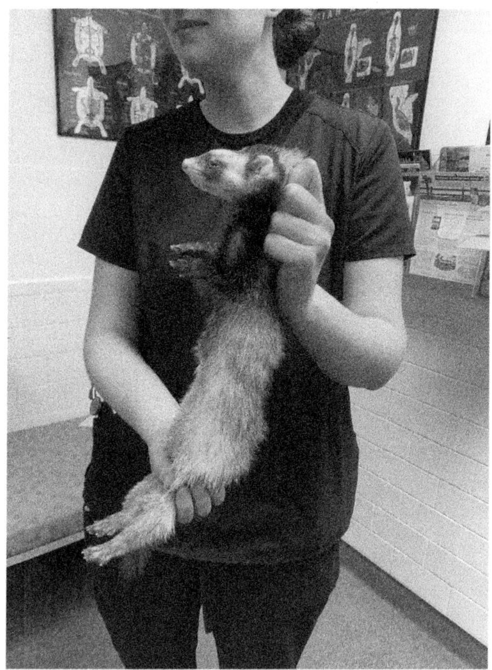

Figure 24.2 Most ferrets can be handled for examination or treatment by holding by the scruff at the back of the neck. *Source:* Courtesy Jennifer Graham.

warning so caution should be taken to prevent bites (Quesenberry and Orcutt 2012). Ferrets often yawn while being scruffed and this allows for a concurrent oral examination. The ear canals should be closely examined with a small otoscope cone and magnification as ear mites are commonly found. If additional restraint is required the ferret can be scruffed while holding around the hips, avoiding pulling on the legs since this often produces more struggling. A distractor treat can be given to help facilitate examinations and restraint using meat-based canned food or a small amount of FerreTone (8-in-1 Pet Products, Islandia, NY) (Chitty 2017a).

24.2.1.4 Vaccination and Routine Healthcare

Ferrets in the United States are commonly vaccinated against CDV and rabies. A series of three CDV vaccinations given at three-week intervals (8, 11, and 14 weeks) with an annual booster is recommended for kits. A two-dose series of CDV vaccine is recommended in unvaccinated adult ferrets with the vaccine administered two to four weeks apart. There have been reports of reversion to virulence from some live canine distemper vaccines in ferrets. There is a licensed canarypox-vectored recombinant CDV vaccine for use in ferrets in the United States called PureVax™ (Merial, Athens, GA). If this is not available, Nobivac DP® (Merck Animal Health, Madison, NJ) diluted with a solvent (not containing leptospirosis) can be used off-label (Chitty 2017b).

Rabies vaccination is required for ferrets in the United States. A licensed product (Imrab-3® or Imrab-3 TF®, Merial, Duluth, GA) is recommended at three months of age with annual boosters. Titers to rabies vaccination develop within 30 days of vaccination (Chitty 2017b; Quesenberry and Orcutt 2012).

Type 1 hypersensitivity reactions or anaphylaxis are commonly associated with vaccine administration in ferrets so shelters should be prepared to monitor for and treat vaccine reactions. Vaccine reactions can range from mild (pruritis, skin erythema) to severe (vomiting, diarrhea, piloerection, hyperthermia, cardiovascular collapse, and death). Vaccine-associated reactions should be reported to the USDA Center for Veterinary Biologics. The authors recommend premedication with diphenhydramine (2 mg/kg intramuscular [IM] or oral [PO]) before vaccination, ideally spacing out vaccines by several days to several weeks, and monitoring ferrets closely for 30 minutes after vaccination. In cases of a vaccine reaction, an antihistamine, epinephrine or a short-acting corticosteroid should be administered if this has not already been done, along with general supportive care measures (Quesenberry and Orcutt 2012).

While endoparasites are not common in ferrets, it is advisable to perform fecal examinations, including direct fecal smears and fecal flotations, on ferrets entering shelter situations, particularly if they are young. Coccidiosis is seen infrequently, as are giardiasis and cryptosporidiosis. Heartworms (*Dirofilaria immitis*) can occur in ferrets in endemic areas. The administration of oral ivermectin once a month is a practical preventive measure (Chitty 2017b; Quesenberry and Orcutt 2012), and topical imidacloprid/moxidectin (Advantage Multi® for Cats, Bayer) has been licensed for use in ferrets as well (See Chapter 18 for more information on heartworm disease).

Ear mites (*Otodectes cynotis*) are common and challenging to detect without a thorough otic exam, so all ferrets presenting in a shelter situation should be carefully screened and routinely treated for this before entering the general population. Ivermectin and selamectin are effective treatments. Flea infestation (*Ctenocephalides* sp.) is possible in ferrets, so all ferrets entering the shelter should be screened for fleas and flea dirt. Ferrets can be treated with products that are safe to use in cats. Lyme disease is not reported in ferrets and ticks are rarely seen (Chitty 2017b; Quesenberry and Orcutt 2012). More information on ear mites and fleas in ferrets can be found later in the section on parasitic diseases in this chapter.

Infectious diseases of ferrets of particular concern in the shelter environment, due to their relatively high prevalence, ease of transmission to other ferrets or other species, and/or zoonotic potential, include bacterial gastroenteritis; ear mites; fleas; CDV; coronavirus; influenza; rabies; and dermatophytosis.

24.2.2 Infectious Diseases in Ferrets: Bacterial

(See Table 24.1 for a list of diseases in ferrets by body systems. "Z" in the table next to a disease indicates it is transmissible to humans.)

24.2.2.1 Bacterial Gastroenteritis (*Campylobacter, Escherichia coli, Salmonella*)

Gram-negative bacteria, including *Campylobacter*, *Escherichia coli*, and *Salmonella* sp., are primarily associated with bacterial gastroenteritis in ferrets, though *Staphylococcus delphini* was reported to cause mucoid diarrhea in kits (Hoefer et al. 2012). Raw diets, stress, lack of hygiene, and overcrowding can predispose to disease (Hoefer et al. 2012), especially because up to 80% of ferrets, in some populations, may be carriers of *Campylobacter jejuni* (Perpinan and Johnson-Delaney 2017).

Clinical signs of bacterial gastroenteritis can include diarrhea (sometimes bloody), dehydration, fever, anorexia, and abdominal pain (Hoefer et al. 2012; Perpinan and Johnson-Delaney 2017). The presence of maternal antibodies in young ferrets can result in self-limiting disease caused by *Campylobacter,* with clinical signs generally seen in ferrets less than six months but rarely in adults (Perpinan and Johnson-Delaney 2017). *E. coli* infection is also seen more commonly in ferrets younger than six months old. The incubation period for *Campylobacter* is less than 24 hours and up to a few days with *E. coli* and *Salmonella*. Duration and severity of disease are dependent on the strain of *E. coli* or *Salmonella*, with systemic disease more commonly seen with these isolates than with *Campylobacter* (Perpinan and Johnson-Delaney 2017). *Campylobacter* can cause intermittent diarrhea for more than a month in infected ferrets; ferrets with *E. coli* and *Salmonella* can have rapidly progressive diarrhea that can result in disseminated intravascular coagulation (DIC) and death within 24 hours of showing signs (Perpinan and Johnson-Delaney 2017).

Bacterial culture and sensitivity (C/S) should be obtained when bacterial enteritis is suspected. *Campylobacter* grows slowly and requires microaerobic conditions and *Salmonella* requires enriched media. Because it can identify virulence factors of *E. coli*, species of *Salmonella*, and avoid culture requirements for *Campylobacter*, polymerase chain reaction (PCR) is often used to diagnose infection (Perpinan and Johnson-Delaney 2017). Because ferrets can be asymptomatic carriers, the detection of bacteria within the intestinal tract is suggestive of infection but not diagnostic for disease. Isolation of bacteria from normally sterile organs (liver, spleen, kidney, etc.) of a deceased ferret is diagnostic for disease (Perpinan and Johnson-Delaney 2017).

Antibiotic therapy should not be delayed in cases of suspected bacterial gastroenteritis. Even though *Campylobacter* infections can be

Table 24.1 Classification of ferret diseases by body system.

System	Symptoms	Etiology
Respiratory		
Bacterial pneumonia – Z	Lethargy, fever, anorexia, weight loss, dyspnea, coughing, nasal discharge	*Streptococcus, E. coli, Klebsiella, Pseudomonas*
Mycoplasmosis	Chronic non-productive cough, hemoptysis, sneezing, labored breathing, and conjunctivitis	*M. molare* and *M. lagogenitalium*
Systemic		
Botulism	Dysphagia, ataxia, ascending paresis, third eyelid prolapse, respiratory paralysis	*Clostridium botulinum types A, B, and C*
Listeriosis – Z	Ataxia, paresis, and paralysis	*Listeria monocytogenes*
Mycobacteriosis – Z	Weight loss, vomiting, diarrhea, lymphadenopathy, splenomegaly, conjunctival lesions, draining tuberculous lesions, and pneumonia	*Mycobacteria bovis, M. avium, M. genavense, M. abscesses, M. triplex*, and *M. celatum*
Heartworms	Anorexia, lethargy, weakness, depression, coughing, dyspnea, cyanosis, pale mucous membranes, and melena	*Dirofilaria immitis*
Gastrointestinal		
Bacterial enteritis – Z	Diarrhea, dehydration fever, anorexia, abdominal pain	*Campylobacter, E. coli, Salmonella*
Proliferative bowel disease	Chronic intermittent diarrhea, weakness, lethargy, weight loss, mucoid, perineal staining, and discolored feces mesenteric lymphadenopathy, thickened bowel loops, and partial rectal prolapse	*Lawsonia intracellularis*
Coccidiosis	Foul-smelling diarrhea, weakness, lethargy, dehydration, rectal prolapse, perineal staining, and tenesmus	*Eimeria* and *Isospora (E. furonis)*
Cryptosporidiosis – Z	Anorexia, weight loss, and diarrhea	*Cryptosporidium parvum*
Giardiasis – Z*	Diarrhea	*Giardia intestinalis*
Helicobacter	Lethargy, anorexia, nausea bruxism, vomiting, dehydration, melena, and emaciation in severe infections. Gastric and duodenal inflammation and ulceration	*Helicobacter mustelae*
Dermatologic		
Ear mites	Head shaking and ear scratching, mild excoriations and crusting around the ears	*Otodectes cynotis*
Fleas	Pruritis, erythemic papules, and alopecia	*Ctenocephalides*

Z-Zoonotic.
Z* Potentially zoonotic.

self-limiting, isolation of affected animals and antibiotic therapy are recommended in a shelter setting to prevent outbreaks and reduce mortality. Chloramphenicol is effective against *E. coli, Salmonella*, and *Campylobacter*; amoxicillin/clavulanic acid combined with a fluoroquinolone or aminoglycoside is also a first-line treatment (Perpinan and Johnson-

Delaney 2017). General supportive care including fluids and supplemental feeding is also recommended. Environmental disinfection with routine sanitation procedures is recommended. Because these infections are potentially zoonotic, immunosuppressed individuals and children should not handle affected ferrets known or suspected to be infected with one of these pathogens.

24.2.2.2 Bacterial Pneumonia

Bacterial pneumonia is characterized by suppurative inflammation and is not a common diagnosis in ferrets. Common bacterial isolates associated with pneumonia in ferrets include *Streptococcus* (including *Streptococcus zooepidemicus), E. coli, Klebsiella pneumoniae, Pseudomonas aeruginosa, Bordetella bronchiseptica, Listeria monocytogenes, Pneumocystis carinii*, and numerous mycobacterial species (Barron and Rosenthal 2012; Richardson and Perpinan 2017). Immunosuppressed individuals will be more at risk of contracting bacterial pneumonia, with routes of exposure including inhalation, aspiration, and hematogenous (Richardson and Perpinan 2017).

Clinical signs noted with bacterial pneumonia include lethargy, fever, anorexia and weight loss, tachypnea, dyspnea, cyanosis, coughing, nasal discharge, and increased lung sounds (Barron and Rosenthal 2012; Richardson and Perpinan 2017). Death from sepsis related to fulminant pneumonia has been reported. Differential diagnoses for these signs include viral and fungal pneumonia, cardiovascular disease, and neoplasia, among others (Barron and Rosenthal 2012; Richardson and Perpinan 2017).

Diagnostics recommended for ferrets presenting with lower respiratory signs include complete blood count (CBC) and chemistry profile, and radiographs; further diagnostics depend on initial findings. Bacterial pneumonia is generally associated with a leukocytosis and neutrophilia +/− left shift. Radiographic findings can include an increased interstitial or alveolar pattern, air bronchograms, and a dependent distribution in cases of aspiration. Tracheal aspirate and bronchiolar lavage can be performed on stable patients under general anesthesia with fluid submitted for culture (aerobic, anaerobic, fungal, mycobacterial, other) and sensitivity based on cytologic results of the wash. Fine needle aspiration (FNA) can be considered in cases of pulmonary consolidation or a mass effect, taking care to avoid iatrogenic pneumothorax (Barron and Rosenthal 2012; Richardson and Perpinan 2017).

Treatment of bacterial pneumonia should include supportive care such as oxygen therapy when warranted, fluid therapy, assisted feeding, and antibiotic therapy. Antibiotic choice can be guided by C/S with quinolones, trimethoprim sulfa, chloramphenicol, cephalosporins, and azithromycin being treatment choices to consider while waiting on C/S results; combination therapy may be necessary. Nebulization, bronchodilators, mucolytics, and coupage may also be helpful (Barron and Rosenthal 2012; Richardson and Perpinan 2017).

Advanced diagnostics and aggressive therapy, while indicated, may not be feasible in the typical shelter setting and careful consideration should be given to balancing individual animal and population level considerations along with available resources. Isolation of affected ferrets is recommended in a shelter setting. Housing ill ferrets away from others of their species as well as from dogs, cats, rabbits, and other common carriers of *B. bronchiseptica* is recommended. While a killed, injectable *B. bronchiseptica* bacterin has been anecdotally reported to prevent bordetellosis in ferrets when used in accordance with recommendation for dogs, modified live intranasal *B. bronchiseptica* is not recommended as it may cause disease in ferrets (Barron and Rosenthal 2012); routine vaccination of ferrets against *B. bronchiseptica* is not recommended in a shelter setting. *K. pneumoniae, P. aeruginosa, L. monocytogenes, B. bronchiseptica,* and mycobacterial species could be of zoonotic concern in immunocompromised humans (Mitchell and Tully 2012).

24.2.2.3 Botulism

Clostridium botulinum types A, B, and C can cause endotoxin release and disease in ferrets, with type C usually being lethal. Contaminated food (particularly canned and meat-based items) is the usual source of *C. botulinum* in ferrets and clinical signs generally occur 12–96 hours after ingestion. Clinical signs can include dysphagia, ataxia, ascending paresis, third eyelid prolapse and eventual respiratory paralysis (Orosz and Johnson-Delaney 2017). Diagnosis is based on the presence of bacteria in stomach contents, feces, or vomitus at necropsy. There is no readily available commercial toxin screening test for this bacterium in ferrets (Orosz and Johnson-Delaney 2017). While botulism would be uncommon in a shelter setting, veterinarians should have this on the differential list for neurologic signs in ferrets as this could occur in an outbreak situation secondary to contaminated food items.

24.2.2.4 Helicobacter mustelae

Virtually all ferrets in the United States are exposed to *Helicobacter mustelae*, a spiral gram-negative rod that has been associated with gastritis and ulcers in ferrets (Hoefer et al. 2012; Perpinan and Johnson-Delaney 2017). Similar to *Helicobacter pylori* in humans, *H. mustelae* requires a microaerophilic environment to grow in culture. Oral administration of *H. mustelae* in ferrets causes colonization, rise in anti-*H. mustelae* antibody titer, and chronic gastritis (Hoefer et al. 2012; Perpinan and Johnson-Delaney 2017). Despite the high rate of infection, most ferrets are asymptomatic for the disease. The disease may become clinically apparent in ferrets stressed with surgery or concurrent disease.

If symptomatic, clinical signs of *H. mustelae* can include lethargy, anorexia, nausea (characterized by hypersalivation and pawing at the mouth), bruxism, vomiting, dehydration, melena, and emaciation in severe infections. Gastric and duodenal inflammation and ulceration can occur, and chronic disease may be associated with gastric adenocarcinoma and lymphoma (Hoefer et al. 2012; Perpinan and Johnson-Delaney 2017). Pale mucous membranes may be evident; though non-specific, splenomegaly and mesenteric lymphadenopathy have been described (Perpinan and Johnson-Delaney 2017).

Routine blood work may show anemia if GI ulceration is present but is otherwise unremarkable. Antibody titers increase with age and chronicity of infection but are not routinely performed in clinical settings. Definitive diagnosis of *Helicobacter* is made by histopathologic examination of silver-stained gastric mucosal samples obtained via endoscopic or surgical biopsy (Hoefer et al. 2012; Perpinan and Johnson-Delaney 2017). Feces, gastric biopsy, and gastric swabs or washes can be submitted for *Helicobacter* culture and/or PCR analysis. Diagnostics other than histopathologic examination are suggestive, but not confirmatory, of disease.

As many GI disorders can improve with antibiotic treatment, response to therapy is not an effective means of diagnosing *Helicobacter* infection. Treatment of *Helicobacter* includes a combination of different drugs (clarithromycin, metronidazole, and bismuth subsalicylate) for three to four weeks to prevent the development of resistance. Other modifications of this protocol can be used, including substitution of amoxicillin or amoxicillin/clavulanic acid for clarithromycin; omeprazole, sucralfate, famotidine, or cimetidine instead of bismuth subsalicylate; substitution of amoxicillin or amoxicillin/clavulanic acid for metronidazole; or a combination of enrofloxacin and bismuth subsalicylate (Hoefer et al. 2012; Perpinan and Johnson-Delaney 2017). Despite fecal excretion of *Helicobacter* increasing with the use of omeprazole, antacids seem to be beneficial in clinical cases. Though infection can theoretically be cleared with appropriate therapy, reinfection can occur at any time. The recurrence of clinical signs despite therapy can indicate *Helicobacter* is not the primary cause of clinical signs (Perpinan and Johnson-Delaney 2017).

Because most ferrets are infected with *Helicobacter*, isolation of affected animals is not a realistic way to control disease in a shelter setting. However, since many other GI diseases can present with similar clinical signs and definitive diagnosis of *Helicobacter* is unlikely to occur in a shelter situation, it is prudent to isolate ferrets with GI signs from asymptomatic animals to reduce the potential for other infectious disease outbreaks. If resources allow, all ferrets entering a shelter situation can be isolated and treated with a *Helicobacter*-specific protocol for three to four weeks prior to introduction to other ferrets in an adoptive home. Finally, the authors believe any chronic GI disease that causes inflammation could theoretically increase the risk of GI neoplasia so a thorough workup, whenever possible, is generally recommended in ferrets showing chronic GI signs.

24.2.2.5 Listeriosis

L. monocytogenes is a ubiquitous gram-positive, non-spore-forming rod that is mildly infectious to ferrets (Mitchell and Tully 2012; Orosz and Johnson-Delaney 2017). Ferrets may act as a source for *L. monocytogenes* or be infected via ingestion of infected food or inhalation. Clinical signs can occur 1–90 days after ingestion and can include ataxia, paresis, and paralysis (Orosz and Johnson-Delaney 2017). Diagnosis is based on culture of the organism. Affected ferrets should be isolated and treated with an antibiotic that penetrates the central nervous system (CNS) such as penicillin or chloramphenicol (Orosz and Johnson-Delaney 2017) and provided appropriate supportive care, or humane euthanasia should be considered. Immunocompromised ferrets and humans are predisposed to contracting *Listeria* and shelters should use routine sanitation measures and minimize exposure of ferrets and other animals to this organism. Raw food diets sold for dogs and cats that may be fed to ferrets have been recalled for *Listeria* contamination (Orosz and Johnson-Delaney 2017).

24.2.2.6 Mycobacteriosis

Species of mycobacteria described to cause infection in ferrets include *Mycobacteria bovis, Mycobacterium avium, Mycobacterium genavense, Mycobacterium abscesses, Mycobacterium triplex*, and *Mycobacterium celatum* (Hoefer et al. 2012; Johnson-Delaney 2017e). Ferrets serve as hosts and sentinels for *M. bovis* in New Zealand (Johnson-Delaney 2017e). Transmission is via ingestion, inhalation of the organisms and ferret-ferret transmission. Transmission from ferrets to other animals (wildlife and livestock as documented to occur in New Zealand) is also possible.

Ferrets with mycobacteriosis may present with signs including weight loss, vomiting, diarrhea, lymphadenopathy, splenomegaly, conjunctival lesions, draining tuberculous lesions, and pneumonia. Diagnosis of mycobacteriosis can be made by acid-fast staining, PCR, or culture of tissue biopsy specimens. Tissues described with granulomatous mycobacterial lesions at necropsy include liver, lungs, lymph nodes, stomach, intestine, and trachea (Hoefer et al. 2012).

Though ferret-human transmission has not been documented, mycobacteria pose a zoonotic risk. Treatment of mycobacteria in ferrets has been described with some apparent success but this is not practical or recommended in a shelter setting. Additionally, if any animal is diagnosed with the disease, any co-housed animals should be considered as exposed and potentially infected. Fortunately, the incidence of mycobacterial infection in pet ferrets is low and likely uncommon in shelter situations.

24.2.2.7 Mycoplasmosis

An outbreak of a novel *Mycoplasma* species has been recently diagnosed in a large breeding facility, with over 8000 ferrets affected. The *Mycoplasma* species identified in the outbreak most closely resembled *Mycoplasma molare* and *Mycoplasma lagogenitalium* though a definitive identification could not be made (Richardson and Perpinan 2017). *Mycoplasma* are generally host-specific, transmitted via inhalation, and cause damage and dysfunction to respiratory epithelial cilia.

Clinical signs in the ferret *Mycoplasma* outbreak included a chronic non-productive cough, hemoptysis, sneezing, labored breathing, and conjunctivitis (Richardson and Perpinan 2017). There was high morbidity but low mortality in the breeding facility outbreak. As with other *Mycoplasma* species, concurrent illness likely contributes to the severity of the disease.

Diagnosis of *Mycoplasma* can be made by cytology, bacterial C/S, and PCR of bronchoalveolar lavage (BAL), oropharyngeal swabs, or postmortem samples. *Mycoplasma* culture requires special media and conditions for growth, so *Mycoplasma*-specific culture should be requested at the time of sample submission. Like *Mycoplasma pulmonis* in rats, *Mycoplasma* in ferrets causes grossly visible multi-focal nodules throughout airways and lung tissue along with lymphoplasmacytic perivascular cuffing and bronchiole-associated lymphoid hyperplasia (Richardson and Perpinan 2017). Based on the author's experience with rats, radiographic changes may not be as obvious in the initial stages. Bronchointerstitial pattern with peribronchial cuffing was reported in a ferret with mycoplasma.

Antibiotics effective against *Mycoplasma* include doxycycline, fluoroquinolones, and azithromycin. General supportive care therapy as described under bacterial pneumonia is also recommended. *Mycoplasma* infections in ferrets may be lifelong.

Mycoplasma should be on the differential list for chronic coughing in ferrets. Coughing ferrets should be segregated from other ferrets in a shelter setting for screening diagnostics and therapy; affected ferrets should ideally remain separated from the general population. Adopters should be informed of the potential for recurrent signs and, in the case of *Mycoplasma* infections, lifelong infection. There is anecdotal information that rabbits can get *M. pulmonis* from infected rats, and it remains unknown if ferrets are also at risk. It is unknown if *Mycoplasma* in ferrets poses a zoonotic risk to humans.

24.2.2.8 Proliferative Bowel Disease (*Lawsonia intracellularis*)

Lawsonia intracellularis is the causative agent for proliferative bowel disease (PBD) in ferrets. *L. intracellularis* causes inflammation of the colonic mucosa and epithelial hyperplasia, resulting in palpably thickened intestinal loops. The same causative agent causes disease in hamsters, swine, rabbits, deer, ratites, and foals (Hoefer et al. 2012). Fecal-oral transmission is the suspected route of transmission and infection is described most frequently in young ferrets between 10 weeks to 6 months old (Hoefer et al. 2012; Perpinan and Johnson-Delaney 2017).

Clinical signs of infected animals include chronic intermittent mucoid diarrhea, weakness, lethargy, weight loss, perineal staining, discolored feces (bile or blood-stained), mesenteric lymphadenopathy, thickened bowel loops, and partial rectal prolapse (Hoefer et al. 2012; Perpinan and Johnson-Delaney 2017). Though the author (JG) is unaware of any studies regarding bacterial shedding in ferrets, if one extrapolates from what is known in other species, it is possible that subclinically infected animals may shed the bacteria. The duration of illness can be 3–18 weeks (Perpinan and Johnson-Delaney 2017). In exposed groups of ferrets, only 1–3% of the population develop signs of disease. Environmental and nutritional stress is thought to contribute to the development of disease (Hoefer et al. 2012).

A presumptive diagnosis of *L. intracellularis* is based on history, clinical signs, and response to therapy. A PCR assay can be used to screen fecal or rectal swabs and colonic biopsy samples (Hoefer et al. 2012). Colonic samples can also be screened via histologic examination, silver stains, or fluorescent-antibody tests (Perpinan and Johnson-Delaney 2017).

Treatment of choice for *L. intracellularis* in affected ferrets is chloramphenicol or metronidazole for 10–14 days. Stress reduction and supportive care as described for bacterial gastroenteritis are also recommended. Because this disease is rarely seen in clinical practice, the incidence in shelter settings is also likely to be low. However, *L. intracellularis* should be a differential for cases of diarrhea and weight loss in young ferrets in shelters.

24.2.3 Infectious Diseases in Ferrets: Parasitic

24.2.3.1 Coccidiosis

Coccidia are protozoal parasites that are rarely associated with apparent clinical disease in ferrets, but outbreaks in high-density populations can cause severe enteric disease and death (Perpinan and Johnson-Delaney 2017). *Eimeria* and *Isospora* species affect ferrets, with *E. furonis* linked to more severe disease (Perpinan and Johnson-Delaney 2017). There can be cross-infection of *Isospora* between dogs/cats/ferrets. Transmission is via the ingestion of sporulated oocysts.

Clinical signs of disease include foul-smelling diarrhea that may appear pasty/gelatinous and contain frank blood or melena. Weakness, lethargy, dehydration, rectal prolapse, perineal staining, and tenesmus can also be seen (Perpinan and Johnson-Delaney 2017). Animals typically recover or die within 5–10 days. Though rare, it is also possible for hepatobiliary coccidiosis to cause severe liver disease in ferrets.

Diagnosis of coccidiosis is made by microscopic examination of direct fecal wet mount or fecal flotation, but false negatives are possible and may not reveal the extent of disease (Perpinan and Johnson-Delaney 2017). Evidence of dehydration and regenerative anemia may be noted on blood work. Necropsy of deceased animals may reveal dilated and thin intestinal walls, nonspecific changes including splenomegaly and hepatic lipidosis, and oocysts and intestinal lesions on histopathologic examination. While large numbers of coccidia in the presence of clinical signs is suggestive of disease, histopathology is needed for definitive diagnosis (Perpinan and Johnson-Delaney 2017) because many animals may shed coccidia without showing any signs of clinical disease. Lesions include epithelial thickening, particularly of the jejunum and ileum, along with lymphoid and granulomatous enteritis with intraepithelial organisms.

Treatment in the face of an outbreak is challenging. Sulfadimethoxine combined with trimethoprim is reported to be partially effective; the effectiveness of amprolium is unknown. Ponazuril has also been suggested as a treatment option in the face of an outbreak and is used in many small mammals at a dose of 10–50 mg/kg orally (PO) once daily for 10 days (Mitchell 2008). Outbreaks of coccidiosis in ferrets have been reported in shelters and breeding facilities and disease can spread rapidly. Decreasing population density and stress may help control the disease.

Coccidiosis is often associated with unsanitary conditions. Though bleach, quaternary ammonium compounds, and heat have been recommended for environmental cleaning (Hoefer et al. 2012), sporulated oocysts are resistant to most disinfectants. It is important to wash areas thoroughly to mechanically remove as many oocysts as possible. Steam cleaning or the application of a 10% ammonia solution or boiling water have been reported as effective to disinfect cages, runs and equipment. Feces must be removed promptly to avoid contamination of food and water bowls, and in-depth insect control is necessary in animal and food areas (Dubey and Greene 2012).

24.2.3.2 Cryptosporidiosis

Cryptosporidium parvum is a 4–6 μm diameter apicomplexan protozoan that exhibits partial acid-fast staining. *C. parvum* can be found in the feces of normal ferrets; stress and immunosuppression can exacerbate clinical signs in an animal that may otherwise have subclinical disease. The transmission route is fecal-oral and the organism is highly contagious between stressed animals. Disease is generally limited to two to three weeks; clinical signs include anorexia, weight loss, and diarrhea caused by small intestinal mucosal damage (Hoefer et al. 2012; Perpinan and Johnson-Delaney 2017). An eosinophilic infiltrate in the laminae propria of the small intestine can be seen in association with this organism (Perpinan and Johnson-Delaney 2017).

Diagnosis can be made by fecal wet mount direct smear or fecal float examination, enzyme linked immunosorbent assay (ELISA), and PCR. Paromomycin at 125–165 mg/kg orally (PO) twice daily (BID) for five days, though not curative, has been recommended along with general supportive care and stress reduction to manage clinical signs associated with cryptosporidiosis (Blagburn 2003). *C. parvum* may pose a zoonotic threat and can infect dogs and cats, so appropriate biosecurity measures should be followed, including the use of masks and gloves when handling affected ferrets or cleaning cages. Environmental oocysts resist most disinfectants used routinely by shelters, including bleach, but can be destroyed with a 5% ammonia solution, 3% hydrogen peroxide for 20 minutes, and temperatures below 32 °F (0 °C) or above 149 °F (65 °C) (Mans and Donnelly 2012). Frequent litter box changes are recommended to decrease the potential for spread of the organism (Hoefer et al. 2012).

24.2.3.3 Dirofilariasis

Heartworm disease caused by *D. immitis*, a parasitic nematode, has been reported in ferrets. Disease can range from asymptomatic infection to sudden death. Ferrets are not likely to serve as a source of transmission to other animals due to their lack of circulating microfilaremia. Please refer to Chapter 18 on Heartworm Disease for more detailed information on the disease in ferrets.

24.2.3.4 Ear Mites

As in dogs and cats, *O. cynotis* is the ear mite affecting ferrets. It is contracted via direct contact with infected animals. Infected ferrets may be asymptomatic or have clinical signs including head shaking and ear scratching. Physical examination findings associated with *Otodectes* infection can include inflammation of the ear canal, intense pruritis during an otic examination, and mild excoriations and crusting around the ears. Neurologic signs are rarely seen. Brown exudate can be normal in ferrets or can be seen with ear-mite infections; microscopic examination of aural debris can be helpful to diagnose this condition. Ear mites are visible with magnification and careful otoscopic examination is a practical way to diagnose this condition in a shelter setting. Because ear mites are very common in ferrets and not always apparent on an otic examination, empiric treatment of all ferrets presenting to the shelter for ear mites is recommended prior to mixing with the general population. The life cycle of *Otodectes* is three weeks, making repeat treatment necessary to resolve infestation with some treatment protocols. Aural topical ivermectin administration (1% ivermectin diluted 1 : 10 in propylene glycol, at a dosage of 400 μg/kg [0.4 mg/kg] of body weight, divided equally between the two ear canals) upon admission with repeat dosing 14 days later is a cost-effective way to manage this parasite. Selamectin has also been used to treat ear mites in ferrets. The ferret's environment, including cages and bedding, should be cleaned and disinfected at the same time to prevent reinfection (Johnson-Delaney 2017f; Orcutt and Tater 2012).

24.2.3.5 Fleas

A variety of flea species, including *Ctenocephalides*, can infest ferrets (Johnson-Delaney 2017f; Orcutt and Tater 2012). Ferrets contract fleas from contaminated environments or by direct contact with an affected animal. Clinical signs can be inapparent or include pruritis, erythemic papules, and alopecia. Though uncommon, flea hypersensitivity is possible in ferrets. The identification of flea or flea excrement on a ferret is diagnostic for this condition. Treatment of the ferret and environment are necessary to resolve this condition. In general, drugs and protocols effective for use in cats are safe and effective in ferrets. Topical pyrethrins, imidacloprid/moxidectin, and selamectin are potential therapy options in ferrets. Shelters should ideally treat affected ferrets upon admission and evaluate for other diseases, particularly adrenal disease, if pruritis is present without signs of external parasites.

24.2.3.6 Giardiasis

Giardiasis in ferrets is caused by *Giardia intestinalis,* a parasitic protozoan. *G. intestinalis* cysts and trophozoites are occasionally found on routine fecal examination in ferrets. If found in association with clinical signs, particularly diarrhea, treatment is warranted. Diagnosis can be made on fecal wet mount direct microscopy or with fecal ELISA testing. Treatment given to ferrets is as in dogs: fenbendazole at 50 mg/kg PO once daily for five days, metronidazole at 25 mg/kg PO twice daily for five days or a combination of the two as described for dogs. Gloves and masks should be worn when handling infected animals since *Giardia* is considered potentially zoonotic. Sanitation of the environment is recommended and many commercially available products, including bleach and quaternary ammonium disinfectants, will be effective (Perpinan and Johnson-Delaney 2017).

24.2.3.7 Sarcoptic Mange

Sarcoptes scabiei mites rarely infest ferrets; the disease is generally contracted from affected dogs or fomites. The author (JG) has seen it most commonly in immunocompromised ferrets exposed to infected dogs. *S. scabiei* is a zoonotic parasite (Johnson-Delaney 2017f; Orcutt and Tater 2012). Ferrets with sarcoptic mange can present with generalized alopecia and intense pruritis or localized disease confined to the feet. Diagnosis can be made via skin scraping but false-negative results with scraping are common. Ivermectin every 7–14 days for three treatments is an option for therapy. Topical or systemic treatment for secondary dermatitis may be required. Diphenhydramine and a nonsteroidal anti-inflammatory drug (NSAID) may help with pruritis. Imidacloprid/moxidectin (1.9–3.3 μg/kg topically every (q) 30 days (d) and selamectin (6–18 mg/kg topically q30d) have been used successfully in dogs with *S. scabiei* and can be considered for off-label use in ferrets. Like therapy in dogs and cats, bedding and the environment should also be addressed when treating mites in ferrets.

24.2.3.8 Toxoplasmosis

Toxoplasmosis is caused by a single-celled protozoan parasite. *Toxoplasma gondii* infection can occur in ferrets as a result of eating raw meat or ingestion of infected cat feces (Orosz and Johnson-Delaney 2017). On a fur farm in New Zealand, 30% of 750 neonatal ferrets died from toxoplasmosis, with no clinical signs and multifocal necrosis found in the lungs, heart, and liver. Clinical signs vary depending on organ infected, may or may not be present, and can include lethargy, anorexia, ophthalmic abnormalities, fever, CNS signs, anemia, hepatitis, respiratory, and GI signs. Diagnosis is made with an ELISA test for IgG and IgM, *T. gondii*-specific antigen testing, or via histopathology. Treatment for toxoplasmosis is sulfonamide (30 mg/kg PO) for at least 14 days and continued until after clinical signs are absent. Pyrimethamine (0.5 mg/kg PO q12h) and sulfadiazine (30 mg/kg PO q12h) can also be used. Toxoplasmosis is unlikely to occur in ferrets in a shelter setting if feeding raw meat is avoided and ferrets are prevented from having access to areas contaminated by cat feces.

24.2.4 Infectious Diseases in Ferrets: Viral

24.2.4.1 Aleutian Disease

Aleutian disease virus (ADV) is a parvovirus that can cause chronic wasting in mink and ferrets (Antinoff and Giovanella 2012; Orosz and Johnson-Delaney 2017). It is not the same parvovirus that infects dogs and cats. Routes of transmission include ingestion and inhalation. The virus is shed in saliva, urine, and feces. The overall prevalence of ADV serologically positive animals in a survey of 446 ferrets was 8.5% (Welchman et al. 1993).

The clinical signs in a ferret with ADV can include ataxia, tremors, ascending paresis, paraplegia or hemiplegia (Antinoff and Giovanella 2012; Orosz and Johnson-Delaney 2017). Splenic and lymph node enlargement may be present. Fecal and urinary incontinence is possible. Signs can be noted as early as 24 hours after infection and persist for several months.

Screening tests for ADV include PCR and counterimmunoelectrophoresis. The ELISA test for ferrets that was available through Avecon Diagnostics Inc. is no longer available. Because normal ferrets may have a high ADV titer but not show signs of disease, a very high titer or paired serology two weeks apart may be more helpful. Though not always present, a hallmark of this disease is a high gamma globulin concentration. A presumptive diagnosis of ADV is made based on compatible clinical signs along with positive results of ADV testing and hypergammaglobulinemia (Antinoff and Giovanella 2012). A definitive diagnosis of ADV is made on histopathologic examination with findings including non-suppurative encephalomyelitis and lymphoplasmacytic infiltrates on tissue samples.

Some ferrets shedding ADV may be asymptomatic with persistent infection or disease may be self-limiting and nonpersistent (Antinoff and Giovanella 2012). Ferrets suspected to have ADV should be isolated from other ferrets. Supportive care measures include supplemental feeding, GI protection, and antibiotics if secondary infection is suspected (Orosz and Johnson-Delaney 2017). Because ADV is an immune-mediated disease, immunosuppressive therapy may be beneficial but is not without risk. A vaccine is not available for this disease in ferrets and euthanasia should be considered for symptomatic ferrets in a shelter setting.

24.2.4.2 Canine Distemper Virus

CDV is a *Morbillivirus* virus in the *Paramyxoviridae* family (Barron and Rosenthal 2012; Richardson and Perpinan 2017). Ferrets are generally exposed to this RNA virus from dogs, though it should be noted that ferrets may also be a source of exposure to dogs in a shelter environment. Infection is usually fatal in ferrets. Transmission is via inhalation or direct contact and the virus remains stable on fomites for up to 20 minutes. The incubation period for CDV in ferrets is usually 7–10 days though it has been reported to be up to 56 days. Shedding occurs seven days after infection.

Clinical signs in the initial stages of infection in ferrets include anorexia, lethargy, photophobia, poor weight gain in young ferrets, pyrexia, and respiratory signs (Barron and Rosenthal 2012; Richardson and Perpinan 2017). A papular dermatitis on the chin may be noted along with dermatitis in the inguinal and perianal area. Generalized pruritis with progression to focal hyperkeratosis is noted in some animals. Progressive signs can include a soiled perineum, mucopurulent oculonasal discharge, pneumonia, hyperkeratosis of the planum nasale and footpads, neurologic signs including seizures and blindness, and death (Barron and Rosenthal 2012; Richardson and Perpinan 2017).

History and clinical signs can be suggestive of infection. Though signs of disease can mimic influenza in the early stages, CDV progresses to a mucopurulent oculonasal discharge after one to two days. Additionally, the presence of dermatitis on the chin and lips is pathognomonic for infection in a ferret showing signs compatible with CDV. Some of the diagnostics that may be helpful in the work-up for CDV include radiographs, blood work, PCR or serologic testing for CDV, fluorescent antibody staining of conjunctival scrapings, and histologic examination and special staining of tissue samples. Radiographs may show changes consistent with pneumonia, including pulmonary congestion or consolidation. Changes in blood work are non-specific and can include nonregenerative anemia, leukopenia, and alpha- and beta-hyperglobulinemia. Because both infected and vaccinated ferrets can have a positive titer on CDV antibody screening, test interpretation is challenging if the vaccine status of the ferret is unknown. Fluorescent antibody staining of conjunctival smears, mucous membrane scrapings, or blood smears can identify CDV antigen; false negatives are common since these tests are generally most useful in the first few days of disease (Barron and Rosenthal 2012). PCR for CDV can be performed on blood, urine, feces, tissue, or deep pharyngeal swabs; false positive results can occur if the ferret was recently vaccinated with a modified-live virus (Barron and Rosenthal 2012). Fluorescent staining of lymph nodes, cerebellum, and bladder epithelium can confirm infection postmortem. Inclusion bodies associated with CDV may be found on histopathologic examination of tracheal epithelium, urinary bladder, skin, GI tract, lymph nodes, spleen, and salivary glands (Barron and Rosenthal 2012).

While supportive care measures are described (Richardson and Perpinan 2017), no treatment is successful in resolving CDV and most infected ferrets will die. Death usually occurs 12–35 days after infection, depending on the strain of CDV. Anti-canine distemper hyperimmune serum may be helpful if given early in the disease, but humane euthanasia is likely the best course of action for CDV-infected ferrets in shelters because of the poor prognosis in individual animals and to minimize the potential of an outbreak. Prevention is by vaccination. Shelters should segregate ferrets from dogs to minimize the potential for exposure to CDV. Though protective titers are not established in ferrets, they are generally assumed to be ≥1 : 50. Ferrets have been shown to have serum neutralizing antibody titers of >1:50 against CDV for >3 years after being vaccinated at 14–16 weeks of age or older (Wagner and Bhardwaj 2012). In case of an outbreak, separate all infected ferrets and vaccinate all healthy unvaccinated ferrets. Because CDV is a labile virus, heat, drying, detergents, and disinfectants are effective against CDV (Barron and Rosenthal 2012).

24.2.4.3 Coronavirus

Clinical presentations of coronavirus in ferrets include a GI form resulting in diarrhea called epizootic catarrhal enteritis (ECE) or ferret enteric coronavirus (FRECV) and a feline infectious peritonitis (FIP)-like presentation with systemic granulomatous inflammation known as ferret systemic coronavirus (FRSCV). The ferret enteric and systemic coronavirus are not identical though closely related, and FRSCV may be a mutated form of FRECV (Perpinan and Johnson-Delaney 2017; Swisher and Lennox 2017).

ECE is a highly transmissible disease that causes diarrhea in ferrets. The virus is shed in saliva and feces and is transmitted via the fecal-oral route. Shedding is intermittent and can be reactivated during times of stress (Hoefer et al. 2012). Older ferrets are generally affected after exposure to young asymptomatic carrier ferrets. Anorexia and lethargy usually occur 48–72 hours after exposure. Vomiting may occur initially and a profuse, odorous, green, watery diarrhea with mucous may follow. Because enteric villi of the intestinal tract can be damaged, maldigestion and malabsorption characterized by seedy stool are evident as time passes. Coronavirus can be detected by reverse transcriptase-polymerase chain reaction (RT-PCR) of feces, saliva, or intestinal tissue samples and differentiate FRECV and FRSCV; RT-PCR that detects feline coronavirus will not detect ferret coronavirus (Perpinan and Johnson-Delaney 2017). Histopathology of the GI tract (jejunum or ileum) with immunohistochemistry (IHC) is required to make a diagnosis of coronavirus, as the presence of the virus alone is not confirmatory for the disease. Histologic changes consist of diffuse lymphocytic enteritis with villus atrophy. Affected ferrets should be isolated until clinical signs resolve and treated symptomatically with fluid therapy, antibiotics for secondary infection, and nutritional support. A short course of steroids and the use of a highly digestible diet may speed recovery. Most ferrets with ECE are symptomatic for a couple of weeks but signs can persist for months. Most commonly used disinfectants will inactivate coronavirus.

FRSCV causes progressive systemic pyogranulomatous disease in ferrets that resembles the dry form of FIP in cats (Hoefer et al. 2012). Ferrets with FRSCV are usually young (<18 months old) and generally present for weight loss, diarrhea, occasional neurologic signs, and have masses evident on abdominal palpation. Elevated body temperature is commonly noted (Swisher and Lennox 2017). The duration of clinical signs averages 67 days and the disease is progressive with a high mortality rate (Hoefer et al. 2012). Diagnosis is made by histopathology and IHC of formalin-fixed tissue samples or RT-PCR of fresh tissue. Blood work generally shows anemia, lymphopenia, and hypergammaglobulinemia. Radiographs commonly reveal severe muscle wasting, loss of serosal detail, splenomegaly, renomegaly, and a mid-abdominal mass effect (Swisher and Lennox 2017). Ultrasound may show evidence of peritonitis, a heterogenous abdominal mass, or a change in echotexture of abdominal lymph nodes. Pyogranulomatous inflammation may be seen on FNA of masses or abdominal lymph nodes. There is no treatment for this condition though palliative care, based on feline FIP protocols has been described (Swisher and Lennox 2017). The prognosis for FRSCV is usually poor, affected animals should be isolated, and euthanasia is likely the most appropriate option in a shelter environment.

24.2.4.4 Influenza

Influenza caused by *Orthomyxoviridae* type A and B viruses can occur in ferrets. Natural outbreaks caused by common influenza A, human strain H1N1, and swine-origin H1N1 have been documented in ferrets. Experimental infection of ferrets with the H3N2 strain of canine influenza virus has been shown to result in seroconversion and detectable shedding. Aerosol exposure to infected dogs did not have the same result, suggesting that interspecies transmission of H3N2 to ferrets is not fully established and further adaptation might be needed (Kim et al. 2013; Lyoo et al. 2015). Nonetheless, it seems prudent to assume that transmission between ferrets and dogs and cats as well as people could occur and to take appropriate biosecurity precautions.

Transmission from ferret to ferret or human to ferret is via aerosol. Febrile ferrets can generally shed virus for three to four days. Depending on the strain, the pathogenicity of influenza is generally low in ferrets, but secondary bacterial infections can occur (Barron and Rosenthal 2012).

Clinical signs of influenza in ferrets can include sneezing, epiphora, muco-serous to mucopurulent nasal discharge, fever, anorexia, conjunctivitis, and photophobia. Enteritis is reported in ferrets on occasion, along with hepatic dysfunction (experimental infections), and hearing loss. Neurologic signs including ataxia, paresis, and torticollis can be seen in more severe infections. Neonatal ferrets with influenza generally develop worse disease than adults and can die of lower airway obstruction (Barron and Rosenthal 2012).

Clinical signs consistent with influenza in an animal with exposure to a sick person or ferret increase the suspicion for this disease. Because clinical signs are like CDV, it is important to determine which pathogen is the cause of signs from a prognostic and population level standpoint. Diagnosis is via immunofluorescent antibody (IFA), radioimmunoassay (RIA), PCR, serology, or viral culture. PCR and antigen detection assays can differentiate Type A and B influenza with a nasopharyngeal swab taken within the first 48–72 hours of showing initial clinical signs. Blood work can show a transient leukopenia. Plasma biochemistry is generally normal but elevations in blood urea nitrogen, creatinine, alanine aminotransferase, potassium, and albumin are possible (Barron and Rosenthal 2012). Postmortem diagnosis is made via histopathology and IHC.

Treatment can include general supportive care and supplemental feeding, bronchodilators, decongestants, and treatment of secondary bacterial infection; antivirals have been used in some situations but are generally not recommended (Richardson and Perpinan 2017). Any ferrets showing signs of infection should be isolated from other animals to minimize the potential of transmission. Routine disinfection is effective in killing the influenza virus. Shelter staff with respiratory signs or fever should wear a mask or avoid contact with ferrets.

24.2.4.5 Rabies

Reports of rabies in ferrets are rare. Ferrets housed outdoors are at more risk of exposure. Dogs, cats, raccoons, foxes, polecats, other land mammals, and bats can transmit the virus to ferrets (Orosz and Johnson-Delaney 2017). The rabies virus, a member of the genus Lyssavirus in the family Rhabdoviridae, is generally transmitted in saliva from bite wounds. The incubation of rabies in ferrets is 28–33 days followed by death 4–5 days later (Antinoff and Giovanella 2012). Clinical signs that may be noted prior to death include behavioral changes, ataxia, paresthesia, and paresis or paralysis. Diagnosis is made at necropsy by virus detection in the CNS or salivary glands. Regulations concerning ferret bite protocol and rabies vaccination vary by state. It is prudent to vaccinate all healthy ferrets in a shelter for rabies before adoption if vaccine history is unknown. The reader is directed to the vaccine recommendations described earlier in this chapter for ferrets, and Chapter 22 for additional information on rabies.

24.2.4.6 Rotavirus

Rotavirus can cause diarrhea in neonatal ferrets between two and eight weeks old, resulting in high morbidity and mortality. Infection in adult ferrets has low morbidity and can cause transient green, mucoid diarrhea (Hoefer et al. 2012). Infection results from contact with affected ferrets or the environment as the virus is transmitted by the fecal-oral route. PCR testing of feces or GI (jejunal and ileal) samples confirms infection with rotavirus. Treatment is with supportive care and antibiotics to manage secondary bacterial infections. Viral particles are stable in feces; bleach is an effective disinfectant for rotavirus (Perpinan and Johnson-Delaney 2017).

24.2.5 Infectious Diseases in Ferrets: Fungal

24.2.5.1 Dermatophytosis

Ferrets are susceptible to infection from *Microsporum canis* and *Trichophyton mentagrophytes*. Ringworm is zoonotic; it is transmitted by direct contact with an infected animal or fomites. Kits and young ferrets are more susceptible to infection and disease can be self-limiting in some cases. Immunosuppressed ferrets are also more susceptible to contracting dermatophytosis (Orcutt and Tater 2012).

Clinical signs of dermatophytosis in ferrets are like those reported in other species. Small papules that spread peripherally may be noted along with areas of alopecia, inflammation, hyperkeratosis, crusting, and broken hair shafts. Lesions are generally non-pruritic (Orcutt and Tater 2012).

M. canis may fluoresce under Wood's lamp. Dermatophytosis is definitively diagnosed by the results of mycotic culture of hair or skin samples. Fungal elements may be seen on microscopic examination of hair samples or histopathologic examination of skin biopsy (Johnson-Delaney 2017f).

Some clinicians report spontaneous regression of disease; however, treatment is generally recommended in a shelter setting. Lime sulfur dips can be used to treat generalized disease. Systemic antifungal therapy is necessary for severe infections and is likely the treatment of choice in combination with lime sulfur dips for treatment in a shelter setting; itraconazole and griseofulvin have been used to manage ringworm in ferrets. It is also very important to thoroughly disinfect the environment using cleaning protocols as described for dogs and cats. The reader is directed to Chapter 20 for additional general information on dermatophytosis.

24.2.5.2 Other Fungal Diseases-Blastomycosis, Coccidioidomycosis, Cryptococcosis

Blastomyces dermatitidis is endemic in the southeastern United States including the Mississippi and Ohio River Valleys. Blastomycosis should be on the differential list for causes of respiratory disease in ferrets who have traveled through or inhabit these regions *Coccidioides immitis* is endemic in the southwestern United States and is the causative agent for coccidioidomycosis in ferrets, manifesting with respiratory and/or systemic signs of illness. *Cryptococcus bacillisporus* and *Cryptococcus neoformans var. grubii* can cause disease in ferrets. Fungal infection usually occurs from environmental exposure. Clinical signs can include rhinitis, pneumonia, pleuritis, chorioretinitis, CNS signs, and dyspnea caused by retropharyngeal or mediastinal lymphadenopathy. Ferrets infected with these diseases are not contagious to other ferrets and the diseases are unlikely to occur in a shelter setting unless a ferret was exposed to the organism prior to entry.

24.3 Rabbits

24.3.1 Anatomy, Handling, Husbandry, and Routine Healthcare

24.3.1.1 Terminology, Anatomy, and Physiology

Leporidae (rabbits and hares) and Ochotonidae (pikas) are the two families in the order Lagomorpha. The order Lagomorpha contains 12 genera and 81 species and is distinguished from the order Rodentia, based on the presence of a second set of upper incisors known as “peg teeth” (Graham 2014; Vella and Donnelly 2012). Jaw movements of rabbits are vertical or transverse. Lagomorphs are hindgut fermenters, herbivorous, and practice cecotrophy. Rabbits are born naked and blind and usually associate in groups, compared to the more solitary hare. Domestic rabbits range in size from 1 kg to over 7 kg and are divided into over 60 fancy and fur breeds with over 500 varieties. The lifespan of rabbits in captivity can reach 19 years (Vella and Donnelly 2012).

The long hind legs of rabbits are well adapted for running, with thick hair on the soles of all the feet instead of footpads. Rabbit skin is very delicate in comparison to other mammals and care needs to be taken when clipping the fur to avoid tears; hair should not be clipped from the plantar aspect of the feet or hocks. Rabbits have scent glands on the underside of the chin, anal glands, and pocket-like inguinal glands on either side of the perianal region that usually contain yellow to brown debris. The intact female, called a doe, has a well-developed dewlap over the throat region. Two to five pairs of mammary glands are found in females. Hearing, smell and touch are well developed and vocalizations in most breeds are minimal. Eyes are laterally positioned providing a circular field of vision. Sensory hairs are positioned around the nose and above the eyes. Rabbits have continuously growing incisor and cheek teeth; the dental formula of rabbits is (I 2/1, C0/0, P 3/2, M 3/3)×2 = 28 (Graham 2014; Vella and Donnelly 2012). Malocclusion and dental disease are common and a thorough oral evaluation is an essential part of the rabbit physical examination.

The GI tract makes up 10–20% of the rabbit's body weight. The cecum holds about 40% of ingesta and is the most prominent organ in the abdominal cavity. The liver contains six lobes and liver lobe torsion is relatively common in rabbits (Graham and Basseches 2014). Rabbits are obligate nasal breathers and upper respiratory disease can cause severe clinical signs. The thoracic cavity of the rabbit is relatively small. The lung lobes of rabbits, three on the left and four on the right, are not divided by connective tissue septa so pneumonia in rabbits is lobar rather than lobular (Vella and Donnelly, 2012). The thymus lies cranioventral to the heart and can persist into adulthood; thymoma, thymic lymphoma, and thymic carcinoma have all been reported in rabbits. The heart of the rabbit is relatively small and has a limited collateral coronary circulation; as such, rabbits are prone to ischemia secondary to coronary vasoconstriction. The fractional excretion of calcium in the urine of rabbits is 45–60%, compared to less than 2% in other species (Vella and Donnelly 2012), making rabbits prone to hypercalciuria and urolithiasis. Rabbits have testes located in a scrotum in front of the penis and lack an os penis. Females have a bicornuate uterus with two cervices. Intact female rabbits have a high incidence of uterine adenocarcinoma.

24.3.1.2 Housing and Husbandry

Rabbits are social animals and can be housed in pairs or small groups if they are neutered and have personalities compatible with conspecifics. Housing rabbits away from dogs, cats, ferrets, and guinea pigs is recommended to avoid exposure of these species to *B. bronchiseptica*. Housing rabbits away from rats may also be prudent to minimize exposure of rabbits to *M. pulmonis*. In addition, they should be housed in an area separate from potential or perceived predators. Sounds and smells from dogs, cats, or ferrets may stress sensitive rabbits.

Rabbits can be housed in cages designed for avian and exotic animals, stainless steel cages designed for dogs and cats, or specially designed hutch cages or enclosures. The floor of the enclosure should have a non-slip surface to avoid injury; a rubberized mat can provide traction and has the added benefit of allowing urine and feces to fall through, preventing soiling of the rabbit. Surfaces that prevent damage to the fur (i.e. solid bottomed caging vs. wire) are preferred, as the fur removal can lead to significant damage to the foot, particularly the hock. When compared to newspaper, straw, shavings, towels, blankets, recycled paper bedding, carpet or foam mats, the type of bedding most protective against the development of pododermatitis in rabbits is hay (Mancinelli et al. 2014).

Care should be taken to avoid overheating rabbits. The ideal housing temperature range for rabbits is 50–70 °F (10–21 °C). If the environmental temperature rises above 80–85 °F (27–29.4 °C), heat stress can occur. Healthy New Zealand white rabbits housed at 107.6 °F (42 °C) and 45 ± 4% relative humidity for one hour, had decreased feed intake lasting five days as well as changes in multiple blood parameters (decreased glucose and cholesterol, and increased triglycerides and blood urea nitrogen [BUN]). Warm areas appropriate for birds or reptiles may cause heat stress in eu- or hyperthermic small mammal animals (Graham and Mader 2012).

The preferred diet for the rabbit is a high-quality, high-fiber (15–16% crude fiber) pelleted diet containing 13–18% (ideally 16%) crude protein, at a rate of 1/4 cup pellets per 2.3 kg body mass divided into two meals per day. The pellets are supplemented with loose hay (mixed grass hay, timothy hay, or high-quality dried grass clippings) ad libitum. Alfalfa hay may be offered throughout the growth stages and should then be discontinued because of its high protein and calcium content. The diet can be supplemented with a small amount of dark fibrous, leafy greens and fresh vegetables (1 cup per 2.3 kg body mass) and small amounts (up to 1 tablespoon per 2.3 kg body mass) of fresh fruit, daily or several times per week. Growing rabbits and females in late gestation may require twice as much food; lactating may consume three times as much food as an adult in maintenance (Graham 2014).

Fresh water must always be available. If water crocks are used, they should be made of a heavy ceramic so they are not easily tipped over. Bowls with high sides are recommended because rabbits tend to hang their dewlaps in the water when they drink. If the sides of the bowl are too low, this chronic wetting can lead to "wet dewlap" disease, which is an easily preventable moist dermatitis that is most often associated with colonization by *Pseudomonas* species. All water containers should be cleaned daily, and water should be refreshed at least once a day (Graham and Mader 2012).

24.3.1.3 Handling

Rabbits are easily stressed; proper handling and housing of rabbits are essential to avoid injury. The rabbit skeleton represents only 7–8% of the body weight (as opposed to 12–13% in cats). With powerful musculature on the hind limbs and the delicate nature of the skeleton, rabbits are prone to fractures of the back and hind limbs. Support of the hindquarters is vital when moving rabbits to prevent injury. Rabbits accustomed to handling can be carried with one hand under the thorax or holding the scruff with the second hand supporting the hindquarters (Figure 24.3). Fractious rabbits should be carried with the head under the handler's arm to minimize stress by covering the eyes; the hindquarters are supported at the same time (Figure 24.4). A rabbit should be placed in its enclosure with its rear facing the back of the cage while supporting the hindquarters to help reduce chances of injury from the rabbit kicking. When examining or placing a rabbit in a cage, a non-slip mat should be used to avoid sliding and injury. Control of the rabbit should always be maintained during transport and examination (Graham and Mader 2012).

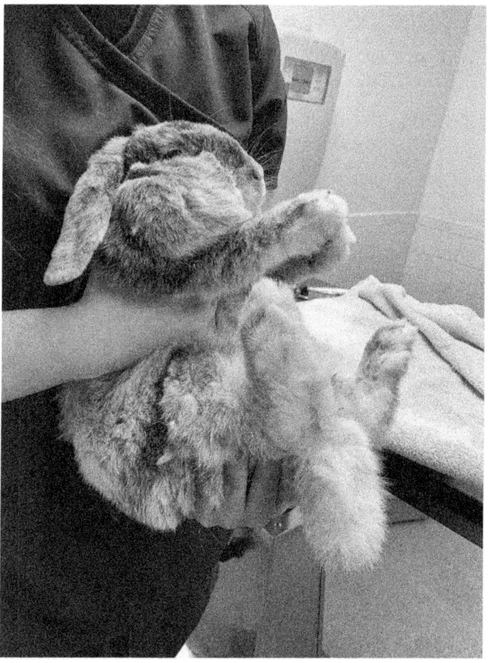

Figure 24.3 Restraint of a rabbit with one hand under its thorax and the other hand supporting its hindquarters. *Source:* Courtesy Jennifer Graham.

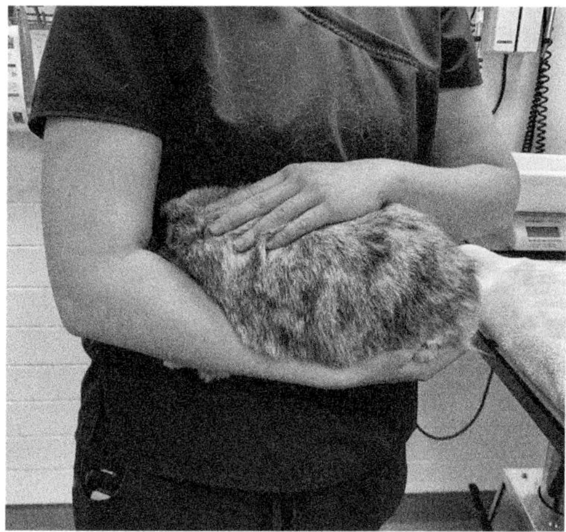

Figure 24.4 Restraint of a stressed rabbit by covering its eyes and supporting its hindquarters. *Source:* Courtesy Jennifer Graham.

A towel can be used to wrap the patient and cover the head to prevent struggling when the rabbit is moved to another location. Similarly, a towel can be wrapped around the rabbit if an assistant is not available to help facilitate physical examination or medication administration (See Figure 24.5). It is important to avoid overheating when using a towel to facilitate handling or examination. As rabbits radiate heat through their ears, covering of the ears should be avoided to minimize the risk of hyperthermia. As an alternative, a hand can be placed over the eyes to calm the rabbit. Rabbits are obligate nasal breathers so care should be taken to avoid obstructing the nostrils with the towel or hand. Though rabbits may appear calm when placed on their backs, research suggests this position induces tonic immobility and is associated with changes in cardiac rate and function, respiratory rate, and increased corticosterone levels in laboratory rabbits. As previously mentioned, it is important for the

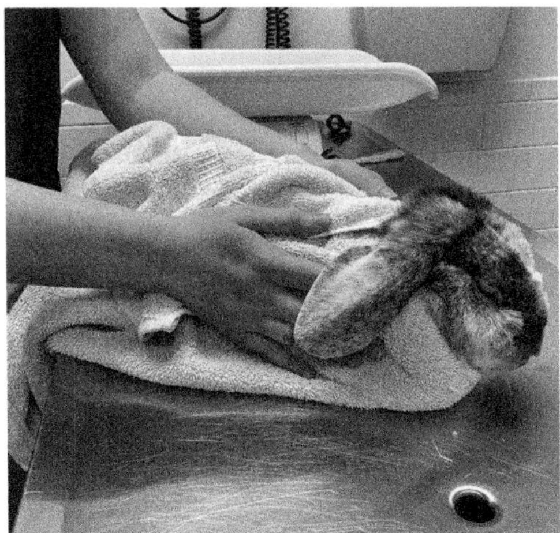

Figure 24.5 To help facilitate examination or medication administration a towel can be wrapped around a rabbit to restrain it. *Source:* Courtesy Jennifer Graham.

rabbit to be kept in areas away from "predator" species such as ferrets, dogs, and cats; noises or smells from these animals may stress the rabbit (Graham and Mader 2012).

24.3.1.4 Vaccination and Routine Healthcare

There are no routine vaccinations recommended for pet rabbits in the United States. In Europe, myxomatosis and Rabbit Viral Hemorrhagic Disease (RVHD) vaccines are recommended for pet rabbits (Graham and Mader 2012). At the time of publication of this text, RVHD has been reported in at least five states in the USA and there is an effort to vaccinate rabbits in areas affected by this disease; therefore, this may become a recommended vaccine for rabbits in the United States in the near future.

The incidence of uterine adenocarcinoma in rabbits older than three years ranges from 50 to 80% in certain breeds; ovariectomy or ovariohysterectomy is recommended in all non-breeding rabbits between six and nine months to reduce the potential for neoplasia (Klaphake and Paul-Murphy 2012). Male rabbits have a low incidence of testicular neoplasia, but neutering may help reduce nuisance behaviors, including urine marking. Rabbits should be screened for evidence of ecto- and endo-parasites prior to or at the point of intake to the shelter. Though fipronil should not be used on rabbits, products that can be safely used on cats (imidacloprid, lufenuron, and selamectin) can generally be used on rabbits. Screening for *Pasteurella multocida* and *Encephalitozoon cuniculi* prior to entering the general rabbit population at a shelter is also a consideration.

Infectious diseases of rabbits of particular concern in the shelter environment, due to their relatively high prevalence, ease of transmission to other rabbits or other species, and/or zoonotic potential, include bacterial respiratory diseases; mites; *E. cuniculi*; *Treponema paraluiscuniculi*; and dermatophytosis.

24.3.2 Infectious Diseases in Rabbits: Bacterial

(See Table 24.2 for a list of diseases in rabbits by body system).

24.3.2.1 Bacterial Enteritis (*E. coli, C. piliforme, L. intracelullaris*)

Bacterial enteritis from enteropathogenic *E. coli* (EPEC) can cause large outbreaks in weaning commercial rabbits, but, though possible, no reports in pet or sheltered rabbits could be found by the author. The bacteria attach to cecal and colonic epithelial cells and cause effacement of the surface microvilli, inhibiting colonic absorption. The severity of disease depends on the age of the rabbit and serotype though mortality can be over 50%. Enteritis caused by *Clostridium piliforme* (Tyzzer's disease), a motile, gram-variable, spore-forming obligate intracellular bacterium, is found in many species of small mammals, including rabbits and guinea pigs. Proliferative enteritis caused by *L. intracellularis*, an intracellular, gram-negative, curved-to-spiraled bacterium, is most often found in swine, but can also be found in rabbits, ferrets, and rodents. Infections in rabbits are most common in weanlings (two to four months) (DeCubellis and Graham 2013; Oglesbee and Jenkins 2012).

Table 24.2 Classification of rabbit diseases by body system.

System	Symptoms	Etiology
Respiratory		
Bacterial upper and lower respiratory disease – Z	Multisystemic-depends on the agent- Pneumonia, pleuritis, nasal exudate, torticollis, ocular discharge, sneezing	*P. multocida, B. bronchiseptica, E. coli, Pseudomonas* sp., *M. pulmonis, Staphylococcus* sp., *Chlamydia*
Systemic		
Encephalitozoonosis – Z	Vestibular dysfunction, urinary incontinence, stiff rear gait, posterior paresis. Also, myocarditis, vasculitis, encephalitis, pneumonitis, hepatitis, nephritis, splenitis, etc.	*Encephalitozoon cuniculi*
Myxomatosis	Swollen eyelids, mucopurulent ocular and nasal discharge, lethargy, seizures. Survivors have edematous nodules on the ears, face, eyelids, and perineum	Myxoma virus
Rabbit Hemorrhagic Disease	Sudden death or fever, anorexia, diarrhea (or constipation), neurologic and other systemic symptoms, including hemorrhage	Calicivirus
Rabies – Z	Anorexia, fever, lethargy, paresis, paralysis, head tremors	Rabies lyssavirus
Herpes simplex (HSV) – Z	Neurologic signs, death	Herpes simplex
Gastrointestinal		
Bacterial enteritis – Z	Signs vary by causative agent. Watery diarrhea, lethargy, anorexia, acute death	*E. coli, C. piliforme, L. intracellularis*
Coccidiosis	Anorexia, diarrhea, abdominal bloating, and icterus	*Eimeria*
Cryptosporidiosis – Z	Diarrhea, anorexia, depression, and dehydration	*Cryptosporidium parvum*
Helminths – Z	Varied	*Passalurus ambiguous, Baylisascaris spp., Taenia*
Rotavirus	Anorexia, dehydration, and green-yellow watery diarrhea	Rotavirus
Dermatologic		
Ear mites	Head shaking, ear drooping, pruritis, "cornflake-like" crusting of the ear canal	*Psoroptes cuniculi*
Fleas	Pruritis, scratching, self-biting and licking, alopecia	*Ctenocephalides canis* and *C. felis*
Lice	Anemia, weight loss, papules, hair loss, pruritis	*Haemodipsus ventricosus*
Cheyletiellosis – Z	Scaly dermatitis, pruritis, alopecia, and broken hairs	*Cheyletiella parasitovorax*
Mites – Z	Vary by agent	*Leporacarus gibbus, Sarcoptes scabiei, Notoedres cati, Demodex cuniculi*

(*Continued*)

Table 24.2 (Continued)

System	Symptoms	Etiology
Rabbit syphilis	Crusty ulcers or edematous papules around the lips, eyelids, nose, and perineal region	*Treponema paraluiscuniculi*
Rabbit (Shope) fibroma	Flat, wart-like tumors on the face, legs, and perineum	Leporipoxvirus
Rabbit (Shope) Papillomavirus	Wart-like keratinized lesions around the ears and eyelids, firm white, moist tumors on legs Dorsal hindfeet	Papillomavirus
Dermatophytosis – Z (ringworm)	Initially pruritic and inflamed lesions that become scabbed, dry, crusty, alopecic lesions on the head, legs, feet, and nail beds	*Trichophyton mentagrophytes, Microsporum* sp.

Z-Zoonotic.

Clinical signs of bacterial enteritis vary depending on the causative agent. *E. coli* can be associated with watery diarrhea. Animals infected with *C. piliforme*, particularly weanlings, progress rapidly from the onset of lethargy, anorexia, and watery diarrhea to acute death. Adults may have a more chronic course. *Lawsonia intracelullaris* infects enteric epithelial cells, causing a proliferative enteropathy marked by diarrhea and wasting (DeCubellis and Graham 2013; Oglesbee and Jenkins 2012). Diagnosis of bacterial enteritis is based on fecal culture and necropsy findings. Necropsy findings with *E. coli* can include characteristic longitudinal "paintbrush" hemorrhages on the cecal wall. A presumptive diagnosis is made by isolation of *E. coli* on fecal cultures because serotyping to confirm that the isolate is an EPEC is not commercially available. Ante-mortem diagnosis of *C. piliforme* is generally not possible because it is an intracellular bacterium that does not grow in culture. At necropsy, infections are marked by patchy necrosis in the liver and proximal colon and degenerative lesions of the myocardium. A presumptive diagnosis of *L. intracellularis* is based on history, clinical signs, and response to therapy. A PCR assay can be used to screen fecal or rectal swabs and colonic biopsy samples. Colonic samples can also be screened via histologic examination, silver stains, or fluorescent-antibody tests (DeCubellis and Graham 2013; Oglesbee and Jenkins 2012).

Treatment for *E. coli* involves supportive care as well as antimicrobial therapy with trimethoprim-sulfamethoxazole or fluoroquinolones pending culture sensitivity results. Treatment has not proven beneficial in cases of *C. piliforme*, but if rabbits are isolated early from symptomatic animals and provided supportive care and a high-fiber diet, the disease may not progress. *L. intracellularis* can be treated with chloramphenicol; macrolide antibiotics used to treat *L. intracellularis* in other species are not recommended for use in rabbits (DeCubellis and Graham 2013; Oglesbee and Jenkins 2012).

General supportive care for bacterial enteritis includes fluids and supplemental feeding. Affected animals should be isolated from the group and other species, and environmental disinfection is recommended. Because other bacterial causes of diarrhea in rabbits include *Salmonella* and *Pseudomonas* sp., routine disinfection methods should be used after handling affected rabbits or cleaning cages. Prevention is best achieved by appropriate disinfection (*C. piliforme* spores are killed with 0.3% sodium hypochlorite solution or 80 °C heat for 30 minutes), good husbandry, and stress reduction, especially during weaning (Oglesbee and Jenkins 2012).

24.3.2.2 Bacterial Respiratory Disease (*P. multocida, B. bronchiseptica, Pseudomonas*, etc.)

Causes of upper and lower respiratory disease in rabbits include *P. multocida, B. bronchiseptica, E. coli, Pseudomonas* sp., *Staphylococcus* sp., *Chlamydia* sp., and others. In a survey of rabbits with signs of upper respiratory disease, *P. multocida* was the most commonly isolated bacteria in greater than 50% of rabbits. Approximately 50% of rabbits also had *B. bronchiseptica*, 28% had *Pseudomonas* sp., and *Staphylococcus* sp. was isolated from 17.4%. A study of 66 rabbits with pulmonary lesions had the following bacteria isolated in order of frequency: *Pasteurella* sp., *E. coli, B. bronchiseptica*, and *P. aeruginosa* (Lennox 2012).

P. multocida is a non–spore-forming, bipolar, gram-negative rod. *P. multocida* is transmitted from acutely infected rabbits via direct contact, fomites, inhalation or wounds. The incubation period of *P. multocida* is about two weeks. The bacteria colonize the nares or cause the production of nasal exudate if the host is unable to resist infection. Snuffles, a common upper respiratory tract disease in domestic rabbits, is caused by a local overgrowth of *P. multocida* in the nasal epithelium. However, cultures of the nasal epithelium are frequently positive for *P. multocida* in clinically normal adult rabbits housed in institutional colonies (40–72%) and conventional rabbitries (28–31%). *P. multocida* can proliferate and spread via the trachea (to the lungs), via the nasolacrimal ducts (to the conjunctiva), via the eustachian tube (to the middle ear, inner ear, and then the brain), or via the bloodstream (septicemia) to the lungs, heart (endocarditis), reproductive organs (orchitis and pyometra-endometritis), skin, and subcutis (subcutaneous abscesses). Pasteurellosis in the lungs can result in fibrinopurulent pneumonia, pleuritis, and cranioventral pulmonary abscesses. Ophthalmic involvement (conjunctivitis, hypopyon, or retrobulbar abscesses) also may be seen with pasteurellosis. Torticollis (head tilt or wry neck) in domestic rabbits is usually caused by the extension of *P. multocida* infection from the nasal cavity to the inner ear via the eustachian tube and middle ear or may arise centrally, in the medulla or cerebellum (Graham 2014; Lennox 2012).

B. bronchiseptica is commonly found in the rabbit respiratory tract, in both asymptomatic rabbits and in association with disease. *B. bronchiseptica* may be a co-pathogen in rabbits and can cause disease in guinea pigs, dogs, cats, and pigs. *Pseudomonas* sp. are a relatively common cause of respiratory disease in rabbits and can affect multiple body systems. *Staphylococcus* sp. are most often secondary invaders in rabbits but have been associated with fibrinous pneumonia and abscesses. *M. pulmonis* was isolated from rabbits with signs of upper respiratory disease; these rabbits were near rats (Lennox 2012).

C/S testing is recommended in rabbits suspected to have respiratory infections because organisms other than *Pasteurella* species may be isolated. Sampling of the external nares may not be reflective of pathogenic organisms in the respiratory tract; deep nasal swab or nasal or tracheal washes are more likely to provide meaningful results. Culture of nasolacrimal duct flush fluid may also be helpful in rabbits with dacryocystitis. Serologic tests, such as ELISA and PCR tests, are available to detect pasteurellosis in rabbits. Radiology may also be a helpful diagnostic tool to consider when working up rabbits with respiratory signs.

Treatment of bacterial respiratory disease is based on C/S results and the location of the infection. Treatment of bacterial pneumonia should include supportive care such as oxygen therapy when warranted, fluid therapy, assisted feeding, and antibiotic therapy. Fluoroquinolone antibiotics, i.e. enrofloxacin at 5–10 mg/kg PO q12h × 14 days, are generally effective in treating pasteurellosis and other respiratory pathogens in rabbits. Other antibiotics such as chloramphenicol have also been used to manage pasteurellosis. In addition, nasolacrimal duct flushing and administration of antibiotics into the duct, such as one drop of ciprofloxacin in each eye every 8–12 hours, is also useful in cases of nasal pasteurellosis.

Though more invasive, rhinotomy with surgical debridement has been suggested as an option to manage granulomatous disease of the nasal cavity that is refractory to antibiotic therapy. Lateral ear canal resection or bulla osteotomy have been used to manage some cases of respiratory disease that cause chronic otitis (Lennox 2012).

Isolation of affected animals is recommended in a shelter setting. Housing rabbits away from dogs, cats, ferrets, and guinea pigs is recommended to avoid exposure of these species to *B. bronchiseptica*. Housing rabbits away from rats may also be prudent to minimize exposure of rabbits to *M. pulmonis*. *P. multocida*, *Pseudomonas* sp., and *B. bronchiseptica* could be of zoonotic concern in immunocompromised humans (Mitchell and Tully 2012).

24.3.3 Infectious Diseases in Rabbits: Parasitic

24.3.3.1 Coccidiosis

Coccidia are the most common parasites of the rabbit GI tract. While they cause significant disease in young (<6 months old) rabbits, they can be incidentally found in adult rabbits. Of the 12 species of the genus *Eimeria*, *Eimeria stiedae* is exclusive to the liver, with the rest causing intestinal disease. Hepatic coccidiosis is ubiquitous in commercial rabbitries and can be fatal in young rabbits by obstructing liver function. Intestinal coccidiosis is common in rabbits of all ages, host-specific, and most often associated with *Elastosis perforans* infection, though *Eimeria magna, Eimeria media*, and *Eimeria irresidua* are also reported. Subclinical infection is common, and disease severity varies with age (worse under six months), species of *Eimeria*, parasite burden, and condition of the rabbit (stress, poor husbandry, poor diet) (DeCubellis and Graham 2013; Oglesbee and Jenkins 2012).

Severe disease with *E. stiedae* is marked by anorexia, diarrhea, abdominal bloating, and icterus. Biochemical tests confirm hepatic disease, with aspartate aminotransferase (AST), alanine transaminase (ALT), bile acids, and total bilirubin elevations. On necropsy, the liver is studded with nodular, encapsulated abscesses. Oocysts can be identified in bile or feces. Clinical signs of significant disease caused by intestinal coccidia, including *E. perforans* include diarrhea with possible mucus or blood, dehydration, and weight loss. Intussusception is a complication of severe disease. The diagnosis of coccidiosis depends on histopathology and/or fecal identification. Molecular assays have been developed to identify intestinal *Eimeria* species (DeCubellis and Graham 2013; Oglesbee and Jenkins 2012).

In addition to supportive care, sulfa drugs are most effective at limiting multiplication until immunity develops. The focus should be on very young, pregnant, or immunocompromised rabbits, as they will be more prone to infection. Sulfadimethoxine (50 mg/kg PO once, then 25 mg/kg PO q24h), trimethoprim-sulfamethoxazole (15–30 mg/kg PO q12-24 h), or ponazuril (30 mg/kg PO q24h) can be used for 10 days of therapy. Amprolium is another option and can be added to drinking water (0.5 ml/pint drinking water for 10 days). Recovering rabbits develop lifelong immunity (Oglesbee and Jenkins 2012). For outbreak control, shelters should minimize stress and use good husbandry practices to keep environments clean.

24.3.3.2 Cryptosporidiosis

C. parvum infects the small intestine and causes a self-limited diarrheal illness (4–5 days duration) in young rabbits (peak, 30–40 days old). Diarrhea is accompanied by anorexia, depression, and dehydration. The organism can be identified on fecal examination or histopathology. Other than supportive care, there is no effective treatment (Oglesbee and Jenkins 2012). Recently, reports of rabbit *Cryptosporidium* species causing zoonotic disease in humans have been reported in several countries; shelter staff are advised to follow appropriate biosecurity procedures, including environmental decontamination as described in the section on Coccidia in ferrets, use of personal protective equipment (PPE), and washing hands following contact with rabbits with diarrhea.

24.3.3.3 Ear Mites

Ear mites (*Psoroptes cuniculi*) are common in rabbits and may cause severe inflammation. Transmission occurs through contact with affected rabbits or fomites; they are not transmissible to other species. *P. cuniculi* has a three-week life cycle and can survive up to three weeks off the host. Clinical signs include head shaking, ear drooping, pruritis, and can progress to "cornflake-like" crusting of the ear canal. In immunocompromised rabbits, inflammation and crusting can become generalized. Otitis media and neurologic signs are occasionally noted in rabbits with deeper infection. Some rabbits may be subclinically infected with mild pruritis noted over a period of years (Orcutt and Tater 2012).

Mites can be seen microscopically, otoscopically, and by the naked eye. Treatment of otoacariasis can be with ivermectin (0.2–0.44 mg/kg PO or subcutaneously (SC)), selamectin (20 mg/kg q7d), or imidacloprid (10 mg/kg)/moxidectin (1 mg/kg). Crusty lesions should not be removed as this is painful, and lesions will resolve with treatment. Environmental cleaning and treatment of contaminated areas with flea products help prevent reinfection. Fipronil and insecticide baths or dips should not be used in rabbits (Orcutt and Tater 2012).

24.3.3.4 Encephalitozoon cuniculi

E. cuniculi is a eukaryotic organism belonging to phylum Microsporidia, kingdom Fungi that causes encephalitozoonosis. International seroprevalence studies show a prevalence of 7.5–84.7% in pet and farmed rabbits. *E. cuniculi* is particularly challenging to manage because the organism can evade humoral-mediated immunity, serologic titer does not correlate with the presence or clinical severity of disease, seroconversion does not result in immunity to disease, and no current treatment recommendations are effective in eliminating the disease. Horizontal and vertical (transplacental) transmission is possible and common routes of infection are via the small intestine (ingestion of urine-contaminated feed) and respiratory tract (spore inhalation). *E. cuniculi* organisms enter host cells primarily by extruding a polar filament to inject an infectious sporoplasm, though phagocytosis of the spore by the host cell has been demonstrated. Brain, kidney, lung, lens, and myocardium are predilection sites for the spores, which are shed via the urine (Fisher and Carpenter 2012).

Vestibular dysfunction (head tilt) in dwarf breeds of domestic rabbits is caused most frequently by *E. cuniculi* (whereas in standard breeds the cause more likely is *P. multocida* or otitis). Though many domestic rabbits infected with *E. cuniculi* are asymptomatic, they may still be shedding infectious organisms. Neurologic signs may include urinary incontinence, stiff rear gait, and posterior paresis. A wide range of symptoms are possible, and *E. cuniculi* infections have been associated with phacouveitis secondary to lens rupture, myocarditis, vasculitis, encephalitis, spinal nerve root inflammation, pneumonitis, hepatitis, nephritis, and splenitis (Fisher and Carpenter 2012). Chronic, recurrent GI signs can also be seen in some rabbits.

A positive encephalitozoon titer with compatible clinical signs suggests but is not conclusive for encephalitozoonosis. Serological testing, including complement fixation, ELISA, India ink immunoreaction, indirect fluorescent antibody, or indirect microagglutination, is commonly used for diagnosis. Immunoglobulin G (IgG) antibody response variation has been demonstrated in rabbit models; it is thought that variations in response may be influenced by exposure load and variation in immune response as serologic titer does not correlate with the presence or severity of clinical signs. A combination of ELISA and protein electrophoresis is useful in the diagnosis of *E. cuniculi* in rabbits. Additionally, more recent work shows improved specificity in diagnosing disease in rabbits when quantitative IgG and IgM antibody titers are run concurrently with C-reactive protein (CRP), available through the University of Miami Avian and Wildlife Laboratory. Beyond postmortem examination, this combination (IgM, IgG, CRP) is the preferred method most clinicians choose for screening rabbits for *E. cuniculi* in clinical practice. A definitive diagnosis of encephalitozoonosis requires histopathologic identification of the organism (Fisher and Carpenter 2012).

No treatment is effective for encephalitozoonosis, though benzimidazoles, including albendazole (7.5–20 mg/kg PO q24h), fenbendazole (20 mg/kg PO q24h), and oxibendazole (15–30 mg/kg PO q24 for seven days, followed by 15 mg/kg PO q24h; the lower dose is preferred by JG) have been shown to help decrease neurologic signs. *In vitro* models are used to evaluate the susceptibility of *E. cuniculi* to various drugs. *In vitro* methods have determined the 50% inhibitory concentrations of fumagillin, thiabendazole, albendazole, oxibendazole, and propamidine isethionate for *E. cuniculi* in rabbit kidney cells. Unfortunately, many of these drugs are potentially toxic to the patient and ultimately do not clear disease.

Cleaning and sanitation are important to limit the transmission of *E. cuniculi*. Most disinfectants inactivate spores, including quaternary ammonium compounds, amphoteric surfactants, phenolic derivatives, alcohols, iodophors, and hydrogen peroxide (Fisher and Carpenter 2012). *E. cuniculi* is an opportunistic infection in immunocompromised humans, making the disease a zoonotic concern. Shelters should inform adopters of the zoonotic nature of this disease and consider screening rabbits for the organism prior to adoption to immunocompromised individuals. Additionally, it is prudent to segregate serologically positive rabbits away from serologically negative rabbits when possible. Any known serologically positive animals should ideally be adopted into households with other serologically positive rabbits to minimize the risk of infection to naïve animals as this organism is intermittently shed.

24.3.3.5 Fleas/Ticks/Lice

Ectoparasites, including fleas, sucking lice, and a wide range of ticks, can infect rabbits. *Ctenocephalides canis* and *Ctenocephalides felis* most commonly infect rabbits, though many other types of fleas can be found on domestic rabbits exposed to wild rabbits. Fleas can be diagnosed based on clinical signs (pruritis, scratching, self-biting, licking, alopecia) and identification of fleas, flea debris, or flea eggs on the rabbit. Fipronil should not be used on rabbits but other products that can be safely used on cats (imidacloprid, lufenuron, and selamectin) can generally be used on rabbits. Some drugs, including selamectin, are metabolized more quickly in rabbits, necessitating different treatment regimens than those used in cats (Fisher and Graham 2018). As for other species, environmental control is also important if fleas are present in areas where animals are housed (Hess and Tater 2012).

Rabbits can be affected by a variety of ixodid and argasid ticks. Ticks are more common in rabbits housed outdoors or with exposure to wild rabbits. Like other species, severe tick infestations can be associated with anemia and transmission of disease. Myxomatosis, papillomatosis, tularemia, Lyme disease, and Rocky Mountain Spotted Fever can be transmitted by ticks. Ticks should be mechanically removed and ivermectin (0.2–0.4 mg/kg) can be used as a treatment for any remaining ticks (Hess and Tater 2012). Tick products for dogs and cat flea and tick collars should not be used on rabbits.

Lice infestations are rare in rabbits, but severe *Haemodipsus ventricosus* infestation can cause anemia, weight loss, papules, hair loss, and pruritis. Additionally, lice can transmit tularemia. Diagnosis can be based on visual examination since lice and eggs are visible with the naked eye. Ivermectin (0.2–0.4 mg/kg q two weeks for two to three treatments PO or SC) can be used to treat lice in rabbits (Hess and Tater 2012).

24.3.3.6 Helminths

Passalurus ambiguous, the rabbit pinworm, is found in most rabbits, but even large parasite burdens are not pathogenic. Adult worms reside in the cecum and colon, and transmission is direct by the ingestion of eggs during cecotrophy. Diagnosis is often routine by identification of worms or eggs in the feces, though identification should not prompt treatment in most cases. When treatment is necessary, i.e. generally if worms are seen in the feces, benzimidazoles such as fenbendazole are effective (Hess and Tater 2012).

Cerebrospinal nematodiasis (neural larval migrans), caused by *Baylisascaris* spp., (*Baylisascaris procyonis, Baylisascaris columnaris)* has been reported in rabbits and may produce fatal or severe neurologic disease. *Baylisascaris* is considered zoonotic and can also cause disease in many other mammals. Rabbits are also an intermediate host for cestodes (i.e. *Taenia spp.*), and the larvae are usually found in the subcutis and skeletal muscle (Hess and Tater 2012). Clinical signs in severe cestode infestations may include diarrhea, bloat, ileus, and severe pain. The rabbit may grow slowly and appear thin despite having a normal appetite. Cestodes can be treated with praziquantel (5–10 mg/kg PO, SC, or IM, repeat in 10 days). Though the treatment of asymptomatic GI cestode infections is generally not warranted in pet rabbits, shelters should consider treatment, especially before adoption, and in obvious cases where tapeworm segments are observed in the feces.

24.3.3.7 Mites

Cheyletiella parasitovorax is the "walking dandruff" mite of rabbits and is contagious to humans and other animals including dogs and cats. This mite lives on the keratin layer of the epidermis and can cause scaly dermatitis, pruritis, alopecia, and broken hairs. Disease tends to be self-limiting but can be severe in young and immunosuppressed rabbits. Diagnosis is based on clinical signs and microscopic identification of mites. Treatment options can include ivermectin (0.2–0.4 mg/kg, repeat in 10–14 days) and selamectin (20 mg/kg, repeat in 14 days); environmental control is also necessary (Hess and Tater 2012).

Leporacarus gibbus is a possibly zoonotic mite of rabbits that is managed similarly to *Cheyletiella*. Other mites, including *S. scabiei, Notoedres cati*, and *Demodex cuniculi* are occasionally found on rabbits. If these mites are found, evaluation for underlying disease-causing immunosuppression is recommended.

24.3.3.8 *Treponema paraluiscuniculi*

Rabbit syphilis, caused by the spirochete *T. paraluiscuniculi*, is a contagious but non-zoonotic venereal disease of rabbits. Transmission occurs through contact with infected skin or between kits and an infected dam. Lesions can be crusty ulcers or edematous papules around the lips, eyelids, nose, and perineal region. Diagnosis is based on history, clinical signs, and identifying the spirochetes in darkfield microscopic examination of scrapings or smears of the skin lesions. Histologic examination with silver stains of skin biopsy sections can also be used for diagnosis but is a low sensitivity test. Serologic testing is available but false negatives are possible. Treatment of rabbit syphilis consists of parenteral benzathine penicillin G/procaine penicillin G (42,000–60,000 U/kg SC q7 days × 3 weeks) or penicillin G procaine (40,000 U/kg IM q24h × 5–7 days) in all exposed rabbits. Enteral penicillins should not be administered to rabbits. The response is rapid; lesions usually regress dramatically after one injection (Hess and Tater 2012).

24.3.4 Infectious Diseases in Rabbits: Viral

24.3.4.1 Myxomatosis

Myxomatosis is a significant disease of European rabbits caused by the myxoma virus. It is transmitted passively by blood-feeding arthropods and is shed via all bodily discharges. Clinical signs vary with the strain of the virus and the nature of the host, with wild rabbits (*Sylvilagus* species) developing benign skin tumors and domestic rabbits (*Orytolagus* species) developing systemic signs including swollen eyelids, and mucopurulent ocular and nasal discharge. Domestic rabbits may be lethargic and have seizures and a high mortality rate, with surviving rabbits developing edematous nodules on the ears, face, eyelids, and perineum. Diagnosis of myxomatosis is based on the clinical signs and pathologic findings (greatly swollen spleen; enlarged, edematous, and often hemorrhagic lymph nodes; hemorrhages; and swollen conjunctiva and nasal mucosa) with a history of myxomatosis in the area. Rabbits generally die so quickly that the diagnosis is often postmortem. Confirmation can be made by electron microscopy, fluorescent antibody, PCR, virus isolation, and antibody levels (ELISA, virus neutralization assays, or complement fixation assays). Intracytoplasmic inclusions may be seen in the epidermis and conjunctival epithelium. This disease has been used as a biological control for the European rabbit in Australia since 1950. No vaccine is commercially available in the United States for mxyomatosis. In the United States, cases of myxomatosis in rabbits have been most commonly reported in Oregon and California. Shelters should minimize contact of domestic rabbits with wild rabbits and arthropods (Hess and Tater 2012).

24.3.4.2 Rotavirus

Rotavirus is a highly infectious cause of GI signs with a high morbidity and variable (generally low) mortality. Weanling rabbits (two to four months) are most susceptible, and disease severity is increased with co-infection with another enteric pathogen. Antibodies to rotavirus are found in laboratory, commercial, and pet rabbits, indicating it can infect most species. Rotavirus infections are marked by anorexia, dehydration, and green-yellow watery diarrhea. The intestines become distended and congested, with petechial hemorrhages, chronic inflammation, and villous atrophy. Diagnosis requires histopathologic examination of the intestine, virus isolation, or antibody detection. Treatment is with supportive care. Though unlikely to affect shelter rabbits, rotavirus should be a differential in cases of diarrhea outbreaks in young rabbits. Affected animals should be isolated, with an emphasis on reducing overcrowding and increasing fiber in the diet.

24.3.4.3 Rabbit Hemorrhagic Disease Virus

Rabbit hemorrhagic disease virus (RHDV) is a calicivirus of the genus *Lagovirus* that affects only European/domestic rabbits. It was first described in China in 1984, and rapidly spread throughout Asia, Australia and New Zealand, and into Europe, with rare outbreaks in the United States and elsewhere. In 1996, the dissemination of rabbit hemorrhagic disease was legalized in Australia as a biological control for rabbits. At the time of publication of this text, RHDV has been reported in at least five states in the USA, with a high likelihood of spread throughout the country.

Transmission is via direct contact with virus shed into urine, feces, respiratory secretions, fomite contamination and intermediate insect vectors. The disease occurs in rabbits over two months of age; neonatal rabbits are resistant to infection. The virus replicates in the liver, causing severe hepatic necrosis and eventual death from DIC. The clinical presentation and course vary from a peracute disease lasting only 12–36 hours followed by sudden death; to an acute or subacute febrile illness with anorexia, diarrhea (or constipation), neurologic and other systemic symptoms lasting a few days to weeks; to a persistent/latent disease with continued virus shedding. Active immunity in recovered rabbits is apparently lifelong. Laboratory studies demonstrate a rapidly worsening lymphopenia and thrombocytopenia, with eventual prolonged prothrombin and thrombin times. At necropsy, there is extensive hepatic necrosis, splenomegaly, pulmonary hemorrhage, and evidence of DIC. Diagnosis is confirmed using specific immunohistochemical stains, electron microscopy, or ELISAs

(Oglesbee and Jenkins 2012). Vaccination programs using attenuated vaccines have had mixed results. A recombinant vaccine has recently been developed and should assist prevention in endemic areas, but no commercially available vaccine for RHDV is currently available in the United States. The virus can be inactivated with 0.5% sodium hypochlorite or 1% formalin. RHDV is a reportable disease with high morbidity (40–100%) and mortality (approaching 100%). There is no treatment. Shelters should immediately notify the state veterinarian in cases of suspected disease outbreaks or suspicious sudden death of a rabbit with no symptoms or with bleeding from the nose, mouth and rectum.

24.3.4.4 Rabbit (Shope) Fibroma Virus and Rabbit (Shope) Papillomavirus

Rabbit (Shope) fibroma virus is a Leporipoxvirus that can infect wild and domestic rabbits. The natural host is the Eastern cottontail rabbit. Shope fibroma virus is transmitted by biting arthropods, including fleas and mosquitoes. The virus causes flat, wart-like tumors on the face, legs, and perineum that are dermal and not attached to subcutaneous tissue. The tumors are easily movable, do not metastasize and usually regress after six months. Diagnosis is based on gross lesions, histopathologic examination, and virus isolation from tumors. Treatment is supportive care and prevention is by minimizing contact of domestic rabbits to infected or wild rabbits and insect vectors (Hess and Tater 2012).

Rabbit (Shope) papillomavirus, also known as cottontail rabbit papillomavirus, is in the Papovaviridae family and is also transmitted by biting arthropods. The virus causes wart-like keratinized lesions on the skin, with lesions generally around the neck and shoulders in wild cottontail rabbits and around the ears and eyelids in domestic rabbits. In naturally infected animals, infection appears as a cutaneous tumor, most commonly on the legs, especially the dorsal surface of the hindfeet. The tumors are firm, white, and moist on the surface and generally persist for up to 150 days and then disappear. In some cases, the tumors can progress to squamous cell carcinoma and metastasize to lymph nodes. Diagnosis is based on the host, clinical signs, and characteristic microscopic appearance and/or virus isolation. Surgical removal of lesions and arthropod control is recommended to prevent disease spread (Hess and Tater 2012).

24.3.4.5 Rabies

Rabies is rarely reported in rabbits but should be considered in cases of rabbits with bites of unknown origin. Nonspecific signs including anorexia, fever, and lethargy have been noted in the initial stages of infection. As the disease progresses, infected rabbits generally display paresis or paralysis and may develop head tremors. Shelters should ensure that any rabbits housed outdoors are protected from contact with wildlife since there is no licensed rabies vaccine available for use in rabbits in the United States (Fisher and Carpenter 2012). See Chapter 22 for more general information about rabies.

24.3.4.6 Herpes Simplex Virus (HSV)

Herpes simplex virus (HSV) encephalitis is rarely reported in rabbits. It is suspected that transmission from humans to rabbits is the most likely route of exposure since spontaneous infections have been reported in rabbits with close contact to humans with herpes labialis. Infection in rabbits has been associated with severe neurologic signs and death. Rabbit caretakers in shelters should be aware of the potential for viral transmission to rabbits, use appropriate sanitation, and minimally handle rabbits during HSV/cold sore outbreaks.

24.3.5 Infectious Diseases in Rabbits: Fungal

24.3.5.1 Dermatophytosis

The most commonly reported mycotic infection in rabbits is ringworm caused by *T. mentagrophytes* and less frequently *Microsporum* sp.

Lesions can be seen around the head, legs, feet, and nail beds. Initially, the infected areas may be pruritic and inflamed, later becoming scabby, dry, crusty, and alopecic. Diagnosis can be made by growth of the fungal organism on dermatophyte culture medium, direct examination of hair shafts mounted with potassium hydroxide, fungal stained skin biopsy samples, or PCR testing (Hess and Tater 2012). Treatment involves antimycotic medications including griseofulvin (12.5–25 mg/kg PO q12–24 h), itraconazole (5–10 mg/kg PO q24h), and terbinafine (10 mg/kg PO q24h), and other drugs considered to be safe for kittens. Treatment should extend to one to two weeks after a negative culture has been obtained. Dips and baths are stressful for rabbits and should be avoided when possible. Shelter employees and the public should be advised of its zoonotic potential. It is also very important to disinfect the environment and cleaning protocols should be used as described in Chapter 20 on dematophytosis in dogs and cats.

24.4 Guinea Pigs

24.4.1 Anatomy, Husbandry, Handling, and Routine Healthcare

24.4.1.1 Terminology, Anatomy, and Physiology

Guinea pigs are considered hystricomorph rodents that produce young that are relatively mature and mobile at the time of birth (precocial). They are monogastric hindgut fermenters with elodont teeth (teeth that continue to erupt throughout the life of the animal.) Guinea pigs lack a tail. Their life span is generally around five to six years (Quesenberry et al. 2012).

An understanding of dental anatomy is important in rodents with elodont teeth. The guinea pig dental formula is 2(I1/1, C0/0, PM1/1, M3/3). If cheek teeth overgrow, it is the result of dental malocclusion from multiple causes including a low fiber diet, congenital malocclusion, or trauma. Due to their anatomic orientation, the maxillary cheek teeth will overgrow into the buccal gingiva, and the mandibular cheek teeth will overgrow axially to entrap the tongue. Guinea pigs have a palatal ostium, which is an opening in the soft palate connecting the oropharynx with the pharynx. Their incisors are white; decreased chewing from low fiber diets results in decreased wear of tooth surfaces and tooth elongation. The diastema is present in guinea pigs between the incisors and the cheek teeth (Quesenberry et al. 2012).

Guinea pigs have a voluminous GI tract with a large cecum for fermentation. They use the "mucous trap" method for colonic separation and coprophagy, in which bacteria from the cecum is trapped in mucous in the colon and then returned to the cecum by anti-peristalsis. This contrasts with the more efficient "wash back" method of lagomorphs (Quesenberry et al. 2012).

Male guinea pigs have prominent accessory sex glands. The coiled vesicular glands may be seen in the abdomen ventral to ureters and should not be mistaken for uterine horns. Inguinal rings are open and there is an os penis. Female guinea pigs have paired uterine horns with a short body and a single cervix. External sexing is easily done by identifying the large scrotal pouch with large testes within. The penis may also be everted from the prepuce by placing pressure at the base. Female guinea pigs have a Y-shaped fold in the perineal tissue, which contains the ventral vulvar and dorsal anal openings.

24.4.1.2 Housing and Husbandry

Guinea pigs are shy but social animals that seek out the company of cohorts. However, they are also prey species and require a secure place to hide. They are somewhat active but do not jump, and therefore do not require a closed top to their enclosure if the walls are at least 10 in. high. Solid cage bottoms are recommended as pododermatitis can develop on wire bottom cages. Additionally, toe and leg fractures can result if a foot slips between cage bars. Guinea pigs are sensitive to heat, but they are cold tolerant. Recommended ambient temperatures for guinea pigs range from 65 to 79 °F; temperatures above 80 °F should be avoided. Low humidity (below 50%) is required for fur health, as matting will occur in wet, warm environments. Bedding should consist of newspaper, shredded paper, straw, or wood shavings (Quesenberry et al. 2012).

Guinea pigs require a dietary source of vitamin C (i.e. pelleted diet manufactured specifically for guinea pigs). They should be fed free-choice high-quality grass hay, guinea pig pellets and a mix of fresh greens and vegetables. Fruits should be given sparingly as the high sugar content can disrupt the cecal microbiome and lead to dysbiosis. Pellets should be selected carefully and should be composed of grass hay. Muesli mix pellets that contain concentrate, cracked corn, dried legumes, dried fruits, seeds, etc., should never be fed to any animal with elodont teeth as these animals rely on high fiber diets to produce adequate chewing to wear tooth length. Guinea pigs are selective feeders and generally will pick out the high concentrate pieces, leaving the high fiber components of the diet behind. This results in more vertical chewing and less lateral chewing, so the teeth can overgrow and lead to myriad dental problems.

24.4.1.3 Handling and Routine Healthcare

Guinea pigs are generally docile and should be handled by fully supporting their weight with one hand while covering their back with the other hand (Figure 24.6). A lightweight towel wrapped snug around the body with the head free (often called a "burrito") can offer additional support when handling more active or resistant guinea pigs.

Guinea pigs' wellness exams must always include a thorough oral examination. An accurate weight and vital parameters (temperature, pulse, respiration rates) should be obtained at the start of any examination. A full examination should include assessment of the eyes, ears, nose, oral cavity, fur, skin, musculoskeletal system, abdominal palpation, and auscultation of the heart, lungs, and GI borborygmi. Attention should be paid to the rectal area of guinea pigs as fecal impactions are common. Routine fecal exams are recommended, but no vaccinations are routinely performed or recommended (Quesenberry et al. 2012).

24.4.2 Infectious Diseases of Guinea Pigs

(See Table 24.3 for a list of diseases in guinea pigs by body system).

24.4.2.1 Respiratory Disease

24.4.2.1.1 Adenoviral Pneumonia Adenoviral pneumonia causes a necrotizing bronchopneumonia with an incubation period of

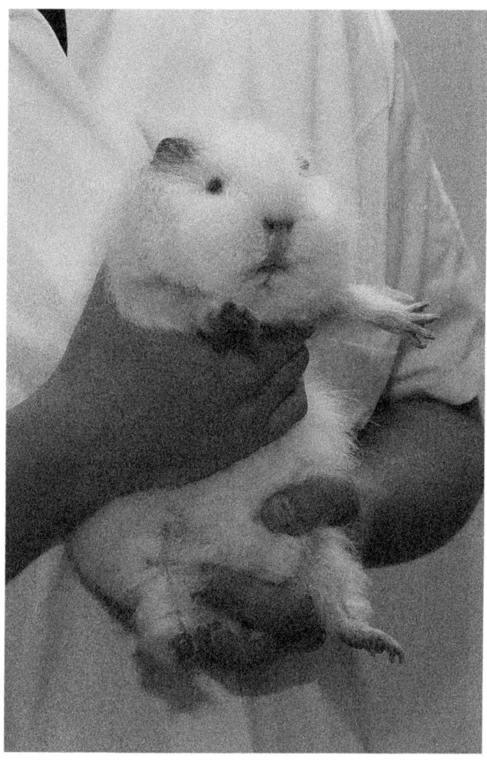

Figure 24.6 Restraint of a guinea pig by fully supporting their weight with one hand while covering their back with the other hand. *Source:* Courtesy N.J. Schoemaker and Yvonne Van Zeeland.

Table 24.3 Classification of Guinea pig diseases by body system.

System	Symptoms	Etiology
Respiratory		
Adenoviral pneumonia	Necrotizing bronchopneumonia, acute death	Adenovirus
Bacterial pneumonia – Z	Ocular/nasal discharge, dyspnea, tachypnea, increased respiratory sounds, sneezing, coughing, depression, anorexia, weight loss, unthrifty appearance, otitis media, deafness, conjunctivitis, abortion	*Bordetella bronchiseptica, Streptococcus pneumoniae, S. pyogenes, Streptobacillus moniliformis, Haemophilus,* and *Klebsiella*
Systemic/Ocular		
Lymphocytic Choriomeningitis Virus (LCMV) – Z	Meningitis and hind-limb paralysis	Arenavirus
Cervical lymphadenitis – Z	Swollen infected lymph nodes, pneumonia, metritis, and septicemia.	*Streptococcus zooepidemicus, Streptobacillus moniliformis*
Inclusion conjunctivitis of guinea pigs (GP-IC) – Z	Keratoconjunctivitis, serous to purulent ocular discharge, conjunctival chemosis, follicular hypertrophy, and uveitis	*Chlamydophila caviae*
Gastrointestinal		
Tyzzer's Disease	Lethargy, anorexia, diarrhea, unkempt appearance, and death	*Clostridium piliforme*
Salmonellosis – Z	Unkempt hair coat, weakness, diarrhea, weight loss, conjunctivitis, and abortion	*Salmonella typhimurium* and *Salmonella enteritidis*
Coccidiosis	Diarrhea	*Eimeria caviae*
Balantidiasis	Diarrhea	*Balantidium caviae*
Cryptosporidium – Z	Failure to gain weight, weight loss, diarrhea, and death	*Cryptosporidium wrairi*
Dermatologic		
Mange – Z	(TC) Severe pruritus with white to yellow crusts, abrasions, and associated inflammation.	*Trixacarus caviae (TC), Chirodiscoides caviae* mites, (also *Sarcoptes muris, Notoedres muris, Mycoptes musculinus)*
Lice	Alopecia, crusts, and unkempt appearance	*Gliricola porcelli* and *Gyropus ovalis*
Fleas	Pruritis, alopecia	*Ctenocephalides felis*
Dermatophytosis (ringworm) – Z	Circular areas of alopecia, erythema, broken hairs, and scaly crusts.	*Trichophyton mentagrophytes, Microsporum canis, M. gypseum*

Z, Zoonotic.

5–10 days (Hawkins and Bishop 2012). Though morbidity is low, mortality is high and guinea pigs may die acutely. This infection is most commonly seen in laboratory populations.

24.4.2.1.2 Bacterial Pneumonia *B. bronchiseptica* is the most common pathogen known to cause pneumonia in guinea pigs (Hawkins and Bishop 2012). *Streptococcus pneumoniae, Streptococcus pyogenes, Streptobacillus moniliformis, Haemophilus,* and *Klebsiella* are other bacterial causes of pneumonia in guinea pigs (Easson 2001). Rabbits, dogs, cats, and nonhuman primates may be asymptomatic carriers of *B. bronchiseptica*. The disease has an approximately one-week incubation period in guinea pigs and is characterized by purulent bronchopneumonia and often fibrino-suppurative pleuritis along with consolidated lung lobes, which is in contrast to the (often mild) upper respiratory signs seen in other species. Clinical signs can be variable and include ocular/nasal discharge, dyspnea, tachypnea, increased respiratory sounds, sneezing, coughing, depression, anorexia, weight loss, unthrifty appearance, otitis media, deafness, conjunctivitis, and abortion. Antimicrobial treatment should ideally be based on bacterial C/S, yet a persistent carrier state may develop and the disease may relapse (Easson 2001). Diagnosis is generally made based on clinical signs, physical examination findings, thoracic radiographs, and C/S of respiratory secretions. Bacterial cultures of nasal or ocular discharge are often inconsistent with tracheal or bronchial isolates, which more accurately reflect causative agents. Supportive care including fluid therapy, vitamin C supplementation, and nutritional support should be initiated; supplemental oxygen, saline nebulization, bronchodilators, and decongestants should be considered as needed.

It is recommended to prevent exposure of guinea pigs to rabbits, dogs, and cats that might be asymptomatic carriers of *Bordetella*. Prevention with an injectable *B. bronchiseptica* vaccine (Bronchicine®, Zoetis, Parsippany, NJ), 0.2 ml SC with a booster two to three weeks later has been used with moderate success in the face of an outbreak (Hawkins and Bishop 2012). While the use of this vaccine is rare in pet guinea pigs in homes, it may be indicated to vaccinate guinea pigs in a shelter environment during times of stress or exposure to *B. bronchiseptica,* but its routine use in all guinea pigs in a shelter setting is not generally recommended.

S. pneumoniae serotypes III, IV, and XIX cause respiratory disease in guinea pigs (Hawkins and Bishop 2012). A major risk factor for the disease is poor husbandry, and infection is often manifested as bronchopneumonia, fibrinopurulent pleuritis, and pericarditis. However, reproductive and neurologic signs have been described less frequently (Quesenberry and Orcutt 2012). Treatment with antibiotics should be based on C/S results. Animals may initially improve but succumb to the disease a few weeks later.

24.4.2.2 Gastrointestinal Disease

24.4.2.2.1 Bacterial Enteritis Bacterial enteritis is a common cause of diarrhea in guinea pigs. Tyzzer's disease (*C. piliforme*) is transmitted by the fecal-oral route and is more commonly seen in young, stressed, or immunocompromised individuals. Risk factors for disease include poor husbandry, overcrowding and other sources of stress, particularly in young animals at the time of weaning. Clinical signs include lethargy, anorexia, diarrhea, unkempt appearance, and death (Hawkins and Bishop 2012). Pathology findings commonly include intestinal inflammation and focal hepatic necrosis. Identification of organisms from liver or intestinal tissue provides the definitive diagnosis, as culture of this organism is not possible on routine media. Treatment is generally unrewarding, so efforts should be focused on disease prevention through sound husbandry practices and stress reduction. Euthanasia may be reasonable based upon the severity of the clinical signs, though treatment with fluid therapy, antimicrobials, and analgesics may be elected in individual cases.

Salmonella typhimurium and *Salmonella enteritidis* are less frequently reported causes of bacterial enteritis in pet guinea pigs, but mortality can be high during an outbreak. Clinical signs may include an unkempt hair coat, weakness, diarrhea, weight loss, conjunctivitis, and abortion. Transmission is by the fecal-oral route. Commonly, contamination of feed or water is the source of infection, and fecal or intestinal C/S testing provide the diagnosis. It is not recommended to treat with antimicrobials as animals can become asymptomatic carriers and *Salmonella* may be zoonotic. If cases are mild, supportive care can be provided, though euthanasia, especially in severe cases, is also reasonable when considering the risk of intermittent shedding of a potentially zoonotic bacterium (Hawkins and Bishop 2012).

24.4.2.2.2 Gastrointestinal Parasitism The most common GI parasites of guinea pigs include *Eimeria caviae, Balantidium caviae,* and *Paraspidodera uncinata*. Clinically significant diarrhea is much more common in juveniles than in adults (Mans and Donnelly 2012). *Cryptosporidium wrairi* can affect young and immunosuppressed individuals, causing failure to gain weight, weight loss, diarrhea, and death (Chrisp et al. 1992). Cryptosporidiosis is a potentially zoonotic disease. Most human cases of cryptosporidiosis are caused by *C. parvum* and *C. hominis*, however *C. felis, C. meleagridis, C. canis, C. suis, C. muris,* and *C. baileyi* can also infect humans. Some individual guinea pigs may recover within four weeks and are considered resistant to infection. Transmission is by the fecal-oral route, and there is no known effective treatment. Biosecurity measures, as previously described in this chapter for managing cryptosporidium in the ferret and rabbit, should be followed. Environmental oocysts can be destroyed with a 5% ammonia solution, 3% hydrogen peroxide for 20 minutes, and temperatures below 32 °F (0 °C) or above 149 °F (65 °C) (Mans and Donnelly 2012).

24.4.2.3 Dermatologic Disease

24.4.2.3.1 Ectoparasitism The most common and severe ectoparasitic dermatitis is caused by the mite *Trixacarus caviae*. Infection is by direct or indirect contact and results in severe pruritus with white to yellow crusts, abrasions, and associated inflammation. Animals may scratch so intensely that the presentation can be confused with seizure activity. Severe scratching often leads to secondary fungal or bacterial infections (Hawkins and Bishop 2012). *T. caviae* is zoonotic and can survive in the environment, which can potentially cause reinfection if appropriate decontamination measures aren't taken. Other common ectoparasites found in guinea pigs include *Chirodiscoides caviae* mites, *Gliricola porcelli* and *Gyropus ovalis* lice, *C. felis* fleas, and rarely *Demodex caviae* (Hawkins and Bishop 2012). Infestation with lice is transmitted by direct contact and usually causes less severe dermatitis. Clinical signs may be mild, but in a heavy infestation, alopecia, crusts, and unkempt appearance may be present. Guinea pigs in contact with rabbits, other rodents, or birds can become infected with other ectoparasites including *Sarcoptes muris, Notoedres muris, Mycoptes musculinus* (Hawkins and Bishop 2012). Direct visualization and identification of ectoparasites or eggs using microscopic examination aids diagnosis. Treatment should be based on the identified organism, but the most commonly used products include ivermectin and selamectin. Ivermectin can be dosed orally or SC, whereas selamectin is administered topically (Eshar and Bdolah-Abram 2012). Flea shampoo and other topical products that are safe for kittens may be used on guinea pigs. Secondary diseases such as inflammation and/or infection should be treated routinely. Inflammation and pruritis can be treated with NSAIDs, antihistamines, and other analgesics if necessary. Secondary infections should be treated with antimicrobials based on C/S. All animals in the enclosure and/or with exposure to affected animals should be treated and the environment disinfected.

24.4.2.3.2 Dermatophytosis Among rodents, dermatophytosis (ringworm) affects guinea pigs most commonly (Pollock 2003). *T. mentagrophytes* is most often identified in clinical cases, but *M. canis* and *M. gypseum* can also infect guinea pigs (Hawkins and Bishop 2012; Pollock 2003). The disease presents similarly to other mammals and is potentially zoonotic. Skin lesions are usually circular areas of alopecia, erythema, broken hairs, and scaly crusts. Dermatophytes infect the epidermis and adnexa, and lesions can be found anywhere on the body. Most commonly, lesions are located on the nose, forehead, pinnae, around the eyes, and on the feet (Pollock 2003). Diagnosis is made based on clinical signs, cytology of hair and skin, and fungal culture. *T. mentagrophytes* does not fluoresce with ultraviolet fluorescent lamp evaluation (Wood's lamp) evaluation, therefore fungal culture is required for an accurate diagnosis. Treatment includes oral antifungal medications (itraconazole, griseofulvin, fluconazole, terbinafine), antifungal shampoos, and topical antifungal lotions or sprays (Hawkins and Bishop 2012). Terbinafine has been shown to be more effective than itraconazole against *Trichophyton* species in rodents (Mieth et al. 1994). The reader is referred to Chapter 20 for further general information on dermatophytosis.

24.4.2.4 Other Conditions

24.4.2.4.1 Bacterial Conjunctivitis Juvenile animals are most commonly affected by conjunctivitis, though any age may be affected. A common pathogen causing bacterial conjunctivitis in guinea pigs is *Chlamydophila caviae*. This is often referred to as inclusion conjunctivitis of guinea pigs (GP-IC) (Lutz-Wohlgroth et al. 2006). Clinical signs include keratoconjunctivitis, serous to purulent ocular discharge, conjunctival chemosis, follicular hypertrophy, and uveitis (Hawkins and Bishop 2012). Diagnosis of GP-IC is achieved by identifying intracytoplasmic inclusions in conjunctival scrapings and *C. caviae* PCR on conjunctival swabs or scrapings (Doerning et al. 1993). *C. caviae* has been identified in rabbits housed with guinea pigs (Hawkins and Bishop 2012). *C. caviae* has zoonotic potential but the infection is often self-limiting within three to four weeks (Lutz-Wohlgroth et al. 2006). Due to the potential for zoonoses and spread within a population of guinea pigs, treatment with a topical tetracycline ophthalmic ointment is often warranted.

24.4.2.4.2 Lymphocytic Choriomeningitis Virus (LCMV) Lymphocytic choriomeningitis virus (LCMV) is an arenavirus that can cause meningitis and hind-limb paralysis. Though more commonly reported in mice, hamsters, and chinchillas, LCMV can less commonly infect guinea pigs. Classic lesions include lymphocytic infiltrates in the choroid plexus and meninges (Hawkins and Bishop 2012). Transmission occurs through inhalation, ingestion, or direct contact with contaminated fluids (urine, saliva, and feces). Transmission can also occur through the placenta of an infected female, and by biting insects. LCMV is zoonotic (Hawkins and Bishop 2012). Euthanasia is often recommended in these cases due to the severity of clinical signs and zoonotic potential.

24.4.2.4.3 Cervical Lymphadenitis Cervical lymphadenitis is a common presentation in guinea pigs. The infection is usually caused by *S. zooepidemicus*, and less commonly by *S. moniliformis*. *S. moniliformis* is zoonotic, while *S. zooepidemicus* is considered part of the normal oropharyngeal and nasal flora of guinea pigs (Hawkins and Bishop 2012). Transmission of these common bacteria can occur between individuals if they don't already harbor the pathogens. Stress in the shelter environment can cause opportunistic infection or recrudescence of chronic infections. Oral abrasions caused by dental malocclusion, rough feed, or bite wounds can lead to invasion of bacteria into soft tissues and cervical lymph nodes. The infected lymph nodes swell, become abscessed, and may rupture. In advanced cases, bacteria can spread systemically, resulting in pneumonia, metritis, and septicemia (Hawkins and Bishop 2012). Clinical signs, Gram's stain, C/S of purulent material or lymph node tissue, and histopathology of tissues all aid in diagnosis (Hawkins and Bishop 2012). Treatment consists of systemic antibiotics based on C/S results and may require surgical removal of the lymph nodes.

24.5 Altricial Rodents (Rats, Mice, Hamsters, and Gerbils)

24.5.1 Anatomy, Husbandry, Handling, and Routine Healthcare

24.5.1.1 Terminology, Anatomy, and Physiology

Rats, mice, hamsters, and gerbils all belong to the group of myomorph rodents, which have the dental formula 2(I1/1, C0/0, PM 0/0, M3/3). These species have young that are born in an undeveloped, helpless state that require care and feeding by the parents (altricial), as well as elodont incisors and anelodont (teeth that grow for a short period and stop erupting) cheek teeth. Most do not vomit due to a strong lower esophageal sphincter. Rats, mice, and gerbils all possess tails longer than their bodies, though the gerbil tail is furred. Hamsters also possess a tail, though it is significantly shorter than other species. All myomorph rodents have large testicles relative to their body size and open inguinal canals, which permit the testicles to move between the abdomen and scrotum. The harderian glands behind the eye produce porphyrin containing secretions that can cause a red tinge to the tears that should not be confused with blood. Rodents are monogastric with a large cecum and colon. Most exhibit coprophagy to provide micronutrients including B vitamins. Since rodents do not possess sweat glands, their ability to withstand heat is limited. The ideal ambient temperature should range from 65 to 77 °F. Sexing is evident in mature animals as the scrotum and testicles are prominent. In younger animals, this is performed by measuring the anogenital distance, which is longer in males than females (Lennox and Bauck 2012).

24.5.1.2 Housing and Husbandry

While rodents are all social to varying degrees, some species do better in groups than others. Rats can live easily in mixed groups, though the introduction of new individuals should always occur in a neutral area. Mice are less social than rats but can be kept in all-female groups. Males tend to be more aggressive when housed with other males, so they are best kept as a single male with females or as a solitary male. The social nature of hamsters can depend on the species, with dwarf hamsters being more social than golden or Chinese hamsters. Gerbils are social in the wild, but in the confines of captivity, their territorial nature can result in aggression and cannibalism. Therefore, it is often best to house gerbils as individuals unless a large enough enclosure can be provided to allow a compatible pair to cohabitate peacefully. Enclosures for all rodents should be escape-proof yet provide adequate ventilation. Elaborate enclosures with tubes and other intricate furniture should be avoided as these may be difficult to disinfect. An ideal enclosure would have easy to access or removable bottoms for cleaning, high sides, large doors to access the animal, and secure locking mechanisms. Cage substrate should consist of shredded paper, pine shavings, or other recycled paper products. Cedar shavings have been anecdotally linked to respiratory and skin disease and should be avoided as a precaution whenever possible. Generally, respiratory irritation and bacteria levels are lower on paper bedding. Most rodents are omnivorous, and a species-specific complete pelleted diet supplemented with fresh foods is recommended. Seed mixtures, while popular, may cause problems due to selective feeding. Individuals may preferentially eat only one type of seed or concentrate; this can result in dietary imbalance and obesity (Lennox and Bauck 2012).

24.5.1.3 Handling

Handling small rodents can be challenging. The technique used will depend on the species, degree of socialization/temperament, and health status of the individual animal. Scruffing tends to work well with small rodents like hamsters, but not on rats. It is important to ensure that enough skin has been grasped, as animals may still be able to reach around and bite. Rats are usually best restrained with gentle hands over the back and around the thorax (Lennox and Bauck 2012). Restraint using the tail, while often used in a laboratory setting, is not recommended with pet rodents as they will be unaccustomed to this. Before handling any rodent, as much information as possible should be obtained by observing the animal in its enclosure. Efforts should be made to prevent biting, as the bite victim may reflexively attempt to dislodge the rodent with a quick action of the hand that may potentially result in harm to the animal. If at any time an animal appears in distress, it should be put back in its enclosure, allowed a break and an alternative restraint strategy should be considered. Sedation can be used for fractious or nervous animals, with care taken with sick or injured individuals (Lennox and Bauck 2012).

24.5.1.4 Routine Healthcare

Wellness examinations are recommended for all pet rodents, with careful attention paid to the presence of any lumps, as masses (mammary, scent gland) are extremely common and best addressed when they are still small. No vaccination or diagnostic testing is routinely performed as part of wellness care for these animals. There is a risk of zoonosis from rodents regarding hantavirus, LCMV, and *S. moniliformis* (rat-bite fever). In addition to utilizing humane and careful handling techniques, special care should be taken to avoid bites and practice good hand hygiene when handling rodents (Lennox and Bauck 2012).

24.5.2 Infectious Diseases of Concern in Rodents in Animal Shelters

(See Table 24.4 for a list of diseases in rodents by body system).

24.5.2.1 Respiratory Disease

24.5.2.1.1 Sendai Virus and Sialodacryoadenitis Virus Sendai virus and Sialodacryoadenitis virus both cause acute respiratory infection, including sneezing, ocular porphyrin staining, conjunctivitis, mild respiratory distress, and keratitis. Infections can affect the upper and lower respiratory tracts. The diseases are generally mild and self-limiting within about two weeks to two months in adults, but neonates and weanlings often die (Brown and Donnelly 2012; Easson 2001). These respiratory viruses are common and often act as co-pathogens with *M. pulmonis* (Graham and Schoeb 2011). When disease expression exceeds the acute timeframe, the cause is most likely concurrent mycoplasma infection (Brown and Donnelly 2012).

Sialodacryoadenitis virus causes inflammation and edema of the cervical salivary glands. The virus is highly contagious and initially presents as rhinitis, followed by necrosis and swelling of the salivary and lacrimal glands. Cervical lymphadenopathy may also occur. Affected rats may be at increased risk of an anesthesia-related complication or death due to reduced airway diameter caused by local swelling. As with most viruses, there is no treatment beyond supportive care. Affected tissues heal within 7–10 days and clinical signs resolve within 30 days (Brown and Donnelly 2012). Sialodacryoadenitis virus can also cause conjunctivitis, keratitis, corneal

Table 24.4 Classification of rodent diseases by body system.

System	Symptoms	Etiology
Respiratory		
Sendai virus	Sneezing, ocular porphyrin staining, conjunctivitis, mild respiratory distress, keratitis	Sendai virus
Sialodacryoadenitis virus	Same as above, also rhinitis, necrosis and swelling of the salivary and lacrimal glands, cervical lymphadenopathy	Sialodacryoadenitis virus
Murine Respiratory Mycoplasmosis (MRM) or chronic respiratory disease (CRD) – Z	Increased respiratory noise, porphyrin staining, sneezing, chattering, labored breathing	*Mycoplasma pulmonis, Streptococcus pneumoniae,* and *Corynebacterium kutscheri*
Pneumonia – Z	Dyspnea, tachypnea, and purulent nasal discharge	*Streptococcus pneumoniae, M. pulmonis*, Sendai virus, CAR bacillus, *Corynebacterium kutscheri*
Gastrointestinal		
Salmonellosis – Z	Diarrhea, anorexia, and weight loss	*Salmonella typhimurium*
"Wet tail"	Hemorrhagic diarrhea, ill thrift, and lethargy acutely, poor growth, diarrhea, hunched posture and palpable abdominal mass subacutely	*Lawsonia intracellularis*
Tyzzer's disease	Lethargy, diarrhea, dehydration, unkempt coats, acute death	*Clostridium piliforme*
Tapeworms – Z	Weight loss, anorexia, death	*Taenia taeniaeformis*
Dermatologic		
Dermatophytosis (ringworm) – Z	Patchy areas of alopecia, crusting, and erythema most common on the face, head, neck, and tail.	*Trichophyton mentagrophytes*
Mange	Thin, greasy coat, pruritis, self-induced dermal ulceration	*Radfordia ensifera*
Mange	Anemia, debilitation, and even death	*Ornithonyssus bacoti*
Staphylococcal dermatitis	Local abscesses, conjunctivitis, dermal ulceration, and other evidence of self-trauma, mainly around face and head	Staphylococcal spp.
Necrotizing dermatitis	Same as above but also necrotic, ulcerated lesions in the shoulder, lumbar, and hip areas	*Streptococcal* spp.

Z, Zoonotic.

ulcers, synechiae, and hyphema. Lesions usually resolve but may progress to chronic keratitis (Brown and Donnelly 2012). Serology can be performed to achieve a definitive diagnosis. Treatment typically includes supportive care except in cases when these viruses occur in conjunction with co-pathogens that may require antimicrobials.

24.5.2.1.2 Murine Respiratory Mycoplasmosis (MRM) Respiratory disease is one of the most significant health problems in pet rats (Brown and Donnelly 2012; Goodman 2004). *M. pulmonis, S. pneumoniae,* and *Corynebacterium kutscheri* are the most common major respiratory pathogens. Sendai virus (paramyxovirus), rat coronavirus (RCV), pneumonia virus of mice (PVM), rat respiratory virus (hantavirus), cilia-associated respiratory (CAR) bacillus, and *Haemophilus* species are considered minor respiratory pathogens that rarely cause clinical disease by themselves. However, the minor respiratory pathogens interact synergistically with the major respiratory pathogens to produce Murine Respiratory Mycoplasmosis (MRM) or chronic respiratory disease (CRD) and bacterial pneumonia, the two major respiratory syndromes in rats and mice (Goodman 2004). Respiratory mycoplasmosis varies in disease expression because of organism, environmental, and host factors that influence the host-pathogen relationship (Brown and Donnelly 2012).

Increased respiratory noise, porphyrin staining, sneezing, chattering, and labored breathing are the most common presenting clinical signs, though initial infection can occur without any clinical signs. Additional clinical signs that may be appreciated include weight loss, hunched posture, ruffled coat, and head tilt (Ganaway et al. 1973). *M. pulmonis* is one of the most common infectious agents in rats and colonizes respiratory epithelium, nasal passages and middle ear. MRM is characterized by chronic pneumonia, suppurative rhinitis, otitis media, and can even spread to visceral organs. Mice tend to develop pulmonary abscesses (Goodman 2004). *M. pulmonis* has also been reported to cause disease in rabbits. MRM is often observed with viral co-infections (Sendai virus, Sialodacryoadenitis virus) and can cause immunosuppression. Infection with MRM causes damage and remodeling of the airway epithelium, colonization of the airways with secondary infections, and chronic airway inflammation (Hardy et al. 2002). Respiratory epithelial dysfunction and infiltration of neutrophils, macrophages, and lymphocytes result (Goodman 2004; Kling 2011).

M. pulmonis is transmitted horizontally by aerosol and direct contact. Vertical transmission can occur in utero, typically at the time of birth (Graham and Schoeb 2011). Infections with *M. pulmonis* persist for the life of the animal and can be exacerbated by myriad factors including vitamin A and E deficiency, increased environmental ammonia (above 19–25 ppm), substrate (cedar or pine), temperature, humidity, exposure to tobacco smoke, and genetic susceptibility of the animal (Goodman 2004; Kling 2011).

Antibiotic therapy may alleviate clinical signs of MRM but does not eliminate the infection. Rats infected with MRM often present with signs of an upper respiratory infection that responds to an initial course of antibiotics. However, given that Mycoplasma is an intracellular bacterium and the infection is not able to be completely cleared, recrudescence usually occurs. Affected rats suffer from chronic bronchopneumonia and bronchiectasis. The chronicity and recrudescent pattern of disease, as well as severity, often increase with age and result in pulmonary fibrosis leading ultimately to right-sided heart disease. In severely affected rats, cor pulmonale may result. Enrofloxacin (10 mg/kg) in combination with doxycycline hyclate (5 mg/kg) is usually helpful in controlling clinical signs, though repeated infections can become refractory to treatment as pulmonary lesions progress. Additional therapies such as nebulization, expectorants, bronchodilators, and NSAIDs are helpful to mitigate clinical signs (Brown and Donnelly 2012).

One author (SEK) has used sildenafil citrate as a pulmonary protectant in cases of MRM. Sildenafil is a phosphodiesterase-V inhibitor that has been used successfully in the treatment of pulmonary hypertension in humans and canines (Bach et al. 2006; Brown et al. 2010; Kellum and Stepien 2007). It is believed that sildenafil has a protective effect on the functional and structural changes in the pulmonary vasculature and lung parenchyma, as well as an anti-inflammatory effect (Lu et al. 2010, Yildirim et al. 2010). This protective effect aids in the mitigation of pulmonary fibrosis and airway thickening and reduces long-term lung changes in rats infected with chronic MRM. Studies using rats as a human model of disease, as well as the clinical experience of one author (EK) in pet rats with MRM suggests that sildenafil has an important role in the long-term treatment and management of MRM (Ganaway et al. 1973; Hardy 2002; Yildirim et al. 2010).

Cardiothoracic auscultation is often insensitive in determining the presence and severity of respiratory disease. Other more specific diagnostic tests are possible and would ideally be performed in order to achieve a diagnosis. However, many of these tests may require sedation and invasive procedures for sample collection or are financially impractical. Therefore, a presumptive diagnosis is often made based on history and clinical signs. Thoracic radiographs may be unremarkable but are useful in helping to rule out other causes of clinical signs such as cardiac disease and neoplasia (Graham and Schoeb 2011). Computed tomography (CT) scan is more sensitive for detecting pulmonary disease and is a useful imaging modality in cases of MRM when resources allow. Serology is the preferred choice for diagnostic testing, as *Mycoplasma* is difficult to grow in a laboratory. Younger rats naturally exposed to *M. pulmonis* may be seronegative for up to four months post-exposure (Brown and Donnelly 2012; Graham and Schoeb 2011).

24.5.2.1.3 Bacterial Pneumonia *S. pneumoniae* is the most common cause of bacterial pneumonia. However, it is seldom the sole infectious agent present, and often is accompanied by *M. pulmonis*, Sendai virus, or CAR bacillus. The disease is more severe in juvenile rats, which may die without any antemortem clinical signs. Mature rats show a more typical disease presentation that includes dyspnea, tachypnea, and purulent nasal discharge. Pneumonia may also be caused by *C. kutscheri*, but is rare and typically only occurs in cases of debilitation or immunosuppression. Diagnosis may be made based on C/S, Gram stain, or cytologic examination of exudate or tracheal wash. Infection can be severe in many cases and progress to septicemia and visceral abscesses. Treatment should include supportive care and antimicrobial therapy, typically beta-lactamase-resistant penicillins.

S. moniliformis is the primary cause of human rat bite fever, a potentially zoonotic disease. Wild and pet rats can harbor this bacterium as it normally inhabits the nasopharynx, middle ear, and respiratory tract (Hill and Brown 2011). It can also be present in urine and blood of infected rats. Rats, mice, and gerbils are usually asymptomatic carriers. Transmission to humans occurs from bites, scratches, or handling infected rat excreta, or ingesting contaminated food or water. Illness can also occur in guinea pigs, non-human primates, and occasionally mice. Clinical signs in infected humans include fever, headache, vomiting, and myalgia, and typically take about seven days after exposure to occur (Hill and Brown 2011). Appropriate handling to reduce risk of bites, attention to hygiene and husbandry to reduce stress, and use of PPE should all be implemented to reduce exposure risk. Whenever an exposure occurs, prompt professional medical attention should be sought.

24.5.2.2 Gastrointestinal Disease

24.5.2.2.1 Bacterial Enteritis *Salmonella* spp., gram negative bacteria, are a common cause of gastroenteritis, and even bacteremia. *S. typhimurium* is the most commonly isolated serotype in human and animal disease (Hill and Brown 2011). An outbreak of multi-drug resistant salmonellosis occurred in 28 humans in 10 states infected with *Salmonella enterica* serotype Typhimurium. The isolate matched a hamster strain, and 22 of the 28 patients reported exposure to pet hamsters, rats, or mice (Swanson et al. 2007). Clinical signs of salmonellosis are rare in infected mice and rats but may include diarrhea, anorexia, and weight loss (Hill and Brown 2011). Salmonellosis causes more severe disease in hamsters, and staff and volunteers should be aware of and take appropriate precautions to limit the potential zoonotic risk of salmonella exposure from rodent feces.

"Wet tail" caused by *L. intracellularis*, is a common pathogen of pet hamsters. This enteritis is more frequently seen in young weanling (four to eight-week-old) hamsters but can affect hamsters of any age in stressful environments (e.g. breeding, over-crowding, etc.) (Fiskett 2011). Transmission is by the fecal-oral route and infection is increased during times of stress, overcrowding, poor nutrition, or concurrent disease. *L. intracellularis* is an intracellular bacterium that causes a proliferative ileitis. This bacterium targets immature, actively dividing enterocytes and inhibits differentiation to mature cells (Fiskett 2011). Infection can spread from the ileum to include the jejunum, cecum, and colon. Due to the aggressive and potentially neoplastic nature of *L. intracellularis,* it has also been referred to as enzootic intestinal adenocarcinoma because the proliferative mucosal cells are often observed penetrating the muscular tunics (Fiskett 2011). Acute infection is characterized by hemorrhagic diarrhea, ill thrift, and lethargy approximately 7–10 days after infection. Clinical presentation of subacute infection includes poor growth, diarrhea, hunched posture suggesting a painful abdomen, and palpable abdominal mass (thickened ileum, abscess, enlarged lymph node). Signs are usually seen 21–30 days after infection. In the chronic state, there may not be any clinical signs, though occasional death and/or abdominal masses may occur. Hamsters showing clinical disease may die within 48 hours (Fiskett 2011).

High mortality (approximately 90%) is associated with this infection, and therefore treatment should be aggressive if it will be pursued; humane euthanasia is a reasonable consideration as well given the poor prognosis (Brown and Donnelly 2012; Fiskett 2011). Treatment should include fluids therapy (oral, subcutaneous, or intraosseous routes), corrective electrolyte replacement, antibiotics, bismuth subsalicylate, and nutritional support. While C/S should ideally guide antimicrobial selection, empiric treatment must be provided given the rapid progression of disease in these small rodents and the difficulty in culturing intracellular bacteria (requires tissue culture). Common antibiotics recommended for the treatment of *L. intracellularis* enteritis include metronidazole, tetracycline, chloramphenicol, enrofloxacin, and trimethoprim-sulfa (Brown and Donnelly 2012; Fiskett 2011). Definitive diagnosis is often made after necropsy and histologic examination, though a fecal PCR assay has been developed to aid ante-mortem diagnosis (Pedersen et al. 2010). Some animals who survive the initial infection may experience subsequent intestinal damage resulting in intestinal obstruction, intussusception, or rectal prolapse (Brown and Donnelly 2012).

While *L. intracellularis* most commonly affects juvenile hamsters, *Clostridium difficile* enterotoxemia is more commonly associated with adult hamster diarrhea. This is often seen several days after the administration of antibiotics, specifically penicillins and lincomycin (Brown and Donnelly 2012). PCR assays for *C. difficile* are highly sensitive and aid diagnosis. Bovine antibodies against toxigenic *C. difficile* have been shown to protect hamsters against experimental antibiotic-associated enterotoxemia when administered orally, though this is not a widely accessible or performed treatment in practice (Lyerly et al. 1991).

Tyzzer's disease, caused by *C. piliforme,* has been described in hamsters and gerbils. Affected rodents typically present with lethargy, diarrhea, dehydration, and unkempt coats. Many may present with acute death. Clinical disease is increased by severe stress, including overcrowding, improper or unsanitary environment, concurrent disease (parasitism), and improper diet. The disease does not usually occur in healthy, immunocompetent animals (Brown and Donnelly 2012). Diagnosis can be made by fecal PCR, or a fecal gram stain can be done to assess for the presence of spore-forming bacteria. While this will not provide a definitive diagnosis, it can help increase the index of suspicion and guide treatment recommendations.

24.5.2.2.2 Taenia taeniaeformis (Tapeworms) *Taenia taeniaeformis* is a tapeworm that can cause non-specific signs including weight loss, anorexia, and death in rodents. This parasite may alter gastric pH and cause a decrease in gastric-acid secretion and hyperplasia of intestinal mucosa (Huynh and Pignon 2013). Parasitic cysts may form in the liver and cause an increase in serum alanine aminotransferase, and/or AST. Additionally, some rats may demonstrate an increase in circulating neutrophils, lymphocytes, and/or eosinophils (Huynh and Pignon 2013). Radiographs and ultrasound may demonstrate hepatic cysts, hepatomegaly, gastric and intestinal mucosal thickening. Infection with this parasite is a risk factor for the development of hepatic sarcoma in rats (Huynh and Pignon 2013). Treatment recommendations are not clear, though praziquantel has been shown to be effective in killing adult and larval stages. Caution should be used when treating encysted larvae, as a severe host immune response may be elicited. The published dose of praziquantel in pet rats is 30 mg/kg PO every 14 days for three treatments. Cats and dogs are the definitive hosts, while rodents and occasionally rabbits act as intermediate hosts. Appropriate biosecurity measures should be used as there is a zoonotic risk to humans handling infected rats and mice (Huynh and Pignon 2013).

24.5.2.3 Dermatologic Disease

24.5.2.3.1 Dermatophytosis *T. mentagrophytes*, the causative agent of ringworm, is uncommon in pet mice and rats. However, disease incidence increases with concurrent ectoparasitism, poor husbandry, and other stressors (Pollock 2003). Lesions, when present, are typical with patchy areas of alopecia, crusting, and erythema most commonly located on the face, head, neck, and tail. Pruritus is usually minimal to absent, and the lesions do not fluoresce under a Wood's lamp (Brown and Donnelly 2012). Proper environmental decontamination for ringworm should be undertaken, and biosecurity measures should be used when handling suspect animals as the disease is zoonotic (See Chapter 20 for more information on dermatophytosis).

24.5.2.3.2 Ectoparasites Rodents infested with ectoparasites generally present with a thin, greasy coat. They may be pruritic and show evidence of self-induced dermal ulceration (Brown and Donnelly 2012). The fur mite, *Radfordia ensifera,* is not usually clinically significant, however heavy infestation may lead to self-trauma and ulcerative dermatitis. *Demodex* species are infrequently seen in pet rats. *Ornithonyssus bacoti*, the tropical rat mite, is often found on rats, mice, gerbils, and hamsters. Heavy infestations cause anemia, debilitation, and even death. Humans can be infested with these mites when the intended animal host is not available. In these situations, it is imperative to identify the animal host of the mites to successfully treat the infestation (Brown and Donnelly 2012; Ellis and Mori 2001; Timm 1988). In mice, the common species of fur mite are *Myobia musculi, M. musculinus,* and *Radfordia affinis. M. musculi* is the most clinically significant species, though infestations typically include more than one species (Brown and Donnelly 2012; Ellis and Mori 2001; Timm 1988). Diagnosis is based on (microscopic) identification of adult mites, nymphs, or eggs on hair shafts. Treatment can be accomplished with ivermectin (SQ or PO) or selamectin (topically). The environment should also be thoroughly decontaminated with pyrethroids or fipronil (Brown and Donnelly 2012).

24.5.2.3.3 Staphylococcal Dermatitis *Staphylococcal* infections are commonly associated with bacterial dermatitis in mice. Risk factors for infection include the strain of mice (nude mice are at increased risk), nutritional deficiency, dermal microbiome, concurrent ectoparasitism, and trauma to skin (Ellis and Mori 2001). Mice present with local abscesses, conjunctivitis, dermal ulceration, and other evidence of self-trauma. Lesions tend to be focused around the face and head. Necrotizing dermatitis presents similarly but is caused by *Streptococcal spp.* (Ellis and Mori 2001). Clinical signs include necrotic, ulcerated lesions in the shoulder, lumbar, and hip areas. Diagnosis for both disease processes is made based on clinical signs, C/S, cytologic examination of skin scrapings, and/or histopathology. Treatment should include eliminating the inciting cause (if identified), debridement and drainage of abscesses, analgesics, and antibiotic therapy based on C/S (Ellis and Mori 2001).

24.6 Conclusion

It is no longer unusual for shelters to receive small mammals and other exotic animals they are not generally accustomed to caring for. This chapter endeavored to present an overview of some of the key anatomic features and general husbandry and handling techniques as well as a brief description of some of the more significant diseases that may be seen in ferrets, rabbits, guinea pigs and rodents housed in shelters. Staff should be trained on how to handle these animals properly, to provide appropriate husbandry and to recognize infectious disease symptoms and other signs of ill health in these animals. Many shelters do not have veterinarians on staff so the prompt recognition of and reporting of health problems to appropriate managers is critical for preventing disease transmission and maintaining effective individual and population welfare. Proper biosecurity precautions should be taken when dealing with (potential) zoonotic diseases and prompt professional medical attention should always be sought when dealing with bite wounds and other disease exposures.

In addition to utilizing the information provided here, the reader is strongly encouraged to consult veterinarians with experience handling these animals as well as current veterinary literature and drug formularies to ensure adherence to the latest standards of care.

References

Antinoff, N. and Giovanella, C.J. (2012). Musculoskeletal and neurologic diseases. In: Ferrets, Rabbits, and Rodents: Clinical Medicine and Surgery, 3e (eds. K.E. Quesenberry and J.W. Carpenter), 132–140. St. Louis: Elsevier.

Bach, J.F., Rozanski, E.A., MacGregor, J. et al. (2006). Retrospective evaluation of sildenafil citrate as a therapy for pulmonary hypertension in dogs. *Journal of Veterinary Internal Medicine* 20: 1132–1135.

Barron, H.W. and Rosenthal, K.L. (2012). Respiratory diseases. In: Ferrets, Rabbits, and Rodents: Clinical Medicine and Surgery, 3e (eds. K.E. Quesenberry and J.W. Carpenter), 78–85. St. Louis: Elsevier.

Blagburn, B. (2003). Current recognition, control and prevention of protozoan parasites affecting dogs and cats. Western Veterinary Conference, Las Vegas, NA.

Brown, C.M. and Donnelly, T. (2012). Chapter 27 – Disease problems of small rodents. In: Ferrets, Rabbits, and Rodents, 3e (eds. J.W. Carpenter and K.E. Quesenberry), 354–372. St. Louis: W.B. Saunders.

Brown, A.J., Davison, E. et al. (2010). Clinical efficacy of sildenafil in treatment of pulmonary arterial hypertension in dogs. *Journal of Veterinary Internal Medicine* 24: 850–854.

Chitty, J.R. (2017a). Physical examination. In: Ferret Medicine and Surgery (ed. C.A. Johnson-Delaney), 75–84. Boca Raton: CRC Press.

Chitty, J.R. (2017b). Ferret preventative care. In: Ferret Medicine and Surgery (ed. C.A. Johnson-Delaney), 85–94. Boca Raton: CRC Press.

Chrisp, C.E., Suckow, M.A., Fayer, R. et al. (1992). Comparison of the host ranges and antigenicity of Cryptosporidium parvum and Cryptosporidium wrairi from Guinea pigs. *The Journal of Protozoology* 39: 406–409.

DeCubellis, J. and Graham, J.E. (2013). Gastrointestinal disease in Guinea pigs and rabbits. *Veterinary Clinics of North America: Exotic Practice* 16: 421–436.

Doerning, B.J., Brammer, D.W., and Rush, H.G. (1993). Pseudomonas aeruginosa infection in a Chinchilla lanigera. *Laboratory Animals* 27: 131–133.

Dubey, J.P. and Greene, C.E. (2012). Chapter 80, Enteric Coccidiosis. In: Infectious Diseases of the Dog and Cat, 4e (ed. C.E. Greene), 833. St. Louis: Elsevier.

Easson, W. (2001). A review of rabbit and rodent production medicine. *Seminars in Avian and Exotic Pet Medicine* 10: 131–139.

Ellis, C. and Mori, M. (2001). Skin diseases of rodents and small exotic mammals. *Veterinary Clinics of North America: Exotic Animal Practice* 4: 493–542.

Eshar, D. and Bdolah-Abram, T. (2012). Comparison of efficacy, safety, and convenience of selamectin versus ivermectin for treatment of Trixacarus caviae mange in pet Guinea pigs (Cavia porcellus). *Journal of the American Veterinary Medical Association* 241: 1056–1058.

Fisher, P.G. and Carpenter, J.W. (2012). Neurologic and musculoskeletal disease. In: Ferrets, Rabbits and Rodents Clinical Medicine and Surgery, 3e (eds. K.E. Quesenberry and J.W. Carpenter), 245–256. St. Louis: Elsevier.

Fisher, P. and Graham, J. (2018). Rabbits. In: Exotic Animal Formulary, 5e (ed. J.W. Carpenter), 494–532. St. Louis: Elsevier.

Fiskett, R.A.M. (2011). Lawsonia intracellularis infection in Hamsters (Mesocricetus auratus). *Journal of Exotic Pet Medicine* 20: 277–283.

Ganaway, J.R., Allen, A.M., Moore, T.D. et al. (1973). Natural infection of germfree rats with Mycoplasma pulmonis. *Journal of Infectious Diseases* 127: 529–537.

Goodman, G. (2004). Infectious respiratory disease in rodents. *In Practice* 26: 200–205.

Graham, J.E. (2014). Lagomorpha (Pikas, Rabbits, and Hares). In: Fowler's Zoo and Wild Animal Medicine Current Therapy 8, 8e (ed. E. Miller), 375–384. St. Louis: Saunders.

Graham, J.E. and Basseches, J. (2014). Liver lobe torsion in rabbits: clinical consequences, diagnosis, and treatment. *Veterinary Clinics of North America: Exotic Practice* 17: 195–202.

Graham, J.E. and Mader, D.R. (2012). Basic approach to veterinary care. In: Ferrets, Rabbits, and Rodents Clinical Medicine and Surgery, 3e (eds. K.E. Quesenberry and J.W. Carpenter), 174–182. St. Louis: Saunders.

Graham, J.E. and Schoeb, T.R. (2011). Mycoplasma pulmonis in rats. *Journal of Exotic Pet Medicine* 20: 270–276.

Hardy, R.D., Jafri, H.S., Olsen, K. et al. (2002). Mycoplasma pneumoniae induces chronic respiratory infection, airway hyperreactivity, and pulmonary inflammation: a murine model of infection-associated chronic reactive airway disease. *Infection and Immunity* 70: 649–654.

Hawkins, M.G. and Bishop, C.R. (2012). Chapter 23 – Disease problems of Guinea pigs. In: Ferrets, Rabbits, and Rodents, 3e (eds. J.W. Carpenter and K.E. Quesenberry), 295–310. Saint Louis: W.B. Saunders.

Hess, L. and Tater, K. (2012). Dermatologic diseases. In: Ferrets, Rabbits, and Rodents Clinical Medicine and Surgery, 3e (eds. K.E. Quesenberry and J.W. Carpenter), 232–244. St. Louis: Elsevier.

Hill, W.A. and Brown, J.P. (2011). Zoonoses of rabbits and rodents. *Veterinary Clinics of North America: Exotic Animal Practice* 14: 519–531.

Hoefer, H.L., Fox, J.G., and Bells, J.A. (2012). Gastrointestinal diseases. In: Ferrets, Rabbits, and Rodents: Clinical Medicine and Surgery (eds. K.E. Quesenberry and J.W. Carpenter), 27–45. St. Louis: Elsevier.

Huynh, M. and Pignon, C. (2013). Gastrointestinal disease in exotic small mammals. *Journal of Exotic Pet Medicine* 22: 118–131.

Johnson-Delaney, C. (2017a). General information. In: Ferret Medicine and Surgery (ed. C. Johnson Delaney), 1–2. Boca Raton: CRC Press.

Johnson-Delaney, C.A. (2017b). Normative data including coat colors. In: Ferret Medicine and Surgery (ed. C.A. Johnson-Delaney), 3–12. Boca Raton: CRC Press.

Johnson-Delaney, C. (2017c). Applied clinical anatomy and physiology. In: Ferret Medicine and Surgery (ed. C. Johnson-Delaney), 13–29. Boca Raton: CRC Press.

Johnson-Delaney, C. (2017d). Ferret behavior, housing, and husbandry. In: Ferret Medicine and Surgery (ed. C. Johnson-Delaney), 31–36. Boca Raton: CRC Press.

Johnson-Delaney, C. (2017e). Nutrition. In: Ferret Medicine and Surgery (ed. C. Johnson-Delaney), 47–64. Boca Raton: CRC Press.

Johnson-Delaney, C.A. (2017f). Disorders of the skin. In: Ferret Medicine and Surgery (ed. C.A. Johnson-Delaney), 325–346. Boca Raton: CRC Press.

Johnson-Delaney, C.A. (2017g). Miscellaneous conditions. In: Ferret Medicine and Surgery (ed. C.A. Johnson-Delaney), 371–376. Boca Raton.pp: CRC Press.

Kellum, H.B. and Stepien, R.L. (2007). Sildenafil citrate therapy in 22 dogs with pulmonary hypertension. *Journal of Veterinary Internal Medicine* 21: 1258–1264.

Kim, H., Song, D., Moon, H. et al. (2013). Inter-and intraspecies transmission of canine influenza virus (H3N2) in dogs, cats, and ferrets. *Influenza and Other Respiratory Viruses* 7 (3): 265–270.

Klaphake, E. and Paul-Murphy, J. (2012). Disorders of the reproductive and urinary systems. In: Ferrets, Rabbits, and Rodents Clinical Medicine and Surgery, 3e (eds. K.E. Quesenberry and J.W. Carpenter), 217–231. St. Louis: Elsevier.

Kling, M.A. (2011). A review of respiratory system anatomy, physiology, and disease in the mouse, rat, hamster, and gerbil. *Veterinary Clinics of North America: Exotic Animal Practice* 14: 287–337.

Lennox, A. (2012). Respiratory disease and pasteurellosis. In: Ferrets, Rabbits, and Rodents Clinical Medicine and Surgery, 3e (eds. K.E. Quesenberry and J.W. Carpenter), 205–216. St. Louis: Elsevier.

Lennox, A.M. and Bauck, L. (2012). Basic anatomy, physiology, husbandry, and clinical techniques. In: Ferrets, Rabbits, and Rodents: Clinical Medicine and Surgery, 3e (eds. K.E. Quesenberry and J.W. Carpenter), 339–353. St. Louis: Elsevier.

Lu, W., Ran, P., Zhang, D. et al. (2010). Sildenafil inhibits chronically hypoxic upregulation of canonical transient receptor potential expression in rat pulmonary arterial smooth muscle. *American Journal of Physiology-Cell Physiology* 298: C114–C123.

Lutz-Wohlgroth, L., Becker, A., Brugnera, E. et al. (2006). Chlamydiales in Guinea-pigs and their zoonotic potential. *Journal of Veterinary Medicine A: Physiology, Pathology and Clinical Medicine* 53: 185–193.

Lyerly, D., Bostwick, E., Binion, S.B. et al. (1991). Passive immunization of hamsters against disease caused by Clostridium difficile by use of bovine immunoglobulin G concentrate. *Infection and Immunity* 59: 2215–2218.

Lyoo, K.S., Kim, J.K., Kang, B. et al. (2015). Comparative analysis of virulence of a novel, avian-origin H3N2 canine influenza virus in various host species. *Virus Research* 195: 135–140.

Mancinelli, E., Keeble, E., Richardson, J. et al. (2014). Husbandry risk factors associated with hock pododermatitis in UK pet rabbits (Oryctolagus cuniculi). *Veterinary Record* 174: 429–436.

Mans, C. and Donnelly, T.M. (2012). Chapter 24 – Disease problems of chinchillas A2. In: Ferrets, Rabbits, and Rodents, 3e (eds. K.E. Quesenberry and J.W. Carpenter), 311–325. St. Louis: W.B. Saunders.

Mieth, H., Leitner, I., and Meingassner, J.G. (1994). The efficacy of orally applied terbinafine, itraconazole and fluconazole in models of experimental trichophytoses. *Journal of Medical and Veterinary Mycology* 32: 181–188.

Mitchell, M.A. (2008). Ponazuril. *Journal of Exotic Pet Medicine* 17 (3): 228–229.

Mitchell, M.A. and Tully, T.N. (2012). Zoonotic diseases. In: Ferrets, Rabbits, and Rodents, Clinical Medicine and Surgery, 3e (eds. K.E. Quesenberry and J.W. Carpenter), 557–565. St. Louis: Elsevier.

Oglesbee, B.L. and Jenkins, J.R. (2012). Gastrointestinal diseases. In: Ferrets, Rabbits, and Rodents Clinical Medicine and Surgery, 3e (eds. K.E. Quesenberry and J.W. Carpenter), 192–204. St. Louis: Elsevier.

Orcutt, C. and Tater, K. (2012). Dermatologic disease. In: Ferrets, Rabbits, and Rodents: Clinical Medicine and Surgery, 3e (eds. K.E. Quesenberry and J.W. Carpenter), 122–140. St. Louis: Elsevier.

Orosz, S. and Johnson-Delaney, C.A. (2017). Disorders of the nervous system. In: Ferret Medicine and Surgery (ed. C.A. Johnson-Delaney), 273–288. Boca Raton: CRC Press.

Pedersen, K.S., Holyoake, P., Stege, H. et al. (2010). Diagnostic performance of different fecal Lawsonia intracellularis – specific polymerase chain reaction assays as diagnostic tests for proliferative enteropathy in pigs: a review. *Journal of Veterinary Diagnostic Investigation* 22: 487–494.

Perpinan, D. and Johnson-Delaney, C.A. (2017). Disorders of the digestive system and liver. In: Ferret Medicine and Surgery (ed. C.A. Johnson-Delaney), 159–190. Boca Raton: CRC Press.

Pollock, C. (2003). Fungal diseases of laboratory rodents. *Veterinary Clinics of North America: Exotic Animal Practice* 6: 401–413.

Powers, L.V. (2012). Basic anatomy, physiology, and husbandry. In: Ferrets, Rabbits, and Rodents: Clinical Medicine and Surgery, 3e (eds. K.E. Quesenberry and J.W. Carpenter), 1–12. St Louis: Elsevier.

Quesenberry, K.E. and Orcutt, C. (2012). Basic approach to veterinary care. In: Ferrets, Rabbits, and Rodents: Clinical Medicine and Surgery, 3e (eds. K.E. Quesenberry and J.W. Carpenter), 13–26. St. Louis: Elsevier.

Quesenberry, K.E., Donnelly, T.M., and Mans, C. (2012). Biology, husbandry, and clinical techniques of Guinea pigs and chinchillas. In: Ferrets, Rabbits, and Rodents: Clinical Medicine and Surgery, 3e (eds. K.E. Quesenberry and J.W. Carpenter), 279–294. St. Louis: Elsevier.

Richardson, J. and Perpinan, D. (2017). Disorders of the respiratory system. In: Ferret Medicine and Surgery (ed. C.A. Johnson-Delaney), 311–324. Boca Raton: CRC Press.

Swanson, S.J., Snider, C., Braden, C.R. et al. (2007). Multidrug-resistant Salmonella enterica serotype Typhimurium associated with pet rodents. *New England Journal of Medicine* 356: 21–28.

Swisher, S. and Lennox, A.M. (2017). Disorders of the hemic, immunological, and lymphatic systems. In: Ferret Medicine and Surgery (ed. C.A. Johnson-Delaney), 237–257. Boca Raton: CRC Press.

Timm, K.I. (1988). Pruritus in Rabbits, Rodents, and Ferrets. *Veterinary Clinics of North America: Small Animal Practice* 18: 1077–1091.

Vella, D. and Donnelly, T.M. (2012). Basic anatomy, physiology, and husbandry. In: Ferrets, Rabbits, and Rodents Clinical Medicine and Surgery, 3e (eds. K.E. Quesenberry and J.W. Carpenter), 157–173. St. Louis: Saunders.

Wagner, R.A. and Bhardwaj, N. (2012). Serum-neutralizing antibody responses to canine distemper virus vaccines in domestic ferrets (Mustela putorius furo). *Journal of Exotic Pet Medicine* 21 (3): 243–247.

Welchman, D.d.B., Oxenham, M., and Done, S. (1993). Aleutian disease in domestic ferrets: diagnostic findings and survey results. *Veterinary Record* 132: 479–484.

Yildirim, A., Ersoy, Y., Ercan, F. et al. (2010). Phosphodiesterase-5 inhibition by sildenafil citrate in a rat model of bleomycin-induced lung fibrosis. *Pulmonary Pharmacology and Therapeutics* 23: 215–221.

Index

Page locators in **bold** indicate tables. Page locators in *italics* indicate figures. This index uses letter-by-letter alphabetization.

b

g

w

y

z